New Insights into Hematologic Malignancies

New Insights into Hematologic Malignancies

Editor: Ted Myers

AMERICAN
MEDICAL PUBLISHERS
www.americanmedicalpublishers.com

AMERICAN
MEDICAL PUBLISHERS
www.americanmedicalpublishers.com

Cataloging-in-Publication Data

New insights into hematologic malignancies / edited by Ted Myers.
p. cm.
Includes bibliographical references and index.
ISBN 979-8-88740-331-1
1. Lymphoproliferative disorders. 2. Lymphomas. 3. Lymphatics--Diseases.
4. Immunological deficiency syndromes. 5. Cell proliferation. 6. Blood--Diseases.
I. Myers, Ted.

RC646.2 .N49 2023
616.42--dc23

American Medical Publishers,
41 Flatbush Avenue,
1st Floor, New York,
NY 11217, USA

ISBN 979-8-88740-331-1 (Hardback)

Contents

Preface

The main aim of this book is to educate learners and enhance their research focus by presenting diverse topics covering this vast field. This is an advanced book which compiles significant studies by distinguished experts in the area of analysis. This book addresses successive solutions to the challenges arising in the area of application, along with it; the book provides scope for future developments.

The branch of medicine that studies the causes, treatment and prevention of blood-related diseases is known as hematology. Hematologic malignancy is a type of cancer that originates in blood-forming tissues such as the bone marrow or in the cells of the immune system. It is caused by cells dividing at an abnormal rate. The three main types of hematologic malignancies include leukemia, lymphoma and multiple myeloma. A cancer that begins in the lymphatic system is called lymphoma. The lymphatic system is an important part of the immune system and it includes lymph nodes, spleen, thymus gland and bone marrow. Lymphoma cancer can affect any part of the lymphatic system. Multiple myeloma is a cancer that originates in the bone marrow. It affects the plasma cells. In multiple myeloma, the plasma cells affected with cancer start building-up in the bone marrow along with the healthy blood cells. Leukemia is a cancer that starts developing in the bone marrow, or blood-forming tissues, or the lymphatic system. The diagnosis includes various blood tests such as complete blood count (CBC) test and electrophoresis blood test. This book includes some of the vital pieces of works being conducted across the world, on various topics related to diagnosis, treatment and control of hematologic malignancies. Students, researchers, hematologists, and all associated with this subject will benefit alike from it.

It was a great honour to edit this book, though there were challenges, as it involved a lot of communication and networking between me and the editorial team. However, the end result was this all-inclusive book covering diverse themes in the field.

Finally, it is important to acknowledge the efforts of the contributors for their excellent chapters, through which a wide variety of issues have been addressed. I would also like to thank my colleagues for their valuable feedback during the making of this book.

Editor

1

Actors on the Scene: Immune Cells in the Myeloma Niche

Patrizia Leone[1], Antonio Giovanni Solimando[1,2], Eleonora Malerba[1], Rossella Fasano[1], Alessio Buonavoglia[1], Fabrizio Pappagallo[1], Valli De Re[3], Antonella Argentiero[2], Nicola Silvestris[1,2], Angelo Vacca[1] and Vito Racanelli[1]*

[1] Department of Biomedical Sciences and Human Oncology, University of Bari Medical School, Bari, Italy, [2] Department of Medical Oncology, IRCCS Istituto Tumori "Giovanni Paolo II" of Bari, Bari, Italy, [3] Bio-Proteomics Facility, Department of Translational Research, Centro di Riferimento Oncologico di Aviano (CRO) IRCCS, Aviano, Italy

***Correspondence:**
Vito Racanelli
vito.racanelli1@uniba.it

Two mechanisms are involved in the immune escape of cancer cells: the immunoediting of tumor cells and the suppression of the immune system. Both processes have been revealed in multiple myeloma (MM). Complex interactions between tumor plasma cells and the bone marrow (BM) microenvironment contribute to generate an immunosuppressive milieu characterized by high concentration of immunosuppressive factors, loss of effective antigen presentation, effector cell dysfunction, and expansion of immunosuppressive cell populations, such as myeloid-derived suppressor cells, regulatory T cells and T cells expressing checkpoint molecules such as programmed cell death 1. Considering the great immunosuppressive impact of BM myeloma microenvironment, many strategies to overcome it and restore myeloma immunosurveillance have been elaborated. The most successful ones are combined approaches such as checkpoint inhibitors in combination with immunomodulatory drugs, anti-monoclonal antibodies, and proteasome inhibitors as well as chimeric antigen receptor (CAR) T cell therapy. How best to combine anti-MM therapies and what is the optimal timing to treat the patient are important questions to be addressed in future trials. Moreover, intratumor MM heterogeneity suggests the crucial importance of tailored therapies to identify patients who might benefit the most from immunotherapy, reaching deeper and more durable responses.

Keywords: multiple myeloma, microenvironment, immune cells, immune checkpoints, immunotherapy

INTRODUCTION

Multiple myeloma (MM) is a malignant plasma cell disease mainly located in the bone marrow (BM) in multiple 'niches'. These provide a microenvironment that promotes tumor survival and progression. Within BM niches, normal and tumor plasma cells can survive for years, even for decades. Moreover, the observation that tumor plasma cells do not grow and expand when cultured alone suggests the huge resilience of these cells within the BM microenvironment (1). The BM milieu consists of a cluster of cells such as immune cells, stromal cells, endothelial cells (ECs), and bone cells, soluble factors (cytokines, chemokines, and growth factors), and non-cellular matrix (2). It is highly vascularized by blood vessels and is a part of the lymphocyte re-circulation network. Cells re-circulating into and out of the BM have the potential to regulate tumor plasma cell growth and progression through a composite array of indirect and direct interactions involving cytokines as well as surface (3) and soluble molecules (4). In this context, the immune system plays a central and multifaceted role.

A multistep development model indicates that MM progresses from a stable premalignant plasma cell clonal expansion termed monoclonal gammopathy of undetermined significance (MGUS). This asymptomatic preneoplastic condition is characterized by a perfect equilibrium between tumor and immune system which allows disease to remain stable and does not develop to MM. Immune cells control, but not eliminate MGUS plasma cells. These findings suggest that malignant transformation depends not only on the features of the tumor cells themselves but also on the surrounding microenvironment and its effects on tumor cells. Complex cancer–immune system interactions generate both pro- and anti-tumor effects whose balance can be altered in favor of an immunosuppressive environment which promote tumor progression (5, 6). On one hand, innate and adaptive immune cells are able to detect tumor plasma cells; tumor-specific cytotoxic T cells can be found in the BM of MGUS and MM patients (7, 8). On the other hand, tumor plasma cells have the ability to promote a tolerant microenvironment and the activation of immunosuppressive mechanisms to counteract effective immune responses. These include impairment of antigen processing and presentation, and T cell response, NK and NKT cell dysfunctions, local recruitment, expansion and activation of immune suppressor cells like T regulatory cells (Tregs) and myeloid derived suppressor cells (MDSCs), and differentiation of the protumoral tumor-associated macrophages and Th17 cells (9–11) (**Figure 1**).

Here we describe interactions between BM tumor plasma cells and different immune cells and provide an overview of the current knowledge on immunotherapeutic strategies.

MYELOMA PLASMA CELL IMMUNOGENICITY

The hallmark of MGUS and MM plasma cells is the production and the surface expression of a monoclonal immunoglobulin (Ig) carrying unique antigenic (idiotypic or Id) determinants in the variable heavy (VH) (12). Thus, the Ig idiotypic structure is a tumor-specific antigen of the myeloma cell clone, distinct from normal cells or normal plasma cells that can be presented as whole molecule on the cell surface or as peptides in the groove of the of major histocompatibility complex (MHC) molecules (13, 14).

Several studies have described idiotype-specific cytotoxic T lymphocytes in MM patients with the capacity to lyse autologous primary tumor plasma cells. Many potential T cell epitopes have been identified within the tumor-derived Ig-VH region, nonetheless, the majority of them didn't trigger high affinity T cell responses (15). Two peptide prediction algorithms, BIMAS and SYFPEITHI, have also confirmed the poor immunogenicity of human idiotypes with a low binding half-life (BIMAS) and a low/intermediate score (SYFPEITHI) on most T cell interaction human leukocyte antigen (HLA) modules (16, 17). Additionally, idiotypic vaccination in MM has been examined in clinical trials where immunologic responses occurred in <50% of patients, and clinical responses have been infrequent (18).

Within the universal tumor antigens, many myeloma-associated antigens (*e.g.* human telomerase reverse transcriptase (hTERT) (19), surviving (20), new york esophageal squamous cell carcinoma 1 (NY-ESO1) (21) mucin-1 (MUC-1) (22), junctional adhesion molecule-A (JAM-A) (23, 24) and the receptor for hyaluronic acid-mediated motility (RHAMM) (25) have been identified as targets recognized by T lymphocytes and used in many vaccination strategies, but in most cases failed to produce clinically meaningful responses. However, many obstacles need to be overcome. The most important one is the myeloma plasma cell escape of tumor-specific immune response. Our group demonstrated that the binding of CD28 expressed on myeloma plasma cells with its ligands CD80/CD86 expressed on BM dendritic cells (DCs) results in downregulation of the expression of proteasome subunits, alteration of the antigen repertoire displayed on myeloma plasma cell surface, and reduced recognition of tumor plasma cells by cytotoxic $CD8^+$ T cells (10).

TUMOR-SPECIFIC CYTOTOXIC $CD8^+$ T CELLS

The mechanisms underlying MGUS to MM progression are incompletely understood. Tumor plasma cell specific $CD8^+$ T cells have been detected in both MGUS and MM patients (8, 26, 27), thereby establishing that there is no tolerance to plasma cell tumors. Nonetheless, in MM, myeloma plasma cell proliferation is not counteracted by $CD8^+$ T cells. These observations have rekindled interest in the immunosurveillance mechanisms of tumor growth (28). Although MM plasma cells do not significantly differ from their premalignant MGUS precursors with respect to cytogenetic abnormalities (29, 30) and gene expression profiles (31), $CD8^+$ T cells have been uncovered to fail to limit the clonal expansion of tumor plasma cells in MM. Our studies have shown that malignant transformation of plasma cells is associated with altered expression of HLA class I antigen processing presenting machinery (APM) components. These alterations are detectable *ex vivo*, occur at the transcriptional level, and, in some cases, are enhanced by IL-6, an essential MM cytokine. For some APM components, changes correlate with the extent of the plasma cells' lysis by $CD8^+$ T cells and with variations in the serum level of the M component in MGUS patients (8). Downregulation of proteasome subunits, in particular, is higher in plasma cells from MM patients than in those from MGUS patients and MM plasma cells are less readily lysed by autologous, *in vitro*-expanded cytotoxic $CD8^+$ T cells than are MGUS plasma cells. This difference in cytotoxicity is evident at the epitope level and is not due to the intrinsic features of $CD8^+$ T cells, given that no difference is observed when $CD8^+$ T cells are tested against HLA-matched target cells that are not plasma cells (8). These findings support the hypothesis that proteasome subunit downregulation decreases expression of tumor antigen peptides on tumor plasma cells, enabling them

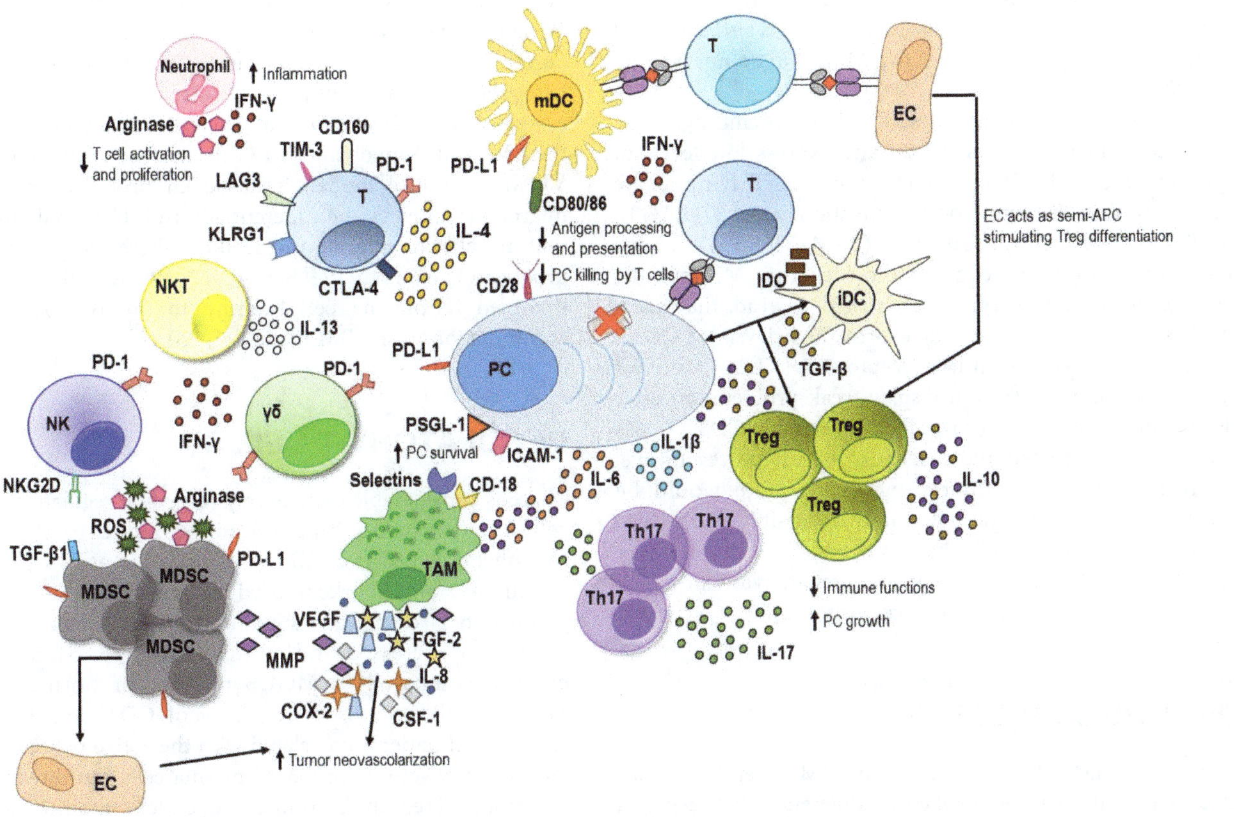

FIGURE 1 | The MM BM microenvironment. On one hand, innate and adaptive immune cells are able to recognize myeloma plasma cells (PC) and generate a weak immune response against tumor. Mature dendritic cells (mDCs) activate tumor-specific T cells that along with natural killer (NK), NKT and gamma delta ($\gamma\delta$) T cells produce low amount of interferon (IFN)-γ. On the other hand, myeloma PCs are able to promote an immunosuppressive microenvironment. They produce immunosuppressive factors including transforming growth factor (TGF)-β, interleukin (IL)-10 and IL-6. PC–immature DC (iDC) interaction stimulates TGF-β production by DC inducing T regulatory (Treg) proliferation with enhancement of levels of TGF-β and IL-10. Immature DCs produce also indoleamine 2,3-dioxygenase (IDO) that causes anergy in activated T cells. The latter exhibits exhaustion markers such as programmed cell death-1 (PD-1), cytotoxic T lymphocyte antigen-4 (CTLA-4), T cell immunoglobulin-3 (TIM-3), and lymphocyte-activation gene 3 (LAG3), and high levels of the senescence markers killer-cell lectin like receptor G1 (KLRG1) and CD160. PD-1 is greatly expressed also by $\gamma\delta$ T cells and NK cells and interacts with its ligand, programmed death ligand 1 (PD-L1), expressed by myeloma PC, DC, and myeloid derived suppressor cells (MDSCs) downregulating immune response. Myeloma PC–mature DC interaction, involving the CD28 receptor and the CD80/CD86 ligands respectively, downregulates proteasome subunit expression in tumor PC and decreases the processing and presentation of tumor antigens thus reducing myeloma PC recognition by cytotoxic CD8$^+$ T cells. Myeloma PC-tumor-associated macrophage (TAM) interaction involving P-selectin glycoprotein ligand 1 (PSGL-1) and intercellular adhesion molecule-1 (ICAM-1) on myeloma PC and E/P selectins and CD18 on TAM confers multidrug resistance to MM PC. Within myeloma niche, TAMs release great amount of IL-6 and IL-10 and contribute to MM-associated neovascularization by vasculogenic mimicry and indirectly by secreting vascular endothelial growth factor (VEGF), IL-8, fibroblast growth factor-2 (FGF-2), metalloproteinases (MMPs), cycloxygenase-2 (COX-2), and colony-stimulating factor-1 (CSF-1). Neutrophils release high amount of IFN-γ that supports their promotion of pro-inflammatory and survival signals within the plasma cell niche and produces arginase that inhibits T cell activation and proliferation. MDSCs also produce high amounts of arginase and reactive oxygen species (ROS) that contribute to T cell suppression, induce anergy of NK cell through membrane-bound TGF-β1 and promote tumor angiogenesis by MMP secretion or direct differentiation into endothelial cells (ECs). Furthermore, ECs can act as semi-professional antigen presenting cells (APCs) stimulating a regulatory tumor-specific T cell population. Within BM, the elevated levels of IL-6, TGF-β, and IL-1β promote T helper IL-17-producing (Th17) cell polarization which release high levels of IL-17 favoring MM plasma cell growth and inhibiting immune system.

to evade CD8$^+$ T cell recognition and killing (10). Moreover, these alterations in the expression of APM components are specific of each premalignant and malignant plasma cell clone, suggesting that the myeloma-specific T cell response can differ from one patient to another. Indeed, CD8$^+$ T cells isolated from MGUS and MM patients can be activated *ex vivo* by DC loaded with autologous but not allogeneic tumor lysates (7, 27, 32). The finding that the impairment of T cell response is restricted to myeloma antigens is supported also by the absence of a clinical T cell immunodeficiency. Myeloma patients show an appropriate T cell immunity against external antigens and do not show an increased incidence of mycobacterial infections or virus associated second malignancies (33).

Some shared antigens have been identified as targets of a spontaneous immune response in MGUS but not MM patients suggesting the capacity of the immune system to recognize premalignant lesions. For instance, the clonogenic CD138$^-$ compartment in MGUS patients expresses SOX2, an embryonal stem cell protein involved in the tumor-initiating potential and self-renewal of tumor cells. The expression of this antigen identifies potential MM progenitors and detection of anti-SOX2 T cells is associated with an improved clinical outcome in patients with asymptomatic plasma cell disorders. SOX2 is also expressed by $CD138^+$ cells in patients with active MM, who do not develop anti-SOX2 immunity (34).

Recent evidence also indicates that MM-specific cytotoxic $CD8^+$ T cells do not express CD28 and express low levels of programmed cell death-1 (PD-1), cytotoxic T lymphocyte antigen-4 (CTLA-4), lymphocyte-activation gene 3 (LAG3), and T cell immunoglobulin-3 (TIM-3) (35). These characteristics further strengthen the idea that MM-specific $CD8^+$ T cells are not anergic or exhausted. Instead, they seem to be "senescent" given that they express high levels of CD57, CD160, and killer-cell lectin like receptor G1 (KLRG1), do not express CD27 and CD28, and display weak proliferation after antigen stimulation (35). So basically, MM-specific $CD8^+$ T cells appear late-differentiated and suspended in a hypo-responsive, non-proliferative state. Interestingly, this state would be telomere-independent and potentially reversible (35) since MM-specific $CD8^+$ T cells have normal-for-age telomere lengths and long-surviving MM patients retain cytotoxic T cell clones with conserved proliferative capacity (36).

$CD4^+$ T HELPER CELLS

The role of $CD4^+$ T helper cells in MM is still unclear; controversial data may be justified by differences between BM and peripheral blood, or by different quantification method (absolute count *versus* percentage), or by changes in Th1/Th2 polarization during the course of the disease. While some authors reported an altered Th1/Th2 balance strongly supported by IL-6, with increased production of Th2 cytokines, such as IL-10 and IL-4 and decreased production of Th1 cytokines, such as IL-2 and IFN-γ (37, 38), others described an elevated Th1/Th2 ratio in MM patients at diagnosis and in refractory phase, pointing towards a close relation to the clinical features (39–41).

Furthermore, increased levels of PD-1 on $CD4^+$ cells have been observed in MM patients with persistent minimal residual disease (MRD) and at relapse compared with T cells of first diagnosed MGUS and MM patient (42). BM myeloma PD-1 expressing $CD4^+$ T cells interact with plasma cells and DCs that display on their surface programmed death ligand 1 (PD-L1) promoting T cell suppression and MM progression (43).

T HELPER 17 CELLS

Elevated levels of interleukin (IL)-6, transforming growth factor (TGF)-β, and IL-1β in myeloma BM microenvironment promote T helper IL-17-producing (Th17) cell polarization with consequent increased of IL-17 levels in BM and peripheral blood of MM patients (36, 44–46). IL-17 induces myeloma cell growth and colony formation *via* IL-17 receptor and inhibits Th1 immune response (45). The amount of Th17 cells in the BM positively correlates with clinicopathological characteristics in MM, like clinical tumor stage, serum lactate dehydrogenase concentration, and serum creatinine concentration (46). In addition, IL-17 plays a role in osteoclast-mediated lytic bone disease (44). Recently, the existence of a direct immunological link between the gut and the BM in MM involving Th17 cells has been proposed. Using a Vk*MYC mouse model, it has been provided that the gut microbiota induces the differentiation of Th17 cells in the gut that are able to migrate to the BM, where they promote MM progression (47). In the BM, IL-17 activates also eosinophils involved in plasma cell homing to the BM and in their accumulation in the BM niche (47, 48).

REGULATORY T CELLS

There is considerable controversy regarding regulatory T (Treg) cell frequency and function in MM due to their source (peripheral blood *versus* BM), differences in assays, purification techniques, and markers used to identify these cells. Treg population is described as reduced and/or dysfunctional (39, 49, 50) or increased and/or functional (36, 51–57) in MM patients compared to MGUS patients or normal controls. Moreover, the increased frequency of $CD4^+$ and $CD8^+$ Treg cells in MM patients correlated with the active phase (54) and a reduced survival (55, 58). MM plasma cells can directly induce functional Treg in a contact dependent manner acting as immature and tolerogenic antigen presenting cells (APCs) (54) as well as in an APC independent manner by the expression of the inducible T cell co-stimulator ligand (ICOSL) (59). It is possible that the mutual and dynamic interactions among cells of the BM microenvironment along with cytokine release modulate the frequency and the suppressive activity of Treg cells. In coculture experiments, cytokines such as IL-10 and TGF-β and human myeloid immature DCs are the most efficacious for induction and expansion of Treg population (60, 61). Tumor cell–immature DC interaction stimulates TGF-β production by DC inducing Treg proliferation (62). Our study demonstrated that EC can act as semi-professional APC stimulating a regulatory tumor-specific $CD8^+$ T cell population with suppressive function within BM of MM patients (11). Moreover, human leukocyte antigen G $(HLA\text{-}G)^+$ T cells with an inhibitory activity comparable to natural Treg can be generated in BM of MM patients after tumor plasma cell–T cell interaction by trogocytosis of immunosuppressive molecules such as HLA-G (63).

$\gamma\delta$ T CELLS

BM MM microenvironment is extremely immunosuppressive and greatly influences gamma delta ($\gamma\delta$) T cells. Indeed, BM derived $V\gamma9V\delta2$ T cells, the main subset of $\gamma\delta$ T cells, become more dysfunctional than those isolated from the peripheral blood of MM patients. The functional exhaustion of BM $V\gamma9V\delta2$ T cells occurs early during disease progression and does not disappear in clinical remission. Upregulation of PD-1 expression on $\gamma\delta$ T cells is already found in MGUS patients and persists in the remission phase and further increases in the relapse (64). One possible explanation is the great concentration of phosphoantigens in the tumor microenvironment and the consequent prolonged TCR engagement. High amounts of isopentenyl pyrophosphate, the prototypic phosphoantigen recognized by Vγ9Vδ2 T cells *via* TCR, are produced by both BM myeloma plasma cells and stromal cells leading to chronic TCR engagement, upregulation of PD-1 expression, and functional exhaustion of $\gamma\delta$ T cells (65). Moreover, many cell subsets including MM plasma cells, myeloid-derived suppressor cells (MDSCs), regulatory T cells (Tregs), and BM-derived stromal cells are implicated in Vγ9Vδ2 T cell hampering through the excessive expression of immune checkpoints (ICP)/ICP-ligands (65).

DENDRITIC CELLS

The role of DC in MM progression is controversial. Some investigators reported impaired functionality and phenotypic profile, while others found that these cells are normal (9). We have demonstrated that BM DCs are functional and play a dual, but opposing role in MM. DCs are concentrated in the BM during the MGUS-to-MM progression and interact with both T cells and myeloma plasma cells. On one hand, DCs are able to uptake apoptotic myeloma plasma cells, mature and process myeloma antigens, cross-present them and successfully activate myeloma-specific BM-infiltrating CD8$^+$ T cells. On the other hand, by using their surface CD80/86 molecules, DCs interact with non-apoptotic tumor plasma cells by the CD28 receptor that is upregulated on their surface, promoting a downregulation of proteasome subunit expression and a consequent escape of myeloma plasma cells from CD8$^+$ T cell recognition and killing (10). Moreover, plasmacytoid DCs promote tumor plasma cell growth, survival, and drug resistance (66) and express high surface levels of programmed death-ligand 1 (PD-L1) conferring T cell and NK cell immune suppression by engaging ICP *via* PD1-PD-L1 signaling axis (67, 68). Myeloid CD141$^+$ DCs also express PD-L1, and the proportion of these cells correlate with the percentage of PD-L1$^+$ plasma cells, suggesting that both cell subsets support anti-tumor T cell response inhibition in MM (68). DCs can also indirectly favor the osteoclastogenesis process by inducing Th17 cell expansion in BM myeloma microenvironment (69) followed by IL-17 accumulation, a potent pro-osteoclastogenic factor (70).

MACROPHAGES

Tumor-associated macrophages (TAMs) constitute an abundant component of myeloma microenvironment that induce myeloma plasma cell survival through both contact-dependent and -independent mechanisms. For instance, a direct physical interaction involving E/P selectins and CD18 on macrophages and P-selectin glycoprotein ligand 1 (PSGL-1) and intercellular adhesion molecule-1 (ICAM-1) on myeloma cells protects plasma cells from drug-induced apoptosis (71–73). Within myeloma niche, after interaction with BM-derived mesenchymal stromal cells, TAMs acquire a secretory profile characterized by a great production of IL-6 and IL-10 and poor production of IL-12 and TNF-α, providing a suitable milieu for myeloma plasma cell growth (74). TAMs also contribute to MM-associated neovascularization by vasculogenic mimicry and indirectly by secreting a wide range of proangiogenic factors, such as vascular endothelial growth factor (VEGF), IL-8, and fibroblast growth factor-2 (FGF-2) as well as metalloproteinases (MMPs), cycloxygenase-2 (COX-2), and colony-stimulating factor-1 (CSF-1). Moreover, they resemble M2-like macrophage population with a reduced cytotoxic capacity for tumor cells and a decreased antigen-presenting capability (75).

A very recent single-cell RNA sequencing study revealed that mature CD14$^+$ monocytes/macrophages lose HLA class II surface expression as early as in the MGUS phase resulting in T cell suppression (76).

NK CELLS

Natural killer (NK) cell differentiation, activation, and cytotoxic ability are strongly compromised during MM progression (77). BM myeloma plasma cells from early-stage patients display low levels of MHC class I molecules and high levels of MHC class I related chain A (MICA) and are readily recognized by NK cells (78). Nevertheless, elevated numbers of NK cells in the BM and blood of MM patients were associated with worse prognoses (79). Myeloma cell recognition and killing by NK cells involve a broad array of activating receptors including the natural killer group 2D (NKG2D), DNAX accessory molecule-1 (DNAM-1), and the natural cytotoxicity receptors (NCR) NKp46, NKp30, and NKp44 (78, 80). Changes in the expression of these NK receptors and NK cell receptor ligands have been observed in BM samples of MGUS and MM patients, suggesting a role of NK cell dysfunction during MGUS-to-MM progression (81). In addition, following an extensive interaction with cytotoxic T and NK cells, myeloma plasma cells obtained from patients with active disease exhibit the MHC class I^{bright}/MICA$^{dim/-}$/CD95$^{dim/-}$ immunophenotype that compromises NK cell function (78, 82, 83). Likewise, the number of effector NK cells localized within the BM progressively decreases during MM growth and correlates with reduced BM NK cell degranulation in MM-bearing mice (84). Moreover, MICA shedding from the surface of myeloma plasma cells may promote downregulation of NKG2D expression on the surface of NK cells weakening the NK-mediated anti-tumor response (83, 85). Defective NK cell functions can be also explained by PD-1 expression on NK cells of MM patients that interact with its ligands PD-L1 on tumor plasma cells downregulating NK cell function (86). Also, the release of soluble factors in the BM microenvironment can influence NK cell activity. For instance, an inflammatory milieu rich in IFN-γ secreted by immune cells strongly increases PD-L1 expression (87). In addition, primary myeloma plasma cells express high levels of HLA-E molecules which bind to the inhibitory NK cell receptor NKG2A hampering NK cell effector functions (80, 88–90).

NKT CELLS

NKT dysfunction has been recognized as potentially important in disease predisposition and progression (91). A progressive decrease of NKT cells and a loss of both peripheral blood and BM NKT cell activity in MM patients have been described by many groups, with disease progression correlating with a reduction of IFN-γ production by NKT cells (26, 92, 93). Likewise, a loss of CD1d expression by myeloma plasma cells has been demonstrated during disease progression with consequent dysfunction of NKT cells (26, 92, 94, 95).

A recent study has demonstrated an enrichment of inflammation-associated lysophosphatidylcholine molecules in MM patient serum compared with healthy donors alongside with an increase of frequency of lisophosphatidylcholine-recognizing CD1d-restricted type II NKT cells. These cells release high amounts of the IL-13, an immunosuppressive cytokine involved in tumor-promoting inflammation and angiogenesis, thus supporting their role in disease progression (96). Furthermore, type II NKT cells may also promote plasma cell differentiation and play a role in the initiation of MM (97, 98).

MYELOID-DERIVED SUPPRESSOR CELLS

In humans, two main subsets of myeloid derived suppressor cells (MDSCs) with the same level of suppressive activity can be identified based on CD14 positivity, granulocyte-MDSCs (G-MDSCs) that are $CD11b^{+}CD14^{-}CD33^{+}CD15^{+}HLA\text{-}DR^{-/low}$ and monocytic-MDSCs (M-MDSCs) that are $CD11b^{+}CD14^{+}CD33^{+}HLA\text{-}DR^{-/low}$ (99). The involvement of these subsets in the pathogenesis of MM is still not clear. Several studies found a significant increase in G-MDSCs in the peripheral blood and BM of newly diagnosed, relapsed, and relapsed/refractory MM patients compared with healthy donors (100–102), while others described an increase of M-MDSCs in first diagnosed and relapsed MM patients compared with those in remission and healthy donors (103, 104). Moreover, the level of M-MDSC correlates with disease progression (104).

Because of their capacity to suppress T cell-mediated immunity, MDSCs play an important role in favoring tumor escape from immunosurveillance (101, 102). MDSCs secrete high amount of arginase which sequestrates L-arginine, an essential amino acid for T cell activity (105). Moreover, MDSCs can inhibit T cell receptor by nitrosylation and reactive oxygen species release (106) and express on their surface high levels of PD-L1 which can interact with PD-1 express on T cells (64).

In addition, MDSCs induce Treg differentiation through TGF-β-dependent and -independent mechanisms involving CD40 or IL-10 and IFN-γ, respectively (100, 106), induce NK cell anergy through membrane-bound TGF-β1 (107, 108), promote tumor angiogenesis by MMP-9 secretion or direct differentiation into EC (109), and stimulate tumor growth through the release of cytokines and growth factors (101).

Using immunocompetent mouse models, it has been demonstrated that MDSC immunosuppression occurs early in MM disease; MDSCs accumulated in the BM of mice as early as one week after tumor inoculation and when these mice were engineered to lose their ability to accumulate MDSC, growth of MM plasma cells was significantly reduced confirming the critical role of MDSC accumulation at early stages of MM progression (102).

NEUTROPHILS

Neutrophils are essential for clearance of extracellular pathogens, as they effectively fight them by releasing cytotoxic granules, toxic enzymes, inflammatory mediators, and reactive oxygen species (110, 111). Thanks to a large number of integrins and molecules expressed on their surface, neutrophils can establish interactions with other immune cells (*e.g.*, T, B, and NK cells, monocytes, macrophages, DCs), can act as weak antigen presenting cells, promote angiogenesis and inflammation, and regulate hematopoiesis (112). In MM, as a consequence of BM infiltration by tumor plasma cells, functional defects of neutrophils including reduced lysozyme activity and increased secretion of the amino acid degrading enzyme, arginase, have been described (113, 114). An involvement of neutrophils in immune suppression *via* IFN-γ signaling has been also revealed since the early asymptomatic phase of MGUS (115). Specifically, Romano et al. (115) have demonstrated that neutrophils from MGUS and MM are chronically activated because of increased signaling through IFN-γ and Toll-like receptors that trigger a chronic inflammatory response *via* STAT protein activation. Compared with neutrophils from healthy patients, neutrophils from MGUS and MM patients show immunosuppressive features. They display an impairment in the FC-γ-receptor I (CD64) mediated phagocytosis under control of IFN-γ and increased secretion of arginase-1, target of STAT proteins (116–118), resulting in inhibition of T cell activation and proliferation (115). Furthermore, during MGUS-to-MM progression, neutrophils progressively enhance the production of IFN-γ in response to MM soluble factors resulting in increased autophagy flux and JAK-2/STAT3 pathway activation, which support their promotion of pro-inflammatory and survival signals within MM niches (119).

In addition, the neutrophil to lymphocyte ratio (NLR) at diagnosis or after 100 days from autologous stem cell transplantation (SCT) can predict outcome in newly diagnosed MM patients treated upfront with novel agents (120–122). Interestingly, NLR could be combined with international staging system (ISS) to better evaluate the risk profile of non-elderly (<65 years) MM patients, to identify patients with poor outcome, and to personalize MM therapy (121).

IMMUNE CHECKPOINTS IN MULTIPLE MYELOMA

The main ICP pathways CTLA-4 and PD-1/PD-L1 have emerged as major immune escape mechanisms in MM. These pathways are crucial in the physiological setting for maintaining the immune equilibrium after the initial T cell response and preventing over-activation of the immune system and tissue damage. Tumor cells upregulate these biologic mechanisms of tolerance and exploit them to elude host immunity (123). Regarding MM, contradictory results exist in this field, due mainly to the different analyzed sources (peripheral blood *versus* BM) suggesting a fundamental role of the local milieu in the regulation of immune ICP cell expression.

Several studies have found an increased number of CTLA4^{+} Treg cells in the BM of MM patients compared with MGUS patients and healthy donors (52, 56, 124), with a correlation between the proportion of cells simultaneously positive for CTLA4 and Foxp3 and the disease stage (54).

PD-1 expression is increased on NK and $\gamma\delta$ T cells isolated from MM patients and correlates with loss of effector cell function (64, 86). CD4^{+} and CD8^{+} T cells express low level of PD-1 in MGUS and newly diagnosed MM patients, suggesting that downregulation of their effector function is partly due to senescence rather than PD-1 mediated exhaustion (35, 124, 125). Paiva et al. have reported increased PD-1 expression levels on CD4^{+} and CD8^{+} T cells only in relapsed or relapsed/refractory MM and in patients with a minimal residual disease (42).

PD-L1 is greatly expressed on plasma cells obtained from MM patients with active, relapsed, and refractory disease, whereas low expression has been found on plasma cells from MGUS patients or healthy donors, suggesting that PD-L1 expression is associated with MM progression and drug resistance (42, 68, 126–128). Moreover, soluble factors such as IFN-γ, IL-6, and indoleamine 2,3-dioxygenase (IDO), detected at high level in myeloma BM microenvironment, upregulate the expression of PD-L1 on myeloma plasma cells (126, 127, 129). PD-L1 is also expressed by other cells of myeloma BM microenvironment, including plasmacytoid DC, NK cells, and MDSCs, according to their immunoregulatory functions (67, 68, 86, 100, 127).

IMMUNOSUPPRESSIVE FACTORS

Along with the crosstalk between tumor plasma cells and BM niche cells, a high concentration of immunosuppressive factors including TGF-β, IL-10, IL-6, and prostaglandin E2 in the MM BM microenvironment promotes tumor propagation and survival and at the same time generates great immune dysfunction (130). In addition, the cellular contact of myeloma plasma cells with BM immature DCs, through CD47–thrombospondin-1 interaction, leads to spontaneous DC fusion and trans-differentiation into osteoclasts (131, 132), which, beside their role in bone lesions, promote suppressive immune BM microenvironment inducing T cell apoptosis by the overexpression of ICP molecules and the release of IDO and APRIL (129). Moreover, IDO causes anergy in activated T cells, induces them to become Treg, and generates a nutritionally depleted niche favoring survival of myeloma cells which have a low proliferative index and are less sensitive to tryptophan depletion (133); APRIL enhances PD-L1 expression on MM cells supplying immune suppression (129). Simultaneously, the establishment of a chronic inflammatory status contributes also to disease progression (134). Increased levels of inflammatory cytokines, such as IL-1, IL-6, IL-12, IL-15, IL-17, IL-18, IL-22, IL-23, TNF-α, and IFN-γ have been revealed in BM serum of MM patients (135), and an eight-gene signature (IL-8, IL-10, IL-17, CCL3, CCL5, VEGFA, EBI3, and NOS2) involved in B-cell inflammation has been described able to distinguish the different phases of disease progression (MGUS/smoldering/symptomatic-MM) with 84% accuracy (134). Moreover, inflammation can lead to high levels of bioactive lipids, such as several species of lysophosphatidylcholine, which can bind to CD1d molecules resulting in dysregulation of lipid-reactive immune cells, activation of CD1d-restricted type II NKT cells, and production of high amount of the immunosuppressive cytokine IL-13 (96).

TARGETING IMMUNE SYSTEM AS AN EFFECTIVE APPROACH TO TREAT MULTIPLE MYELOMA

Considering the great immunosuppressive impact of BM myeloma microenvironment, many strategies to overcome it and restore myeloma immunosurveillance have been elaborated (**Figure 2**). Autologous SCT following myeloablative treatment allows the introduction of a new immune system and has significantly contributed to improve survival of MM patients in the last 15 years (136). Unfortunately, the graft *versus*-myeloma (GvM) response is usually weak and most patients relapse. An alternative is the adoptive therapy with BM infiltrating lymphocytes enriched in myeloma-specific T cells that enhances the anti-tumor immunity, but has a poor durability of the clinical response (137), or the allogeneic SCT which provides a new T cell repertoire, triggers a potent GvM response, but it is limited by the high transplant-related mortality (138).

The emergence of ICP blockade therapies over the last decade raised great interest also in MM. Despite at first, *in vitro* and *in vivo* studies showed that PD-1/PD-L1 blockade enhanced T and NK cell mediated anti-myeloma immune responses (42, 64, 86, 139–141) suggesting that ICP inhibition may be a promising therapeutic strategy against MM, clinical trials have provided unsatisfactory results (125). A possible explanation is that myeloma-specific T cells have an anergic or senescent phenotype rather than an exhausted phenotype, a prerequisite for the success of ICP blockade therapies.

Current lines of evidence indicate that the senescent phenotype could be reversed by immunomodulatory drugs

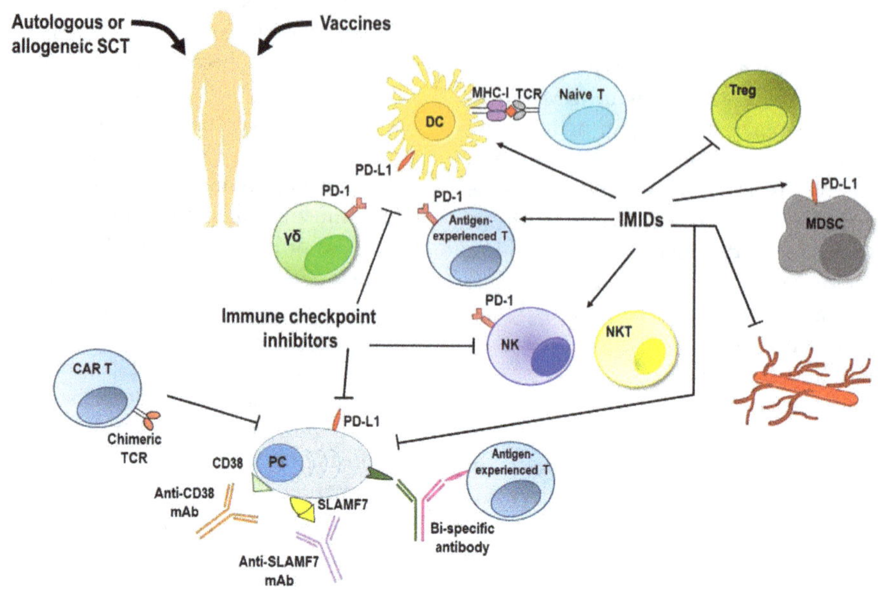

FIGURE 2 | Targeting immune system to induce anti-MM responses. MM immunosuppressive microenvironment remains the major hurdle to achieve a long lasting response along with low toxicity. Vaccination strategies have shown no clear clinical efficacy. Autologous and allogeneic stem cell transplantation (SCT) following myeloablative treatment allows introduction of a new immune system, but generates a very weak anti-tumor immune response. Immune checkpoint inhibitors, immunomodulatory drugs (IMiDs), and monoclonal antibodies (mAbs) used as single agents provided unsatisfactory results. Immunotherapy with adoptively transferred chimeric antigen receptor (CAR) T cells and new bi-specific antibodies are currently being tested in clinical trials, and initial results have been encouraging. Moreover, newer approaches based on the combination of immunotherapeutic strategies are achieving promising results with acceptable safety and durable responses. DC, dendritic cells; *γδ*, gamma delta T cells; MDSC, myeloid derived suppressor cells; MHC-I, major histocompatibility complex-class I; NK, natural killer cells; NKT, natural killer T cells; PC, plasma cells; PD-1, programmed cell death-1; PD-L1, programmed death ligand 1; SLAMF7, family member 7 of the signaling lymphocytic activation molecule; TCR, T cell receptor; Treg, regulatory T cells.

(IMiDs), thalidomide, and its analogs lenalidomide and pomalidomide, or histone deacetylase inhibitors (35). Besides their direct anti-tumor effects (142), IMiDs promote immune activation including functional enhancement of T, NK, and NKT cells, increase of Th1 cytokine production, reduction of Treg activity, improvement of DC maturation and functions, and enhancement of anti-MM antibody dependent cell-mediated cytotoxicity (ADCC) (143–145). Therefore, IMiDs exert anti-angiogenic and anti-inflammatory effects and can disrupt plasma cell–BM microenvironment interactions (146). Interestingly, *in vitro* studies have demonstrated that lenalidomide treatment reduces PD-1 expression on T and NK cells and PD-L1 expression on tumor plasma cells and MDSCs (86) suggesting that IMiDs could enhance the effect of the ICP inhibitor (139). Indeed, combined therapeutic strategies with IMiDs and ICP inhibitors achieved promising results with acceptable safety and durable responses. A phase II study (NCT02289222) combining the anti-PD-1 pembrolizumab with pomalidomide and low-dose dexamethasone in 48 patients with relapsed/refractory MM resulted in an objective response of 60% including stringent complete response/complete response (8%), very good partial response (19%), and partial response (33%), with a median duration of response of 14.7 months (147). Next phase III studies of pembrolizumab in combination with pomalidomide and dexamethasone (NCT02576977) or lenalidomide and dexamethasone (NCT02579863) have been halted by the US Food and Drug Administration because of unsatisfactory results in terms of objective response and high mortality (148). A phase I trial of the anti-PD-1 nivolumab in combination with IMiDs, daratumumab, and proteasome inhibitors uncovered this combined therapy to be effective with a low toxicity profile in highly pretreated and refractory MM patients (149). Further clinical studies are ongoing to investigate the efficacy and the toxicity of nivolumab in combination with other anti-myeloma drugs in earlier stages of disease and in low-risk MM patients. In addition, clinical trials of anti-PD-L1 monoclonal antibodies (mAbs) (atezolizumab and durvalumab) alone or in combination with other anti-myeloma agents are highly expected (150).

The use of mAbs targeting CD38, daratumumab, and isatuximab is also potentially useful for treatment of relapsed/refractory MM who have received two or more prior lines of therapy (151–153). The effect of drugs alone is enhanced by the addition of IMiDs or proteasome inhibitors. Phase III trials comparing the combination of daratumumab with bortezomib and dexamethasone or lenalidomide and dexamethasone *versus* the drugs alone showed improved progression-free survival and overall response (154–157). The improvement of response and progression-free survival with acceptable safety has been recently achieved also in newly-diagnosed transplant-eligible patients by using daratumumab in combination with bortezomib, thalidomide, and dexamethasone (158).

The ICARIA-MM phase III study comparing the combination of isatuximab, pomalidomide, and dexamethasone *versus* pomalidomide and dexamethasone alone in relapsed/refractory MM patients revealed that isatuximab in the combination regimen increased the number of patients achieving a response and significantly improved the strength of response and the median progression-free survival (159).

Alternative strategies include the use of agents to disrupt BM-myeloma cell interactions. One of these agents is elotuzumab, a humanized mAb that binds to SLAMF7 (family member 7 of the signaling lymphocytic activation molecule), an immunomodulatory receptor expressed on several hematopoietic cells, including myeloma cells and NK cells (160–162). A phase I, multicenter, open-label, dose escalation study of elotuzumab showed a favorable toxicity profile but no objective responses with stable disease reported in 26% of patients (163). However, the combination of elotuzumab with pomalidomide and dexamethasone revealed a significant improvement over pomalidomide and dexamethasone alone in treatment outcomes of relapsed/refractory MM patients. Specifically, the overall response rate was higher in the elotuzumab group (53%) than in the control group (26%) with a better progressionfree survival mainly observed in patients pretreated with at least four prior lines of therapy or patients who were considered as having highrisk disease on the basis of International Myeloma Working Group Criteria (164).

Immunotherapy with adoptively transferred chimeric antigen receptor (CAR) T cells targeting myeloma-associated antigens is currently being tested in clinical trials and initial results have been encouraging. A new effective therapy for MM is the use of anti-B cell maturation antigen (BCMA) CAR T cells. Treatment of relapsed/refractory MM patients provided promising results with a high overall response. However, the durability of this response was limited and even patients with initial complete response finally relapsed. Moreover, toxicities included cytokine release syndrome, and neurotoxicity has been reported (165, 166). The main mechanism of resistance to CAR T cell therapy is the evasion of fully differentiated tumor cells expressing lower levels of BCMA. Recently, the SLAM receptor CD229/LY9 has been used as potential target for chimeric antigen receptor (CAR) T cell therapy in MM due to its strong and broader expression on the surface of BM plasma cells from MM and MGUS patients and on chemotherapy-resistant myeloma precursor cells (167–169). CD229 CAR T cells displayed a strong and persistent activity against MM *in vitro* and *in vivo*. They efficiently killed not only terminally differentiated MM plasma cells, but also memory B cells and MM propagating cells (170).

Other immunotherapies including new bi-specific antibodies, which brings tumor cells into contact with immune effector cells, *e.g.*, T cells and NK cells, and vaccines in combination with mAbs or checkpoint inhibitors are still in early-stage clinical trials (150). To date, bi-specific antibodies have been evaluated in relapsed/refractory MM patients with promising results (171).

FUTURE DIRECTIONS

Our knowledge about mechanisms behind MM immunosuppression and sustenance of disease progression has advanced considerably. Crosstalk between immune cells and tumor endothelium regulates the entry and egress of immune cells within BM contributing to tumor immune surveillance and, at the same time, promoting angiogenesis, MM dissemination, and tumor growth (3, 11, 172, 173). Therefore, combination of canonical anti-angiogenesis treatments with immunomodulatory drugs may enhance the success of cancer immunotherapy. Moreover, it is clear that MM consists of several different genetic subtypes, and it is important to account for this when designing therapeutic regimens. A range of features including patient's immune profile, patient's baseline risk stratification, genetic mutations, disease biology, and imaging findings should be taken into account and integrated with each other to design tailored therapies targeting patients who might benefit the most from immunotherapy (174). New technologies for multi-dimensional measurement (for instance combination of single-cell RNA sequencing, genomic, immunophenotyping) of immune cells and proteins might help to build an "immunogram" to evaluate immune status and cancer-immune interactions in individual patients and thereby predict capacity to respond to immunotherapeutic strategies (76, 175).

Actually, along with immune-based approaches, the gene editing technology has emerged. Specifically, CRISPR-Cas9 technique can be used to detect necessary genes for MM plasma cells and genes involved in drug resistance, to explore the mechanism of drug action and to develop immunotherapy and screening for new drug targets (176).

Current research reveals that CRISPR/Cas9 is an efficient gene knockout platform to improve efficacy and safety of CAR T cells (177–179). Rupp et al. produced CD19-specific CAR T cells that were deficient in PD-1 using PD-1 disruption mediated by CRISPR/Cas9. The destruction of PD-1 increased CAR T cell ability to kill tumor cells *in vitro* (180). Based on these findings, CRISPR/Cas9 holds great promise for the treatment of MM.

AUTHOR CONTRIBUTIONS

Conceptualization: PL, AGS, and VR. Writing: PL. Data curation: PL, AGS, EM, RF, AB, FP, VDR, and AA. Funding: VR. Supervision: NS, AV, and VR. All authors contributed to the article and approved the submitted version.

REFERENCES

1. Hughes V. Microenvironment: Neighbourhood watch. *Nature* (2011) 480 (7377):S48–9. doi: 10.1038/480S48a
2. Kawano Y, Moschetta M, Manier S, Glavey S, Görgün GT, Roccaro AM, et al. Targeting the bone marrow microenvironment in multiple myeloma. *Immunol Rev* (2015) 263(1):160–72. doi: 10.1111/imr.12233
3. Solimando AG, Da Via MC, Leone P, Borrelli P, Croci GA, Tabares P, et al. Halting the vicious cycle within the multiple myeloma ecosystem: blocking JAM-A on bone marrow endothelial cells restores the angiogenic homeostasis and suppresses tumor progression. *Haematologica* (2020) haematol.2019.239913. doi: 10.3324/haematol.2019.239913
4. Balakumaran A, Robey PG, Fedarko N, Landgren O. Bone marrow microenvironment in myelomagenesis: its potential role in early diagnosis. *Expert Rev Mol Diagn* (2010) 10(4):465–80. doi: 10.1586/erm.10.31
5. Quezada SA, Peggs KS, Simpson TR, Allison JP. Shifting the equilibrium in cancer immunoediting: from tumor tolerance to eradication. *Immunol Rev* (2011) 241(1):104–18. doi: 10.1111/j.1600-065X.2011.01007.x
6. Schreiber RD, Old LJ, Smyth MJ. Cancer immunoediting: integrating immunity's roles in cancer suppression and promotion. *Science (N Y NY)* (2011) 331(6024):1565–70. doi: 10.1126/science.1203486
7. Dhodapkar MV, Krasovsky J, Osman K, Geller MD. Vigorous premalignancy-specific effector T cell response in the bone marrow of patients with monoclonal gammopathy. *J Exp Med* (2003) 198(11):1753–7. doi: 10.1084/jem.20031030
8. Racanelli V, Leone P, Frassanito MA, Brunetti C, Perosa F, Ferrone S, et al. Alterations in the antigen processing-presenting machinery of transformed plasma cells are associated with reduced recognition by CD8+ T cells and characterize the progression of MGUS to multiple myeloma. *Blood* (2010) 115(6):1185–93. doi: 10.1182/blood-2009-06-228676
9. Guillerey C, Nakamura K, Vuckovic S, Hill GR, Smyth MJ. Immune responses in multiple myeloma: role of the natural immune surveillance and potential of immunotherapies. *Cell Mol Life Sci: CMLS* (2016) 73 (8):1569–89. doi: 10.1007/s00018-016-2135-z
10. Leone P, Berardi S, Frassanito MA, Ria R, De Re V, Cicco S, et al. Dendritic cells accumulate in the bone marrow of myeloma patients where they protect tumor plasma cells from CD8+ T-cell killing. *Blood* (2015) 126(12):1443–51. doi: 10.1182/blood-2015-01-623975
11. Leone P, Di Lernia G, Solimando AG, Cicco S, Saltarella I, Lamanuzzi A, et al. Bone marrow endothelial cells sustain a tumor-specific CD8+ T cell subset with suppressive function in myeloma patients. *Oncoimmunology* (2019) 8(1):e1486949. doi: 10.1080/2162402X.2018.1486949
12. Mellstedt H, Holm G, Björkholm M. Multiple myeloma, Waldenström's macroglobulinemia, and benign monoclonal gammopathy: characteristics of the B cell clone, immunoregulatory cell populations and clinical implications. *Adv Cancer Res* (1984) 41:257–89. doi: 10.1016/s0065-230x(08)60018-4
13. Bogen B, Weiss S. Processing and presentation of idiotypes to MHC-restricted T cells. *Int Rev Immunol* (1993) 10(4):337–55. doi: 10.3109/08830189309061709
14. Weiss S. Bogen B. B-lymphoma cells process and present their endogenous immunoglobulin to major histocompatibility complex-restricted T cells. *Proc Natl Acad Sci U S A* (1989) 86(1):282–6. doi: 10.1073/pnas.86.1.282
15. Brown RD, Ho PJ. Detection of malignant plasma cells in the bone marrow and peripheral blood of patients with multiple myeloma. *Methods Mol Biol (Clifton NJ)* (2002) 179:85–91. doi: 10.1385/1-59259-238-4:085
16. Hansson L, Rabbani H, Fagerberg J, Osterborg A. Mellstedt H. T-cell epitopes within the complementarity-determining and framework regions of the tumor-derived immunoglobulin heavy chain in multiple myeloma. *Blood* (2003) 101(12):4930–6. doi: 10.1182/blood-2002-04-1250
17. Sze DMY, Brown RD, Yuen E, Gibson J, Ho J, Raitakari M, et al. Clonal cytotoxic T cells in myeloma. *Leuk Lymphoma* (2003) 44(10):1667–74. doi: 10.1080/1042819031000097438
18. Bogen B, Ruffini PA, Corthay A, Fredriksen AB, Frøyland M, Lundin K, et al. Idiotype-specific immunotherapy in multiple myeloma: suggestions for future directions of research. *Haematologica* (2006) 91(7):941–8.
19. Maecker B, von Bergwelt-Baildon MS, Anderson KS, Vonderheide RH, Anderson KC, Nadler LM, et al. Rare naturally occurring immune responses to three epitopes from the widely expressed tumour antigens hTERT and CYP1B1 in multiple myeloma patients. *Clin Exp Immunol* (2005) 141 (3):558–62. doi: 10.1111/j.1365-2249.2005.02879.x
20. Grube M, Moritz S, Obermann EC, Rezvani K, Mackensen A, Andreesen R, et al. CD8+ T cells reactive to survivin antigen in patients with multiple myeloma. *Clin Cancer Res* (2007) 13(3):1053–60. doi: 10.1158/1078-0432.CCR-06-1722
21. Szmania S, Tricot G, van Rhee F. NY-ESO-1 immunotherapy for multiple myeloma. *Leuk Lymphoma* (2006) 47(10):2037–48. doi: 10.1080/10428190600742292
22. Treon SP, Maimonis P, Bua D, Young G, Raje N, Mollick J, et al. Elevated soluble MUC1 levels and decreased anti-MUC1 antibody levels in patients with multiple myeloma. *Blood* (2000) 96(9):3147–53.
23. Kelly KR, Espitia CM, Zhao W, Wendlandt E, Tricot G, Zhan F, et al. Junctional adhesion molecule-A is overexpressed in advanced multiple myeloma and determines response to oncolytic reovirus. *Oncotarget* (2015) 6(38):41275–89. doi: 10.18632/oncotarget.5753
24. Solimando AG, Brandl A, Mattenheimer K, Graf C, Ritz M, Ruckdeschel A, et al. JAM-A as a prognostic factor and new therapeutic target in multiple myeloma. *Leukemia* (2018) 32(3):736–43. doi: 10.1038/leu.2017.287
25. Schmitt M, Schmitt A, Rojewski MT, Chen J, Giannopoulos K, Fei F, et al. RHAMM-R3 peptide vaccination in patients with acute myeloid leukemia, myelodysplastic syndrome, and multiple myeloma elicits immunologic and clinical responses. *Blood* (2008) 111(3):1357–65. doi: 10.1182/blood-2007-07-099366
26. Dhodapkar MV, Geller MD, Chang DH, Shimizu K, Fujii S-I, Dhodapkar KM, et al. A reversible defect in natural killer T cell function characterizes the progression of premalignant to malignant multiple myeloma. *J Exp Med* (2003) 197(12):1667–76. doi: 10.1084/jem.20021650
27. Dhodapkar MV, Krasovsky J, Olson K. T cells from the tumor microenvironment of patients with progressive myeloma can generate strong, tumor-specific cytolytic responses to autologous, tumor-loaded dendritic cells. *Proc Natl Acad Sci United States America* (2002) 99 (20):13009–13. doi: 10.1073/pnas.202491499
28. Finn OJ. Premalignant lesions as targets for cancer vaccines. *J Exp Med* (2003) 198(11):1623–6. doi: 10.1084/jem.20031787
29. Fonseca R, Bailey RJ, Ahmann GJ, Rajkumar SV, Hoyer JD, Lust JA, et al. Genomic abnormalities in monoclonal gammopathy of undetermined significance. *Blood* (2002) 100(4):1417–24.
30. Kuehl WM, Bergsagel PL. Multiple myeloma: evolving genetic events and host interactions. *Nat Rev Cancer* (2002) 2(3):175–87. doi: 10.1038/nrc746
31. Zhan F, Hardin J, Kordsmeier B, Bumm K, Zheng M, Tian E, et al. Global gene expression profiling of multiple myeloma, monoclonal gammopathy of undetermined significance, and normal bone marrow plasma cells. *Blood* (2002) 99(5):1745–57. doi: 10.1182/blood.v99.5.1745
32. Wen Y-J, Min R, Tricot G, Barlogie B, Yi Q. Tumor lysate-specific cytotoxic T lymphocytes in multiple myeloma: promising effector cells for immunotherapy. *Blood* (2002) 99(9):3280–5. doi: 10.1182/blood.v99.9.3280
33. Joshua D, Suen H, Brown R, Bryant C, Ho PJ, Hart D, et al. The T Cell in Myeloma. *Clin Lymphoma Myeloma Leuk* (2016) 16(10):537–42. doi: 10.1016/j.clml.2016.08.003
34. Spisek R, Kukreja A, Chen L-C, Matthews P, Mazumder A, Vesole D, et al. Frequent and specific immunity to the embryonal stem cell-associated antigen SOX2 in patients with monoclonal gammopathy. *J Exp Med* (2007) 204(4):831–40. doi: 10.1084/jem.20062387
35. Suen H, Brown R, Yang S, Weatherburn C, Ho PJ, Woodland N, et al. Multiple myeloma causes clonal T-cell immunosenescence: identification of potential novel targets for promoting tumour immunity and implications for checkpoint blockade. *Leukemia* (2016) 30(8):1716–24. doi: 10.1038/leu.2016.84
36. Bryant C, Suen H, Brown R, Yang S, Favaloro J, Aklilu E, et al. Long-term survival in multiple myeloma is associated with a distinct immunological profile, which includes proliferative cytotoxic T-cell clones and a favourable Treg/Th17 balance. *Blood Cancer J* (2013) 3:e148. doi: 10.1038/bcj.2013.34
37. Frassanito MA, Cusmai A, Dammacco F. Deregulated cytokine network and defective Th1 immune response in multiple myeloma. *Clin Exp Immunol* (2001) 125(2):190–7. doi: 10.1046/j.1365-2249.2001.01582.x
38. Sharma A, Khan R, Joshi S, Kumar L, Sharma M. Dysregulation in T helper 1/T helper 2 cytokine ratios in patients with multiple myeloma. *Leuk Lymphoma* (2010) 51(5):920–7. doi: 10.3109/10428191003699563

39. Feng P, Yan R, Dai X, Xie X, Wen H, Yang S. The alteration and clinical significance of Th1/Th2/Th17/Treg cells in patients with multiple myeloma. *Inflammation* (2015) 38(2):705–9. doi: 10.1007/s10753-014-9980-4
40. Murakami H, Ogawara H, Hiroshi H. Th1/Th2 cells in patients with multiple myeloma. *Hematol (Amsterdam Netherlands)* (2004) 9(1):41–5. doi: 10.1080/10245330310001652437
41. Ogawara H, Handa H, Yamazaki T, Toda T, Yoshida K, Nishimoto N, et al. High Th1/Th2 ratio in patients with multiple myeloma. *Leuk Res* (2005) 29 (2):135–40. doi: 10.1016/j.leukres.2004.06.003
42. Paiva B, Azpilikueta A, Puig N, Ocio EM, Sharma R, Oyajobi BO, et al. PD-L1/PD-1 presence in the tumor microenvironment and activity of PD-1 blockade in multiple myeloma. *Leukemia* (2015) 29(10):2110–3. doi: 10.1038/leu.2015.79
43. Dhodapkar MV, Sexton R, Das R, Dhodapkar KM, Zhang L, Sundaram R, et al. Prospective analysis of antigen-specific immunity, stem-cell antigens, and immune checkpoints in monoclonal gammopathy. *Blood* (2015) 126 (22):2475–8. doi: 10.1182/blood-2015-03-632919
44. Noonan K, Marchionni L, Anderson J, Pardoll D, Roodman GD, Borrello I. A novel role of IL-17-producing lymphocytes in mediating lytic bone disease in multiple myeloma. *Blood* (2010) 116(18):3554–63. doi: 10.1182/blood-2010-05-283895
45. Prabhala RH, Pelluru D, Fulciniti M, Prabhala HK, Nanjappa P, Song W, et al. Elevated IL-17 produced by TH17 cells promotes myeloma cell growth and inhibits immune function in multiple myeloma. *Blood* (2010) 115 (26):5385–92. doi: 10.1182/blood-2009-10-246660
46. Shen C-J, Yuan Z-H, Liu Y-X, Hu G-Y. Increased Numbers of T Helper 17 Cells and the Correlation with Clinicopathological Characteristics in Multiple Myeloma. *J Int Med Res* (2012) 40(2):556–64. doi: 10.1177/147323001204000217
47. Calcinotto A, Brevi A, Chesi M, Ferrarese R, Garcia Perez L, Grioni M, et al. Microbiota-driven interleukin-17-producing cells and eosinophils synergize to accelerate multiple myeloma progression. *Nat Commun* (2018) 9(1):4832. doi: 10.1038/s41467-018-07305-8
48. Chu VT, Fröhlich A, Steinhauser G, Scheel T, Roch T, Fillatreau S, et al. Eosinophils are required for the maintenance of plasma cells in the bone marrow. *Nat Immunol* (2011) 12(2):151–9. doi: 10.1038/ni.1981
49. Gupta R, Ganeshan P, Hakim M, Verma R, Sharma A, Kumar L. Significantly reduced regulatory T cell population in patients with untreated multiple myeloma. *Leuk Res* (2011) 35(7):874–8. doi: 10.1016/j.leukres.2010.11.010
50. Prabhala RH, Neri P, Bae JE, Tassone P, Shammas MA, Allam CK, et al. Dysfunctional T regulatory cells in multiple myeloma. *Blood* (2006) 107 (1):301–4. doi: 10.1182/blood-2005-08-3101
51. Beyer M, Kochanek M, Giese T, Endl E, Weihrauch MR, Knolle PA, et al. In vivo peripheral expansion of naive CD4+CD25high FoxP3+ regulatory T cells in patients with multiple myeloma. *Blood* (2006) 107(10):3940–9. doi: 10.1182/blood-2005-09-3671
52. Braga WMT, da Silva BR, de Carvalho AC, Maekawa YH, Bortoluzzo AB, Rizzatti EG, et al. FOXP3 and CTLA4 overexpression in multiple myeloma bone marrow as a sign of accumulation of CD4(+) T regulatory cells. *Cancer Immunol Immunother: CII* (2014) 63(11):1189–97. doi: 10.1007/s00262-014-1589-9
53. Feyler S, von Lilienfeld-Toal M, Jarmin S, Marles L, Rawstron A, Ashcroft AJ, et al. CD4(+)CD25(+)FoxP3(+) regulatory T cells are increased whilst CD3(+)CD4(-)CD8(-)alphabetaTCR(+) Double Negative T cells are decreased in the peripheral blood of patients with multiple myeloma which correlates with disease burden. *Br J Haematol* (2009) 144(5):686–95. doi: 10.1111/j.1365-2141.2008.07530.x
54. Frassanito MA, Ruggieri S, Desantis V, Di Marzo L, Leone P, Racanelli V, et al. Myeloma cells act as tolerogenic antigen-presenting cells and induce regulatory T cells in vitro. *Eur J Haematol* (2015) 95(1):65–74. doi: 10.1111/ejh.12481
55. Giannopoulos K, Kaminska W, Hus I, Dmoszynska A. The frequency of T regulatory cells modulates the survival of multiple myeloma patients: detailed characterisation of immune status in multiple myeloma. *Br J Cancer* (2012) 106(3):546–52. doi: 10.1038/bjc.2011.575
56. Muthu Raja KR, Kubiczkova L, Rihova L, Piskacek M, Vsianska P, Hezova R, et al. Functionally suppressive CD8 T regulatory cells are increased in patients with multiple myeloma: a cause for immune impairment. *PLoS One* (2012) 7(11):e49446. doi: 10.1371/journal.pone.0049446
57. Wang J-N, Cao X-X, Zhao A-L, Cai H, Wang X, Li J. Increased activated regulatory T cell subsets and aging Treg-like cells in multiple myeloma and monoclonal gammopathy of undetermined significance: a case control study. *Cancer Cell Int* (2018) 18:187. doi: 10.1186/s12935-018-0687-8
58. Alrasheed N, Lee L, Ghorani E, Henry JY, Conde L, Chin M, et al. Marrow-Infiltrating Regulatory T Cells Correlate with the Presence of Dysfunctional CD4+PD-1+ Cells and Inferior Survival in Patients with Newly Diagnosed Multiple Myeloma. *Clin Cancer Res* (2020) 26(13):3443–54. doi: 10.1158/1078-0432.CCR-19-1714
59. Feyler S, Scott GB, Parrish C, Jarmin S, Evans P, Short M, et al. Tumour cell generation of inducible regulatory T-cells in multiple myeloma is contact-dependent and antigen-presenting cell-independent. *PLoS One* (2012) 7(5): e35981. doi: 10.1371/journal.pone.0035981
60. Banerjee DK, Dhodapkar MV, Matayeva E, Steinman RM, Dhodapkar KM. Expansion of FOXP3high regulatory T cells by human dendritic cells (DCs) in vitro and after injection of cytokine-matured DCs in myeloma patients. *Blood* (2006) 108(8):2655–61. doi: 10.1182/blood-2006-03-011353
61. Levings MK, Gregori S, Tresoldi E, Cazzaniga S, Bonini C, Roncarolo MG. Differentiation of Tr1 cells by immature dendritic cells requires IL-10 but not CD25+CD4+ Tr cells. *Blood* (2005) 105(3):1162–9. doi: 10.1182/blood-2004-03-1211
62. Ghiringhelli F, Puig PE, Roux S, Parcellier A, Schmitt E, Solary E, et al. Tumor cells convert immature myeloid dendritic cells into TGF-beta-secreting cells inducing CD4+CD25+ regulatory T cell proliferation. *J Exp Med* (2005) 202(7):919–29. doi: 10.1084/jem.20050463
63. Brown R, Kabani K, Favaloro J, Yang S, Ho PJ, Gibson J, et al. CD86+ or HLA-G+ can be transferred via trogocytosis from myeloma cells to T cells and are associated with poor prognosis. *Blood* (2012) 120(10):2055–63. doi: 10.1182/blood-2012-03-416792
64. Castella B, Foglietta M, Sciancalepore P, Rigoni M, Coscia M, Griggio V, et al. Anergic bone marrow Vγ9Vδ2 T cells as early and long-lasting markers of PD-1-targetable microenvironment-induced immune suppression in human myeloma. *Oncoimmunology* (2015) 4(11):e1047580. doi: 10.1080/2162402X.2015.1047580
65. Castella B, Foglietta M, Riganti C, Massaia M. Vγ9Vδ2 T Cells in the Bone Marrow of Myeloma Patients: A Paradigm of Microenvironment-Induced Immune Suppression. *Front Immunol* (2018) 9:1492. doi: 10.3389/fimmu.2018.01492
66. Chauhan D, Singh AV, Brahmandam M, Carrasco R, Bandi M, Hideshima T, et al. Functional interaction of plasmacytoid dendritic cells with multiple myeloma cells: a therapeutic target. *Cancer Cell* (2009) 16(4):309–23. doi: 10.1016/j.ccr.2009.08.019
67. Ray A, Das DS, Song Y, Richardson P, Munshi NC, Chauhan D, et al. Targeting PD1-PDL1 immune checkpoint in plasmacytoid dendritic cell interactions with T cells, natural killer cells and multiple myeloma cells. *Leukemia* (2015) 29(6):1441–4. doi: 10.1038/leu.2015.11
68. Sponaas A-M, Moharrami NN, Feyzi E, Standal T, Holth Rustad E, Waage A, et al. PDL1 Expression on Plasma and Dendritic Cells in Myeloma Bone Marrow Suggests Benefit of Targeted anti PD1-PDL1 Therapy. *PLoS One* (2015) 10(10):e0139867. doi: 10.1371/journal.pone.0139867
69. Dhodapkar KM, Barbuto S, Matthews P, Kukreja A, Mazumder A, Vesole D, et al. Dendritic cells mediate the induction of polyfunctional human IL17-producing cells (Th17-1 cells) enriched in the bone marrow of patients with myeloma. *Blood* (2008) 112(7):2878–85. doi: 10.1182/blood-2008-03-143222
70. Kotake S, Udagawa N, Takahashi N, Matsuzaki K, Itoh K, Ishiyama S, et al. IL-17 in synovial fluids from patients with rheumatoid arthritis is a potent stimulator of osteoclastogenesis. *J Clin Invest* (1999) 103(9):1345–52. doi: 10.1172/JCI5703
71. Kim J, Denu RA, Dollar BA, Escalante LE, Kuether JP, Callander NS, et al. Macrophages and mesenchymal stromal cells support survival and proliferation of multiple myeloma cells. *Br J Haematol* (2012) 158(3):336–46. doi: 10.1111/j.1365-2141.2012.09154.x
72. Zheng Y, Cai Z, Wang S, Zhang X, Qian J, Hong S, et al. Macrophages are an abundant component of myeloma microenvironment and protect myeloma cells from chemotherapy drug-induced apoptosis. *Blood* (2009) 114 (17):3625–8. doi: 10.1182/blood-2009-05-220285

73. Zheng Y, Yang J, Qian J, Qiu P, Hanabuchi S, Lu Y, et al. PSGL-1/selectin and ICAM-1/CD18 interactions are involved in macrophage-induced drug resistance in myeloma. *Leukemia* (2013) 27(3):702–10. doi: 10.1038/leu.2012.272
74. Kim J, Hematti P. Mesenchymal stem cell-educated macrophages: a novel type of alternatively activated macrophages. *Exp Hematol* (2009) 37 (12):1445–53. doi: 10.1016/j.exphem.2009.09.004
75. Berardi S, Ria R, Reale A, De Luisi A, Catacchio I, Moschetta M, et al. Multiple myeloma macrophages: pivotal players in the tumor microenvironment. *J Oncol* (2013) 2013:183602. doi: 10.1155/2013/183602
76. Zavidij O, Haradhvala NJ, Mouhieddine TH, Sklavenitis-Pistofidis R, Cai S, Reidy M, et al. Single-cell RNA sequencing reveals compromised immune microenvironment in precursor stages of multiple myeloma. *Nat Cancer* (2020) 1:493–506. doi: 10.1038/s43018-020-0053-3
77. Dosani T, Carlsten M, Maric I, Landgren O. The cellular immune system in myelomagenesis: NK cells and T cells in the development of myeloma [corrected] and their uses in immunotherapies. *Blood Cancer J* (2015) 5: e306. doi: 10.1038/bcj.2015.32
78. Carbone E, Neri P, Mesuraca M, Fulciniti MT, Otsuki T, Pende D, et al. NKG2D, and natural cytotoxicity receptors regulate multiple myeloma cell recognition by natural killer cells. *Blood* (2005) 105(1):251–8. doi: 10.1182/blood-2004-04-1422
79. García-Sanz R, González M, Orfão A, Moro MJ, Hernández JM, Borrego D, et al. Analysis of natural killer-associated antigens in peripheral blood and bone marrow of multiple myeloma patients and prognostic implications. *Br J Haematol* (1996) 93(1):81–8. doi: 10.1046/j.1365-2141.1996.4651006.x
80. El-Sherbiny YM, Meade JL, Holmes TD, McGonagle D, Mackie SL, Morgan AW, et al. The requirement for DNAM-1, NKG2D, and NKp46 in the natural killer cell-mediated killing of myeloma cells. *Cancer Res* (2007) 67 (18):8444–9. doi: 10.1158/0008-5472.CAN-06-4230
81. Costello RT, Boehrer A, Sanchez C, Mercier D, Baier C, Le Treut T, et al. Differential expression of natural killer cell activating receptors in blood versus bone marrow in patients with monoclonal gammopathy. *Immunology* (2013) 139(3):338–41. doi: 10.1111/imm.12082
82. Bernal M, Garrido P, Jiménez P, Carretero R, Almagro M, López P, et al. Changes in activatory and inhibitory natural killer (NK) receptors may induce progression to multiple myeloma: implications for tumor evasion of T and NK cells. *Hum Immunol* (2009) 70(10):854–7. doi: 10.1016/j.humimm.2009.07.004
83. Jinushi M, Vanneman M, Munshi NC, Tai Y-T, Prabhala RH, Ritz J, et al. MHC class I chain-related protein A antibodies and shedding are associated with the progression of multiple myeloma. *Proc Natl Acad Sci U S A* (2008) 105(4):1285–90. doi: 10.1073/pnas.0711293105
84. Ponzetta A, Benigni G, Antonangeli F, Sciumè G, Sanseviero E, Zingoni A, et al. Multiple Myeloma Impairs Bone Marrow Localization of Effector Natural Killer Cells by Altering the Chemokine Microenvironment. *Cancer Res* (2015) 75(22):4766–77. doi: 10.1158/0008-5472.CAN-15-1320
85. von Lilienfeld-Toal M, Frank S, Leyendecker C, Feyler S, Jarmin S, Morgan R, et al. Reduced immune effector cell NKG2D expression and increased levels of soluble NKG2D ligands in multiple myeloma may not be causally linked. *Cancer Immunol Immunother: CII* (2010) 59(6):829–39. doi: 10.1007/s00262-009-0807-3
86. Benson DM, Bakan CE, Mishra A, Hofmeister CC, Efebera Y, Becknell B, et al. The PD-1/PD-L1 axis modulates the natural killer cell versus multiple myeloma effect: a therapeutic target for CT-011, a novel monoclonal anti-PD-1 antibody. *Blood* (2010) 116(13):2286–94. doi: 10.1182/blood-2010-02-271874
87. Garcia-Diaz A, Shin DS, Moreno BH, Saco J, Escuin-Ordinas H, Rodriguez GA, et al. Interferon Receptor Signaling Pathways Regulating PD-L1 and PD-L2 Expression. *Cell Rep* (2017) 19(6):1189–201. doi: 10.1016/j.celrep.2017.04.031
88. Fauriat C, Just-Landi S, Mallet F, Arnoulet C, Sainty D, Olive D, et al. Deficient expression of NCR in NK cells from acute myeloid leukemia: Evolution during leukemia treatment and impact of leukemia cells in NCRdull phenotype induction. *Blood* (2007) 109(1):323–30. doi: 10.1182/blood-2005-08-027979
89. Sarkar S, van Gelder M, Noort W, Xu Y, Rouschop KMA, Groen R, et al. Optimal selection of natural killer cells to kill myeloma: the role of HLA-E and NKG2A. *Cancer Immunol Immunother: CII* (2015) 64(8):951–63. doi: 10.1007/s00262-015-1694-4
90. Tognarelli S, Wirsching S, von Metzler I, Rais B, Jacobs B, Serve H, et al. Enhancing the Activation and Releasing the Brakes: A Double Hit Strategy to Improve NK Cell Cytotoxicity Against Multiple Myeloma. *Front Immunol* (2018) 9:2743. doi: 10.3389/fimmu.2018.02743
91. Dhodapkar MV. MGUS to myeloma: a mysterious gammopathy of underexplored significance. *Blood* (2016) 128(23):2599–606. doi: 10.1182/blood-2016-09-692954
92. Nur H, Fostier K, Aspeslagh S, Renmans W, Bertrand E, Leleu X, et al. Preclinical evaluation of invariant natural killer T cells in the 5T33 multiple myeloma model. *PLoS One* (2013) 8(5):e65075. doi: 10.1371/journal.pone.0065075
93. Pasiarski M, Grywalska E, Kosmaczewska A, Góźdź S, Steckiewicz P, Garus B, et al. Assessment of peripheral blood and bone marrow T, NK, NKT and dendritic cells in patients with multiple myeloma. *Postepy Higieny I Medycyny Doswiadczalnej (Online)* (2015) 69:1435–42.
94. Chan AC, Neeson P, Leeansyah E, Tainton K, Quach H, Prince HM, et al. Natural killer T cell defects in multiple myeloma and the impact of lenalidomide therapy. *Clin Exp Immunol* (2014) 175(1):49–58. doi: 10.1111/cei.12196
95. Spanoudakis E, Hu M, Naresh K, Terpos E, Melo V, Reid A, et al. Regulation of multiple myeloma survival and progression by CD1d. *Blood* (2009) 113 (11):2498–507. doi: 10.1182/blood-2008-06-161281
96. Chang DH, Deng H, Matthews P, Krasovsky J, Ragupathi G, Spisek R, et al. Inflammation-associated lysophospholipids as ligands for CD1d-restricted T cells in human cancer. *Blood* (2008) 112(4):1308–16. doi: 10.1182/blood-2008-04-149831
97. Nair S, Boddupalli CS, Verma R, Liu J, Yang R, Pastores GM, et al. Type II NKT-TFH cells against Gaucher lipids regulate B-cell immunity and inflammation. *Blood* (2015) 125(8):1256–71. doi: 10.1182/blood-2014-09-600270
98. Nair S, Sng J, Boddupalli CS, Seckinger A, Chesi M, Fulciniti M, et al. Antigen-mediated regulation in monoclonal gammopathies and myeloma. *JCI Insight* (2018) 3(8):e98259. doi: 10.1172/jci.insight.98259
99. Peranzoni E, Zilio S, Marigo I, Dolcetti L, Zanovello P, Mandruzzato S, et al. Myeloid-derived suppressor cell heterogeneity and subset definition. *Curr Opin Immunol* (2010) 22(2):238–44. doi: 10.1016/j.coi.2010.01.021
100. Favaloro J, Liyadipitiya T, Brown R, Yang S, Suen H, Woodland N, et al. Myeloid derived suppressor cells are numerically, functionally and phenotypically different in patients with multiple myeloma. *Leuk Lymphoma* (2014) 55(12):2893–900. doi: 10.3109/10428194.2014.904511
101. Görgün GT, Whitehill G, Anderson JL, Hideshima T, Maguire C, Laubach J, et al. Tumor-promoting immune-suppressive myeloid-derived suppressor cells in the multiple myeloma microenvironment in humans. *Blood* (2013) 121(15):2975–87. doi: 10.1182/blood-2012-08-448548
102. Ramachandran IR, Martner A, Pisklakova A, Condamine T, Chase T, Vogl T, et al. Myeloid-derived suppressor cells regulate growth of multiple myeloma by inhibiting T cells in bone marrow. *J Immunol (Baltimore Md: 1950)* (2013) 190(7):3815–23. doi: 10.4049/jimmunol.1203373
103. Brimnes MK, Vangsted AJ, Knudsen LM, Gimsing P, Gang AO, Johnsen HE, et al. Increased level of both CD4+FOXP3+ regulatory T cells and CD14 +HLA-DR$^-$/low myeloid-derived suppressor cells and decreased level of dendritic cells in patients with multiple myeloma. *Scand J Immunol* (2010) 72(6):540–7. doi: 10.1111/j.1365-3083.2010.02463.x
104. Wang Z, Zhang L, Wang H, Xiong S, Li Y, Tao Q, et al. Tumor-induced CD14+HLA-DR (-/low) myeloid-derived suppressor cells correlate with tumor progression and outcome of therapy in multiple myeloma patients. *Cancer Immunol Immunother: CII* (2015) 64(3):389–99. doi: 10.1007/s00262-014-1646-4
105. Rodriguez PC, Quiceno DG, Zabaleta J, Ortiz B, Zea AH, Piazuelo MB, et al. Arginase I production in the tumor microenvironment by mature myeloid cells inhibits T-cell receptor expression and antigen-specific T-cell responses. *Cancer Res* (2004) 64(16):5839–49. doi: 10.1158/0008-5472.CAN-04-0465
106. Serafini P, Borrello I, Bronte V. Myeloid suppressor cells in cancer: recruitment, phenotype, properties, and mechanisms of immune suppression. *Semin Cancer Biol* (2006) 16(1):53–65. doi: 10.1016/j.semcancer.2005.07.005

107. Lazarova M, Steinle A. Impairment of NKG2D-Mediated Tumor Immunity by TGF-beta. *Front Immunol* (2019) 10:2689. doi: 10.3389/fimmu.2019.02689
108. Li H, Han Y, Guo Q, Zhang M, Cao X. Cancer-Expanded Myeloid-Derived Suppressor Cells Induce Anergy of NK Cells through Membrane-Bound TGF-β1. *J Immunol* (2009) 182(1):240–9. doi: 10.4049/jimmunol.182.1.240
109. Yang L, DeBusk LM, Fukuda K, Fingleton B, Green-Jarvis B, Shyr Y, et al. Expansion of myeloid immune suppressor Gr+CD11b+ cells in tumor-bearing host directly promotes tumor angiogenesis. *Cancer Cell* (2004) 6 (4):409–21. doi: 10.1016/j.ccr.2004.08.031
110. Cossio I, Lucas D, Hidalgo A. Neutrophils as regulators of the hematopoietic niche. *Blood* (2019) 133(20):2140–8. doi: 10.1182/blood-2018-10-844571
111. Tamassia N, Bianchetto-Aguilera F, Arruda-Silva F, Gardiman E, Gasperini S, Calzetti F, et al. Cytokine production by human neutrophils: Revisiting the "dark side of the moon". *Eur J Clin Invest* (2018) 48(Suppl 2):e12952. doi: 10.1111/eci.12952
112. Mayadas TN, Cullere X, Lowell CA. The multifaceted functions of neutrophils. *Annu Rev Pathol* (2014) 9:181–218. doi: 10.1146/annurev-pathol-020712-164023
113. Karle H, Hansen NE, Plesner T. Neutrophil defect in multiple myeloma. Studies on intraneutrophilic lysozyme in multiple myeloma and malignant lymphoma. *Scand J Haematol* (1976) 17(1):62–70.
114. Romano A, Parrinello NL, La Cava P, Tibullo D, Giallongo C, Camiolo G, et al. PMN-MDSC and arginase are increased in myeloma and may contribute to resistance to therapy. *Expert Rev Mol Diagn* (2018) 18 (7):675–83. doi: 10.1080/14737159.2018.1470929
115. Romano A, Parrinello NL, Simeon V, Puglisi F, La Cava P, Bellofiore C, et al. High-density neutrophils in MGUS and multiple myeloma are dysfunctional and immune-suppressive due to increased STAT3 downstream signaling. *Sci Rep* (2020) 10(1):1983. doi: 10.1038/s41598-020-58859-x
116. Munera V, Popovic PJ, Bryk J, Pribis J, Caba D, Matta BM, et al. Stat 6-dependent induction of myeloid derived suppressor cells after physical injury regulates nitric oxide response to endotoxin. *Ann Surg* (2010) 251(1):120–6. doi: 10.1097/SLA.0b013e3181bfda1c
117. Vasquez-Dunddel D, Pan F, Zeng Q, Gorbounov M, Albesiano E, Fu J, et al. STAT3 regulates arginase-I in myeloid-derived suppressor cells from cancer patients. *J Clin Invest* (2013) 123(4):1580–9. doi: 10.1172/JCI60083
118. Waight JD, Netherby C, Hensen ML, Miller A, Hu Q, Liu S, et al. Myeloid-derived suppressor cell development is regulated by a STAT/IRF-8 axis. *J Clin Invest* (2013) 123(10):4464–78. doi: 10.1172/JCI68189
119. Puglisi F, Parrinello NL, Giallongo C, Cambria D, Camiolo G, Bellofiore C, et al. Plasticity of High-Density Neutrophils in Multiple Myeloma is Associated with Increased Autophagy Via STAT3. *Int J Mol Sci* (2019) 20 (14):3548. doi: 10.3390/ijms20143548
120. Romano A, Laura Parrinello N, Cerchione C, Letizia Consoli M, Parisi M, Calafiore V, et al. and LMR ratio in newly diagnosed MM patients treated upfront with novel agents. *Blood Cancer J* (2017) 7(12):649. doi: 10.1038/s41408-017-0019-6
121. Romano A, Parrinello NL, Consoli ML, Marchionni L, Forte S, Conticello C, et al. Neutrophil to lymphocyte ratio (NLR) improves the risk assessment of ISS staging in newly diagnosed MM patients treated upfront with novel agents. *Ann Hematol* (2015) 94(11):1875–83. doi: 10.1007/s00277-015-2462-4
122. Solmaz Medeni S, Acar C, Olgun A, Acar A, Seyhanli A, Taskiran E, et al. Can Neutrophil-to-Lymphocyte Ratio, Monocyte-to-Lymphocyte Ratio, and Platelet-to-Lymphocyte Ratio at Day +100 be used as a prognostic marker in Multiple Myeloma patients with autologous transplantation? *Clin Transplant* (2018) 32(9):e13359. doi: 10.1111/ctr.13359
123. Gajewski TF, Schreiber H, Fu Y-X. Innate and adaptive immune cells in the tumor microenvironment. *Nat Immunol* (2013) 14(10):1014–22. doi: 10.1038/ni.2703
124. Zelle-Rieser C, Thangavadivel S, Biedermann R, Brunner A, Stoitzner P, Willenbacher E, et al. T cells in multiple myeloma display features of exhaustion and senescence at the tumor site. *J Hematol Oncol* (2016) 9 (1):116. doi: 10.1186/s13045-016-0345-3
125. Suen H, Brown R, Yang S, Ho PJ, Gibson J, Joshua D. The failure of immune checkpoint blockade in multiple myeloma with PD-1 inhibitors in a phase 1 study. *Leukemia* (2015) 29(7):1621–2. doi: 10.1038/leu.2015.104
126. Liu J, Hamrouni A, Wolowiec D, Coiteux V, Kuliczkowski K, Hetuin D, et al. Plasma cells from multiple myeloma patients express B7-H1 (PD-L1) and increase expression after stimulation with IFN-{gamma} and TLR ligands via a MyD88-, TRAF6-, and MEK-dependent pathway. *Blood* (2007) 110 (1):296–304. doi: 10.1182/blood-2006-10-051482
127. Tamura H, Ishibashi M, Yamashita T, Tanosaki S, Okuyama N, Kondo A, et al. Marrow stromal cells induce B7-H1 expression on myeloma cells, generating aggressive characteristics in multiple myeloma. *Leukemia* (2013) 27(2):464–72. doi: 10.1038/leu.2012.213
128. Yousef S, Marvin J, Steinbach M, Langemo A, Kovacsovics T, Binder M, et al. Immunomodulatory molecule PD-L1 is expressed on malignant plasma cells and myeloma-propagating pre-plasma cells in the bone marrow of multiple myeloma patients. *Blood Cancer J* (2015) 5:e285. doi: 10.1038/bcj.2015.7
129. An G, Acharya C, Feng X, Wen K, Zhong M, Zhang L, et al. Osteoclasts promote immune suppressive microenvironment in multiple myeloma: therapeutic implication. *Blood* (2016) 128(12):1590–603. doi: 10.1182/blood-2016-03-707547
130. Pratt G, Goodyear O, Moss P. Immunodeficiency and immunotherapy in multiple myeloma. *Br J Haematol* (2007) 138(5):563–79. doi: 10.1111/j.1365-2141.2007.06705.x
131. Kukreja A, Radfar S, Sun B-H, Insogna K, Dhodapkar MV. Dominant role of CD47-thrombospondin-1 interactions in myeloma-induced fusion of human dendritic cells: implications for bone disease. *Blood* (2009) 114 (16):3413–21. doi: 10.1182/blood-2009-03-211920
132. Tucci M, Ciavarella S, Strippoli S, Brunetti O, Dammacco F, Silvestris F. Immature dendritic cells from patients with multiple myeloma are prone to osteoclast differentiation in vitro. *Exp Hematol* (2011) 39(7):773–83.e1. doi: 10.1016/j.exphem.2011.04.006
133. Nair JR, Rozanski CH, Lee KP. Under one roof: The bone marrow survival niche for multiple myeloma and normal plasma cells. *Oncoimmunology* (2012) 1(3):388–9. doi: 10.4161/onci.18746
134. Botta C, Di Martino MT, Ciliberto D, Cucè M, Correale P, Rossi M, et al. A gene expression inflammatory signature specifically predicts multiple myeloma evolution and patients survival. *Blood Cancer J* (2016) 6(12): e511. doi: 10.1038/bcj.2016.118
135. Musolino C, Allegra A, Innao V, Allegra AG, Pioggia G, Gangemi S. Inflammatory and Anti-Inflammatory Equilibrium, Proliferative and Antiproliferative Balance: The Role of Cytokines in Multiple Myeloma. *Mediators Inflamm* (2017) 2017:1852517. doi: 10.1155/2017/1852517
136. Rajkumar SV. Multiple myeloma: 2020 update on diagnosis, risk-stratification and management. *Am J Hematol* (2020) 95(5):548–67. doi: 10.1002/ajh.25791
137. Noonan KA, Huff CA, Davis J, Lemas MV, Fiorino S, Bitzan J, et al. Adoptive transfer of activated marrow-infiltrating lymphocytes induces measurable antitumor immunity in the bone marrow in multiple myeloma. *Sci Trans Med* (2015) 7(288):288ra78. doi: 10.1126/scitranslmed.aaa7014
138. Bensinger W. Allogeneic stem cell transplantation for multiple myeloma. *Hematology/Oncology Clinics North Am* (2014) 28(5):891–902. doi: 10.1016/j.hoc.2014.06.001
139. Görgün G, Samur MK, Cowens KB, Paula S, Bianchi G, Anderson JE, et al. Lenalidomide Enhances Immune Checkpoint Blockade-Induced Immune Response in Multiple Myeloma. *Clin Cancer Res* (2015) 21(20):4607–18. doi: 10.1158/1078-0432.CCR-15-0200
140. Hallett WHD, Jing W, Drobyski WR, Johnson BD. Immunosuppressive effects of multiple myeloma are overcome by PD-L1 blockade. *Biol Blood Marrow Transplant* (2011) 17(8):1133–45. doi: 10.1016/j.bbmt.2011.03.011
141. Kearl TJ, Jing W, Gershan JA, Johnson BD. Programmed death receptor-1/programmed death receptor ligand-1 blockade after transient lymphodepletion to treat myeloma. *J Immunol (Baltimore Md: 1950)* (2013) 190(11):5620–8. doi: 10.4049/jimmunol.1202005
142. Hideshima T, Chauhan D, Shima Y, Raje N, Davies FE, Tai YT, et al. Thalidomide and its analogs overcome drug resistance of human multiple myeloma cells to conventional therapy. *Blood* (2000) 96(9):2943–50.
143. Costa F, Vescovini R, Bolzoni M, Marchica V, Storti P, Toscani D, et al. Lenalidomide increases human dendritic cell maturation in multiple myeloma patients targeting monocyte differentiation and modulating mesenchymal stromal cell inhibitory properties. *Oncotarget* (2017) 8 (32):53053–67. doi: 10.18632/oncotarget.18085
144. Galustian C, Meyer B, Labarthe M-C, Dredge K, Klaschka D, Henry J, et al. The anti-cancer agents lenalidomide and pomalidomide inhibit the

proliferation and function of T regulatory cells. *Cancer Immunol Immunother: CII* (2009) 58(7):1033–45. doi: 10.1007/s00262-008-0620-4
145. Luptakova K, Rosenblatt J, Glotzbecker B, Mills H, Stroopinsky D, Kufe T, et al. Lenalidomide enhances anti-myeloma cellular immunity. *Cancer Immunol Immunother: CII* (2013) 62(1):39–49. doi: 10.1007/s00262-012-1308-3
146. Quach H, Ritchie D, Stewart AK, Neeson P, Harrison S, Smyth MJ, et al. Mechanism of action of immunomodulatory drugs (IMiDS) in multiple myeloma. *Leukemia* (2010) 24(1):22–32. doi: 10.1038/leu.2009.236
147. Badros A, Hyjek E, Ma N, Lesokhin A, Dogan A, Rapoport AP, et al. Pembrolizumab, pomalidomide, and low-dose dexamethasone for relapsed/refractory multiple myeloma. *Blood* (2017) 130(10):1189–97. doi: 10.1182/blood-2017-03-775122
148. Costa F, Das R, Kini Bailur J, Dhodapkar K, Dhodapkar MV. Checkpoint Inhibition in Myeloma: Opportunities and Challenges. *Front Immunol* (2018) 9:2204. doi: 10.3389/fimmu.2018.02204
149. Thanendrarajan S, Puryear J, Schinke CD, van Rhee F, Zangari M, Mathur P, et al. Nivolumab for Treatment of Advanced, Refractory, High-Risk Multiple Myeloma. *Blood* (2017) 130.
150. Soekojo CY, Ooi M, de Mel S, Chng WJ. Immunotherapy in Multiple Myeloma. *Cells* (2020) 9(3):601. doi: 10.3390/cells9030601
151. Lokhorst HM, Plesner T, Laubach JP, Nahi H, Gimsing P, Hansson M, et al. Targeting CD38 with Daratumumab Monotherapy in Multiple Myeloma. *N Engl J Med* (2015) 373(13):1207–19. doi: 10.1056/NEJMoa1506348
152. Lonial S, Weiss BM, Usmani SZ, Singhal S, Chari A, Bahlis NJ, et al. Daratumumab monotherapy in patients with treatment-refractory multiple myeloma (SIRIUS): an open-label, randomised, phase 2 trial. *Lancet (Lond Engl)* (2016) 387(10027):1551–60. doi: 10.1016/S0140-6736(15)01120-4
153. Mikhael J, Richter J, Vij R, Cole C, Zonder J, Kaufman JL, et al. A dose-finding Phase 2 study of single agent isatuximab (anti-CD38 mAb) in relapsed/refractory multiple myeloma. *Leukemia* (2020). doi: 10.1038/s41375-020-0857-2
154. Dimopoulos MA, Oriol A, Nahi H, San-Miguel J, Bahlis NJ, Usmani SZ, et al. Daratumumab, Lenalidomide, and Dexamethasone for Multiple Myeloma. *N Engl J Med* (2016) 375(14):1319–31. doi: 10.1056/NEJMoa1607751
155. Mateos M-V, González-Calle V. Timing of treatment of smoldering myeloma: early treatment. *Blood Adv* (2018) 2(21):3045–9. doi: 10.1182/bloodadvances.2018021220
156. Palumbo A, Chanan-Khan A, Weisel K, Nooka AK, Masszi T, Beksac M, et al. Daratumumab, Bortezomib, and Dexamethasone for Multiple Myeloma. *N Engl J Med* (2016) 375(8):754–66. doi: 10.1056/NEJMoa1606038
157. Spencer A, Lentzsch S, Weisel K, Avet-Loiseau H, Mark TM, Spicka I, et al. Daratumumab plus bortezomib and dexamethasone versus bortezomib and dexamethasone in relapsed or refractory multiple myeloma: updated analysis of CASTOR. *Haematologica* (2018) 103(12):2079–87. doi: 10.3324/haematol.2018.194118
158. Moreau P, Attal M, Hulin C, Arnulf B, Belhadj K, Benboubker L, et al. Bortezomib, thalidomide, and dexamethasone with or without daratumumab before and after autologous stem-cell transplantation for newly diagnosed multiple myeloma (CASSIOPEIA): a randomised, open-label, phase 3 study. *Lancet (Lond Engl)* (2019) 394(10192):29–38. doi: 10.1016/S0140-6736(19)31240-1
159. Attal M, Richardson PG, Rajkumar SV, San-Miguel J, Beksac M, Spicka I, et al. Isatuximab plus pomalidomide and low-dose dexamethasone versus pomalidomide and low-dose dexamethasone in patients with relapsed and refractory multiple myeloma (ICARIA-MM): a randomised, multicentre, open-label, phase 3 study. *Lancet (Lond Engl)* (2019) 394(10214):2096–107. doi: 10.1016/S0140-6736(19)32556-5
160. Balasa B, Yun R, Belmar NA, Fox M, Chao DT, Robbins MD, et al. Elotuzumab enhances natural killer cell activation and myeloma cell killing through interleukin-2 and TNF-α pathways. *Cancer Immunol Immunother: CII* (2015) 64(1):61–73. doi: 10.1007/s00262-014-1610-3
161. Cannons JL, Tangye SG, Schwartzberg PL. SLAM family receptors and SAP adaptors in immunity. *Annu Rev Immunol* (2011) 29:665–705. doi: 10.1146/annurev-immunol-030409-101302
162. Collins SM, Bakan CE, Swartzel GD, Hofmeister CC, Efebera YA, Kwon H, et al. Elotuzumab directly enhances NK cell cytotoxicity against myeloma via CS1 ligation: evidence for augmented NK cell function complementing ADCC. *Cancer Immunol Immunother: CII* (2013) 62(12):1841–9. doi: 10.1007/s00262-013-1493-8
163. Zonder JA, Mohrbacher AF, Singhal S, van Rhee F, Bensinger WI, Ding H, et al. A phase 1, multicenter, open-label, dose escalation study of elotuzumab in patients with advanced multiple myeloma. *Blood* (2012) 120(3):552–9. doi: 10.1182/blood-2011-06-360552
164. Dimopoulos MA, Dytfeld D, Grosicki S, Moreau P, Takezako N, Hori M, et al. Elotuzumab plus Pomalidomide and Dexamethasone for Multiple Myeloma. *N Engl J Med* (2018) 379(19):1811–22. doi: 10.1056/NEJMoa1805762
165. Cohen AD, Garfall AL, Stadtmauer EA, Melenhorst JJ, Lacey SF, Lancaster E, et al. B cell maturation antigen-specific CAR T cells are clinically active in multiple myeloma. *J Clin Invest* (2019) 129(6):2210–21. doi: 10.1172/JCI126397
166. Raje N, Berdeja J, Lin Y, Siegel D, Jagannath S, Madduri D, et al. Anti-BCMA CAR T-Cell Therapy bb2121 in Relapsed or Refractory Multiple Myeloma. *New Engl J Med* (2019) 380(18):1726–37. doi: 10.1056/NEJMoa1817226
167. Carulli G, Buda G, Azzarà A, Ciancia EM, Sammuri P, Domenichini C, et al. CD229 Expression on Bone Marrow Plasma Cells from Patients with Multiple Myeloma and Monoclonal Gammopathies of Uncertain Significance. *Acta Haematol* (2016) 135(1):11–4. doi: 10.1159/000380939
168. Muccio VE, Saraci E, Gilestro M, Gattei V, Zucchetto A, Astolfi M, et al. Multiple myeloma: New surface antigens for the characterization of plasma cells in the era of novel agents. *Cytometry Part B Clin Cytometry* (2016) 90(1):81–90. doi: 10.1002/cyto.b.21279
169. Yousef S, Kovacsovics-Bankowski M, Salama ME, Bhardwaj N, Steinbach M, Langemo A, et al. CD229 is expressed on the surface of plasma cells carrying an aberrant phenotype and chemotherapy-resistant precursor cells in multiple myeloma. *Hum Vaccines Immunother* (2015) 11(7):1606–11. doi: 10.1080/21645515.2015.1046658
170. Radhakrishnan SV, Luetkens T, Scherer SD, Davis P, Vander Mause ER, Olson ML, et al. CD229 CAR T cells eliminate multiple myeloma and tumor propagating cells without fratricide. *Nat Commun* (2020) 11(1):798. doi: 10.1038/s41467-020-14619-z
171. Zhou X, Einsele H, Danhof S. Bispecific Antibodies: A New Era of Treatment for Multiple Myeloma. *J Clin Med* (2020) 9(7). doi: 10.3390/jcm9072166
172. Da Via MC, Solimando AG, Garitano-Trojaola A, Barrio S, Munawar U, Strifler S, et al. CIC Mutation as a Molecular Mechanism of Acquired Resistance to Combined BRAF-MEK Inhibition in Extramedullary Multiple Myeloma with Central Nervous System Involvement. *Oncologist* (2020) 25(2):112–8. doi: 10.1634/theoncologist.2019-0356
173. Lamanuzzi A, Saltarella I, Desantis V, Frassanito MA, Leone P, Racanelli V, et al. Inhibition of mTOR complex 2 restrains tumor angiogenesis in multiple myeloma. *Oncotarget* (2018) 9(29):20563–77. doi: 10.18632/oncotarget.25003
174. Solimando AG, Da Vià MC, Cicco S, Leone P, Di Lernia G, Giannico D, et al. High-Risk Multiple Myeloma: Integrated Clinical and Omics Approach Dissects the Neoplastic Clone and the Tumor Microenvironment. *J Clin Med* (2019) 8(7). doi: 10.3390/jcm8070997
175. Blank CU, Haanen JB, Ribas A, Schumacher TN. CANCER IMMUNOLOGY. The "cancer immunogram". *Science* (2016) 352(6286):658–60. doi: 10.1126/science.aaf2834
176. Hong L, Zhang C, Jiang Y, Liu H, Huang H, Guo D. Therapeutic status and the prospect of CRISPR/Cas9 gene editing in multiple myeloma. *Future Oncol (Lond Engl)* (2020) 16(16):1125–36. doi: 10.2217/fon-2019-0822
177. Beauvais D, Danhof S, Hayden PJ, Einsele H, Yakoub-Agha I. Clinical data, limitations and perspectives on chimeric antigen receptor T-cell therapy in multiple myeloma. *Curr Opin Oncol* (2020) 32(5):418–26. doi: 10.1097/CCO.0000000000000667
178. Liu X, Zhang Y, Cheng C, Cheng AW, Zhang X, Li N, et al. CRISPR-Cas9-mediated multiplex gene editing in CAR-T cells. *Cell Res* (2017) 27(1):154–7. doi: 10.1038/cr.2016.142
179. Nerreter T, Letschert S, Götz R, Doose S, Danhof S, Einsele H, et al. Super-resolution microscopy reveals ultra-low CD19 expression on myeloma cells that triggers elimination by CD19 CAR-T. *Nat Commun* (2019) 10(1):3137. doi: 10.1038/s41467-019-10948-w

180. Rupp LJ, Schumann K, Roybal KT, Gate RE, Ye CJ, Lim WA, et al. CRISPR/Cas9-mediated PD-1 disruption enhances anti-tumor efficacy of human chimeric antigen receptor T cells. *Sci Rep* (2017) 7(1):737. doi: 10.1038/s41598-017-00462-8

2

WNT Signaling in Hematological Malignancies

Michela Frenquelli[1,2*] *and Giovanni Tonon*[2,3*]

[1] B-cell Neoplasia Unit, Division of Experimental Oncology, IRCCS San Raffaele Scientific Institute, Milan, Italy, [2] Functional Genomics of Cancer Unit, Division of Experimental Oncology, IRCCS San Raffaele Scientific Institute, Milan, Italy, [3] Center for Omics Sciences (COSR), IRCCS San Raffaele Scientific Institute, Milan, Italy

***Correspondence:**
Michela Frenquelli
frenquelli.michela@hsr.it
Giovanni Tonon
tonon.giovanni@hsr.it

The role of the WNT signaling pathway in key cellular processes, such as cell proliferation, differentiation and migration is well documented. WNT signaling cascade is initiated by the interaction of WNT ligands with receptors belonging to the Frizzled family, and/or the ROR1/ROR2 and RYK families. The downstream signaling cascade results in the activation of the canonical β-catenin dependent pathway, ultimately leading to transcriptional control of cell proliferation, or the non-canonical pathway, mainly acting on cell migration and cell polarity. The high level of expression of both WNT ligands and WNT receptors in cancer cells and in the surrounding microenvironment suggests that WNT may represent a central conduit of interactions between tumor cells and microenviroment. In this review we will focus on WNT pathways deregulation in hematological cancers, both at the ligand and receptor levels. We will review available literature regarding both the classical β-catenin dependent pathway as well as the non-canonical pathway, with particular emphasis on the possible exploitation of WNT aberrant activation as a therapeutic target, a notion supported by preclinical data.

Keywords: multiple myeloma, WNT, ROR2, Wnt/b-catenin, microenvironment

INTRODUCTION

The WNT signaling pathway is central for development and homeostasis within tissues. The WNT signaling cascade is initiated by the interaction of WNT proteins (lipid-modified secreted glycoproteins) with various receptors and co-receptors whose activation elicit several processes, such as cell proliferation, differentiation, apoptosis, polarity, migration and invasion (1, 2).

WNT proteins are evolutionary conserved and in mammals WNT family genes comprise 19 members. These secreted, cystein-rich proteins exert their effects through the interaction with the Frizzled family of proteins (consisting of 10 members). Frizzled (FZD) are seven-pass transmembrane, and each FZD protein contains a cysteine-rich domain (CRD) with approximately 10 cysteine residues, essential for the binding to WNT proteins (3, 4).

Apart from FZD, other proteins are involved in WNT recognition: the co-receptor low-density lipoprotein receptor-related proteins (LRP 5 and 6), the receptor Tyr kinase-like orphan receptor family (ROR1 and ROR2), the Receptor Tyrosine Kinase (RYK) and the protein Tyr kinase 7 (PTK7).

The WNT pathway is broadly divided into canonical (β-catenin-dependent) and non-canonical (β-catenin-independent), depending on the agonists, the receptors and the intracellular players involved. Given the high number of both WNT ligands and receptors, the possible combinations are numerous, making its regulation exceedingly complex. The activation of either signaling pathway is receptor and ligand dependent and yet is also influenced by the cellular context. As an approximation, certain WNTs (WNT1, WNT3A and WNT8) activate the canonical β-catenin-dependent WNT signaling pathway by preferentially binding to FZD receptor coupled to LRP5/6 co-receptors. Conversely, WNT5A and WNT11 preferentially bind to ROR1, ROR2 and RYK receptors and are predominantly involved in the β-catenin-independent, non-canonical pathway.

Irrespectively from the signaling branch activated upon binding of WNT ligands to FZD or other receptors, the signal is commonly transduced to a protein called Disheveled (DVL) that represents the molecular hub executing both the canonical and non-canonical pathways (5). How can the same DVL protein be involved in different signaling pathways? The molecular wiring underlying this behaviour remains unknown, but various mechanisms have been proposed to confer specificity to DVL activity, including different phosphorylation events on DVL or the establishment of alternative interactions between DVL and its protein partners. This latter hypothesis is supported by the presence of three conserved domains in DVL protein (namely DIX, DEP and PDZ) which mediate its interaction with effector proteins involved in different signaling branches. Indeed, it has been suggested that DIX and PDZ domains are implicated in the activation of β-catenin signaling, whereas DEP and PDZ are preferentially engaged in the interactions with proteins (e.g. Daam1, Prickle) that trigger the non-canonical signaling pathway (6).

WNT/β-CATENIN SIGNALING

As mentioned earlier, FZD proteins act as main receptors for WNT ligands, together with the co-receptor LRP5/6.

In the absence of exogenous WNT, the pathway is maintained in the "off" state by the so-called "β-catenin destruction complex". This multiprotein complex, composed by Axin, β-catenin, APC, GSK3 and CK1, keeps β-catenin at low levels by phosphorylating it, and thus marking it for recognition by β-TRCP ubiquitin ligase, leading to its subsequent ubitiquination and degradation (7, 8). When a WNT molecule binds to FZD, it induces the phosphorylation of LRP6 (9), and the association of DVL proteins to the receptor. Both these events that are required for initiation of the signaling cascade resulting in the exposure of DVL's DIX domain that works as a docking site for Axin pulling it away from the destruction complex. Moreover, the cytoplasmic tail of LRP5/6 contains several PPPSPxS domains that can bind Axin and become a competing substrate for GSK3. As a result, the destruction complex is disassembled and β-catenin is no longer marked for destruction. Therefore, β-catenin accumulates in the cytoplasm and then translocates in the nucleus (10), where it associates with the TCF/LEF transcription factors and activates the transcription of target genes such as Myc, Cyclin D1, Survivin and MMP (11) mainly implicated in the regulation of cell proliferation (**Figure 1**).

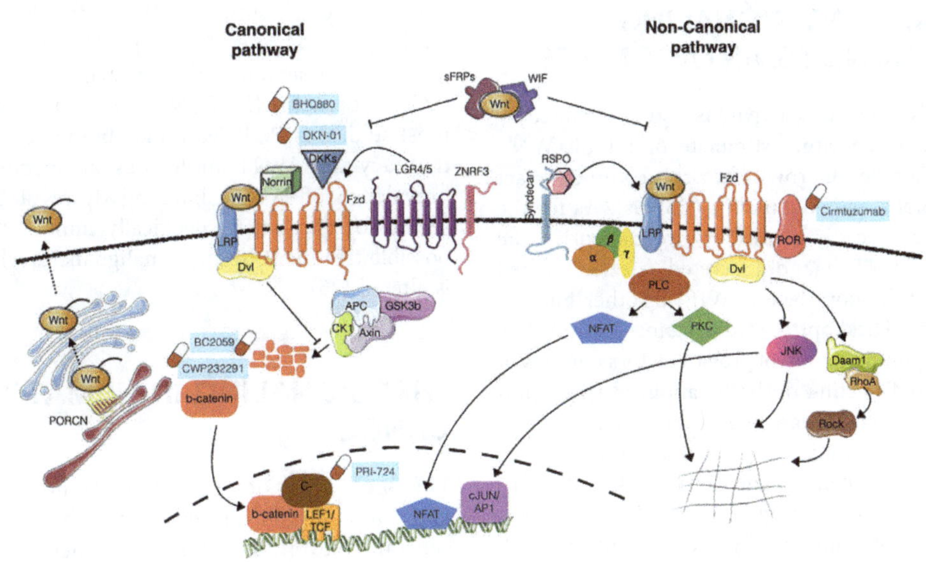

FIGURE 1 | WNT pathaway signaling. Schematic representation of canonical (β-catenin dependent) and non-canonical (β-catenin independent) WNT signaling. WNT ligand interaction with FZD receptors together with LRP5/6 co-receptors inhibits the activity of the "destruction complex" (composed by Axin, APC, CK1 and GSK3β), allowing the stabilization of β-catenin, its translocation into the nucleus and the transcriptional activation of target genes. The activation of the non-canonical pathway involves additional co-receptors (e.g. ROR1 and ROR2) and is mediated by small GTPases RhoA, Daam1 and ROCK, acting on cytoskeleton remodelling, or PLC, JNK and NFAT, acting on transcriptional activity. Further layers of regulation of the pathway are exerted at the level of WNT ligands modification/secretion (mainly through PRCN), engagement of additional activator proteins (Norrin, Syndecans, RSPO, LGR4/5, ZNRF3) or the presence of antagonists (DKK, WIF, sFRPs). Compounds under clinical evaluation are indicated next to the appropriate target. Images have been created with Servier Medical Art (https://smart.servier.com/).

NON-CANONICAL WNT SIGNALING

The interactions of other WNT ligands (such as WNT5A and WNT11) and receptors (including ROR1 and ROR2) results in the activation of alternative signaling routes different from the canonical β-catenin dependent pathway, known as WNT non-canonical pathways. The first example of a non-canonical pathway is the Planar Cell Polarity (PCP)/Jun N-terminal kinase (JNK) signaling cascade that involves the activation of JNK, Rho, Rac and Rho kinase (ROCK) proteins (12). In this context, WNT ligand binding to FZD receptor stimulates the recruitment of DVL, which contrarily to what happens in the canonical-pathway, interacts with DAAM1 (Disheveled associated activator of morphogenesis 1) thereby stimulating Rac and Rho small GTPases and JNK, whose activation results in actin polymerization and cytoskeletal modifications (13) (**Figure 1**). In addition to the PCP pathway, another significant noncanonical pathway is the WNT/Ca^{2+} pathway, characterized by an increase in the intracellular calcium level as a result of WNT binding. This pathway subsequently activates heterotrimeric G proteins and Phospholipase-C (PLC) which hydrolyses membrane phospholipids to di-acyl glycerol and inositol 1,4,5-triphosphate (IP3). This neo-generated IP3 causes the release of calcium from the endoplasmic reticulum which activates Protein kinase C (PKC) and ultimately activating calcineurin and NFAT transcription factor, thus regulating transcriptional programs involved in cell fate and cell migration (14) (**Figure 1**).

REGULATION OF WNT SIGNALING BY ADDITIONAL AGONISTS/ANTAGONISTS

The fine-tuning of WNT signaling activity is also determined by additional proteins that can either stimulate or inhibit WNT pathway. Two major families of growth factors are known to act as WNT agonists: Norrin, and R-spondins (RSPOs). As for the antagonists they can be broadly divided in two categories: the one interfering with WNT ligand (Secreted frizzled-related proteins- sFPRs, Wnt inhibitory factor- WIF) or other binding to the receptor complex (Dickkopf-related proteins- DKKs) (15).

WNT agonists: R-Spondin family of growth factors consists of 4 members (RSPO1 to 4), acting on both canonical (β-catenin dependent) and non-canonical signaling. Their mechanism of action is still controversial but it is suggested that RSPO proteins bind to leuchin-rich G protein 4 and 5 (LRG-4 and 5) to sequester ZNRF3, an E3 ubiquitin ligase involved in the turn-over of Fz-LRP6 receptor complex. By sequestering ZNRF3, RSPO-LRG interaction induces the accumulation of the receptor complex on the cell surface, thus enhancing WNT signaling (16). RSPOs can also amplify non-canonical PCP signaling, likely through the interaction of RSPO/Syndecans with WNT/Fz (17).

Another secreted factor capable of enhancing WNT activation is Norrin which was described to interact with Fz4 (18, 19) and to specifically activate canonical signaling.

WNT antagonists: The largest family of secreted WNT inhibitors is represented by sFRPs. In humans, it comprises five members (sFRP1-5), all sharing a conserved CRD at the N-terminus. They act binding WNT ligands and preventing their interaction with the receptor, although mouse sFRP3 has been shown to interact with FZD8 (20), suggesting an additional mode of inhibition (21). They potentially bind to different WNT proteins, so they can inhibit both canonical and non-canonical signaling.

WNT Inhibitor factor 1 (WIF-1) is another secreted factor that acts binding to WNT ligands and preventing their interaction with the receptors. In this way, WIF-1 can inhibit both canonical and non-canonical signaling.

Lastly, the DKK family includes four members (DKK1 to 4), with DDK1, 2 and 4 binding to LRP5/6 and inhibiting the canonical β-catenin pathway. DDK3 does not seem to bind to LRP5/6 and is likely acting on a different pathway such as the TGF-β one (22).

AN ADDITIONAL LAYER OF REGULATION: SECRETION OF WNT LIGANDS

WNTS are secreted proteins exerting their function on a short- or long-range gradient in the neighboring cells. Their proper secretion and release in the extracellular space represents an additional level of signaling modulation. Indeed, WNT proteins need indeed to be posttranslational modified in order to be exported and to be biologically active. One of the most crucial modification is acylation, critical for the transportation from the Golgi to the cell surface (23) and for the correct and efficient binding to FZD receptors (24). WNT acylation occurs through the concerted action of three enzymes: stearoyl CoA desaturase (SCD), porcupine (PORCN) and Notum. Of these enzymes, the most studied is PORCN, a membrane-bound O-acyltransferase that acylates WNT molecules at specific sites. Given the prevalence of WNT signaling dysregulation in cancer, the search for drugs that specifically inhibit PORCN represents a possible treatment in those malignancies where WNT signaling is altered (25).

WNT SIGNALING IN HEMATOLOGICAL CANCER

The high level of expression of both WNT ligands and WNT receptors in cancer suggests that WNT may represent a central conduit of interactions between tumor cells and the microenvironment. Although most of the studies of WNT involvement in cancer come from solid tumors, WNT signaling deregulation has also been observed in hematological cancers.

WNT ligands are normally expressed in the hematopoietic stem cells (HSC) compartment and the surrounding microenvironment, and WNT signaling is crucial for HSC self-renewal and homeostasis (26), as well as for the maturation of hematopoietic progenitors (27). The normal hemopoiesis is maintained through the balance between extracellular factors (WNT ligands, agonists and antagonists), cell surface receptors, cytoplasmic components (adapters, destruction complex components etc.) and nuclear factors. Deregulation in any of the involved partners involved could cause hematopoietic disorders.

Aberrant WNT signaling has been reported for example in acute myeloid leukemia (AML). Common chromosomal translocations found in AML (AML1–ETO, PML–RARα and MLL–AF9) result in the stimulation of WNT signaling in AML cells (28, 29), inducing expression of WNT target genes and increasing proliferation. Moreover hyper-activation of the WNT pathway has also been associated to the overexpression of FZD4 (30) and pakoglobin (31). Other evidences suggest that modulation of endogenous WNT antagonists, such as DKK1 and DKK2 (32, 33) or SFRP (34) in AML patients increase the activity of WNT pathway and correlates with adverse clinical outcome.

In chronic myelogenous leukaemia (CML), increased levels of nuclear β- catenin were detected, thus enhancing the self-renewal capacity of CML cells both *in vitro* (35) and in animal models (36). Both canonical and non-canonical WNT signaling seem to be involved in the resistance to the tyrosine-kinase inhibitor Imatinib and in CML relapse as suggested by preclinical data on CML mouse models (37, 38).

WNT pathway deregulation is suggested to exert a crucial role in acute lymphoblastic leukemias (ALL) as well. In T-ALL, that is strictly dependent on Notch pathway alterations, a pivotal role for canonical WNT signaling has been postulated, based on the high expression of β-catenin, its cofactor LEF1 (39) and on the increased proliferation observed in cells expressing high levels of LEF1 (40). In B-ALL, elevated levels of WNT16 have been found in E2A-PBX1 translocated leukemias (41). Moreover, WNT2B, WNT5A, WNT10B and WNT16B ligands, FZD7 and FZD8 receptors and LRP5/6 co-receptors are overexpressed at different levels in B-ALL (42).

Aberrant WNT signaling is not only involved in the development of leukemias originating from the stem cell compartments, but it is also observed in disorders originating from mature cells.

Dysregulated WNT signaling has also been implicated in the development of Multiple Myeloma (MM). Indeed, β- catenin is often overexpressed and constitutively activated in MM cells, impacting on cell proliferation (43). Moreover, different WNT ligands are expressed in the bone-marrow microenvironment of MM patients, acting both in an autocrine and paracrine manner (44). As a result of these alterations, activation of both the canonical and non-canonical pathways has been observed, hence modulating proliferation capacity (45), migration/invasion (46, 47) and resistance to therapy (48). In this frame, we have recently shown that overexpression of the ROR2 receptor mediates myeloma cells interactions with the bone marrow and its depletion *in vivo* results in detachment of myeloma cells from their niche and delays disease progression. We also demonstrated, using *in vitro* and *ex vivo* 3D-culture systems, that ROR2 exerts a pivotal role in the adhesion of cancer cells to the microenvironment, mainly through the PI3K-AKT pathway, and that genetic and pharmacological inhibition of the AKT pathway is able to reduce ROR2-induced adhesion of malignant cells to bone marrow components (46). Deregulation of WNT pathway, also in terms of WNT antagonist expression, such SFRP2 and DKK1, also has relevant effects on the shaping of bone-marrow niche microenvironment, contributing to alter bone homeostasis and resulting in osteolytic bone disease (49, 50).

In chronic lymphocytic leukemia (CLL) several components of the WNT pathway have been found deregulated: WNT3, WNT5B, WNT6, WNT10A, WNT14, and WNT16, as well as the WNT receptor FZD3, are highly expressed in CLL when compared with normal B cells (51–53). Moreover, soluble inhibitors of the WNT pathway (DKKs and SFRPs) are downregulated (54, 55), further potentiating WNT signaling. More importantly the ROR1 receptor is specifically expressed in malignant CLL cells and not in normal B cells and has been implicated in both proliferation and migration of CLL cells (56, 57).

Aberrant WNT signaling can also be found also in lymphomas. Indeed, elevated levels of nuclear β-catenin have been detected in primary samples of different lymphoma sub-types, even in the absence of mutations in APC or β-catenin (58–60), suggesting that the pathway is activated by autocrine or paracrine mechanisms. Indeed, many WNT components are dysregulated in different type of lymphoma. For example, in Mantle Cell lymphoma (MCL) gene expression profiling studies revealed increased expression of FZD7, APC, LRP5, AXIN1and DVL3 (61).

DISCUSSION

Targeting WNT Pathway: Is This the Way?

Many players of both the canonical and non-canonical WNT signaling are deregulated in hematological cancers, making the WNT pathway an interesting therapeutic opportunity for blood cancers. In this context, candidate drugs can act on WNT signaling pathway at different levels. The ideal druggable targets are both WNT ligands and the receptors or co-receptors, as they are easily accessible for a small compound. However, also intracellular mediators at different signaling levels or additional regulators of WNT pathways (extracellular regulators like DKKs or sFRPs or regulators of WNT secretion like PORCN) have been proposed as possible targets. In this section we report the main therapeutic agents targeting the WNT pathway and currently under clinical trials for the treatment of hematological malignancies (https://clinicaltrials.gov/, summarized in **Table 1**).

The most advanced clinical application of inhibitors of the WNT family is represented by the monoclonal antibody Cirmtuzumab, targeting the WNT receptor ROR1, that is overexpressed in CLL. Preclinical studies performed with Cirmtuzumab have shown excellent results in terms of induction of apoptosis and inhibition of cell migration both in *in vitro* and *in vivo* models of CLL (62, 63) and phase I clinical trial (NCT02860676) with this monoclonal antibody confirmed

TABLE 1 | WNT pathway targeting under clinical investigation.

Drug	Target- mechanism of action	Stage of drug development	Clinical trial identifier	Disease
Cirmtuzumab	Anti -ROR1 monoclonal antibody	Phase 1	NCT02222688 NCT02860676	CLL
Cirmtuzumab/Cirmtuzumab+ Ibrutinib	Anti -ROR1 monoclonal antibody+ BTK inhibitor	Phase 1b/2	NCT03088878	CLL, SLL, MCL
Cirmtuzumab/Cirmtuzumab+ Venetoclax	Anti -ROR1 monoclonal antibody+ Bcl2 inhibitor	Phase 2	NCT04501939	CLL
ROR1R-CAR-T Cell Infusion	Killing of ROR1+ cells	Phase 1	NCT02194374	CLL, SLL
VLS-101	Use ROR1 antibody to recognize malignant cells, then killed by the drug MMAE	Phase 1	NCT03833180	CLL, MCL, FL, MZL, DLBCL, RS, BL, LL, T-NHL, ALL, AML, WM
PRI-724	Disrupt the interaction of β-catenin and CBP	Phase 1/2	NCT01606579	AML, CML
CWP232291	Inhibits β-catenin transcriptional activity	Phase 1	NCT01398462	AML, CML, Myelodiplastic syndrome, Myelofibrosis
CWP232291/CWP232291+ Lenalidomide and Dexamethasone	Inhibits β-catenin transcriptional activity+ Immunomodulators	Phase 1a/1b	NCT02426723	MM
CWP232291/CWP232291+ ara-C/ cytarabine	Inhibits β-catenin transcriptional activity	Phase 1/2	NCT03055286	AML
AEB071	PKC inhibitor	Phase 1	NCT01402440	DLBCL
AEB071/AEB071+ Everolimus	PKC inhibitor+ immunosuppressor	Phase 1	NCT01854606	DLBCL
AEB071	PKC inhibitor	Phase 2	NCT02285244	PML, MCL, SLL, CLL, RS
DKN-01	Inhibits DKK1	Phase 1	NCT01457417	MM
DKN-01/DKN-01+ Lenalidomide/ Dexamethasone	Inhibits DKK1	Phase 1	NCT01711671	MM
BHQ880+ Bortezomib and dexamethasone	Monoclonal antibody to DKK1	Phase 2	NCT01337752	MM
BHQ880/BHQ880+ zoledronic acid	Monoclonal antibody to DKK1	Phase 1	NCT00741377	MM
BHQ880	Monoclonal antibody to DKK1	Phase 2	NCT01302886	Smoldering MM
Dendritic cell DKK1 vaccine	DKK1	Early Phase 1	NCT03591614	MGUS, Smoldering MM, MM

CLL, Chronic Lymphocytic Leukemia; MCL, Mantle Cell Lymphoma; FL, Follicular Lymphoma; MZL, Marginal Zone Lymphoma; DLBCL, Diffuse Large B-cell Lymphoma; RS, Richter Syndrome; BL, Burkitt Lymphoma; LL, Lymphoplasmacytoid Lymphoma; T-NHL, T-cell Non-Hodgkin Lymphoma; ALL, Acute Lymphoid Leukemia; AML, Acute Myeloid Leukemia; WM, Waldenstrom Macroglobulinemia; SLL, Small Lymphocytic Leukemia; PML, Pro-myelocytic Leukemia; MM, Multiple Myeloma; MGUS, Monoclonal Gammopathy on unknown significance.

its safety and biological activity of Cirmtuzumab, even if a clear clinical benefit was not evident (64). Other clinical trials aimed to test the efficacy of this promising compound in different combination settings are currently ongoing (NCT03088878 Phase 1b/II clinical trial in combination with Ibrutinib) or planned (NCT04501939 phase II trial in combination with Venetoclax).

Promising results were also obtained with PRI-724/C-82 compound, a C-EBP/β-catenin inhibitor, on different models of leukemia (including T-ALL, AML and CML) also in the context of drug resistant cells (37, 65). A phase 1/2 clinical study with this candidate drug (NCT01606579) has been performed on AML and CML patients has been conducted, although the results are not available yet.

Another interesting molecule that impacts on WNT-β-catenin signaling is the CWP232291 inhibitor. This molecule targets β -catenin for degradation, thus inhibiting its signaling and exerting anti-apoptotic and anti-proliferative activities. CWP232291 is currently in use in different clinical trials in AMLs and MM, and it was recently reported that this compound is well tolerated and shows encouraging clinical activity (66).

Moreover, another β-catenin inhibitor, BC2059, was shown to reduce proliferation and induce apoptosis on both MM primary samples and cell lines, alone or in combination with proteasome inhibitors, and to delay tumor growth *in vivo* (67).

As previously mentioned, it is possible to interfere with WNT signaling activation also by targeting extracellular regulators of the pathway. The example of DKK1, that has been exploited as therapeutic target especially in MM, is paradigmatic of how the WNT pathway may represent a real communication route between cells of the microenvironment and tumor cells. Indeed, MM-secreted DKK1 is indeed mainly active on osteoblasts, preventing their differentiation and contributing to the development of osteolytic lesions. The targeting of DKK1 could be achieved through the treatment with the DKN-01 inhibitor, in a phase I trial (NCT01711671 and NCT01457417) or with the anti-DKK1 monoclonal antibody BHQ880, which has been included in an already completed phase 1 (NCT01302886) and phase 2 trials (NCT01337752 and NCT00741377) showing potential clinical activity in myeloma patients (68). DKK1 has also been exploited in an immunotherapy setting in a myeloma mouse model (69) and also with primary myeloma samples (70), and an early phase 1 study (NCT03591614) is going to start soon.

CONCLUSIONS

In this review we tried to focus on the specific aberrations affecting the WNT pathway in different hematological cancer and how these aberrations could be exploited as therapeutic targets, developing drugs and compounds with specific effects on that particular biological process. If on the one hand the presence of many WNT components (19 WNT ligands and more than 15 receptors) offers several possibilities of tackling the pathway (though the problem of redundancy still remains), on the other hand the fact that WNT signaling is essential for many processes in development and homeostasis poses several challenges on the side of drug specificity and safety. The considerable bulk of knowledge accrued so far and the initial testing of several compounds impinging on this pathway suggest that the WNT network is both a crucial mediator of cancer cell survival and proliferation as well as an enticing target for new drugs. Nevertheless, much effort is still active on the identification of peculiar abnormalities and on the way to specifically target them, with the final aim of exploiting the WNT pathway alterations to stratify patients and provide novel tools to be exploited in a personalized medicine setting.

AUTHOR CONTRIBUTIONS

MF wrote the manuscript. GT reviewed and wrote the manuscript. All authors contributed to the article and approved the submitted version.

REFERENCES

1. Clevers H. Wnt/β-Catenin Signaling in Development and Disease. *Cell* (2006) 127:469–80. doi: 10.1016/j.cell.2006.10.018
2. van Amerongen R, Nusse R. Towards an integrated view of Wnt signaling in development. *Development* (2009) 136:3205–14. doi: 10.1242/dev.033910
3. Wu CH, Nusse R. Ligand receptor interactions in the Wnt signaling pathway in Drosophila. *J Biol Chem* (2002) 277:41762–9. doi: 10.1074/jbc.M207850200
4. Voloshanenko O, Gmach P, Winter J, Kranz D, Boutros M. Mapping of Wnt-Frizzled interactions by multiplex CRISPR targeting of receptor gene families. *FASEB J* (2017) 31:4832–44. doi: 10.1096/fj.201700144R
5. Gao C, Chen Y. Dishevelled : The hub of Wnt signaling. *Cell Signal* (2010) 22:717–27. doi: 10.1016/j.cellsig.2009.11.021
6. Wharton KA. Runnin' with the Dvl: Proteins that associate with Dsh/Dvl and their significance to Wnt signal transduction. *Dev Biol* (2003) 253:1–17. doi: 10.1006/dbio.2002.0869
7. Gammons M, Bienz M. Multiprotein complexes governing Wnt signal transduction. *Curr Opin Cell Biol* (2018) 51:42–9. doi: 10.1016/j.ceb.2017.10.008
8. van Kappel EC, Maurice MM. Molecular regulation and pharmacological targeting of the β-catenin destruction complex. *Br J Pharmacol* (2017) 174:4575–88. doi: 10.1111/bph.13922
9. Niehrs C, Shen J. Regulation of Lrp6 phosphorylation. *Cell Mol Life Sci* (2010) 67:2551–62. doi: 10.1007/s00018-010-0329-3
10. Anthony CC, Robbins DJ, Ahmed Y, Lee E. Nuclear Regulation of Wnt/β-Catenin Signaling: It's a Complex Situation. *Genes (Basel)* (2020) 11:886. doi: 10.3390/genes11080886
11. Cadigan KM, Waterman ML. TCF/LEFs and Wnt signaling in the nucleus. *Cold Spring Harb Perspect Biol* (2012) 4:a007906. doi: 10.1101/cshperspect.a007906
12. Butler MT, Wallingford JB. Planar cell polarity in development and disease. *Nat Rev Mol Cell Biol* (2017) 18:375–88. doi: 10.1038/nrm.2017.11
13. Hall A. Rho GTPases and the control of cell behaviour. *Biochem Soc Trans* (2005) 33:891–5. doi: 10.1042/BST20050891
14. De A. Wnt/Ca 2 signaling pathway: A brief overview. *Acta Biochim Biophys Sin (Shanghai)* (2011) 43:745–56. doi: 10.1093/abbs/gmr079
15. Cruciat CM, Niehrs C. Secreted and transmembrane Wnt inhibitors and activators. *Cold Spring Harb Perspect Biol* (2013) 5(3):a015081. doi: 10.1101/cshperspect.a015081
16. Hao HX, Xie Y, Zhang Y, Zhang O, Oster E, Avello M, et al. ZNRF3 promotes Wnt receptor turnover in an R-spondin-sensitive manner. *Nature* (2012) 485:195–202. doi: 10.1038/nature11019
17. Ohkawara B, Glinka A, Niehrs C. Rspo3 Binds Syndecan 4 and Induces Wnt/PCP Signaling via Clathrin-Mediated Endocytosis to Promote Morphogenesis. *Dev Cell* (2011) 20:303–14. doi: 10.1016/j.devcel.2011.01.006
18. Wang Y, Rattner A, Zhou Y, Williams J, Smallwood PM, Nathans J. Norrin/Frizzled4 signaling in retinal vascular development and blood brain barrier plasticity. *Cell* (2012) 151:1332–44. doi: 10.1016/j.cell.2012.10.042
19. Ke J, Harikumar KG, Erice C, Chen C, Gu X, Wang L, et al. Structure and function of Norrin in assembly and activation of a Frizzled 4-Lrp5/6 complex. *Genes Dev* (2013) 27:2305–19. doi: 10.1101/gad.228544.113
20. Bafico A, Gazit A, Pramila T, Finch PW, Yaniv A, Aaronson SA. Interaction of frizzled related protein (FRP) with Wnt ligands and the frizzled receptor suggests alternative mechanisms for FRP inhibition of Wnt signaling. *J Biol Chem* (1999) 274:16180–7. doi: 10.1074/jbc.274.23.16180
21. Xavier CP, Melikova M, Chuman Y, Üren A, Baljinnyam B, Rubin JS. Secreted Frizzled-related protein potentiation versus inhibition of Wnt3a/β-catenin signaling. *Cell Signal* (2014) 26:94–101. doi: 10.1016/j.cellsig.2013.09.016
22. Romero D, Al-Shareef Z, Gorroño-Etxebarria I, Atkins S, Turrell F, Chhetri J, et al. Dickkopf-3 regulates prostate epithelial cell acinar morphogenesis and prostate cancer cell invasion by limiting TGF-β-dependent activation of matrix metalloproteases. *Carcinogenesis* (2016) 37:18–29. doi: 10.1093/carcin/bgv153
23. Port F, Basler K. Wnt Trafficking: New Insights into Wnt Maturation, Secretion and Spreading. *Traffic* (2010) 11:1265–71. doi: 10.1111/j.1600-0854.2010.01076.x
24. Janda CY, Garcia KC. Wnt acylation and its functional implication in Wnt signalling regulation. *Biochem Soc Trans* (2015) 43:211–6. doi: 10.1042/BST20140249
25. Torres VI, Godoy JA, Inestrosa NC. Modulating Wnt signaling at the root: Porcupine and Wnt acylation. *Pharmacol Ther* (2019) 198:34–45. doi: 10.1016/j.pharmthera.2019.02.009
26. Malhotra S, Kincade PW. Wnt-Related Molecules and Signaling Pathway Equilibrium in Hematopoiesis. *Cell Stem Cell* (2009) 4:27–36. doi: 10.1016/j.stem.2008.12.004
27. Staal FJT, Luis TC, Tiemessen MM. WNT signalling in the immune system: WNT is spreading its wings. *Nat Rev Immunol* (2008) 8:581–93. doi: 10.1038/nri2360

28. Müller-Tidow C, Steffen B, Cauvet T, Tickenbrock L, Ji P, Diederichs S, et al. Translocation Products in Acute Myeloid Leukemia Activate the Wnt Signaling Pathway in Hematopoietic Cells. *Mol Cell Biol* (2004) 24:2890-904. doi: 10.1128/mcb.24.7.2890-2904.2004
29. Lane SW, Wang YJ, Lo Celso C, Ragu C, Bullinger L, Sykes SM, et al. Differential niche and Wnt requirements during acute myeloid leukemia progression. *Blood* (2011) 118:2849–56. doi: 10.1182/blood-2011-03-345165
30. Tickenbrock L, Hehn S, Sargin B, Choudhary C, Bäumer N, Buerger H, et al. Activation of Wnt signalling in acute myeloid leukemia by induction of Frizzled-4. *Int J Oncol* (2008) 33:1215–21. doi: 10.3892/ijo_00000111
31. Morgan RG, Pearn L, Liddiard K, Pumford SL, Burnett AK, Tonks A, et al. γ-Catenin is overexpressed in acute myeloid leukemia and promotes the stabilization and nuclear localization of β-catenin. *Leukemia* (2013) 27:336-43. doi: 10.1038/leu.2012.221
32. Valencia A, Román-Gómez J, Cervera J, Such E, Barragán E, Bolufer P, et al. Wnt signaling pathway is epigenetically regulated by methylation of Wnt antagonists in acute myeloid leukemia. *Leukemia* (2009) 23:1658–66. doi: 10.1038/leu.2009.86
33. Griffiths EA, Gore SD, Hooker C, McDevitt MA, Karp JE, Smith BD, et al. Acute myeloid leukemia is characterized by Wnt pathway inhibitor promoter hypermethylation. *Leuk Lymphoma* (2010) 51:1711–9. doi: 10.3109/10428194.2010.496505
34. Jost E, Schmid J, Wilop S, Schubert C, Suzuki H, Herman JG, et al. Epigenetic inactivation of secreted Frizzled-related proteins in acute myeloid leukaemia. *Br J Haematol* (2008) 142:745–53. doi: 10.1111/j.1365-2141.2008.07242.x
35. Jamieson CHM, Ailles LE, Dylla SJ, Muijtjens M, Jones C, Zehnder JL, et al. Granulocyte-macrophage progenitors as candidate leukemic stem cells in blast-crisis CML. *N Engl J Med* (2004) 351:657–67. doi: 10.1056/NEJMoa040258
36. Zhao C, Blum J, Chen A, Kwon HY, Jung SH, Cook JM, et al. Loss of β-Catenin Impairs the Renewal of Normal and CML Stem Cells In Vivo. *Cancer Cell* (2007) 12:528–41. doi: 10.1016/j.ccr.2007.11.003
37. Heidel FH, Bullinger L, Feng Z, Wang Z, Neff TA, Stein L, et al. Genetic and pharmacologic inhibition of β-catenin targets imatinib-resistant leukemia stem cells in CML. *Cell Stem Cell* (2012) 10:412–24. doi: 10.1016/j.stem.2012.02.017
38. Gregory MA, Phang TL, Neviani P, Alvarez-Calderon F, Eide CA, O'Hare T, et al. Wnt/Ca(2+)/NFAT Signaling Maintains Survival of Ph(+) Leukemia Cells upon Inhibition of Bcr-Abl. *Cancer Cell* (2010) 18:74–87. doi: 10.1016/j.ccr.2010.04.025
39. Ng OH, Erbilgin Y, Firtina S, Celkan T, Karakas Z, Aydogan G, et al. Deregulated WNT signaling in childhood T-cell acute lymphoblastic leukemia. *Blood Cancer J* (2014) 4:e192. doi: 10.1038/bcj.2014.12
40. Guo X, Zhang R, Liu J, Li M, Song C, Dovat S, et al. Characterization of LEF1 high expression and novel mutations in adult acute lymphoblastic leukemia. *PloS One* (2015) 10(5):e0125429. doi: 10.1371/journal.pone.0125429
41. Mcwhirter JR, Neuteboom STC, Wancewicz EV, Monia BP, Downing JR, Murre C. Oncogenic homeodomain transcription factor E2A-Pbx1 activates a novel WNT gene in pre-B acute lymphoblastoid leukemia. *Proc Natl Acad Sci U S A* (1999) 96:11464–9. doi: 10.1073/pnas.96.20.11464
42. Khan NI, Bradstock KF, Bendall LJ. Activation of Wnt/β-catenin pathway mediates growth and survival in B-cell progenitor acute lymphoblastic leukaemia. *Br J Haematol* (2007) 138:338–48. doi: 10.1111/j.1365-2141.2007.06667.x
43. Derksen PWB, Tjin E, Meijer HP, Klok MD, Mac Gillavry HD, Van Oers MHJ, et al. Illegitimate WNT signaling promotes proliferation of multiple myeloma cells. *Proc Natl Acad Sci U S A* (2004) 101:6122–7. doi: 10.1073/pnas.0305855101
44. Mahtouk K, Moreaux J, Hose D, Rème T, Meissner T, Jourdan M, et al. Growth factors in multiple myeloma: a comprehensive analysis of their expression in tumor cells and bone marrow environment using Affymetrix microarrays. *BMC Cancer* (2010) 10:198. doi: 10.1186/1471-2407-10-198
45. van Andel H, Kocemba KA, Spaargaren M, Pals ST. Aberrant Wnt signaling in multiple myeloma: molecular mechanisms and targeting options. *Leukemia* (2019) 33:1063–75. doi: 10.1038/s41375-019-0404-1
46. Frenquelli M, Caridi N, Antonini E, Storti F, Viganò V, Gaviraghi M, et al. The WNT receptor ROR2 drives the interaction of multiple myeloma cells with the microenvironment through AKT activation. *Leukemia* (2020) 34:257–70. doi: 10.1038/s41375-019-0486-9
47. Qiang YW, Walsh K, Yao L, Kedei N, Blumberg PM, Rubin JS, et al. Wnts induce migration and invasion of myeloma plasma cells. *Blood* (2005) 106:1786–93. doi: 10.1182/blood-2005-01-0049
48. Bjorklund CC, Ma W, Wang ZQ, Davis RE, Kuhn DJ, Kornblau SM, et al. Evidence of a role for activation of Wnt/β-catenin signaling in the resistance of plasma cells to lenalidomide. *J Biol Chem* (2011) 286:11009–20. doi: 10.1074/jbc.M110.180208
49. Kaiser M, Mieth M, Liebisch P, Oberländer R, Rademacher J, Jakob C, et al. Serum concentrations of DKK-1 correlate with the extent of bone disease in patients with multiple myeloma. *Eur J Haematol* (2008) 80:490–4. doi: 10.1111/j.1600-0609.2008.01065.x
50. Terpos E, Ntanasis-Stathopoulos I, Gavriatopoulou M, Dimopoulos MA. Pathogenesis of bone disease in multiple myeloma: From bench to bedside. *Blood Cancer J* (2018) 8:7. doi: 10.1038/s41408-017-0037-4
51. Kaucká M, Plevová K, Pavlová Š, Janovská P, Mishra A, Verner J, et al. The planar cell polarity pathway drives pathogenesis of chronic lymphocytic leukemia by the regulation of b-lymphocyte migration. *Cancer Res* (2013) 73:1491–501. doi: 10.1158/0008-5472.CAN-12-1752
52. Poppova L, Janovska P, Plevova K, Radova L, Plesingerova H, Borsky M, et al. Decreased WNT3 expression in chronic lymphocytic leukaemia is a hallmark of disease progression and identifies patients with worse prognosis in the subgroup with mutated IGHV. *Br J Haematol* (2016) 175:851–9. doi: 10.1111/bjh.14312
53. Janovská P, Bryja V. Wnt signalling pathways in chronic lymphocytic leukaemia and B-cell lymphomas. *Br J Pharmacol* (2017) 174:4701–15. doi: 10.1111/bph.13949
54. Moskalev EA, Luckert K, Vorobjev IA, Mastitsky SE, Gladkikh AA, Stephan A, et al. Concurrent epigenetic silencing of wnt/β-catenin pathway inhibitor genes in B cell chronic lymphocytic leukaemia. *BMC Cancer* (2012) 12:213. doi: 10.1186/1471-2407-12-213
55. Pei L, Choi JH, Liu J, Lee EJ, McCarthy B, Wilson JM, et al. Genome-wide DNA methylation analysis reveals novel epigenetic changes in chronic lymphocytic leukemia. *Epigenetics* (2012) 7:567–78. doi: 10.4161/epi.20237
56. Cui B, Ghia EM, Chen L, Rassenti LZ, DeBoever C, Widhopf GF, et al. High-level ROR1 associates with accelerated disease progression in chronic lymphocytic leukemia. *Blood* (2016) 128:2931–40. doi: 10.1182/blood-2016-04-712562
57. Aghebati-Maleki L, Shabani M, Baradaran B, Motallebnezhad M, Majidi J, Yousefi M. Receptor tyrosine kinase-like orphan receptor 1 (ROR-1): An emerging target for diagnosis and therapy of chronic lymphocytic leukemia. *BioMed Pharmacother* (2017) 88:814–22. doi: 10.1016/j.biopha.2017.01.070
58. Zhang D, O'Neil MF, Cunningham MT, Fan F, Olyaee M, Li L. Abnormal Wnt signaling and stem cell activation in reactive lymphoid tissue and low-grade marginal zone lymphoma. *Leuk Lymphoma* (2010) 51:906–10. doi: 10.3109/10428191003695645
59. Gelebart P, Anand M, Armanious H, Peters AC, Bard JD, Amin HM, et al. Constitutive activation of the Wnt canonical pathway in mantle cell lymphoma. *Blood* (2008) 112:5171–9. doi: 10.1182/blood-2008-02-139212
60. Ge X, Lv X, Feng L, Liu X, Wang X. High expression and nuclear localization of β-catenin in diffuse large B-cell lymphoma. *Mol Med Rep* (2012) 5:1433–7. doi: 10.3892/mmr.2012.835
61. Rizzatti EG, Falcão RP, Panepucci RA, Proto-Siqueira R, Anselmo-Lima WT, Okamoto OK, et al. Gene expression profiling of mantle cell lymphoma cells reveals aberrant expression of genes from the PI3K-AKT, WNT and TGFβ signalling pathways. *Br J Haematol* (2005) 130:516–26. doi: 10.1111/j.1365-2141.2005.05630.x
62. Yu J, Chen L, Cui B, Wu C, Choi MY, Chen Y, et al. Cirmtuzumab inhibits Wnt5a-induced Rac1 activation in chronic lymphocytic leukemia treated with ibrutinib. *Leukemia* (2017) 31:1333–9. doi: 10.1038/leu.2016.368
63. Choi MY, Widhopf GF, Wu CCN, Cui B, Lao F, Sadarangani A, et al. Pre-clinical Specificity and Safety of UC-961, a First-In-Class Monoclonal Antibody Targeting ROR1. *Clin Lymphoma Myeloma Leuk* (2015) 15:S167-9. doi: 10.1016/j.clml.2015.02.010
64. Choi MY, Widhopf GF, Ghia EM, Kidwell RL, Hasan MK, Yu J, et al. Phase I Trial: Cirmtuzumab Inhibits ROR1 Signaling and Stemness Signatures in Patients with Chronic Lymphocytic Leukemia. *Cell Stem Cell* (2018) 22:951-959.e3. doi: 10.1016/j.stem.2018.05.018

65. Zhou H, Mak PY, Mu H, Mak DH, Zeng Z, Cortes J, et al. Combined inhibition of β-catenin and Bcr–Abl synergistically targets tyrosine kinase inhibitor-resistant blast crisis chronic myeloid leukemia blasts and progenitors in vitro and in vivo. *Leukemia* (2017) 31(10):2065–74. doi: 10.1038/leu.2017.87
66. Lee JH, Faderl S, Pagel JM, Jung CW, Yoon SS, Pardanani AD, et al. Phase 1 study of CWP232291 in patients with relapsed or refractory acute myeloid leukemia and myelodysplastic syndrome. *Blood Adv* (2020) 4:2032–43. doi: 10.1182/bloodadvances.2019000757
67. Savvidou I, Khong T, Cuddihy A, McLean C, Horrigan S, Spencer A. β-catenin inhibitor BC2059 is efficacious as monotherapy or in combination with proteasome inhibitor bortezomib in multiple myeloma. *Mol Cancer Ther* (2017) 16:1765–78. doi: 10.1158/1535-7163.MCT-16-0624
68. Iyer SP, Beck JT, Stewart AK, Shah J, Kelly KR, Isaacs R, et al. A Phase IB multicentre dose-determination study of BHQ880 in combination with anti-myeloma therapy and zoledronic acid in patients with relapsed or refractory multiple myeloma and prior skeletal-related events. *Br J Haematol* (2014) 167:366–75. doi: 10.1111/bjh.13056
69. Lu C, Meng S, Jin Y, Zhang W, Li Z, Wang F, et al. A novel multi-epitope vaccine from MMSA-1 and DKK1 for multiple myeloma immunotherapy. *Br J Haematol* (2017) 178:413–26. doi: 10.1111/bjh.14686
70. Li R, Zheng C, Wang Q, Bi E, Yang M, Hou J, et al. Identification of an immunogenic DKK1 long peptide for immunotherapy of human multiple myeloma. *Haematologica* (2020) 20:haematol.2019.236836. doi: 10.3324/haematol.2019.236836. haematol.2019.236836.

3

Exosomes in the Pathogenesis and Treatment of Multiple Myeloma in the Context of the Bone Marrow Microenvironment

Tianzeng Chen[1], *Maria Moscvin*[1] *and Giada Bianchi*[1,2*]

[1] *Division of Hematology, Department of Medicine, Brigham and Women's Hospital, Boston, MA, United States,* [2] *Harvard Medical School, Boston, MA, United States*

***Correspondence:**
Giada Bianchi
gbianchi1@BWH.HARVARD.EDU

Multiple myeloma (MM), the second most common hematological malignancy, is an incurable cancer of plasma cells. MM cells diffusely involves the bone marrow (BM) and establish a close interaction with the BM niche that in turn supports MM survival, proliferation, dissemination and drug resistance. In spite of remarkable progress in understanding MM biology and developing drugs targeting MM in the context of the BM niche, acquisition of multi-class drug resistance is almost universally inevitable. Exosomes are small, secreted vesicles that have been shown to mediate bidirectional transfer of proteins, lipids, and nucleic acids between BM microenvironment and MM, supporting MM pathogenesis by promoting angiogenesis, osteolysis, and drug resistance. Exosome content has been shown to differ between MM patients and healthy donors and could potentially serve as both cancer biomarker and target for novel therapies. Furthermore, the natural nanostructure and modifiable surface properties of exosomes make them good candidates for drug delivery or novel immunomodulatory therapy. In this review we will discuss the current knowledge regarding exosome's role in MM pathogenesis and its potential role as a novel biomarker and therapeutic tool in MM.

Keywords: exosome, multiple myeloma (MM), bone marrow, microenvironment, pathogenesis, emerging roles

INTRODUCTION

Multiple myeloma is the second most common hematological malignancy in the Western world after non-Hodgkin lymphoma, accounting for approximately 13% of all hematological cancers (1). About 32,270 new cases of MM and 12,830 MM-related deaths are expected in 2020 (2). Although autologous stem-cell transplantation and agents targeting both MM and the BM niche, such as immunomodulatory drugs (IMiDs), proteasome inhibitors, and monoclonal antibodies, have profoundly extended the overall survival of MM patients, the disease remains incurable (3). Multiclass relapsed/refractory MM patients face a dismal prognosis with limited therapeutic options, and thus there is an urgent need to understand better the biology of MM and explore new therapeutic approaches (4).

MM is characterized by end organ damage caused by monoclonal expansion of malignant plasma cells within the BM, associated with an excess of monoclonal protein in the blood or urine

(5). Recent data show that MM consistently progresses from a precursor state of monoclonal gammopathy of undetermined significance (MGUS) or smoldering multiple myeloma (SMM) (6, 7). The facts that the primary oncogenic mutations observed in MM patients are already present in MGUS or SMM and that genomic landscape appears remarkably similar across the plasma cell disorder spectrum, suggest that the BM microenvironment may play a crucial role in disease progression from an asymptomatic state to malignant neoplasms (8, 9).

It has been widely demonstrated that the BM microenvironment promotes tumor growth, angiogenesis, and osteolysis (9). Among various interactions within the bone marrow, recent studies reveal that exosomes are important cross-talking mediators during tumor growth and progression (10). Exosomes are small (30-100nm diameter) membrane vesicles generated in multivesicular endosomes (MVEs) and released upon the fusion of MVEs with cell membrane (11, 12). These nano vesicles are secreted by most cell types under both physiological and pathological conditions, mediating local and systemic cell-to-cell communication through selective transfer of mRNA, non-coding RNA (ncRNA), proteins, and lipids (13, 14). There is a growing interest in understanding how exosomes contribute to MM pathogenesis and if they could be use as a therapeutic vehicle in MM treatment.

EXOSOME BIOGENESIS

Exosome biogenesis starts in the endosomal system as endosomes accumulate intraluminal vesicles and mature into multivescular endosomes (MVEs or MVBs) (15, 16). During the process, cargo macromolecules including lipids, proteins, and nucleic acids are clustered and recruited *via* ESCRT (endosomal sorting complex required for transport)–dependent or ESCRT-independent mechanisms (12, 15). Once matured, MVEs that are not destined for degradation are transported along microtubules and docked to the plasma membrane, after which exosomes are released upon the fusion of MVEs and the plasma membrane (12, 16). When exosomes reach the recipient cells, they exert their effects by binding to the cell surface and triggering downstream intracellular signaling; by fusing directly with the plasma membrane to deliver cargos; or by being internalized through pathways such as endocytosis and phagocytosis (12).

Exosomes were initially thought to be means for cells to eliminate unwanted materials, but they are now considered more as biological active entities that play a role in intercellular communication and contribute to many physiological and pathological functions (16–19). In recent reports, exosomes have been shown to be an important element mediating cell recruitment, immunosuppressive effects, and horizontal transfer of genetic information either locally or systemically to ensure continuous crosstalk between the tumor and its microenvironment (18, 20). Emerging evidence supports that MM-derived exosomes (MM-EXs) reprogram recipient cell functions in the BM to modulate and mold a pro-tumor environment capable of supporting disease progression (21). MM-EXs affect the function of several components of the BM milieu, including natural killer (NK) cells, myeloid-derived suppressor cell (MDSC), mesenchymal stem cells (MSC), endothelial cells, osteoblast (OB), and osteoclast (OC) (**Figure 1**). Exosome signaling is bidirectional and bone marrow stromal cells (BMSCs)-derived exosomes (BMSC-EXs) have been shown to induce MM growth, survival, and drug resistance (22).

EXOSOMES ROLE IN MM PATHOGENESIS

Roccaro et al. demonstrated that BMSC-EXs obtained from MM patients promoted tumor growth while BMSC-EXs from healthy donors inhibited MM cell proliferation (23, 24). Exosome profiling showed MM-BMSC-EXs expressed a lower level of tumor-suppressive factor miRNA-15a, and a higher level of chemokine C-C motif ligand (CCL) 2, interleukin (IL) 6, and fibronectin, which play a crucial role in MM pathogenesis and tumor progression (24). A distinct study similarly confirmed the difference in exosomal content between normal and MM in the 5T33 murine model (25). BMSC selectively transferred certain proteins into MM cells that induced p38, p53, c-Jun N-terminal kinase (JNK), and Akt pathways to promote MM cell survival (25). Interestingly, Wang et al. also reported that exosomes obtained from both normal donor and MM patient BMSCs induced drug resistance of human MM cells. They proposed that BMSC-EXs-mediated upregulation of anti-apoptotic B-cell lymphoma (Bcl)-2 and downregulation of apoptotic Caspase 9 and Caspase 3 in MM cells inhibited spontaneous and bortezomib-induced apoptosis (25). Recently, a study showed that BMSC-derived exosomes from PI-resistant MM patients transferred PSMA3 and PSMA3 Antisense RNA1 to MM cells, causing increased proteasome activity and thus mediating PI resistance (26).

Rather than a one-way order, the mutual communication between MM and BMSC cells *via* exosomes enables a feedback loop in the BM microenvironment to support MM progression. Our group showed that co-culture of MM induced HDAC3 expression in BMSC cells, while HDAC3 knock down in BMSC lead to quantitative and qualitative changes in secreted exosomes that contributed to MM cell growth arrest (27). Moreover, De Veirman et al. examined the miRNA changes in human MSC after culture with conditioned medium of MM cells and found 19 dysregulated miRNAs, including upregulated miR-146a. They further demonstrated that exosomes transferred miR-146a from MM cells into MSC. In return, the overexpression of miR-146a in MSC increased the secretion of cytokines and chemokines including C-X-C motif chemokine ligand (CXCL) 1, CXCL10, IL6, IL8, CCL2, and CCL5, resulting in the enhancement of MM cell viability and migration (28).

Uptake of BMSC-derived exosomes by MDSCs in MM patients results in accelerated tumor growth and generation of an immunosuppressive BM milieu. An *in vitro* study showed that BMSC-derived exosomes induced the survival and expansion of MDSCs through activating signal transducer and activator of transcription (STAT) 3 and STAT1 pathways and increasing the

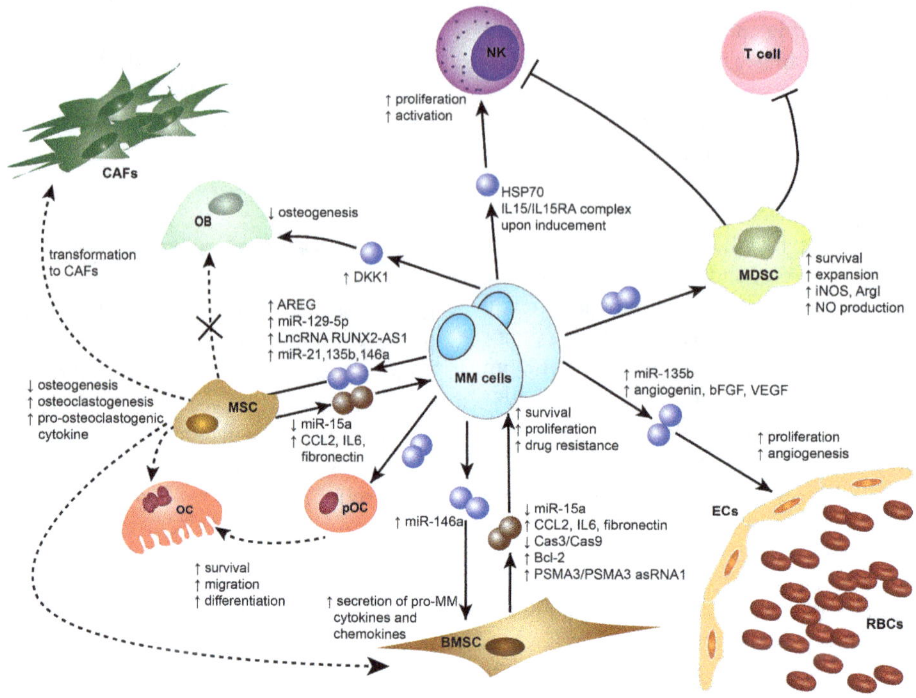

FIGURE 1 | Exosomes mediate cross-cell communication in the multiple myeloma (MM) bone marrow microenvironment (BMM). Tumor-derived exosomes remodel stromal cells, affect osteogenesis, induce angiogenesis, and help create an immunosuppressive microenvironment. Small dark blue spheres represent MM-derived exosomes and brown spheres represent MSC/BMSC-derived exosomes contribute to MM survival, proliferation, and drug resistance. Dotted arrows indicate differentiation, whereas solid arrows indicate effects on a target cell. Cells and associated effects are shown. BMSC, Bone marrow stromal cell; CAF, Cancer-associated fibroblast; ECs, Endothelial cells; MSC, Mesenchymal stem cell; MDSC, myeloid-derived suppressor cells; NK, Natural killer cell; OB, Osteoblast; OC, Osteoclast; pOC, Pre-osteoclast cell; RBCs, Red blood cells. AREG, amphiregulin; ArgI arginase 1; bFGF, basic fibroblast growth factor; Bcl-2, B-cell lymphoma 2; Cas3, Caspase-3; Cas9, Caspase-9; CCL2, chemokine C-C motif ligand 2; HSP70, Heat Shock Protein 70; IL6, Interleukin 6; IL15 Interleukin 15; IL15RA IL15 Receptor Subunit Alpha; iNOS, Inducible nitric oxide synthase; NO, Nitric oxide; PSMA3, Proteasome subunit alpha type-3; PSMA3 asRNA1, PSMA3 antisense RNA1; VEGF, Vascular endothelial growth factor; LncRNA RUNX2-AS1, Long non-coding RNA Runt-related transcription factor 2 antisense RNA1.

anti-apoptotic proteins B-cell lymphoma-extra large (Bcl-xL) and induced myeloid leukemia cell differentiation protein Mcl-1 (29). The same group also showed that exosomes from BMSCs further activated MDSCs *in vivo* to increase their nitric oxide production, which contributed to the inhibition of T cells (29, 30). They later showed that MM-EXs also activated STAT3 in MDSCs to express high levels of both arginase 1 and inducible nitric oxide synthase, which enhanced T-cell suppression (31).

EXOSOME IMPACT ON BM MICROENVIRONMENT REMODELING

Osteolysis is a common characteristic of MM resulting from a disrupted equilibrium between OBs and OCs, which are responsible for new bone apposition and bone resorption, respectively to guarantee adequate bone mass (32, 33). Exosomes in the BM have been shown to contribute to this pro-OC microenvironment, resulting in impaired bone formation and MM-related bone disease. Emerging evidence suggests that exosomal ncRNAs play an important role in this regard (34, 35).

Raimondi et al. were the first to show that exosomes derived from MM cells and MM patient's sera directly influenced OCs differentiation and function. MM-EXs not only supported migration of pre-osteoclast cells (pOCs) through the increasing of C-X-C chemokine receptor type 4 expressions, but also induced their differentiation into multinuclear OCs with specific OCs markers such as cathepsin K, matrix metalloproteinases 9 (MMP9), and tartrate-resistant acid phosphatase (TRAP). Besides promoting their bone resorptive activity, MM-EXs suppressed apoptosis of pOCs and enhanced their survival by activating the Akt pathway (36). Recent studies confirmed those observations and further explored the effective contents in MM-EXs and their mechanisms to exert functions on MSCs. LncRNA RUNX2 antisense RNA 1 (RUNX2-AS1), amphiregulin, and miR-129-5p were identified to be specifically enriched in MM-EXs. Upon internalization of the exosomes by MSC, these molecules reduced RUNX2 splicing efficiency, activated the epidermal EGFR pathway, and downregulated the expression of the transcription factor Sp1, respectively (37–39). Each pathway has been demonstrated to decrease the osteogenic potential of MSCs, increase osteoclastogenesis, and contribute to osteoblast deficiency. A new study also identified UPR (unfolded protein response)-related signaling molecules in MM-EXs that were proposed to induce osteoclastogenesis through activation of the XBP1/IRE1α

axis (40). Additionally, MM-EXs promoted secretion of pro-osteoclastogenic cytokine IL8 and IL6 *via* APE1/NF-κB pathway and suppressed osteoblastic differentiation proteins Runt-related transcription factor 2 (Runx2), Osterix and osteocalcin (38, 39, 41). Exosomes derived from 5TGM1, murine MM cells also demonstrated the ability to block osteoblast differentiation and functionality *in vitro*. Faict and colleagues suggested that the transfer of dickkopf WNT signaling pathway inhibitor 1 (DKK1) triggered inactivation of the Wnt signaling pathway that lead to a reduction in Runx2, Osterix, and Collagen 1A1 in osteoblasts (42).

Several studies indicated that soluble factors from MM cells stimulated the overexpression of miR-135b in MSCs, which was associated with the negative regulation of MSCs osteogenesis and their impaired osteogenic differentiation ability in MM patients (43). Umezu et al. later showed that exosomes from chronic hypoxia-resistant MM (HR-MM) cells, which mimicked tumor cells from the BM, were highly enriched in miR-135b (44). They provided new evidence that exosomal miR-135b directly suppressed factor inhibiting HIF-1 (FIH-1) to accelerate hypoxia-inducible factor (HIF)-1 transcriptional activity in endothelial cells and attributed to hypoxia-driven accelerated tube formation (44, 45). As BM is highly vascularized and naturally hypoxic and the MM-infiltrated BM even more hypoxic due to the massive proliferation of MM cells, exosomes target it primarily to increase angiogenesis (46, 47). Using the same HR-MM model both *in vitro* and *in vivo*, Umezu demonstrated that miR-340 from healthy BMSC exosomes inhibited angiogenesis *via* the hepatocyte growth factor/c-MET (HGF/c-MET) signaling pathway in endothelial cells. However, BMSC exosomes from older donors with senescent profiles were less effective in reducing angiogenesis (48). In murine models, Wang et al. confirmed a strong pro-angiogenic effect of MM-EXs and identified multiple angiogenic factors as cargo proteins, including angiogenin, basic fibroblast growth factor (bFGF), and vascular endothelial growth factor (VEGF) (31, 49). They further demonstrated that MM-EXs enhanced phosphorylation of Stat3, JNKs, and p53 in endothelial cells and directly facilitate their growth (31).

DIAGNOSTIC AND PROGNOSTIC ROLE OF EXOSOMES

Accurate diagnosis and prognosis with a close monitor of disease progression are essential in designing appropriate therapy for patients. There are significant research interests in identifying biomarkers and other non-invasive approaches for diagnosis and disease classification to facilitate patient follow up and care. As previously shown, exosomes are actively secreted by cells and can be isolated from the peripheral blood, making them suitable candidates as biomarkers (50). Proteomic characterization of exosomes secreted by different MM cell lines revealed that they contained a common pattern of proteins and thus could potentially represent an important tool to detect low burden disease (51). Exosomal lncRNA profiling distinguished MM and MGUS patients from healthy donors (14, 52). MicroRNAs are also important components of exosomes, delivering tumor-promoting messages and impacting signaling and protein expression in target cells (53). A study of circulating exosomal miRNAs isolated from the serum of 156 patients identified 22 miRNAs expressed at a significantly lower level in MM patients compared to healthy individuals. Among those, let-7b and miR-18a were significantly associated with both progression-free survival and overall survival. Patients characterized by lower exosomal let-7b and miR-18a levels were more likely to present with high stage in the International Staging System and have a poor outcome (54). Another study found that miR-129-5p, which targeted OBs differentiation markers, was enriched in exosomes from MM patients compared to those from SMM patients, suggesting exosomes may be a useful marker of disease progression (39). Higher expression of exosomal miR-214 detected in osteoporotic patients also suggested exosome's potential as a biomarker for MM bone diseases (34, 35). Further validation in other independent MM patient cohorts will explore the potential of circulating exosomal miRNAs to improve the prognostic and risk stratification.

Tools to predict drug resistance are becoming increasingly important in the era of personalized medicine. Zhang et al. focused on the predictive value of exosomal miRNA for primary or acquired drug resistance in MM patients. They analyzed 204 patients data and discovered that exosomal miR-16-5p, miR-15a-5p and vmiR-20a-5p, miR-17-5p were downregulated in patients resistant to bortezomib (55). Another study identified circulating exosomal PSMA3 and PSMA3-AS1 as clinically relevant biomarkers correlated with PI resistance. Newly diagnosed, MM patients with a low exosomal expression of PSMA3 and PSMA3-AS1 were sensitive to bortezomib, whereas patients with a high expression responded poorly (26).

Allogeneic hematopoietic stem cell transplantation (HSCT) is a treatment strategy that can be carefully considered in young patients with aggressive MM as a tool to achieve long-term disease remission. However, transplant-related complications, primarily acute and chronic graft-vs-host disease (GVHD) are a substantial cause of morbidity and mortality (56). Lia et al. conducted an exploratory study of 41 MM patients undergoing allogeneic HSCT to investigate exosomal surface antigens as potential predicative biomarkers for acute GVHD. CD146 correlated with a 60% increased risk of developing GVHD, whereas CD31 and CD140-α with a 40% and 60%, respectively, reduced risk (57).

EXOSOME-RELATED TARGETS AND THERAPIES

Exosomes are important message carriers that contribute to generate a tumor permissive microenvironment in the BM. A number of studies have investigated the therapeutic potential of targeting exosome secretion in MM. In murine MM models, sphingomyelinase inhibitor GW4869 blocked exosome secretion, preventing exosome-mediated bone lesions and increasing cortical bone volume. Importantly, GW4869 also strongly synergized with bortezomib in mediating anti-myeloma activity, suggesting that perturbation of exosomes can directly affect MM survival and proliferation (37, 42). However, ceramide C6 (C6-cer), an exogenous ceramide supplement, dose-dependently increased MM exosome secretion but inhibited cell proliferation and induced apoptosis (58). Interestingly, after C6-cer treatment, Cheng et al. detected decreased levels of tumor suppressive miRs including miR 202, miR 16, miR 29b, and miR 15a in MM cells and increased levels of these miRs in exosomes. While discrepancy of alterations in intracellular miRs and MM proliferation and apoptosis upon C6-cer treatment still requires further investigation, they demonstrated that those MM-EXs with elevated tumor-suppressive miRs exhibited paracrine effects on recipient MM cells that suppress tumor growth (58).

Apart from targeting exosome secretion, disrupting interactions between exosomes and recipient cells to prevent exosome uptake or content loading also has therapeutic value. Purushothaman et al. discovered that heparan sulfate plays a dual role in exosome-cell interaction, capturing fibronectin on exosomes and acting as a receptor for fibronectin on target cells. Fibronectin-mediated binding of exosomes to target cells can trigger signaling pathways like p38 and pERK and downstream expression of DKK-1 and MMP-9, two molecules with well-known roles in MM progression (59). They further showed that removal of heparan sulfate with bacterial heparitinase or using antibody specific for the Hep-II heparin-binding domain of fibronectin dramatically inhibits exosome-target cell interaction (59). The heparin-derived compound Roneparstat significantly inhibited interactions between exosomes and the target cells with a high safety profile in a phase 1 clinical trial (NCT01764880) (60). While the efficacy of Roneparstat still needs more investigation, interfering with fibronectin-heparan sulfate interactions to suppress exosome-mediated cross talk provides a novel insight to target myeloma tumor growth or progression.

However, despite the tumor-promoting and immunosuppressive effects of exosomes discussed previously, some studies showed that exosomes displaying high levels of heat shock protein 70 (HSP70) could boost NK cell responses (61). A study demonstrated that upon doxorubicin and melphalan treatment, MM cells significantly increased released exosomes that could stimulate interferon gamma (IFNγ) production, probably through mechanisms involving toll-like receptor (TLR) 2 and HSP70-dependent activation of the NF-κB pathway (62). Another study indicated that low doses of doxorubicin and melphalan could induce senescence to boost the expression of IL15/IL15RA complex on the surface of MM cells and their exosomes, promoting NK cell activation and proliferation (63). Therefore, suitable chemotherapeutic regimens may target and modulate exosomes to elicit anti-myeloma immune response. Tumor-derived exosomes as a source of tumor antigens for vaccines have also been explored. Xie et al. showed that membrane-bound HSP70-engineered myeloma cell-derived exosomes were able to induce DCs maturation and stimulate efficient CD4+ Th1, CD8+ CTL, and NK-mediated antitumor immunity. Membrane-bound HSP70 functioned both as an antigenic peptide chaperone and a danger signal that triggered DCs and therefore contributed significant adjuvant effects to exosome-based antitumor vaccine (64).

Besides providing novel therapeutic targets, the natural nanostructure and modifiable surface properties of exosomes make them a good candidate for drug delivery or immunomodulatory therapy. Knowing that cancer cells have selective sensitivity to TNF-related apoptosis-inducing ligand (TRAIL), Rivoltini et al. genetically modified cells to express TRAIL that could be subsequently embedded in secreted exosomes (65, 66). Those TRAIL-armed exosomes induced potent target cell apoptosis *in vitro* and controlled cancer progression when directly injected into tumor lesion. Though TRAIL exosomes had a preferential interaction with TRAIL-death receptor (DR) 5, *in vivo* study still showed increased areas of necrosis together with augmented levels of dead cells even in MM cells expressing other DR (66). Moreover, TRAIL exosomes can be easily produced in large amounts and stored before administration, making this a versatile, off-the-shelf therapeutic approach. Given their high stability in body fluids and natural delivery functions, TRAIL exosomes can also be loaded with drugs and genetic material and delivered to cancer cells through uptake process to elicit antitumor effects. Researchers are also exploring exosome-mimetic nanovesicles of similar sizes, morphologic features, and targeting abilities to replace exosomes in drug delivery (67, 68). With rapid technology advancement, engineering exosomes or their mimics to carry tumor-suppressive molecules or signals will, alone or in combination with other therapeutic approaches, contribute to innovative and effective MM treatment regimens.

CONCLUSIONS AND FUTURE PERSPECTIVE

Despite tremendous progress in the treatment of MM, this remains an incurable disease. It is well established that the BM microenvironment supports tumor in multiple aspects, while accumulating evidences demonstrate that exosomes plays a crucial role in the microenvironment network. Through selective transfer of mRNA, ncRNA, proteins, and lipids, exosomes are shown to mediate cell-to-cell communication and promote MM proliferation, drug resistance, immunosuppression, osteolysis, and angiogenesis. Recent studies are also investigating exosomes as potential biomarkers for MM diagnosis and predictive markers of drug response. In addition, the natural nanostructure of exosomes and their capacity to deliver molecules to target cells make them excellent drug carrier. Overall, exosomes offer the opportunity to both deepen our understanding of the molecular mechanism of MM pathogenesis and to provide a potential useful biomarker and therapeutic strategy in MM.

AUTHOR CONTRIBUTIONS

TC and GB conceived the project, wrote the initial draft, and finalized the manuscript. MM contributed to modifications of the initial draft. All authors contributed to the article and approved the submitted version.

REFERENCES

1. Palumbo A, Anderson K. Multiple myeloma. *N Engl J Med* (2011) 364:1046–60. doi: 10.1056/NEJMra1011442
2. Siegel RL, Miller KD, Jemal A. Cancer statistics, 2020. *CA A Cancer J Clin.* (2020) 70:7–30. doi: 10.3322/caac.21590
3. Kumar SK, Rajkumar SV, Dispenzieri A, Lacy MQ, Hayman SR, Buadi FK, et al. Improved survival in multiple myeloma and the impact of novel therapies. *Blood* (2008) 111(5):2516–20. doi: 10.1182/blood-2007-10-116129
4. Bianchi G, Ghobrial IM. Molecular mechanisms of effectiveness of novel therapies in multiple myeloma. *Leuk Lymphoma* (2013) 54(2):229–41. doi: 10.3109/10428194.2012.706287
5. Hideshima T, Mitsiades C, Tonon G, Richardson PG, Anderson KC. Understanding multiple myeloma pathogenesis in the bone marrow to identify new therapeutic targets. *Nat Rev Cancer* (2007) 7(8):585–98. doi: 10.1038/nrc2189
6. Landgren O. Monoclonal gammopathy of undetermined significance and smolderingmultiple myeloma: biological insights and early treatment strategies. *Hematol Am Soc Hematol Educ Program* (2013) 2013:478–87. doi: 10.1182/asheducation-2013.1.478
7. Manier S, Kawano Y, Bianchi G, Roccaro AM, Ghobrial IM. Cell autonomous and microenvironmental regulation of tumor progression in precursor states of multiple myeloma. *Curr Opin Hematol* (2016) 23(4):426–33. doi: 10.1097/MOH.0000000000000259
8. Bianchi G, Munshi NC. Pathogenesis beyond the cancer clone(s) in multiplemyeloma. *Blood* (2015) 125(20):3048–58. doi: 10.1182/blood-2014-11-568881
9. Lemaire M, Deleu S, De Bruyne E, Van Valckenborgh E, Menu E, Vanderkerken K. The Microenvironment and Molecular Biology of the Multiple Myeloma Tumor. *Adv Cancer Res* (2011) 110:19–42. doi: 10.1016/B978-0-12-386469-7.00002-5. Elsevier Inc.
10. Wang J, Faict S, Maes K, De Bruyne E, Van Valckenborgh E, Schots R, et al. Extracellular vesicle cross-talk in the bone marrow microenvironment: Implications in multiple myeloma. *Oncotarget* (2016) 7(25):38927–45. doi: 10.18632/oncotarget.7792
11. Théry C, Ostrowski M, Segura E. Membrane vesicles as conveyors of immune responses. *Nat Rev Immunol* (2009) 9(8):581–93. doi: 10.1038/nri2567
12. Van Niel G, D'Angelo G, Raposo G. Shedding light on the cell biology of extracellular vesicles. *Nat Rev Mol Cell Biol [Internet]* (2018) 19(4):213–28. doi: 10.1038/nrm.2017.125
13. Yang C, Robbins PD. The roles of tumor-derived exosomes in cancerpathogenesis. *Clin Dev Immunol* (2011) 2011:842849. doi: 10.1155/2011/842849
14. Raimondo S, Urzì O, Conigliaro A, Raimondi L, Amodio N, Alessandro R. Emerging insights on the biological impact of extracellularvesicle-associated ncRNAs in multiple Myeloma. *Non-coding RNA* (2020) 6(3):30. doi: 10.3390/ncrna6030030
15. Colombo M, Raposo G, Théry C. Biogenesis, Secretion, and Intercellular Interactions of Exosomes and Other Extracellular Vesicles. *Annu Rev Cell Dev Biol* (2014) 30(1):255–89. doi: 10.1146/annurev-cellbio-101512-122326
16. Hessvik NP, Llorente A. Current knowledge on exosome biogenesis and release. *Cell Mol Life Sci* (2018) 75(2):193–208. doi: 10.1007/s00018-017-2595-9
17. Johnstone RM, Adam M, Hammond JR, Orr L, Turbide C. Vesicle formation during reticulocyte maturation. Association of plasma membrane activities with released vesicles (exosomes). *J Biol Chem* (1987) 262(19):9412–20.
18. Peinado H, Lavotshkin S, Lyden D. The secreted factors responsible for pre-metastatic niche formation: Old sayings and new thoughts. *Semin Cancer Biol* (2011) 21(2):139–46. doi: 10.1016/j.semcancer.2011.01.002
19. Yáñez-Mó M, Siljander PRM, Andreu Z, Zavec AB, Borràs FE, Buzas EI, et al. Biological properties of extracellular vesicles and their physiological functions. *J Extracell Vesicles* (2015) 4(2015):27066. doi: 10.3402/jev.v4.27066
20. Ratajczak J, Wysoczynski M, Hayek F, Janowska-Wieczorek A, Ratajczak MZ. Membrane-derived microvesicles: Important and underappreciated mediators of cell-to-cell communication. *Leukemia* (2006) 20(9):1487–95. doi: 10.1038/sj.leu.2404296
21. Boyiadzis M, Whiteside TL. The emerging roles of tumor-derived exosomes in hematological malignancies. *Leukemia* (2017) 31(6):1259–68. doi: 10.1038/leu.2017.91
22. Moloudizargari M, Abdollahi M, Asghari MH, Zimta AA, Neagoe IB, Nabavi SM. The emerging role of exosomes in multiple myeloma. *Blood Rev* (2019) 38:100595. doi: 10.1016/j.blre.2019.100595
23. Li M, Xia B, Wang Y, James You M, Zhang Y. Potential therapeutic roles of exosomes in multiple myeloma: A systematic review. *J Cancer* (2019) 10 (24):6154–60. doi: 10.7150/jca.31752
24. Roccaro AM, Sacco A, Maiso P, Azab AK, Tai Y, Reagan M, et al. BM mesenchymal stromal cell – derived exosomes facilitate multiple myeloma progression Find the latest version : BM mesenchymal stromal cell – derived exosomes facilitate multiple myeloma progression. *J Clin Invest* (2013) 123 (4):1542–55. doi: 10.1172/JCI66517
25. Wang J, Hendrix A, Hernot S, Lemaire M, De Bruyne E, Van Valckenborgh E, et al. Bone marrow stromal cell-derived exosomes as communicators in drug resistance in multiple myeloma cells. *Blood* (2014) 124(4):555–66. doi: 10.1182/blood-2014-03-562439
26. Xu H, Han H, Song S, Yi N, Qian C, Qiu Y, et al. Exosome-transmitted PSMA3 and PSMA3-AS1 promote proteasome inhibitor resistance in multiple myeloma. *Clin Cancer Res* (2019) 25(6):1923–35. doi: 10.1158/1078-0432.CCR-18-2363
27. Ho M, Chen T, Liu J, Dowling P, Hideshima T, Zhang L, et al. Targeting histone deacetylase 3 (HDAC3) in the bone marrow microenvironment inhibits multiple myeloma proliferation by modulating exosomes and IL-6 trans-signaling. *Leukemia* (2020) 34(1):196–209. doi: 10.1038/s41375-019-0493-x
28. De Veirman K, Wang J, Xu S, Leleu X, Himpe E, Maes K, et al. Induction of miR-146a by multiple myeloma cells in mesenchymal stromal cells stimulates their pro-tumoral activity. *Cancer Lett* (2016) 377(1):17–24. doi: 10.1016/j.canlet.2016.04.024
29. Wang J, De Veirman K, De Beule N, Maes K, De Bruyne E, Van Valckenborgh E, et al. The bone marrow microenvironment enhances multiple myeloma progression by exosome-mediated activation of myeloid-derived suppressor cells. *Oncotarget* (2015) 6(41):43992–4004. doi: 10.18632/oncotarget.6083
30. Gabrilovich DI, Nagaraj S. Myeloid-derived suppressor cells as regulators of the immune system. *Nat Rev Immunol* (2009) 9(3):162–74. doi: 10.1038/nri2506
31. Wang J, De Veirman K, Faict S, Frassanito MA, Ribatti D, Vacca A, et al. Multiple myeloma exosomes establish a favourable bone marrow microenvironment with enhanced angiogenesis and immunosuppression. *J Pathol* (2016) 239(2):162–73. doi: 10.1002/path.4712
32. Harada SI, Rodan GA. Control of osteoblast function and regulation of bone mass. *Nature* (2003) 423(6937):349–55. doi: 10.1038/nature01660
33. Hameed A, Brady JJ, Dowling P, Clynes M, O'Gorman P. Bone Disease in Multiple Myeloma: Pathophysiology and Management. *Cancer Growth Metastasis* (2014) 7:33–42. doi: 10.4137/CGM.s16817
34. Raimondi L, De Luca A, Giavaresi G, Raimondo S, Gallo A, Taiana E, et al. Non-Coding RNAs in Multiple Myeloma Bone Disease Pathophysiology. *Non-Coding RNA* (2020) 6(3):37. doi: 10.3390/ncrna6030037
35. Morelli E, Gullà A, Rocca R, Federico C, Raimondi L, Malvestiti S, et al. The non-coding RNA landscape of plasma celldyscrasias. *Cancers (Basel)* (2020) 12(2):320. doi: 10.3390/cancers12020320
36. Raimondi L, De Luca A, Amodio N, Manno M, Raccosta S, Taverna S, et al. Involvement of multiple myeloma cell-derived exosomes in osteoclast differentiation. *Oncotarget* (2015) 6(15):13772–89. doi: 10.18632/oncotarget.3830
37. Li B, Xu H, Han H, Song S, Zhang X, Ouyang L. Exosome-mediated transfer of lncRUNX2-AS1 from multiple myelomacells to MSCs contributes to osteogenesis. *Oncogene* (2018) 37:5508–19. doi: 10.1038/s41388-018-0359-0
38. Raimondo S, Saieva L, Vicario E, Pucci M, Toscani D, Manno M, et al. Multiple myeloma-derived exosomes are enriched of amphiregulin (AREG) and activate the epidermal growth factor pathway in the bone microenvironment leading toosteoclastogenesis. *J Hematol Oncol* (2019) 12 (1):2. doi: 10.1186/s13045-018-0689-y
39. Raimondo S, Urz O, Conigliaro A, Bosco L, Parisi S, Carlisi M, et al. Extracellular Vesicle microRNAs Contribute to the OsteogenicInhibition of Mesenchymal Stem Cells in Multiple Myeloma. *Cancers (Basel)* (2020) 12 (2):449. doi: 10.3390/cancers12020449
40. Raimondi L, De Luca A, Fontana S, Amodio N, Costa V, Carina V, et al. Multiple myeloma-derived extracellular vesicles induceosteoclastogenesis through the activation of the XBP1/IRE1α axis. *Cancers (Basel)* (2020) 12 (8):2167. doi: 10.3390/cancers12082167

41. Liu Z, Liu H, Li Y, Shao Q, Chen J, Song J, et al. Multiple myeloma- derived exosomes inhibit osteoblastic differentiation and improve IL-6 secretion of BMSCs from multiple myeloma. *J Investig Med* (2020) 68(1):45–51. doi: 10.1136/jim-2019-001010
42. Faict S, Muller J, De Veirman K, De Bruyne E, Maes K, Vrancken L, et al. Exosomes play a role in multiple myeloma bone disease and tumor development by targeting osteoclasts and osteoblasts. *Blood Cancer J* (2018) 8(11):105. doi: 10.1038/s41408-018-0139-7
43. Xu S, Santini GC, De Veirman K, Vande Broek I, Leleu X, De A, et al. Upregulation of miR-135b Is Involved in the Impaired Osteogenic Differentiation of Mesenchymal Stem Cells Derived from Multiple Myeloma Patients. *PLoS ONE* (2013) 8:(11):e79752. doi: 10.1371/journal.pone.0079752
44. Umezu T, Tadokoro H, Azuma K, Yoshizawa S, Ohyashiki K, Ohyashiki JH. Exosomal miR-135b shed from hypoxic multiple myeloma cells enhances angiogenesis by targeting factor-inhibiting HIF-1. *Blood* (2014) 124(25):3748–57. doi: 10.1182/blood-2014-05-576116
45. Fan G. Hypoxic exosomes promote angiogenesis Platelets: balancing the septic triad. *Blood* (2015) 124(25):3669–71. doi: 10.1182/blood-2014-10-607846
46. Ramasamy SK. Structure and Functions of Blood Vessels and Vascular Niches in Bone. *Stem Cells Int* (2017) 2017:5046953. doi: 10.1155/2017/5046953
47. Ohyashiki JH, Umezu T, Ohyashiki K. Exosomes promote bone marrow angiogenesis in hematologic neoplasia: The role of hypoxia. *Curr Opin Hematol* (2016) 23(3):268–73. doi: 10.1097/MOH.0000000000000235
48. Umezu T, Imanishi S, Azuma K, Kobayashi C, Yoshizawa S, Ohyashiki K, et al. Replenishing exosomes from older bone marrow stromal cells withmiR-340 inhibits myeloma-related angiogenesis. *Blood Adv* (2017) 1(13):812–23 doi: 10.1182/bloodadvances.2016003251
49. Jakob C, Sterz J, Zavrski I, Heider U, Kleeberg L, Fleissner C, et al. Angiogenesis in multiple myeloma. *Eur J Cancer* (2006) 42(11):1581–90. doi: 10.1016/j.ejca.2006.02.017
50. Canella A, Harshman SW, Radomska HS, Freitas MA, Pichiorri F. The potential diagnostic power of extracellular vesicle analysis for multiple myeloma. *Expert Rev Mol Diagn* (2016) 16(3):277–84. doi: 10.1586/14737159.2016.1132627
51. Harshman SW, Canella A, Ciarlariello PD, Rocci A, Agarwal K, Smith EM, et al. Characterization of Multiple Myeloma Vesicles by Label-Free Relative Quantitation. *Proteomics* (2013) 13:3013–29. doi: 10.1002/pmic.201300142
52. Sedlarikova L, Bollova B, Radova L, Brozova L, Jarkovsky J, Almasi M, et al. Circulating exosomal long noncoding RNA PRINS—First findings in monoclonal gammopathies. *Hematol Oncol* (2018) 36(5):786–91. doi: 10.1002/hon.2554
53. Melo SA, Sugimoto H, O'Connell JT, Kato N, Villanueva A, Vidal A, et al. Cancer Exosomes Perform Cell-Independent MicroRNA Biogenesis and Promote Tumorigenesis. *Cancer Cell* (2014) 26(5):707–21. doi: 10.1016/j.ccell.2014.09.005
54. Manier S, Liu CJ, Avet-Loiseau H, Park J, Shi J, Campigotto F, et al. Prognostic role of circulating exosomal miRNAs in multiple myeloma. *Blood* (2017) 129 (17):2429–36. doi: 10.1182/blood-2016-09-742296
55. Zhang L, Pan L, Xiang B, Zhu H, Wu Y, Chen M, et al. Potential role of exosome-associated microRNA panels and in vivo environment to predict drug resistance for patients with multiple myeloma. *Oncotarget* (2016) 7 (21):30876–91. doi: 10.18632/oncotarget.9021
56. Hammami MB, Talkin R, Al-Taee AM, Schoen MW, Goyal SD, Lai J-P. Autologous Graft-Versus-Host Disease of the Gastrointestinal Tract in Patients With Multiple Myeloma and Hematopoietic Stem Cell Transplantation. *Gastroenterol Res* (2018) 11(1):52–7. doi: 10.14740/gr925w
57. Lia G, Brunello L, Bruno S, Carpanetto A, Omedè P, Festuccia M, et al. Extracellular vesicles as potential biomarkers of acute graft-vs-host disease. *Leukemia* (2018) 32(3):765–73. doi: 10.1038/leu.2017.277
58. Cheng Q, Li X, Wang Y, Dong M, Zhan FH, Liu J. The ceramide pathway is involved in the survival, apoptosis and exosome functions of human multiple myeloma cells in vitro. *Acta Pharmacol Sin* (2018) 39(4):561–8. doi: 10.1038/aps.2017.118
59. Purushothaman A, Bandari SK, Liu J, Mobley JA, Brown EA, Sanderson RD. Fibronectin on the surface of myeloma cell-derived exosomes mediates exosome-cell interactions. *J Biol Chem* (2016) 291(4):1652–63. doi: 10.1074/jbc.M115.686295
60. Galli M, Chatterjee M, Grasso M, Specchia G, Magen H, Einsele H, et al. Phase I study of the heparanase inhibitor International Staging System stage. *Haematologica* (2018) 103(10):e469–72. doi: 10.3324/haematol.2017.182865
61. Gastpar R, Gehrmann M, Bausero MA, Asea A, Gross C, Schroeder JA, et al. Heat shock protein 70 surface-positive tumor exosomes stimulate migratory and cytolytic activity of natural killer cells. *Cancer Res* (2005) 65(12):5238–47. doi: 10.1158/0008-5472.CAN-04-3804
62. Vulpis E, Cecere F, Molfetta R, Soriani A, Fionda C, Peruzzi G. Genotoxic stress modulates the release of exosomes from multiple myeloma cells capable of activating NK cell cytokine production: Role of HSP70 / TLR2 / NF-kB axis. *Oncoimmunology* (2017) 6(3):e1279372. doi: 10.1080/2162402X.2017.1279372
63. Borrelli C, Ricci B, Vulpis E, Fionda C, Ricciardi MR, Petrucci MT, et al. Drug-Induced Senescent Multiple Myeloma Cells Elicit NK CellProliferation by Direct or Exosome-Mediated IL15 Trans-Presentation. *Cancer Immunol Res* (2018) 6(7):860–9. doi: 10.1158/2326-6066.CIR-17-0604
64. Xie Y, Bai O, Zhang H, Yuan J, Zong S, Chibbar R, et al. Membrane-bound HSP70-engineered myeloma cell-derived exosomes stimulate more efficient CD8+ CTL- and NK-mediated antitumour immunity than exosomes released from heat-shocked tumour cells expressing cytoplasmic HSP70. *J Cell Mol Med* (2010) 14(11):2655–66. doi: 10.1111/j.1582-4934.2009.00851.x
65. Lemke J, Von Karstedt S, Zinngrebe J, Walczak H. Getting TRAIL back on track for cancer therapy. *Cell Death Differ* (2014) 21(9):1350–64. doi: 10.1038/cdd.2014.81
66. Rivoltini L, Chiodoni C, Squarcina P, Tortoreto M, Villa A, Vergani B, et al. TNF-related apoptosis-inducing ligand (trail)-armed exosomes deliver proapoptotic signals to tumor site. *Clin Cancer Res* (2016) 22(14):3499–512. doi: 10.1158/1078-0432.CCR-15-2170
67. Jang SC, Kim OY, Yoon CM, Choi DS, Roh TY, Park J, et al. Bioinspired exosome-mimetic nanovesicles for targeted delivery of chemotherapeutics to malignant tumors. *ACS Nano* (2013) 7(9):7698–710. doi: 10.1021/nn402232g
68. Wu JY, Ji AL, Wang ZX, Qiang GH, Qu Z, Wu JH, et al. Exosome-Mimetic Nanovesicles from Hepatocytes promote hepatocyte proliferation in vitro and liver regeneration in vivo. *Sci Rep* (2018) 8(1):2471. doi: 10.1038/s41598-018-20505-y

4

Mitochondrial Bioenergetics at the Onset of Drug Resistance in Hematological Malignancies

Alessandro Barbato[1], Grazia Scandura[2], Fabrizio Puglisi[1], Daniela Cambria[1], Enrico La Spina[2], Giuseppe Alberto Palumbo[3], Giacomo Lazzarino[4], Daniele Tibullo[5], Francesco Di Raimondo[2], Cesarina Giallongo[3] and Alessandra Romano[6*]*

[1] Department of Clinical and Experimental Medicine, University of Catania, Catania, Italy, [2] Department of General Surgery and Medical-Surgical Specialties, University of Catania, Catania, Italy, [3] Department of Medical, Surgical Sciences and Advanced Technologies G.F. Ingrassia, University of Catania, Catania, Italy, [4] Saint Camillus International University of Health and Medical Sciences, Rome, Italy, [5] Department of Biotechnological and Biomedical Sciences, University of Catania, Catania, Italy, [6] Department of Surgery and Medical Specialties, University of Catania, Catania, Italy

****Correspondence:***
Daniele Tibullo
d.tibullo@unict.it
Alessandra Romano
sandrina.romano@gmail.com

The combined derangements in mitochondria network, function and dynamics can affect metabolism and ATP production, redox homeostasis and apoptosis triggering, contributing to cancer development in many different complex ways. In hematological malignancies, there is a strong relationship between cellular metabolism, mitochondrial bioenergetics, interconnections with supportive microenvironment and drug resistance. Lymphoma and chronic lymphocytic leukemia cells, e.g., adapt to intrinsic oxidative stress by increasing mitochondrial biogenesis. In other hematological disorders such as myeloma, on the contrary, bioenergetics changes, associated to increased mitochondrial fitness, derive from the adaptive response to drug-induced stress. In the bone marrow niche, a reverse Warburg effect has been recently described, consisting in metabolic changes occurring in stromal cells in the attempt to metabolically support adjacent cancer cells. Moreover, a physiological dynamic, based on mitochondria transfer, between tumor cells and their supporting stromal microenvironment has been described to sustain oxidative stress associated to proteostasis maintenance in multiple myeloma and leukemia. Increased mitochondrial biogenesis of tumor cells associated to acquisition of new mitochondria transferred by mesenchymal stromal cells results in augmented ATP production through increased oxidative phosphorylation (OX-PHOS), higher drug resistance, and resurgence after treatment. Accordingly, targeting mitochondrial biogenesis, electron transfer, mitochondrial DNA replication, or mitochondrial fatty acid transport increases therapy efficacy. In this review, we summarize selected examples of the mitochondrial derangements in hematological malignancies, which provide metabolic adaptation and apoptosis resistance, also supported by the crosstalk with tumor microenvironment. This field promises a rational design to improve target-therapy including the metabolic phenotype.

Keywords: OX-PHOS, mitochondria, multiple myeloma, acute myeloid leukemia, chronic lymphatic leukemia, lymphoma

INTRODUCTION

Since the first description by Rudolf Albrecht von Kölliker in 1857, scientists have explored the essential roles of mitochondria in cell biology, as the powerhouse of the cells able to produce comparing weight to weight, thousands of times more energy per second as compared to sun production (1). Mitochondria can fuel cellular energy demands by using as substrate pyruvate, arising from glycolysis or lipolysis coupled to β-oxidation of fatty acids (FA), in the oxidative-phosphorylation (OX-PHOS) process coupled to the electron transport chain (ETC).

The combined derangements in mitochondria network function and dynamics can affect metabolism and ATP production, redox homeostasis and apoptosis triggering, contributing to cancer development in many different complex ways (2). In cancer, there is a gap in knowledge about the protein composition, structure and dynamics of lipid droplet–mitochondria structures and how bidirectional FAs exchange occur, even if the strong relationship between cellular metabolism, mitochondrial bioenergetics, and tumorigenesis development is an established emerging hallmark (2, 3).

There is a growing evidence that the metabolic reprogramming required in cancers to fuel the increased energy demand is coupled to the increased ability to evade apoptosis (2, 4). Modulating ATP availability might be an essential strategy in inducing cell resistance and sustaining cancer progression and growth (4). Recent findings have demonstrated that cancer cells take advantage of high OXPHOS, including leukemias, lymphomas, pancreatic ductal adenocarcinoma, melanoma, and endometrial carcinoma (5–16), while mitochondria can modulate their morphology regulating the intrinsic apoptotic pathway and participating in the resistance of cancer cells to apoptotic stimuli (17–27).

In this review, we will summarize the most advanced body of knowledge about the mitochondrial derangements in hematological malignancies which provide metabolic adaptation and apoptosis resistance, with a particular focus on the implication of novel relevant targets to reduce the risk of recurrence (**Figure 1**).

MITOCHONDRIA AND CANCER CELL BIOENERGETICS

Mitochondria and ATP Production: The Oxidative-Phosphorylation Process

The oxidative-phosphorylation (OX-PHOS) process is the electron transfer chain (ETC) driven by substrate oxidation (e.g pyruvate) coupled to the synthesis of ATP through an electrochemical transmembrane gradient. OX-PHOS is carried in the internal mitochondrial membrane (IMM) where four big multi-protein complexes, that contain flavins, iron-sulfur clusters, heme proteins, copper (Cu) structures, are organized to provide energy transformations in the ETC, namely Complex I, Complex II, Complex III Complex IV, as described in recent review for more details (20–22, 28–30), which operate together to generate water and a proton gradient, in presence of oxygen. The energy accumulated in the form of electrochemical proton gradient is used by F0-F1 ATP synthase (called Complex V also) to produce ATP from ADP and phosphate (4, 28, 31, 32).

Complex I (NADH–CoQ reductase), the largest respiratory complex, catalyzes the electron transfer from NADH to the CoQ

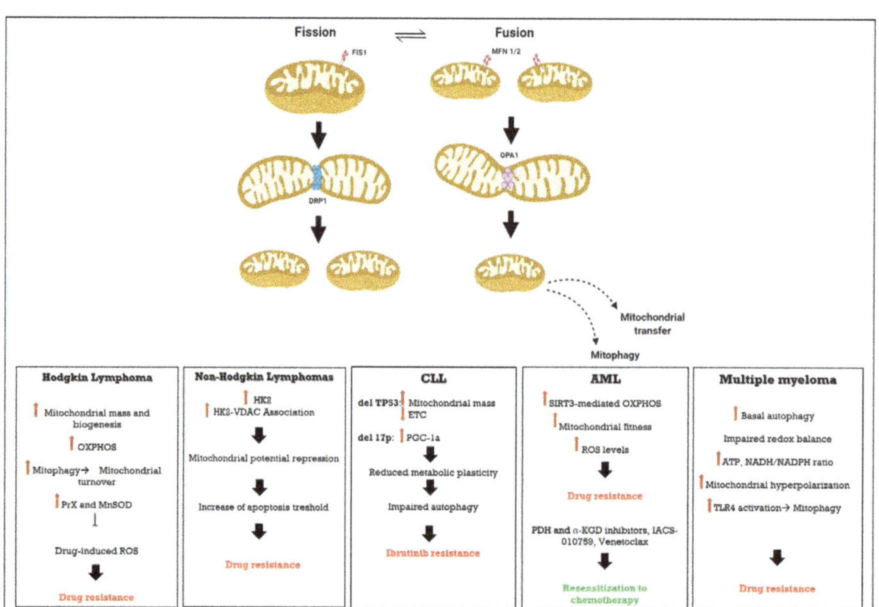

FIGURE 1 | Schematic representation of Mitochondrial involvement in drug restistance in hematological malignancies.

(ubiquinone), thus to regenerate NAD^+ levels oxidizing the NADH, which is formed both during the tricarboxylic acid (TCA) cycle and β-oxidation of fatty acids (31, 33). Complex moves four protons from the mitochondrial matrix to the intermembrane space generating a potential decrease of 360 mV (33).

Complex II (succinate dehydrogenase or succinate-ubiquinone oxidoreductase), a membrane-bound component of the Krebs cycle, permits the oxidation of the metabolite succinate to fumarate, transferring two protons to CoQ, trough the FAD/FADH2 coenzymes, thus to coupling the ETC and TCA cycle (34, 35).

Complex III (coenzyme Q: cytochrome c-oxidoreductase) catalyzes the reduction of cytochrome c, provides two protons to the CoQH2, originating from complex I and II to regenerate the CoQ, and pumps 4 protons from the mitochondrial matrix to the intermembrane space. The resulting so-called *Q cycle* allows the formation of a proton gradient across the membrane: oxidation of CoQ pumps four protons into the intermembrane space (positive side), two protons are taken up from the matrix (negative side) and two electrons are transferred from the ubiquinol to the ubiquinone, *via* two cytochrome c intermediates, to complete the cytochrome c reduction (36).

Complex IV (cytochrome c oxidase) transfers electrons from cytochrome c to oxygen to generate water and a proton gradient; its assembly and deregulation has been extensively reviewed recently (37).

Complex V consists of two main subunits: F0 is the transmembrane unit that works like a proton-driven turbine; F1 is the catalytic subunit located on the mitochondrial matrix side (38).

As a whole, OX-PHOS couples energy demands to the structural integrity of mitochondria within the cells. The membrane potential is essential for mitochondrial functions for cell survival and is well used by cancer cells to trigger molecular changes to make mitochondria network more efficient to provide energy requirements and resilience to changes in the redox status, induced by increased proliferation rate, and consequent increased nucleotide and lipid synthesis and/or drug exposure.

Mitochondria Network and Response to Dynamic Energy Demand: Fusion, Lipid Droplets (LDs) Trafficking, and Fission

Mitochondria are small organelles devoted to homeostasis and redox status maintenance within the cell, through cellular respiration, with consequent ATP production, heat production, biosynthesis of lipids and iron-containing prosthetic group heme enzymes, and apoptosis control (39, 40). These processes happen simultaneously in different compartments, identifiable by ultrastructural hallmarks, including double lipid membranes and inner membrane folds forming "cristae". The outer mitochondrial membrane (OMM) is a double phospholipid membrane separating the inside of the organelle from the rest of the cell while the inner mitochondrial membrane (IMM), separates the inter-membrane space from the central matrix, the site of the electron transport chain (ETC). The IMM and the OMM enclose the intermembrane space (IMS) of mitochondria.

The adaptation of mitochondrial morphology to cellular bioenergetics occurs at IMM by remodeling of mitochondrial cristae (5, 17, 41). The number of mitochondria in the cell and their distribution in the mitochondrial networks is regulated by two interconnected and highly dynamic processes: the fusion, which allows the merge of two mitochondria into one, and the fission, which allows the division of one mitochondrion in two daughter mitochondria, in response to ATP request or to release of cytochrome C, leading to cell death (18, 20–22, 42).

In metabolic active cells, mitochondrial fusion is tightly regulated by three GTP-ase enzymes of the dynamin superfamily: Mfn1 (Mitofusin-1), Mfn2 (Mitofusin-2), localized on the OMM, and OPA1 (optic atrophy 1), associated with the IMM.

In highly-energy demanding cells not all mitochondria work with the same efficiency (43, 44) and a balance between fluctuating energy demands, energy storage in LDs and utilization in mitochondria is required. Indeed, "peridroplet" mitochondria, characterized by elevated Krebs cycle activity but low FA oxidation capacity, support LDs biogenesis and protect the cell from lipotoxicity, while non-lipid droplet-bound cytoplasmic mitochondria are addressed to FA oxidation and energy production (43). The presence of two kind of mitochondria networks become relevant when starvation occurs and autophagy, which leads to bulk release of FAs, is triggered. In these scenarios, LDs provide a lipid buffering system that sequesters FAs released during the autophagic degradation of membranous organelles, reducing mitochondria lipotoxicity. In turn, FAs are removed by cytoplasmatic lipases to enable their transfer to mitochondria to provide an "on-demand" source of fatty acids for bulk ATP production (44), only in highly fused peridroplet mitochondria. If mitochondrial fusion is prevented, FAs could not be efficiently metabolized and are re-associated with LDs and fluxed. Thus, relevant to cancer metabolism, mitochondrial fusion dynamics ensures maximum oxidative metabolism and avoids FA toxicity in starved cells (44). As shown in murine brown adipose cells, lack of Mfn2 induces LDs accumulation and mitochondrial dysfunction (45). Indeed, mitochondrial fusion is required for β-oxidation of fatty acids (FA) and mitochondrial respiration (46); otherwise, LDs accumulate and FA efflux into neighboring cells (44).

The trafficking of FA between mitochondria and LDs is bidirectional, regulated by the lipid droplet-coating proteins PLIN1 and PLIN5 that, if overexpressed, promote clustering of mitochondria around LDs, by binding Mfn2 (43). In basal state, Plin1 and Plin5 participate to accumulate palmitate into triglycerides to limit its utilization by the mitochondria, by inhibiting hydrolysis and stabilizing the lipid droplet. In starvation, as consequence of protein kinase A-stimulated triggering, LD hydrolysis inhibition is lifted, and FAs are released from LDs to undergo β-oxidation in mitochondria (47, 48). This is associated to a transcriptional signaling, as well. Indeed, in response to starvation-induced lipolysis and protein kinase A-dependent translocation and enrichment of PLIN5 in the nucleus, transcriptional complexes with sirtuin 1 (SIRT1) and peroxisome proliferator-activated receptor γ co-activator 1α (PGC1α) can activate Nrf2-ARE system and promote transcription of target genes involved in mitochondrial biogenesis and oxidative metabolism (49). Finally, during starvation and autophagy activation, LDs can remove damaged lipids and proteins from mitochondria, to delay mitochondria fission and apoptosis triggering (43, 44, 49–52).

In resting cells, when metabolic requirements are reduced or when there is an insult leading to increased oxidative stress (e.g., oxidative damage, overcharge of ROS levels), mitochondrial fission is carried out by multi proteins machineries, such as the GTP-molecules Fis1 (Mitochondrial fission protein 1), which is integrated into the OMM, and Drp1 (Dynamin-related protein 1). Fis1 allows Drp1 to shuttle from the cytosol to the OMM, where it forms a ring that drives the division of the organelle, changing its function and structure, including mitochondrial outer membrane permeabilization, calcium influx and cytochrome c release. The resulting modifications occurring in both proteins and lipids damage mitochondria structures and induce the collapse of the mitochondrial membrane potential. The increased number of fragmented organelles in the mitochondrial network can then to be removed by a specialized form of autophagy, called mitophagy (13, 22, 26, 42, 53). Thus, mitophagy It plays a major role in maintaining a proper mitochondrial turnover by degrading damaged organelles and promoting a stable cellular pool of excellent working organelles (20, 27, 54), leading to ineffectiveness of drugs impairing mitochondrial function and consequently to chemotherapy resistance in cancer.

Warburg Effect and its Relationship to Mitochondrial Metabolism

In cancer cells, the rate of glucose uptake is dramatically increased with consequent high secretion of lactate to support malignant cell proliferation. This process, known as Warburg Effect, occurs in the presence of oxygen and performing mitochondria (55). Indeed, in the recent decade it has been demonstrated that while glycolysis is drastically increased in tumor cells, mitochondria fitness continues to operate normally (PMID: 25277420). This upregulation of glycolysis is not just for ATP production, but also for synthesis of biomass and the production of NADPH to reduce ROS and oxidative stress.

A symbiotic relationship exists among tumor and cancer-associated fibroblasts (CAFs). In this "two-compartment" model, cancer cells and CAFs become metabolically coupled (reverse Warburg effect). High production of ROS in tumor cells promotes the oxidative stress in CAFs inducing their metabolic reprogramming associated to increased aerobic glycolysis and production of energy-rich fuels such as pyruvate, lactate and fatty acids, which in turn support the OX-PHOS in cancer cells (56). Conversely, cancer cells take up these energy-rich metabolites, which in turn enter in the tricarboxylic acid (TCA) pathway, sustain ATP production by OX-PHOS, and in overall increase cell fitness for cell growth and migration (57–63).

Relevant for hematological malignancies, in the bone marrow there is a physiological dynamic, inverse metabolic state, based on mitochondria transfer, between hematopoietic stem and progenitor cells and their supporting stromal microenvironment during quiescence, proliferation and differentiation of these two populations (64, 65), in response to lactate in the extracellular space (66).

This mitochondrial transfer has been described to sustain oxidative stress associated to proteostasis maintenance in multiple myeloma (67, 68) and acute myeloid leukemia, associated to drug resistance and disease recurrence (39, 69–74).

INCREASED OX-PHOS IN HODGKIN LYMPHOMA IS ASSOCIATED TO REVERSE WARBURG EFFECT PROMOTING DRUG RESISTANCE

Hodgkin lymphoma (HL) is a hematopoietic neoplasm generated from B-cells, affecting secondary lymphoid tissues such as lymph nodes and spleen. Despite recent advances in the biological knowledge and targeted therapy, almost a quarter of lymphoma patients relapse, due to the complex interactions between residual neoplastic cells and the microenvironment, and the emergence of metabolic adaptive responses which mediate drug resistance and contribute to clonal selection, at different times and in the different sites of the same patient (75–79).

In classic HL (cHL) a few neoplastic cells (Hodgkin and Reed-Stenberg HRS cells) are surrounded by an inflammatory microenvironment of accessory myeloid and lymphoid cells (80–86). Compared to the normal counterpart of B cells deriving from (post-)germinal center (GC) cells, HRS have more mitochondrial mass, e.g., more TOMM20 (Transporter of the outer mitochondrial membrane 20) and mitochondrial biogenesis proteins, upregulate some OX-PHOS key proteins (11), have dismal lactate production (87), but increased expression of lactate importer MCT1 (monocarboxylate transporter 1) (11). As consequence, HRS metabolic profile is characterized by high ATP production, as consequence of high OX-PHOS (87).

Increased OX-PHOS is associated to increased basal autophagy flux and increased mitochondrial turnover *via* mitophagy, which provides to maintain high quality mitochondria and metabolic intermediates conveying drug resistance (88). Carbon skeletons can be further provided by the supportive microenvironment, since the surrounding cells in HL exhibit high-glycolytic activity, associated to increased lactate dehydrogenase activity and lactate release, with increased lactate exporter MCT4 expression (11). The induction of Warburg effect in the microenvironment and the reverse Warburg effect in HRS cells could mediate drug resistance to chemotherapy drugs that disrupt OX-PHOS function such as doxorubicin or affect the cellular redox state (11, 89).

Drugs commonly used in the first-line treatment, such as bleomycin, doxorubicine, and vinblastine, part of ABVD regimen (85, 90–92), generate large amount of reactive oxygen species, causing oxidative stress and apoptosis (93), but increasing at the same time the expression of antioxidant enzymes that could contribute to chemoresistance in HRS cells. Bur et al., assessed expression of peroxiredoxin (Prx) II, Prx III, Prx V, Prx VI, and manganese superoxide dismutase (MnSOD) in 99 cases of uniformly treated HL. Prxs I–VI participate in cellular antioxidant defense by reducing alkyl hydroperoxides and hydrogen peroxide to the corresponding alcohol and water, while MnSOD catalyzes the dismutation of superoxide to hydrogen peroxide and oxygen and is the most important antioxidant enzyme in mitochondria, where oxidative stress is most evident under physiological circumstances, owing to oxidative phosphorylation (94). Data reported by Bur *et al.*, suggest that the induction of mitochondrial located antioxidant enzymes (MnSOD and Prx III) in both HRS cells and in reactive cellular infiltrate is significantly induced in the most aggressive cases. The evidence of a low rate of complete response to ABVD treatment in patients with low Prx V expression is therefore in line with the role of oxidative stress in the mechanism of action of these drugs. More precisely, all patients with low cytoplasmic Prx V expression in RS cells achieved CR, whereas the CR rate was highly low in those with high cytoplasmic Prx V expression in RS cells (95). Thanks to their mitochondria, HRS can sustain substantial amount of oxidative stress, and, in line with this, mitochondrial Prx V expression is related to a poor response to ABVD chemotherapy.

The reverse Warburg effect in cHL could be overcome by drugs which target glycolysis in the microenvironment (e.g., arsenic or metformin) which become synergic with other agents directed against the crosstalk between neoplastic cells and the environment, like check-point inhibitors (96, 97). The high-glycolytic activity in HL microenvironment is clinically relevant, since and associated to prognostic meaning of 18-FDG-PET persistent positivity after first cycles of chemotherapy (81–83, 98).

Taken together these data reflect the high involvement of mitochondria in the resistance to the drugs commonly used for the treatment of cHL, making them a highly favorable target for therapeutic manipulation *via* biguanides and metformin (99).

OX-PHOS IDENTIFIES METABOLIC SUBTYPES OF B-CELL NON-HODGKIN LYMPHOMAS

Non-Hodgkin lymphoma (NHL) includes quite heterogeneous group of blood neoplasms that differ for metabolism, cell of origin, clinical course, and response to treatment (79, 100–102). The relationship between metabolic pathway differences and drug resistance has led to an increasing interest in metabolic mechanisms important for lymphoma cells surviving.

A recent *in vitro* study about nine different B cell NHL cell lines has revealed their capacity to use glucose or glutamine as source of energy to sustain high proliferative rate. The capacity to use different substrates is related to differences in metabolic pathways. Particularly, glutamine-addicted cells use mitochondrial metabolism, while glucose-addicted cells have glycolytic metabolism also in presence of oxygen (Warburg effect), while cells that can use glutamine or glucose equally have a higher metabolic plasticity that allows them to use one or another pathway depending on the substrates availability (103).

In diffuse large B cell lymphoma (DLBCL), metabolic diversity is related to different expression profiles identified as a three-consensus cluster today used for DLBCL classification: B cell receptor (BCR)/proliferation cluster (BRC-DLBCL), oxidative phosphorylation cluster (OX-PHOS DLBCL), and host response (HR) cluster (102). Indeed, BCR-DLBCLs shows a higher expression of many component of the BCR signaling (102, 104, 105) and it is linked to the downstream PI3K/AKT/mTORC1 pathway involved in regulation of pro-survival factors, glucose acquisition, and glycolysis flux activation (14, 106, 107). Conversely, OX-PHOS DLBCLs shows an increase in mitochondrial activity and mitochondrial fatty acid oxidation (14). However, lymphoma cells show an important metabolic plasticity, and acute inhibition of BCR signaling increases glutamine catabolism fuelling the TCA cycle and palmitate-induced mitochondrial oxygen consumption (14). Increased contribution of mitochondria for energy production is related to differential activity or efficiency of mitochondrial ETC complexes which are encoded by nuclear and mitochondrial independently transcribed and translated genomes, with the exception of complex II (9, 14). The high expression of components of mitochondrial translation machinery is fundamental for OX-PHOS cells maintenance, so inhibition of mitochondrial translation machinery causes ROS production responsible of cell death (9). Moreover, lymphoma cell lines are able to regulate their metabolic activity in relation of oxygen availability. Indeed, OX-PHOS DLBCL can become resistant to hypoxic stress thanks to an increasing of Hexokinase II (HK2) expression upon eIF4E1 and HIF1α regulation, related to a high involvement of glycolysis pathway (108, 109). Gu and colleagues found that rituximab resistance in cell lines of lymphoma (110, 111) was associated to the impaired glucose metabolism, due to overexpression of HK2, which interacts with the protein of the mitochondrial outer membrane VDAC (voltage-dependent anion channel), to repress the mitochondrial membrane potential and increase the mitochondrial apoptosis threshold (112). Targeting HK2 resulted in decreased mitochondrial membrane potential, ATP production, cell viability, and re-sensitization to chemotherapy agents, suggesting that overexpression of HK2 could be a novel potential therapeutic target in rituximab-refractory lymphomas (111). Analysis of expression profile of newly diagnosed DLBCL has showed that glyceraldehyde-3-phosphate dehydrogenase (GAPDH) is related to metabolic profile of lymphoma cells. Particularly, GAPDH expression is significantly correlated with the percentage of ATP generated from glycolysis, so low GAPDH level is related to oxygen consumption in OX-PHOS -DLBCL while high GAPDH level is related to lactate production in BCR-DLBCLs. Moreover, the increased activation of mTORC1 activity in

OX-PHOS-DLBCL is associated with the increase in glutamine transport rate, reduction of intracellular metabolites involved in glycolysis (G6P, G3P, and lactate) and non-oxidative arm of the pentose phosphate pathway (113).

The not-uniform metabolic behavior of DLBLC has clinical implications: first, the limited role of early PET positivity during treatment, that could reflect residual glycolytic activity of neoplastic versus microenvironment cells, based on cell of origin; second, the suboptimal results of lymphoma treatment, as shown by the association between relation between gene expression related to mitochondrial energetic function and R-CHOP resistance (113); third, the metabolic rewiring associated to the residual activity of the B-cell receptor. Casola and colleagues demonstrated that the two lymphoma clusters have a different fitness. Indeed, BCR^{+} cell lines have a higher competitive fitness than BCR^{-} counterparts thanks to BCR/PI3Kδ axis activation, which induces glycogen synthase kinase-3β phosphorylation (114) and regulates the transcriptional program, under MYC control, for the expression of OX-PHOS genes, which use carbon-skeleton of glutamine to fuel TCA cycle. Indeed, the competitive advantage of BCR- clones on BCR+ clones was due to increased glutamine catabolism, that could be observed also in absence of BCR/PI3Kδ axis through a constitutive activation of RAS/MAPK pathway (115).

METABOLIC REWIRING IN CHRONIC LYMPHATIC LEUKEMIA

Chronic Lymphocytic leukemia (CLL) is due to the clonal expansion and accumulation of malignant B-cell lymphocytes in the blood stream and in homing tissues, such as bone marrow and lymphoid organs. Circulating CLL lymphocytes are quiescent and dependent on intrinsic survival factors and proliferate when they enter homing tissues, revealing a challenge for the design of therapeutic interventions that target intrinsic survival pathways (116). Circulating and homing require a plastic metabolic rewiring that allows cells to modify their metabolism and fulfill the requirements needed to sustain survival, differentiation or proliferation (117, 118). To this end, the number of mitochondria, the total mitochondrial mass, biogenesis, bioenergetics (basal, maximal, and ATP-linked respiration rates), membrane potential and ROS are increased in CLL cells compared to naïve B-lymphocytes (119). As discussed above, also CLL cells use preferentially the reverse Warburg effect, relying primarily on OX-PHOS for generating energy (120). Clinically relevant, 18-FDG-PET is not always informative to evaluate disease burden and it is indicated only when Richter's Syndrome or transformation to another aggressive B-cell lymphoma is suspected (121).

Using NanoString technology, it was shown that CLL lymphocytes display heightened expression of mitochondrial IDH3 and citrate transporter (SLC25A1) which yield α-ketoglutarate from isocitrate and cytoplasmic export of citrate respectively (122). ZAP-70+ CLL cells exhibited significantly higher bioenergetics than B lymphocytes or ZAP-70- CLL cells and were more sensitive to the uncoupler, carbonyl cyanide-p-trifluoro-methoxyphenylhydrazone (FCCP). Univariable and multivariable linear regression analysis demonstrated that ZAP-70+ predicted increased maximal respiration. ZAP-70+ is a surrogate for B cell receptor (BCR) activation and can be targeted by ibrutinib, which is a clinically approved Bruton's tyrosine kinase (BTK) inhibitor. Ibrutinib-treated patients exhibit decreased oxygen consumption rates (OCR) of CLL cells. similar to control B lymphocytes, suggesting that drug treatment resets the mitochondrial bioenergetics (117). Increased OX-PHOS is a resistance mechanism to BCL-2 inhibitor venetoclax, suggesting that the implementation of combinatorial therapy with metabolic modulators may overcome drug resistance (123).

MITOCHONDRIAL FITNESS MEDIATES RESISTANCE TO BORTEZOMIB IN MULTIPLE MYELOMA

Multiple Myeloma (MM) is a neoplastic plasma cell disorder characterized by a complex array of clinical manifestations, including hypercalcemia, renal dysfunction, anemia, and bone lesions (collectively known as CRAB symptoms), in a wide spectrum of clinical variants ranging from benign MGUS and smoldering/indolent MM, to more aggressive, disseminated forms of MM and plasma cell leukemia (124). There is no a unique driver genetic event in MM onset, but a complex variety of chromosomal and genomic rearrangements (125), occurring at different timepoints in response to external driving forces (e.g., exposure to microbes, chronic antigen stimulation, oxidative stress). Among the most frequent mutated genes, FAM46C has been involved in both mitochondrial and bioenergetics dysfunction associated to drug resistance (126), proteostasis (127), and disease onset.

Physiologically, in the plasma cell (PCs) ontogeny, immunoglobulin synthesis and survival of competitive clones relies on preserved cell bioenergetics. In response to increased poli-ubiquitinated proteins requiring autophagy triggering (128), long-lived PCs robustly engage pyruvate-dependent respiration and rely on OX-PHOS whereas their short-lived counterparts could not (129). Thus, the transition from plasmablast to short-lived and long-lived PCs is associated to increased autophagy fluxes to allow removal of damaged mitochondria and lipid droplets accumulation to maintain protein and lipid homeostasis (44). Several groups have recently showed that integrity of mitochondrial function relies on p62 to limit oxidative stress, and conversely, lack of p62 is associated with inhibited complex I mitochondrial respiration. As consequence, reduced efficiency of electron transport chain (ETC) is associated to metabolic derangement inducing pentose phosphate pathway and increased cytosolic reduced glutathione (GSH) levels. Conversely, complex I inhibition resulted in lower mitochondrial membrane potential and higher cytosolic ROS production. Pharmacological activation of transcription factor Nrf2 increased mitochondrial NADH levels and restored mitochondrial membrane potential in p62-deficient cells (130).

Relying on the detoxifying mitochondrial function is consequence of other two aberrant metabolic changes occurring in MM: the oxidative stress, consequence of the aberrant protein synthesis of incomplete immunoglobulins with defective glycosylation (131), and the lack of glutamine synthetase which confers increased ammonium production and requires nitrates detoxification (132).

In relapsed and refractory patients MM PCs overexpress mitochondrial biogenesis signatures regulated by the cellular iron content (133). The consequent loss of integrity of redox balance, with the nuclear compartmentalization of heme-oxygenase 1 is associated to drug resistance and genomic instability (134). MM can intake iron to increase their scavenger antioxidant-related genes and mitochondrial mass. Iron trafficking, by modifying energetic metabolism of cancer cells and impairing inflammatory status of macrophages in the microenvironment, is a critical regulator to reshape the MM tumor niche (135). However, to make the picture more complex, MM cell lines are characterized by distinct ferritin levels, which directly correlate with bortezomib resistance and pre-treatment with ferric ammonium citrate (FAC) decreased bortezomib sensitivity *in vitro* (135).

Bioenergetics changes, associated to increased mitochondrial biomass and function, can be elicited as part of the adaptive response to treatment (135–138). In vitro, human MM cell lines resistant to bortezomib or dexamethasone have higher concentrations of ATP, NADH/NADPH ratio, associated to hyperpolarization of mitochondrial membrane leading to impaired drug response (137, 139). In vitro, pre-treament with the OX-PHOS inhibitor tigecycline can increase bortezomib sensitivity (Alejandra Ortiz-Ruiz, ASH 2019, poster 4408) (140). Similarly, inhibition of PGC-1α (SR18292), relevant for OX-PHOS, significantly impaired the proliferation and survival of MM cells due to the energy exhaustion and oxidative damage (141). These and other preclinical studies confirm OX-PHOS as possible targets for sensitization to chemotherapy treatment in MM (142), including the efficacy of Venetoclax (BCL-2 inhibitor) that could be used independently from the genetic lesion (143). Further steps could include a metabolic classification of MM subtypes based on mitochondria number and OX-PHOS quantification (143).

Our group has recently disclosed that TLR4 acts as a mitochondria protective factor against bortezomib-induced mitochondria damage and apoptosis (144). Targeting TLR4 signaling in bortezomib resistant cells damages mitochondrial fitness and increases mitophagy leading to apoptosis. As TLR4 pathway is also activated in MM mesenchymal stromal cells (MSCs) driving their commitment toward a pro-inflammatory and pro-tumor behavior (145), TLR4 inhibition could be an adjuvant therapy to interrupt the self-reinforcing stromal changes in MM microenvironment. Taken together, changes in microenvironment composition (146) and REDOX status can affect sensitivity to novel agents (147) and should be taken in account in designing novel combinations.

MITOCHONDRIAL METABOLISM DEPENDENCY IN ACUTE MYELOID LEUKEMIA AND NOVEL THERAPEUTIC TARGETS

Acute myeloid leukemia (AML) is a heterogeneous disease characterized by a blockade in differentiation of hematopoietic stem cells with a clonal proliferation of myeloid blast in BM and peripheral blood. Due to the high relapse rate and poor clinical outcome, overcoming chemoresistance remains the most important goal in AML patients. Changes in cell metabolism and metabolic adaptation are a hallmark of many cancers, including AML, supporting tumor initiation, growth, and response to therapeutics. The discovery of enzymes deficiency and mutations in key metabolic enzymes has highlighted the importance of metabolism in cancer biology and how these changes might constitute a weakness for cancer treatment.

A study carried out by Chen et al., reported that some metabolites such as pyruvate and lactate were specifically enriched in the serum of patients at diagnosis compared to healthy controls and demonstrated prognostic value in cytogenetically normal AML (CN-AML) patients as it could predict poor survival for these patients (148). Interestingly, deletions of the two glycolytic enzymes PKM2 and LDHA, which catalyze the production of cytosolic pyruvate and lactate, respectively, inhibit leukemia initiation *in vivo* in AML mice models.

It has also been reported that a wide percentage of AML patients are deficient in arginosuccinate synthetase-1 (ASS1), an enzyme that allows the conversion of citrulline and aspartate into argininosuccinate (149). The loss of ASS1 has also been found in other tumor types where it is required to support cell proliferation and nucleotide synthesis by sustaining the intracellular aspartate level (150). A decrease in ASS1 can also lead to a dependence on arginine, which has been explored as a potential vulnerability in different cancer types, including AML (151).

Recent advances in cancer genetics have found mutations in the isocitrate dehydrogenase 1 (*IDH1)* and 2 (*IDH2) genes* occur frequently in a variety of human cancers, including AML. Wild-type IDH1 and IDH2 are important metabolic enzymes catalyzing the oxidative decarboxylation of isocitrate to generate α-ketoglutarate (αKG) and CO2. IDH1 represents the peroxisomes and cytosol isoform, while IDH2 is localized in mitochondria. The common function of IDH1/2 active-site mutations is a new enzyme activity that catalyzes the conversion of αKG to D-2-hydroxyglutarate (D2HG). Under physiological conditions, cellular D2HG accumulation is limited due to the actions of the endogenous D2HG dehydrogenase (D2HGDH), which catalyzes the reverse reaction from D2HG to αKG.

D2HG has been demonstrated to inhibit αKG-dependent dioxygenases that are involved in the regulation of epigenetics and differentiation and is thought to induce epigenetic dysfunction inhibiting normal cellular differentiation. Specifically, elevated D2HG levels competitively inhibit αKG-dependent lysine demethylases, resulting in elevated levels of histone methylation in a variety of cell line models (152, 153). Consequently, inhibition of cellular differentiation by D2HG is thought to promote the pathological self-renewal of stem-like progenitor cells, which may create a cellular state prone to malignant transformation.

Evidence from AML patients and preclinical models strongly suggests that *IDH1* and *IDH2* mutations are oncogenic drivers of AML and myelodysplastic syndrome and that targeting IDH mutant neomorphic activity in this context may provide therapeutic benefit by promoting the differentiation of malignant myeloid cells. Research attempts have been made to identify small molecule inhibitors of mutant IDH enzymes and to develop these molecules as drugs for anti-cancer therapy (153).

In addition to targeting metabolic enzymes, targeting OX-PHOS turned out to be a promising strategy to improve the treatment outcomes of AML. Indeed, leukemic cells have higher copy number of mitochondrial DNA, more mitochondria and increased oxygen consumption in comparison to normal hematopoietic stem cells, without a concomitant increase in respiratory chain complex activity, which confers increased susceptibility to oxidative stress (154). Acquisition of chemoresistance is associated to a shift toward a high OX-PHOS status characterized by increased mitochondrial fitness and high levels of ROS (155). Mechanistically, this can be due to increased SIRT3 expression, which significantly decreased nicotinamide adenine dinucleotide phosphate (NADP)/reduced NADP ratio and increased reduced glutathione/oxidized glutathione ratio, associated to OX-PHOS induction (156).

For those cancers, like AML, that rely on OX-PHOS, its inhibition could represent an effective therapeutic strategy. In solid cancers OH-PHOS inhibitors, including biguanides and metformin, are currently under investigation in several trials, designed to evaluate the combination of metformin with chemotherapy, as recently reviewed (157, 158). Several drugs, including biguanides, metformin, atovaquone, and arsenic trioxide, are used at clinical level for non-oncologic indications, but growing evidences indicate their potential use as OX-PHOS inhibitors (8). The detrimental effect of metformin is emerging in AML, alone (159) or in combination with cytarabine (160), and Venetoclax induced cell-cycle arrest leading to clinical trials.

CPI-613, designated as orphan drug for the treatment of peripheral T-cell lymphoma, is a lipoate analog that blocks pyruvate dehydrogenase (PDH) and α-ketoglutarate dehydrogenase (KGDH), induces collapse of mitochondrial function associated to large, tumor-specific production of mitochondrial ROS (161). Based on encouraging results in phase I clinical studies (162, 163), a phase III randomized study is ongoing in the setting of refractory/relapsing AML to compare the efficacy of standard chemotherapy supplemented or not with CPI-613. Similarly, phase I trials disclosed promising results using IACS-010759, is an ECT inhibitor, acting against complex I in AML and NHL (164).

Taken together, ongoing trials in AML and other hematological malignancies show that targeting OX-PHOS is a promising strategy to induce a metabolic rewiring leading to chemo-sensitization.

CONCLUSIONS

Mitochondria play many important roles in cell functions and homeostasis, including the production of ATP, the release of death-promoting factors upon apoptotic stimuli and a variety of metabolic pathways. Contrary to conventional wisdom, functional mitochondria are essential for cancer cells. Although mutations in mitochondrial genes are common in cancer cells, they do not inactivate mitochondrial energy metabolism but rather alter the mitochondrial bioenergetic and biosynthetic state. These alterations activate out-of-context programs that are important in the onset and the development of malignancies. However, different cancer cell types undergo different bioenergetic alterations, some to more glycolytic and others to more oxidative, depending in part on the developmental state of the cell undergoing neoplastic transformation (165).

In most hematological malignancies, cancer cells show greater basal mitochondrial activity compared to healthy counterparts leading to higher levels of oxidative stress. ROS, adaptation to ROS, and mitochondrial biogenesis appear to form a self-amplifying feedback loop to sustain recurrence, as shown in CLL (119). However, in other settings, like MM, bioenergetics of tumor cells can change, as consequence of increased mitochondrial biomass and function, as part of the adaptive response to drug-induced stress (139).

In particular, interactions between cancer cells and surrounding microenvironment highly affect the growth, metabolism, metastasis and progression of cancer. The so-called reverse Warburg effect has been proposed to reconsider bioenergetics of cancer cells and stromal cells become metabolically coupled (56, 58, 59). In a vicious circle, neoplastic cells induce oxidative stress in neighboring microenvironment to undergo aerobic glycolysis and generate high level of energy-rich fuels (such as pyruvate, ketone bodies, fatty acids, and lactate) that fuel mitochondrial OX-PHOS in cancer cells and are utilized for efficient ATP production (56). In addition, microenvironment can contribute through horizontal mitochondrial transfer, when neoplastic cells become incapable of aerobic respiration due to defective or deleted mtDNA (166), Taking up functional mitochondria derived from the microenvironment can increase mitochondrial mass to improve metabolic fitness of neoplastic cells and conferring drug resistance.

It is probably that in next years "*mitochondrial medicine*" will play an active role to design effective therapeutic strategies to target the interplay between microenvironment and neoplastic cells to tailor the metabolic phenotype and not only the genomic aberrancies, with novel targets for selective anti-cancer therapy.

AUTHOR CONTRIBUTIONS

AB, GS, CG, and AR designed the paper and wrote the manuscript. FP and FR reviewed literature about myeloma. DC and ES reviewed literature about lymphoma. GP reviewed literature about AML. GL and DT reviewed literature about OX-PHOS targeting. All authors contributed to the article and approved the submitted version.

REFERENCES

1. Schatz G. The Magic Garden. *Annu Rev Biochem* (2007) 76:673–8. doi: 10.1146/annurev.biochem.76.060806.091141
2. Vakifahmetoglu-Norberg H, Ouchida AT, Norberg E. The role of mitochondria in metabolism and cell death. *Biochem Biophys Res Commun* (2017) 482:426–31. doi: 10.1016/j.bbrc.2016.11.088
3. Frezza C, Gottlieb E. Mitochondria in cancer: not just innocent bystanders. *Semin Cancer Biol* (2009) 19:4–11. doi: 10.1016/j.semcancer.2008.11.008
4. Moreno-Sánchez R, Rodríguez-Enríquez S, Marín-Hernández A, Saavedra E. Energy metabolism in tumor cells. *FEBS J* (2007) 274:1393–418. doi: 10.1111/j.1742-4658.2007.05686.x
5. Field CS, Baixauli F, Kyle RL, Puleston DJ, Cameron AM, Sanin DE, et al. Mitochondrial Integrity Regulated by Lipid Metabolism Is a Cell-Intrinsic Checkpoint for Treg Suppressive Function. *Cell Metab* (2020) 31:422–37.e5. doi: 10.1016/j.cmet.2019.11.021
6. Panuzzo C, Jovanovski A, Pergolizzi B, Pironi L, Stanga S, Fava C, et al. Mitochondria: A Galaxy in the Hematopoietic and Leukemic Stem Cell Universe. *Int J Mol Sci* (2020) 21:3298. doi: 10.3390/ijms21113928
7. Zhang L, Yao Y, Zhang S, Liu Y, Guo H, Ahmed M, et al. Metabolic reprogramming toward oxidative phosphorylation identifies a therapeutic target for mantle cell lymphoma. *Sci Transl Med* (2019) 11(491):eaau1667. doi: 10.1126/scitranslmed.aau1167
8. Ashton TM, McKenna WG, Kunz-Schughart LA, Higgins GS. Oxidative Phosphorylation as an Emerging Target in Cancer Therapy. *Clin Cancer Res* (2018) 24:2482–90. doi: 10.1158/1078-0432.CCR-17-3070
9. Norberg E, Lako A, Chen PH, Stanley IA, Zhou F, Ficarro SB, et al. Differential contribution of the mitochondrial translation pathway to the survival of diffuse large B-cell lymphoma subsets. *Cell Death Differ* (2017) 24:251–62. doi: 10.1038/cdd.2016.116
10. Gooptu M, Whitaker-Menezes D, Sprandio J, Domingo-Vidal M, Lin Z, Uppal G, et al. Mitochondrial and glycolytic metabolic compartmentalization in diffuse large B-cell lymphoma. *Semin Oncol* (2017) 44:204–17. doi: 10.1053/j.seminoncol.2017.10.002
11. Mikkilineni L, Whitaker-Menezes D, Domingo-Vidal M, Sprandio J, Avena P, Cotzia P, et al. Hodgkin lymphoma: A complex metabolic ecosystem with glycolytic reprogramming of the tumor microenvironment. *Semin Oncol* (2017) 44:218–25. doi: 10.1053/j.seminoncol.2017.10.003
12. Sewastianik T, Szydlowski M, Jablonska E, Bialopiotrowicz E, Kiliszek P, Gorniak P, et al. FOXO1 is a TXN- and p300-dependent sensor and effector of oxidative stress in diffuse large B-cell lymphomas characterized by increased oxidative metabolism. *Oncogene* (2016) 35:5989–6000. doi: 10.1038/onc.2016.126
13. Giménez-Cassina A, Danial NN. Regulation of mitochondrial nutrient and energy metabolism by BCL-2 family proteins. *Trends Endocrinol Metab* (2015) 26:165–75. doi: 10.1016/j.tem.2015.02.004
14. Caro P, Kishan AU, Norberg E, Stanley IA, Chapuy B, Ficarro SB, et al. Metabolic signatures uncover distinct targets in molecular subsets of diffuse large B cell lymphoma. *Cancer Cell* (2012) 22:547–60. doi: 10.1016/j.ccr.2012.08.014
15. Flis K, Irvine D, Copland M, Bhatia R, Skorski T. Chronic myeloid leukemia stem cells display alterations in expression of genes involved in oxidative phosphorylation. *Leuk Lymphoma* (2012) 53:2474–8. doi: 10.3109/10428194.2012.696313
16. Shahruzaman SH, Fakurazi S, Maniam S. Targeting energy metabolism to eliminate cancer cells. *Cancer Manag Res* (2018) 10:2325–35. doi: 10.2147/CMAR.S167424
17. Cogliati S, Frezza C, Soriano ME, Varanita T, Quintana-Cabrera R, Corrado M, et al. Mitochondrial Cristae Shape Determines Respiratory Chain Supercomplexes Assembly and Respiratory Efficiency. *Cell* (2013) 155:160–71. doi: 10.1016/j.cell.2013.08.032
18. Maycotte P, Marín-Hernández A, Goyri-Aguirre M, Anaya-Ruiz M, Reyes-Leyva J, Cortés-Hernández P. Mitochondrial dynamics and cancer. *Tumour Biol* (2017) 39:1010428317698391. doi: 10.1177/1010428317698391
19. Humphries BA, Cutter AC, Buschhaus JM, Chen YC, Qyli T, Palagama DSW, et al. Enhanced mitochondrial fission suppresses signaling and metastasis in triple-negative breast cancer. *Breast Cancer Res* (2020) 22:60. doi: 10.1186/s13058-020-01301-x
20. Chan DC. Mitochondrial Dynamics and Its Involvement in Disease. *Annu Rev Pathol* (2020) 15:235–59. doi: 10.1146/annurev-pathmechdis-012419-032711
21. Farmer T, Naslavsky N, Caplan S. Tying trafficking to fusion and fission at the mighty mitochondria. *Traffic* (2018) 19:569–77. doi: 10.1111/tra.12573
22. Herst PM, Rowe MR, Carson GM, Berridge MV. Functional Mitochondria in Health and Disease. *Front Endocrinol (Lausanne)* (2017) 8:296. doi: 10.3389/fendo.2017.00296
23. Chen H, Chan DC. Mitochondrial Dynamics in Regulating the Unique Phenotypes of Cancer and Stem Cells. *Cell Metab* (2017) 26:39–48. doi: 10.1016/j.cmet.2017.05.016
24. Morciano G, Pedriali G, Sbano L, Iannitti T, Giorgi C, Pinton P. Intersection of mitochondrial fission and fusion machinery with apoptotic pathways: Role of Mcl-1. *Biol Cell* (2016) 108:279–93. doi: 10.1111/boc.201600019
25. Babbar M, Sheikh MS. Metabolic Stress and Disorders Related to Alterations in Mitochondrial Fission or Fusion. *Mol Cell Pharmacol* (2013) 5:109–33.
26. Rehman J, Zhang HJ, Toth PT, Zhang Y, Marsboom G, Hong Z, et al. Inhibition of mitochondrial fission prevents cell cycle progression in lung cancer. *FASEB J* (2012) 26:2175–86. doi: 10.1096/fj.11-196543
27. Figge MT, Reichert AS, Meyer-Hermann M, Osiewacz HD. Deceleration of fusion-fission cycles improves mitochondrial quality control during aging. *PLoS Comput Biol* (2012) 8:e1002576. doi: 10.1371/journal.pcbi.1002576
28. Mills EL, Kelly B, O'Neill LAJ. Mitochondria are the powerhouses of immunity. *Nat Immunol* (2017) 18:488–98. doi: 10.1038/ni.3704
29. Vyas S, Zaganjor E, Haigis MC. Mitochondria and Cancer. *Cell* (2016) 166:555–66. doi: 10.1016/j.cell.2016.07.002
30. Ulivieri C. Cell death: insights into the ultrastructure of mitochondria. *Tissue Cell* (2010) 42:339–47. doi: 10.1016/j.tice.2010.10.004
31. Sazanov LA. The mechanism of coupling between electron transfer and proton translocation in respiratory complex I. *J Bioenerg Biomembr* (2014) 46:247–53. doi: 10.1007/s10863-014-9554-z
32. Buttgereit F, Brand MD. A hierarchy of ATP-consuming processes in mammalian cells. *Biochem J* (1995) 312(Pt 1):163–7. doi: 10.1042/bj3120163
33. Urra FA, Muñoz F, Lovy A, Cárdenas C. The Mitochondrial Complex(I)ty of Cancer. *Front Oncol* (2017) 7:118. doi: 10.3389/fonc.2017.00118
34. Kluckova K, Bezawork-Geleta A, Rohlena J, Dong L, Neuzil J. Mitochondrial complex II, a novel target for anti-cancer agents. *Biochim Biophys Acta* (2013) 1827:552–64. doi: 10.1016/j.bbabio.2012.10.015
35. Cecchini G. Function and structure of complex II of the respiratory chain. *Annu Rev Biochem* (2003) 72:77–109. doi: 10.1146/annurev.biochem.72.121801.161700
36. Bleier L, Dröse S. Superoxide generation by complex III: from mechanistic rationales to functional consequences. *Biochim Biophys Acta* (2013) 1827:1320–31. doi: 10.1016/j.bbabio.2012.12.002
37. Dennerlein S, Rehling P. Human mitochondrial COX1 assembly into cytochrome c oxidase at a glance. *J Cell Sci* (2015) 128:833–7. doi: 10.1242/jcs.161729
38. Jonckheere AI, Smeitink JA, Rodenburg RJ. Mitochondrial ATP synthase: architecture, function and pathology. *J Inherit Metab Dis* (2012) 35:211–25. doi: 10.1007/s10545-011-9382-9
39. Wang J, Liu X, Qiu Y, Shi Y, Cai J, Wang B, et al. Cell adhesion-mediated mitochondria transfer contributes to mesenchymal stem cell-induced chemoresistance on T cell acute lymphoblastic leukemia cells. *J Hematol Oncol* (2018) 11:11. doi: 10.1186/s13045-018-0554-z
40. Wang C, Youle RJ. The role of mitochondria in apoptosis*. *Annu Rev Genet* (2009) 43:95–118. doi: 10.1146/annurev-genet-102108-134850

41. Soultawi C, Fortier Y, Soundaramourty C, Estaquier J, Laforge M. Mitochondrial Bioenergetics and Dynamics During Infection. *Exp Suppl* (2018) 109:221–33. doi: 10.1007/978-3-319-74932-7_5
42. Xie LL, Shi F, Tan Z, Li Y, Bode AM, Cao Y. Mitochondrial network structure homeostasis and cell death. *Cancer Sci* (2018) 109:3686–94. doi: 10.1111/cas.13830
43. Benador IY, Veliova M, Mahdaviani K, Petcherski A, Wikstrom JD, Assali EA, et al. Mitochondria Bound to Lipid Droplets Have Unique Bioenergetics, Composition, and Dynamics that Support Lipid Droplet Expansion. *Cell Metab* (2018) 27:869–85.e6. doi: 10.1016/j.cmet.2018.03.003
44. Rambold AS, Cohen S, Lippincott-Schwartz J. Fatty acid trafficking in starved cells: regulation by lipid droplet lipolysis, autophagy, and mitochondrial fusion dynamics. *Dev Cell* (2015) 32:678–92. doi: 10.1016/j.devcel.2015.01.029
45. Boutant M, Kulkarni SS, Joffraud M, Ratajczak J, Valera-Alberni M, Combe R, et al. Mfn2 is critical for brown adipose tissue thermogenic function. *EMBO J* (2017) 36:1543–58. doi: 10.15252/embj.201694914
46. Koundouros N, Poulogiannis G. Reprogramming of fatty acid metabolism in cancer. *Br J Cancer* (2020) 122:4–22. doi: 10.1038/s41416-019-0650-z
47. Zhu Y, Ren C, Zhang M, Zhong Y. Perilipin 5 Reduces Oxidative Damage Associated With Lipotoxicity by Activating the PI3K/ERK-Mediated Nrf2-ARE Signaling Pathway in INS-1 Pancreatic β-Cells. *Front Endocrinol (Lausanne)* (2020) 11:166. doi: 10.3389/fendo.2020.00166
48. Wang H, Sreenivasan U, Hu H, Saladino A, Polster BM, Lund LM, et al. Perilipin 5, a lipid droplet-associated protein, provides physical and metabolic linkage to mitochondria. *J Lipid Res* (2011) 52:2159–68. doi: 10.1194/jlr.M017939
49. Jarc E, Petan T. Lipid Droplets and the Management of Cellular Stress. *Yale J Biol Med* (2019) 92:435–52.
50. Voisin P, Bernard M, Bergès T, Regnacq M. Amino acid starvation inhibits autophagy in lipid droplet-deficient cells through mitochondrial dysfunction. *Biochem J* (2020) 477(18):3613–23. doi: 10.1042/BCJ20200551
51. Li Y, Zong WX, Ding WX. Recycling the danger via lipid droplet biogenesis after autophagy. *Autophagy* (2017) 13:1995–7. doi: 10.1080/15548627.2017.1371394
52. Klecker T, Braun RJ, Westermann B. Lipid Droplets Guard Mitochondria during Autophagy. *Dev Cell* (2017) 42:1–2. doi: 10.1016/j.devcel.2017.06.018
53. Simula L, Nazio F, Campello S. The mitochondrial dynamics in cancer and immune-surveillance. *Semin Cancer Biol* (2017) 47:29–42. doi: 10.1016/j.semcancer.2017.06.007
54. Mai S, Muster B, Bereiter-Hahn J, Jendrach M. Autophagy proteins LC3B, ATG5 and ATG12 participate in quality control after mitochondrial damage and influence lifespan. *Autophagy* (2012) 8:47–62. doi: 10.4161/auto.8.1.18174
55. Liberti MV, Locasale JW. The Warburg Effect: How Does it Benefit Cancer Cells? *Trends Biochem Sci* (2016) 41:211–8. doi: 10.1016/j.tibs.2015.12.001
56. Fu Y, Liu S, Yin S, Niu W, Xiong W, Tan M, et al. The reverse Warburg effect is likely to be an Achilles' heel of cancer that can be exploited for cancer therapy. *Oncotarget* (2017) 8:57813–25. doi: 10.18632/oncotarget.18175
57. Martinez-Outschoorn U, Sotgia F, Lisanti MP. Tumor microenvironment and metabolic synergy in breast cancers: critical importance of mitochondrial fuels and function. *Semin Oncol* (2014) 41:195–216. doi: 10.1053/j.seminoncol.2014.03.002
58. Witkiewicz AK, Whitaker-Menezes D, Dasgupta A, Philp NJ, Lin Z, Gandara R, et al. Using the "reverse Warburg effect" to identify high-risk breast cancer patients: stromal MCT4 predicts poor clinical outcome in triple-negative breast cancers. *Cell Cycle* (2012) 11:1108–17. doi: 10.4161/cc.11.6.19530
59. Sotgia F, Whitaker-Menezes D, Martinez-Outschoorn UE, Flomenberg N, Birbe RC, Witkiewicz AK, et al. Mitochondrial metabolism in cancer metastasis: visualizing tumor cell mitochondria and the "reverse Warburg effect" in positive lymph node tissue. *Cell Cycle* (2012) 11:1445–54. doi: 10.4161/cc.19841
60. Martinez-Outschoorn UE, Pavlides S, Howell A, Pestell RG, Tanowitz HB, Sotgia F, et al. Stromal-epithelial metabolic coupling in cancer: integrating autophagy and metabolism in the tumor microenvironment. *Int J Biochem Cell Biol* (2011) 43:1045–51. doi: 10.1016/j.biocel.2011.01.023
61. Martinez-Outschoorn UE, Pavlides S, Whitaker-Menezes D, Daumer KM, Milliman JN, Chiavarina B, et al. Tumor cells induce the cancer associated fibroblast phenotype via caveolin-1 degradation: implications for breast cancer and DCIS therapy with autophagy inhibitors. *Cell Cycle* (2010) 9:2423–33. doi: 10.4161/cc.9.12.12048
62. Bonuccelli G, Whitaker-Menezes D, Castello-Cros R, Pavlides S, Pestell RG, Fatatis A, et al. The reverse Warburg effect: glycolysis inhibitors prevent the tumor promoting effects of caveolin-1 deficient cancer associated fibroblasts. *Cell Cycle* (2010) 9:1960–71. doi: 10.4161/cc.9.10.11601
63. Pavlides S, Whitaker-Menezes D, Castello-Cros R, Flomenberg N, Witkiewicz AK, Frank PG, et al. The reverse Warburg effect: aerobic glycolysis in cancer associated fibroblasts and the tumor stroma. *Cell Cycle* (2009) 8:3984–4001. doi: 10.4161/cc.8.23.10238
64. Golan K, Wellendorf A, Takihara Y, Kumari A, Khatib-Massalha E, Kollet O, et al. Mitochondria Transfer from Hematopoietic Stem and Progenitor Cells to Pdgfrα+/Sca-1-/CD48dim BM Stromal Cells Via CX43 Gap Junctions and AMPK Signaling Inversely Regulate ROS Generation in Both Cell Populations. *Blood* (2016) 128:5–5. doi: 10.1182/blood.V128.22.5.5
65. Maryanovich M, Zaltsman Y, Ruggiero A, Goldman A, Shachnai L, Zaidman SL, et al. An MTCH2 pathway repressing mitochondria metabolism regulates haematopoietic stem cell fate. *Nat Commun* (2015) 6:7901. doi: 10.1038/ncomms8901
66. Khatib-Massalha E, Bhattacharya S, Massalha H, Biram A, Golan K, Kollet O, et al. Lactate released by inflammatory bone marrow neutrophils induces their mobilization via endothelial GPR81 signaling. *Nat Commun* (2020) 11:3547. doi: 10.1038/s41467-020-17402-2
67. Boise LH, Shanmugam M. Stromal Support of Metabolic Function through Mitochondrial Transfer in Multiple Myeloma. *Cancer Res* (2019) 79:2102–3. doi: 10.1158/0008-5472.CAN-19-0500
68. Marlein CR, Piddock RE, Mistry JJ, Zaitseva L, Hellmich C, Horton RH, et al. CD38-Driven Mitochondrial Trafficking Promotes Bioenergetic Plasticity in Multiple Myeloma. *Cancer Res* (2019) 79:2285–97. doi: 10.1158/0008-5472.CAN-18-0773
69. Burt R, Dey A, Aref S, Aguiar M, Akarca A, Bailey K, et al. Activated stromal cells transfer mitochondria to rescue acute lymphoblastic leukemia cells from oxidative stress. *Blood* (2019) 134:1415–29. doi: 10.1182/blood.2019001398
70. Kolba MD, Dudka W, Zaręba-Kozioł M, Kominek A, Ronchi P, Turos L, et al. Tunneling nanotube-mediated intercellular vesicle and protein transfer in the stroma-provided imatinib resistance in chronic myeloid leukemia cells. *Cell Death Dis* (2019) 10:817. doi: 10.1038/s41419-019-2045-8
71. Rodriguez AM, Nakhle J, Griessinger E, Vignais ML. Intercellular mitochondria trafficking highlighting the dual role of mesenchymal stem cells as both sensors and rescuers of tissue injury. *Cell Cycle* (2018) 17:712–21. doi: 10.1080/15384101.2018.1445906
72. Griessinger E, Moschoi R, Biondani G, Peyron JF. Mitochondrial Transfer in the Leukemia Microenvironment. *Trends Cancer* (2017) 3:828–39. doi: 10.1016/j.trecan.2017.10.003
73. Marlein CR, Zaitseva L, Piddock RE, Robinson SD, Edwards DR, Shafat MS, et al. NADPH oxidase-2 derived superoxide drives mitochondrial transfer from bone marrow stromal cells to leukemic blasts. *Blood* (2017) 130:1649–60. doi: 10.1182/blood-2017-03-772939
74. Moschoi R, Imbert V, Nebout M, Chiche J, Mary D, Prebet T, et al. Protective mitochondrial transfer from bone marrow stromal cells to acute myeloid leukemic cells during chemotherapy. *Blood* (2016) 128:253–64. doi: 10.1182/blood-2015-07-655860
75. Rasche L, Kortüm KM, Raab MS, Weinhold N. The Impact of Tumor Heterogeneity on Diagnostics and Novel Therapeutic Strategies in Multiple Myeloma. *Int J Mol Sci* (2019) 20:1248. doi: 10.3390/ijms20051248
76. Araf S, Wang J, Korfi K, Pangault C, Kotsiou E, Rio-Machin A, et al. Genomic profiling reveals spatial intra-tumor heterogeneity in follicular lymphoma. *Leukemia* (2018) 32:1261–5. doi: 10.1038/s41375-018-0043-y
77. Rasche L, Chavan SS, Stephens OW, Patel PH, Tytarenko R, Ashby C, et al. Spatial genomic heterogeneity in multiple myeloma revealed by multi-region sequencing. *Nat Commun* (2017) 8:268. doi: 10.1038/s41467-017-00296-y
78. Mithraprabhu S, Khong T, Ramachandran M, Chow A, Klarica D, Mai L, et al. Circulating tumour DNA analysis demonstrates spatial mutational heterogeneity that coincides with disease relapse in myeloma. *Leukemia* (2017) 31:1695–705. doi: 10.1038/leu.2016.366

79. Opinto G, Vegliante MC, Negri A, Skrypets T, Loseto G, Pileri SA, et al. The Tumor Microenvironment of DLBCL in the Computational Era. *Front Oncol* (2020) 10:351. doi: 10.3389/fonc.2020.00351
80. Romano A, Parrinello NL, Chiarenza A, Motta G, Tibullo D, Giallongo C, et al. Immune off-target effects of Brentuximab Vedotin in relapsed/refractory Hodgkin Lymphoma. *Br J Haematol* (2019) 185:468–79. doi: 10.1111/bjh.15801
81. Agostinelli C, Gallamini A, Stracqualursi L, Agati P, Tripodo C, Fuligni F, et al. The combined role of biomarkers and interim PET scan in prediction of treatment outcome in classical Hodgkin's lymphoma: a retrospective, European, multicentre cohort study. *Lancet Haematol* (2016) 3:e467–79. doi: 10.1016/S2352-3026(16)30108-9
82. Romano A, Parrinello NL, Vetro C, Tibullo D, Giallongo C, La Cava P, et al. The prognostic value of the myeloid-mediated immunosuppression marker Arginase-1 in classic Hodgkin lymphoma. *Oncotarget* (2016) 7:67333–46. doi: 10.18632/oncotarget.12024
83. Romano A, Parrinello NL, Vetro C, Forte S, Chiarenza A, Figuera A, et al. Circulating myeloid-derived suppressor cells correlate with clinical outcome in Hodgkin Lymphoma patients treated up-front with a risk-adapted strategy. *Br J Haematol* (2015) 168:689–700. doi: 10.1111/bjh.13198
84. Vetro C, Romano A, Ancora F, Coppolino F, Brundo MV, Raccuia SA, et al. Clinical Impact of the Immunome in Lymphoid Malignancies: The Role of Myeloid-Derived Suppressor Cells. *Front Oncol* (2015) 5:104. doi: 10.3389/fonc.2015.00104
85. Romano A, Vetro C, Caocci G, Greco M, Parrinello NL, Di Raimondo F, et al. Immunological deregulation in classic hodgkin lymphoma. *Mediterr J Hematol Infect Dis* (2014) 6:e2014039. doi: 10.4084/mjhid.2014.039
86. Tiacci E, Döring C, Brune V, van Noesel CJ, Klapper W, Mechtersheimer G, et al. Analyzing primary Hodgkin and Reed-Sternberg cells to capture the molecular and cellular pathogenesis of classical Hodgkin lymphoma. *Blood* (2012) 120:4609–20. doi: 10.1182/blood-2012-05-428896
87. Birkenmeier K, Dröse S, Wittig I, Winkelmann R, Käfer V, Döring C, et al. Hodgkin and Reed-Sternberg cells of classical Hodgkin lymphoma are highly dependent on oxidative phosphorylation. *Int J Cancer* (2016) 138:2231–46. doi: 10.1002/ijc.29934
88. Birkenmeier K, Moll K, Newrzela S, Hartmann S, Dröse S, Hansmann ML. Basal autophagy is pivotal for Hodgkin and Reed-Sternberg cells' survival and growth revealing a new strategy for Hodgkin lymphoma treatment. *Oncotarget* (2016) 7:46579–88. doi: 10.18632/oncotarget.10300
89. Yadav N, Kumar S, Marlowe T, Chaudhary AK, Kumar R, Wang J, et al. Oxidative phosphorylation-dependent regulation of cancer cell apoptosis in response to anticancer agents. *Cell Death Dis* (2015) 6:e1969. doi: 10.1038/cddis.2015.305
90. Romano A, Parrinello NL, Vetro C, Chiarenza A, Cerchione C, Ippolito M, et al. Prognostic meaning of neutrophil to lymphocyte ratio (NLR) and lymphocyte to monocyte ration (LMR) in newly diagnosed Hodgkin lymphoma patients treated upfront with a PET-2 based strategy. *Ann Hematol* (2018) 97:1009–18. doi: 10.1007/s00277-018-3276-y
91. Gallamini A, Tarella C, Viviani S, Rossi A, Patti C, Mulé A, et al. Early Chemotherapy Intensification With Escalated BEACOPP in Patients With Advanced-Stage Hodgkin Lymphoma With a Positive Interim Positron Emission Tomography/Computed Tomography Scan After Two ABVD Cycles: Long-Term Results of the GITIL/FIL HD 0607 Trial. *J Clin Oncol* (2018) 36:454–62. doi: 10.1200/JCO.2017.75.2543
92. Gallamini A, Di Raimondo F, La Nasa G, Romano A, Borra A, Greco M. Standard therapies versus novel therapies in Hodgkin lymphoma. *Immunol Lett* (2013) 155:56–9. doi: 10.1016/j.imlet.2013.09.011
93. Aggarwal V, Tuli HS, Varol A, Thakral F, Yerer MB, Sak K, et al. Role of Reactive Oxygen Species in Cancer Progression: Molecular Mechanisms and Recent Advancements. *Biomolecules* (2019) 9(11):735. doi: 10.3390/biom9110735
94. Rabilloud T, Heller M, Gasnier F, Luche S, Rey C, Aebersold R, et al. Proteomics analysis of cellular response to oxidative stress. Evidence for in vivo overoxidation of peroxiredoxins at their active site. *J Biol Chem* (2002) 277:19396–401. doi: 10.1074/jbc.M106585200
95. Bur H, Haapasaari KM, Turpeenniemi-Hujanen T, Kuittinen O, Auvinen P, Marin K, et al. Oxidative stress markers and mitochondrial antioxidant enzyme expression are increased in aggressive Hodgkin lymphomas. *Histopathology* (2014) 65:319–27. doi: 10.1111/his.12389
96. Vial G, Detaille D, Guigas B. Role of Mitochondria in the Mechanism(s) of Action of Metformin. *Front Endocrinol* (2019) 10:294. doi: 10.3389/fendo.2019.00294
97. Chukkapalli V, Gordon LI, Venugopal P, Borgia JA, Karmali R. Metabolic changes associated with metformin potentiates Bcl-2 inhibitor, Venetoclax, and CDK9 inhibitor, BAY1143572 and reduces viability of lymphoma cells. *Oncotarget* (2018) 9:21166–81. doi: 10.18632/oncotarget.24989
98. Casasnovas RO, Bouabdallah R, Brice P, Lazarovici J, Ghesquieres H, Stamatoullas A, et al. PET-adapted treatment for newly diagnosed advanced Hodgkin lymphoma (AHL2011): a randomised, multicentre, non-inferiority, phase 3 study. *Lancet Oncol* (2019) 20:202–15. doi: 10.1016/S1470-2045(18)30784-8
99. Cunha Júnior AD, Pericole FV, Carvalheira JBC. Metformin and blood cancers. *Clinics (Sao Paulo)* (2018) 73:e412s. doi: 10.6061/clinics/2018/e412s
100. Alizadeh AA, Eisen MB, Davis RE, Ma C, Lossos IS, Rosenwald A, et al. Distinct types of diffuse large B-cell lymphoma identified by gene expression profiling. *Nature* (2000) 403:503–11. doi: 10.1038/35000501
101. Jaffe ES, Harris NL, Stein H, Isaacson PG. Classification of lymphoid neoplasms: the microscope as a tool for disease discovery. *Blood* (2008) 112:4384–99. doi: 10.1182/blood-2008-07-077982
102. Monti S, Savage KJ, Kutok JL, Feuerhake F, Kurtin P, Mihm M, et al. Molecular profiling of diffuse large B-cell lymphoma identifies robust subtypes including one characterized by host inflammatory response. *Blood* (2005) 105:1851–61. doi: 10.1182/blood-2004-07-2947
103. Liu X, Wang L, Jiang W, Lu W, Yang J, Yang W. B cell lymphoma with different metabolic characteristics show distinct sensitivities to metabolic inhibitors. *J Cancer* (2018) 9:1582–91. doi: 10.7150/jca.24331
104. Chen L, Monti S, Juszczynski P, Ouyang J, Chapuy B, Neuberg D, et al. SYK inhibition modulates distinct PI3K/AKT- dependent survival pathways and cholesterol biosynthesis in diffuse large B cell lymphomas. *Cancer Cell* (2013) 23:826–38. doi: 10.1016/j.ccr.2013.05.002
105. Chen L, Monti S, Juszczynski P, Daley J, Chen W, Witzig TE, et al. SYK-dependent tonic B-cell receptor signaling is a rational treatment target in diffuse large B-cell lymphoma. *Blood* (2008) 111:2230–7. doi: 10.1182/blood-2007-07-100115
106. Doughty CA, Bleiman BF, Wagner DJ, Dufort FJ, Mataraza JM, Roberts MF, et al. Antigen receptor-mediated changes in glucose metabolism in B lymphocytes: role of phosphatidylinositol 3-kinase signaling in the glycolytic control of growth. *Blood* (2006) 107:4458–65. doi: 10.1182/blood-2005-12-4788
107. Broecker-Preuss M, Becher-Boveleth N, Bockisch A, Dührsen U, Müller S. Regulation of glucose uptake in lymphoma cell lines by c-MYC- and PI3K-dependent signaling pathways and impact of glycolytic pathways on cell viability. *J Transl Med* (2017) 15:158. doi: 10.1186/s12967-017-1258-9
108. Bhalla K, Jaber S, Nahid MN, Underwood K, Beheshti A, Landon A, et al. Role of hypoxia in Diffuse Large B-cell Lymphoma: Metabolic repression and selective translation of HK2 facilitates development of DLBCL. *Sci Rep* (2018) 8:744. doi: 10.1038/s41598-018-25251-9
109. Nakajima K, Kawashima I, Koshiisi M, Kumagai T, Suzuki M, Suzuki J, et al. Glycolytic enzyme hexokinase II is a putative therapeutic target in B-cell malignant lymphoma. *Exp Hematol* (2019) 78:46–55.e3. doi: 10.1016/j.exphem.2019.09.023
110. Czuczman MS, Olejniczak S, Gowda A, Kotowski A, Binder A, Kaur H, et al. Acquirement of rituximab resistance in lymphoma cell lines is associated with both global CD20 gene and protein down-regulation regulated at the pretranscriptional and posttranscriptional levels. *Clin Cancer Res* (2008) 14:1561–70. doi: 10.1158/1078-0432.CCR-07-1254
111. Gu JJ, Singh A, Xue K, Mavis C, Barth M, Yanamadala V, et al. Up-regulation of hexokinase II contributes to rituximab-chemotherapy resistance and is a clinically relevant target for therapeutic development. *Oncotarget* (2017) 9 (3):4020–33. doi: 10.18632/oncotarget.23425
112. Wilson JE. Isozymes of mammalian hexokinase: structure, subcellular localization and metabolic function. *J Exp Biol* (2003) 206:2049–57. doi: 10.1242/jeb.00241
113. Chiche J, Reverso-Meinietti J, Mouchotte A, Rubio-Patiño C, Mhaidly R, Villa E, et al. GAPDH Expression Predicts the Response to R-CHOP, the Tumor

Metabolic Status, and the Response of DLBCL Patients to Metabolic Inhibitors. *Cell Metab* (2019) 29:1243–57.e10. doi: 10.1016/j.cmet.2019.02.002
114. Yang K, Chen Z, Gao J, Shi W, Li L, Jiang S, et al. The Key Roles of GSK-3β in Regulating Mitochondrial Activity. *Cell Physiol Biochem* (2017) 44:1445–59. doi: 10.1159/000485580
115. Varano G, Raffel S, Sormani M, Zanardi F, Lonardi S, Zasada C, et al. The B-cell receptor controls fitness of MYC-driven lymphoma cells via GSK3β inhibition. *Nature* (2017) 546:302–6. doi: 10.1038/nature22353
116. Messmer BT, Messmer D, Allen SL, Kolitz JE, Kudalkar P, Cesar D, et al. In vivo measurements document the dynamic cellular kinetics of chronic lymphocytic leukemia B cells. *J Clin Invest* (2005) 115:755–64. doi: 10.1172/JCI23409
117. Roy Chowdhury S, Bouchard EDJ, Saleh R, Nugent Z, Peltier C, Mejia E, et al. Mitochondrial Respiration Correlates with Prognostic Markers in Chronic Lymphocytic Leukemia and Is Normalized by Ibrutinib Treatment. *Cancers (Basel)* (2020) 12(3):650. doi: 10.3390/cancers12030650
118. Roy Chowdhury S, Banerji V. Targeting Mitochondrial Bioenergetics as a Therapeutic Strategy for Chronic Lymphocytic Leukemia. *Oxid Med Cell Longev* (2018) 2018:2426712. doi: 10.1155/2018/2426712
119. Jitschin R, Hofmann AD, Bruns H, Giessl A, Bricks J, Berger J, et al. Mitochondrial metabolism contributes to oxidative stress and reveals therapeutic targets in chronic lymphocytic leukemia. *Blood* (2014) 123:2663–72. doi: 10.1182/blood-2013-10-532200
120. Galicia-Vázquez G, Aloyz R. Metabolic rewiring beyond Warburg in chronic lymphocytic leukemia: How much do we actually know? *Crit Rev Oncol Hematol* (2019) 134:65–70. doi: 10.1016/j.critrevonc.2018.12.003
121. Vaisitti T, Gaudino F, Ouk S, Moscvin M, Vitale N, Serra S, et al. Targeting metabolism and survival in chronic lymphocytic leukemia and Richter syndrome cells by a novel NF-κB inhibitor. *Haematologica* (2017) 102:1878–89. doi: 10.3324/haematol.2017.173419
122. Owen OE, Kalhan SC, Hanson RW. The key role of anaplerosis and cataplerosis for citric acid cycle function. *J Biol Chem* (2002) 277:30409–12. doi: 10.1074/jbc.R200006200
123. Guièze R, Liu VM, Rosebrock D, Jourdain AA, Hernández-Sánchez M, Martinez Zurita A, et al. Mitochondrial Reprogramming Underlies Resistance to BCL-2 Inhibition in Lymphoid Malignancies. *Cancer Cell* (2019) 36:369–84.e13. doi: 10.1016/j.ccell.2019.08.005
124. Romano A, Parrinello NL, Simeon V, Puglisi F, La Cava P, Bellofiore C, et al. High-density neutrophils in MGUS and multiple myeloma are dysfunctional and immune-suppressive due to increased STAT3 downstream signaling. *Sci Rep* (2020) 10:1983. doi: 10.1038/s41598-020-58859-x
125. Maura F, Bolli N, Angelopoulos N, Dawson KJ, Leongamornlert D, Martincorena I, et al. Genomic landscape and chronological reconstruction of driver events in multiple myeloma. *Nat Commun* (2019) 10:3835. doi: 10.1101/388611
126. Zhu YX, Shi CX, Bruins LA, Jedlowski P, Wang X, Kortüm KM, et al. Loss of FAM46C Promotes Cell Survival in Myeloma. *Cancer Res* (2017) 77:4317–27. doi: 10.1158/0008-5472.CAN-16-3011
127. Herrero AB, Quwaider D, Corchete LA, Mateos MV, García-Sanz R, Gutiérrez NC. FAM46C controls antibody production by the polyadenylation of immunoglobulin mRNAs and inhibits cell migration in multiple myeloma. *J Cell Mol Med* (2020) 24:4171–82. doi: 10.1111/jcmm.15078
128. Pengo N, Scolari M, Oliva L, Milan E, Mainoldi F, Raimondi A, et al. Plasma cells require autophagy for sustainable immunoglobulin production. *Nat Immunol* (2013) 14:298–305. doi: 10.1038/ni.2524
129. Lam TT, Zhu H, Guan Y, Holmes EC. Genomic Analysis of the Emergence, Evolution, and Spread of Human Respiratory RNA Viruses. *Annu Rev Genomics Hum Genet* (2016) 17:193–218. doi: 10.1146/annurev-genom-083115-022628
130. Bartolome F, Esteras N, Martin-Requero A, Boutoleau-Bretonniere C, Vercelletto M, Gabelle A, et al. Pathogenic p62/SQSTM1 mutations impair energy metabolism through limitation of mitochondrial substrates. *Sci Rep* (2017) 7:1666. doi: 10.1038/s41598-017-01678-4
131. Glavey SV, Manier S, Natoni A, Sacco A, Moschetta M, Reagan MR, et al. The sialyltransferase ST3GAL6 influences homing and survival in multiple myeloma. *Blood* (2014) 124:1765–76. doi: 10.1182/blood-2014-03-560862
132. Bolzoni M, Chiu M, Accardi F, Vescovini R, Airoldi I, Storti P, et al. Dependence on glutamine uptake and glutamine addiction characterize myeloma cells: a new attractive target. *Blood* (2016) 128:667–79. doi: 10.1182/blood-2016-01-690743
133. Zhan X, Yu W, Franqui-Machin R, Bates ML, Nadiminti K, Cao H, et al. Alteration of mitochondrial biogenesis promotes disease progression in multiple myeloma. *Oncotarget* (2017) 8:111213–24. doi: 10.18632/oncotarget.22740
134. Tibullo D, Barbagallo I, Giallongo C, Vanella L, Conticello C, Romano A, et al. Heme oxygenase-1 nuclear translocation regulates bortezomibinduced cytotoxicity and mediates genomic instability in myeloma cells. *Oncotarget* (2016) 7:28868–80. doi: 10.18632/oncotarget.7563
135. Camiolo G, Barbato A, Giallongo C, Vicario N, Romano A, Parrinello NL, et al. Iron regulates myeloma cell/macrophage interaction and drives resistance to bortezomib. *Redox Biol* (2020) 36:101611. doi: 10.1016/j.redox.2020.101611
136. Soriano GP, Besse L, Li N, Kraus M, Besse A, Meeuwenoord N, et al. Proteasome inhibitor-adapted myeloma cells are largely independent from proteasome activity and show complex proteomic changes, in particular in redox and energy metabolism. *Leukemia* (2016) 30:2198–207. doi: 10.1038/leu.2016.102
137. Thompson RM, Dytfeld D, Reyes L, Robinson RM, Smith B, Manevich Y, et al. Glutaminase inhibitor CB-839 synergizes with carfilzomib in resistant multiple myeloma cells. *Oncotarget* (2017) 8:35863–76. doi: 10.18632/oncotarget.16262
138. Song IS, Kim HK, Lee SR, Jeong SH, Kim N, Ko KS, et al. Mitochondrial modulation decreases the bortezomib-resistance in multiple myeloma cells. *Int J Cancer* (2013) 133:1357–67. doi: 10.1002/ijc.28149
139. Tibullo D, Giallongo C, Romano A, Vicario N, Barbato A, Puglisi F, et al. Mitochondrial Functions, Energy Metabolism and Protein Glycosylation are Interconnected Processes Mediating Resistance to Bortezomib in Multiple Myeloma Cells. *Biomolecules* (2020) 10:696. doi: 10.3390/biom10050696
140. Ma R, Zhang Y, Wang W, Wu J, Yang Q, Xu W, et al. Inhibition of autophagy enhances the antitumour activity of tigecycline in multiple myeloma. *J Cell Mol Med* (2018) 22:5955–63. doi: 10.1111/jcmm.13865
141. Xiang Y, Fang B, Liu Y, Yan S, Cao D, Mei H, et al. SR18292 exerts potent antitumor effects in multiple myeloma via inhibition of oxidative phosphorylation. *Life Sci* (2020) 256:117971. doi: 10.1016/j.lfs.2020.117971
142. Aminzadeh-Gohari S, Weber DD, Vidali S, Catalano L, Kofler B, Feichtinger RG. From old to new — Repurposing drugs to target mitochondrial energy metabolism in cancer. *Semin Cell Dev Biol* (2020) 98:211–23. doi: 10.1016/j.semcdb.2019.05.025
143. Bajpai R, Sharma A, Achreja A, Edgar CL, Wei C, Siddiqa AA, et al. Electron transport chain activity is a predictor and target for venetoclax sensitivity in multiple myeloma. *Nat Commun* (2020) 11:1228. doi: 10.1038/s41467-020-15051-z
144. Giallongo C, Tibullo D, Puglisi F, Barbato A, Vicario N, Cambria D, et al. Inhibition of TLR4 Signaling Affects Mitochondrial Fitness and Overcomes Bortezomib Resistance in Myeloma Plasma Cells. *Cancers (Basel)* (2020) 12 (8):1999. doi: 10.3390/cancers12081999
145. Giallongo C, Tibullo D, Camiolo G, Parrinello NL, Romano A, Puglisi F, et al. TLR4 signaling drives mesenchymal stromal cells commitment to promote tumor microenvironment transformation in multiple myeloma. *Cell Death Dis* (2019) 10:704. doi: 10.1038/s41419-019-1959-5
146. Romano A, Parrinello NL, La Cava P, Tibullo D, Giallongo C, Camiolo G, et al. PMN-MDSC and arginase are increased in myeloma and may contribute to resistance to therapy. *Expert Rev Mol Diagn* (2018) 18 (7):675–83. doi: 10.1080/14737159.2018.1470929
147. Barbagallo I, Giallongo C, Volti GL, Distefano A, Camiolo G, Raffaele M, et al. Heme Oxygenase Inhibition Sensitizes Neuroblastoma Cells to Carfilzomib. *Mol Neurobiol* (2019) 56(2):1451–60. doi: 10.1007/s12035-018-1133-6
148. Chen W-L, Wang J-H, Zhao A-H, Xu X, Wang Y-H, Chen T-L, et al. A distinct glucose metabolism signature of acute myeloid leukemia with prognostic value. *Blood* (2014) 124:1645–54. doi: 10.1182/blood-2014-09-602706
149. Miraki-Moud F, Ghazaly E, Ariza-McNaughton L, Hodby KA, Clear A, Anjos-Afonso F, et al. Arginine deprivation using pegylated arginine deiminase has activity against primary acute myeloid leukemia cells in vivo. *Blood* (2015) 125:4060–8. doi: 10.1182/blood-2014-10-608133

150. Rabinovich S, Adler L, Yizhak K, Sarver A, Silberman A, Agron S, et al. Diversion of aspartate in ASS1-deficient tumours fosters de novo pyrimidine synthesis. *Nature* (2015) 527:379–83. doi: 10.1038/nature15529
151. Waitkus MS, Diplas BH, Yan H. Biological Role and Therapeutic Potential of IDH Mutations in Cancer. *Cancer Cell* (2018) 34(2):186–95. doi: 10.1016/j.ccell.2018.04.011
152. Chowdhury R, Yeoh KK, Tian YM, Hillringhaus L, Bagg EA, Rose NR, et al. The oncometabolite 2-hydroxyglutarate inhibits histone lysine demethylases. *EMBO Rep* (2011) 12:463–9. doi: 10.1038/embor.2011.43
153. Xu W, Yang H, Liu Y, Yang Y, Wang PP, Kim SHH, et al. Oncometabolite 2-hydroxyglutarate is a competitive inhibitor of α-ketoglutarate-dependent dioxygenases. *Cancer Cell* (2011) 19:17–30. doi: 10.1016/j.ccr.2010.12.014
154. Sriskanthadevan S, Jeyaraju DV, Chung TE, Prabha S, Xu W, Skrtic M, et al. AML cells have low spare reserve capacity in their respiratory chain that renders them susceptible to oxidative metabolic stress. *Blood* (2015) 125:2120–30. doi: 10.1182/blood-2014-08-594408
155. Farge T, Saland E, de Toni F, Aroua N, Hosseini M, Perry R, et al. Chemotherapy-Resistant Human Acute Myeloid Leukemia Cells Are Not Enriched for Leukemic Stem Cells but Require Oxidative Metabolism. *Cancer Discov* (2017) 7:716–35. doi: 10.1158/2159-8290.CD-16-0441
156. Ma J, Liu B, Yu D, Zuo Y, Cai R, Yang J, et al. SIRT3 deacetylase activity confers chemoresistance in AML via regulation of mitochondrial oxidative phosphorylation. *Br J Haematol* (2019) 187:49–64. doi: 10.1111/bjh.16044
157. Nayak AP, Kapur A, Barroilhet L, Patankar MS. Oxidative Phosphorylation: A Target for Novel Therapeutic Strategies Against Ovarian Cancer. *Cancers (Basel)* (2018) 10(9):337. doi: 10.3390/cancers10090337
158. Castelli G, Pelosi E, Testa U. Emerging Therapies for Acute Myelogenus Leukemia Patients Targeting Apoptosis and Mitochondrial Metabolism. *Cancers (Basel)* (2019) 11(2):260. doi: 10.3390/cancers11020260
159. Green AS, Chapuis N, Maciel TT, Willems L, Lambert M, Arnoult C, et al. The LKB1/AMPK signaling pathway has tumor suppressor activity in acute myeloid leukemia through the repression of mTOR-dependent oncogenic mRNA translation. *Blood* (2010) 116:4262–73. doi: 10.1182/blood-2010-02-269837
160. Vitkevičienė A, Janulis V, Žučenka A, Borutinskaitė V, Kaupinis A, Valius M, et al. Oxidative phosphorylation inhibition induces anticancerous changes in therapy-resistant-acute myeloid leukemia patient cells. *Mol Carcinog* (2019) 58:2008–16. doi: 10.1002/mc.23092
161. Stuart SD, Schauble A, Gupta S, Kennedy AD, Keppler BR, Bingham PM, et al. A strategically designed small molecule attacks alpha-ketoglutarate dehydrogenase in tumor cells through a redox process. *Cancer Metab* (2014) 2:4. doi: 10.1186/2049-3002-2-4
162. Pardee TS, Lee K, Luddy J, Maturo C, Rodriguez R, Isom S, et al. A phase I study of the first-in-class antimitochondrial metabolism agent, CPI-613, in patients with advanced hematologic malignancies. *Clin Cancer Res* (2014) 20:5255–64. doi: 10.1158/1078-0432.CCR-14-1019
163. Pardee TS, Anderson RG, Pladna KM, Isom S, Ghiraldeli LP, Miller LD, et al. A Phase I Study of CPI-613 in Combination with High-Dose Cytarabine and Mitoxantrone for Relapsed or Refractory Acute Myeloid Leukemia. *Clin Cancer Res* (2018) 24:2060–73. doi: 10.1158/1078-0432.CCR-17-2282
164. Molina JR, Sun Y, Protopopova M, Gera S, Bandi M, Bristow C, et al. An inhibitor of oxidative phosphorylation exploits cancer vulnerability. *Nat Med* (2018) 24:1036–46. doi: 10.1038/s41591-018-0052-4
165. Wallace DC. Mitochondria and cancer. *Nat Rev Cancer* (2012) 12:685–98. doi: 10.1038/nrc3365
166. Guerra F, Arbini AA, Moro L. Mitochondria and cancer chemoresistance. *Biochim Biophys Acta Bioenerg* (2017) 1858:686–99. doi: 10.1016/j.bbabio.2017.01.012

5

Game of Bones: How Myeloma Manipulates its Microenvironment

Tyler Moser-Katz[1], Nisha S. Joseph[1], Madhav V. Dhodapkar[1], Kelvin P. Lee[2] and Lawrence H. Boise[1]*

[1] *Department of Hematology and Medical Oncology, Winship Cancer Institute, Emory University, Atlanta, GA, United States,*
[2] *Department of Immunology, Roswell Park Cancer Institute, Buffalo, NY, United States*

***Correspondence:**
Lawrence H. Boise
lboise@emory.edu

Multiple myeloma is a clonal disease of long-lived plasma cells and is the second most common hematological cancer behind Non-Hodgkin's Lymphoma. Malignant transformation of plasma cells imparts the ability to proliferate, causing harmful lesions in patients. In advanced stages myeloma cells become independent of their bone marrow microenvironment and form extramedullary disease. Plasma cells depend on a rich array of signals from neighboring cells within the bone marrow for survival which myeloma cells exploit for growth and proliferation. Recent evidence suggests, however, that both the myeloma cells and the microenvironment have undergone alterations as early as during precursor stages of the disease. There are no current therapies routinely used for treating myeloma in early stages, and while recent therapeutic efforts have improved patients' median survival, most will eventually relapse. This is due to mutations in myeloma cells that not only allow them to utilize its bone marrow niche but also facilitate autocrine pro-survival signaling loops for further progression. This review will discuss the stages of myeloma cell progression and how myeloma cells progress within and outside of the bone marrow microenvironment.

Keywords: multiple myeloma, bone marrow microenviroment, MGUS, smoldering myeloma, myeloma therapy

INTRODUCTION

Multiple myeloma (MM) is defined as a clonal proliferation of malignant plasma cells, and it accounts for roughly 10% of all hematological cancers (1). Myeloma cells retain numerous features of plasma cell biology including a reliance on signals within the bone marrow microenvironment (2). Interestingly, myeloma's precursor states share the same genetic alterations observed in symptomatic MM patients in both the plasma cells and the microenvironment (3, 4). In advanced stages, myeloma cells can extravasate from the bone marrow leading to extramedullary plasmacytomas and/or circulating plasma cells in the blood (5). Currently, there are ~70 patient-derived myeloma cell lines (HMCL), representing the most advanced stage of myeloma progression whereby myeloma cells survive independently of the bone marrow microenvironment. To this effect, myeloma cells can be compared to an expansive civilization that strategically taps the resources of its niche and when left unchecked will colonize and overtake its host. The malignant cells compete in a "Game of Bones" against the host's innate defenses and utilize the microenvironment in as a means of gaining an advantage. This review will examine progression of disease from asymptomatic precursor states to MM while shining a light on the changes myeloma cells induce in themselves and within the microenvironment to enable such progression. It will also address the signals that allow myeloma to survive independently of the bone marrow microenvironment in their quest for further growth and expansion.

SPECTRUM OF PLASMA CELL DYSCRASIAS

Multiple Myeloma

Historically, establishing the diagnosis of multiple myeloma required both documented bone marrow plasmacytosis (BMPC) ≥10% or an extramedullary plasmacytoma with evidence of end organ damage defined by the CRAB criteria (elevated serum calcium levels, renal insufficiency, anemia, and lytic bone disease). However, in 2014, the International Myeloma Working Group (IMWG) revised the diagnostic criteria to include ultra high-risk patients previously classified as having pre-myeloma or SMM given the ~80% risk of progression to symptomatic disease at two years. These risk factors include BMPC ≥60%, involved to uninvolved serum free light chain ratio >100, and >1 focal lesion on whole body MRI or PET-CT (6–9).

Management and therapy selection for myeloma patients can be determined based on risk stratification. Previously, the International Staging System (ISS) divided disease burden of myeloma into three stages. Serum levels of beta-2 microglobulin (ß2M) and albumin were determined to be the most accurate predictors of disease burden and median survival. Stage I is defined as ß2M < 3.5 mg/L and serum albumin ≥ 3.5 g/dL. In Stage III, ß2M ≥ 5.5 mg/L and serum albumin < 3.5 g/dL. Stage II refers to the intermediate stage of neither Stage I or III (10, 11). Recognizing the important role cytogenetics play in risk stratification, revised ISS (R-ISS) was recently developed still utilizing the ISS, but incorporating both serum lactate dehydrogenase (LDH) levels as well as high risk cytogenetics defined by IgH-MMSET/FGFR3 [t(4,14)] translocations, IgH-MAF [t(14,16)] translocations, and deletion of the p arm of chromosome 17 (del17p) (**Table 1**).

Outside of the R-ISS risk stratification model, there are additional favorable and adverse risk factors that aid clinicians

TABLE 1 | Defining stages of myeloma.

MGUS				
	Risk Factors	Risk Group	Risk of progression at 20 years (%)	Reference
	(1) Serum M-protein <1.5 g/dL; (2) non-IgG subtype (IgM or IgA); (3) serum FLC ratio <0.26 or >1.65)	Low-risk (0 factors)	5	
		Low-intermediate risk (any 1 abnormal factor)	21	
		High-intermediate risk (any 2 abnormal factors)	37	
		High-risk (all 3 factors abnormal)	58	Rajkumar et al. (Lancet Oncology, 2014)
SMM				
Mayo 2018 model	Risk Factors	Risk Group	Risk of progression at 2 years (%)	
	(1) M-protein >2 g/dL, (2) BMPC >20%, (3) FLC ratio >20	Low-risk (0 factors)	5	
		Intermediate risk (1 factor)	17	
		High risk (2-3 factors)	46	Lakshman et al. (BCJ, 2018)
IMWG 2019 model	(1) M-protein >2 g/dL, (2) BMPC >20%, (3) FLC ratio >20 (4) HR-CTG			
		Low (0 factors)	3.7	
		Low-Intermediate (1 factor)	25	
		Intermediate-High (2 factors)	49	
		High (3+ factors)	72	San Miguel et al. (JCO, 2019)
MM				
	Criteria	Stage	Median OS (months)	
ISS	B2M<3.5, Alb >3.5	1	62	
	Not meeting criteria for either ISS 1 or 3	2	44	
	B2M >5.5	3	29	Griepp et al. (J. ASCO, 2005)
R-ISS	ISS stage 1 without HR-CTG and LDH WNL	1	Not reached	
	Not meeting criteria for either R-ISS 1 or 3	2	83	
	ISS stage 3 with either LDH >ULN and HR-CTG	3	43	Palumbo et al. (J. ASCO, 2015)

MGUS, monoclonal gammopathy of undetermined significance; SMM, smoldering multiple myeloma; MM, multiple myeloma; BMPC, bone marrow plasma cells; OS, overall survival; ISS, International Staging System; R-ISS, revised ISS; B2M, beta2-microglobulin; Alb, Albumin; FLC, free light chain; LDH, lactate dehydrogenase; HR-CTG, high risk cytogenetics; WNL, within normal limit; ULN, upper limit of normal.

in appropriate stratification and subsequent treatment of myeloma patients. These factors include additional cytogenetic features, presence of extramedullary disease, gene expression profiling, and plasma cell proliferation. Standard risk myeloma encompasses 80 to 85% of newly diagnosed myeloma (NDMM) patients and portends good prognosis with a median overall survival (OS) not reached at 10 years (12). Cytogenetic features indicative of standard risk disease includes trisomies of chromosomes 3, 5, 7, 9, 11, 15, 19, and 21 that is referred to as hyperdiploidy as well as IgH-Cyclin D1 [t(11,14)], and IgH-Cyclin D3 [t(6,14)] translocations. High risk patients encompass 15 to 20% of NDMM patients and have median OS of 5 years (13). In addition to high risk cytogenetic features previously described, additional markers of aggressive disease include complex karyotype, defined as three or more changes on standard karyotype analysis. Another marker of high risk disease is amplification of the q arm of chromosome 1 (amp1q). Co-occurrence of 1q gain with other high risk markers portends poor prognosis, and patients with >4 copies of 1q are at very high risk for progression following initial treatment (14). Another marker of high risk includes the least common IgH translocation with MAFB [t(14,20)] which makes up <1% of myeloma patients (13). High risk myeloma patients are also identified by disease burden (ISS stage III), proliferation (BMPC labelling index ≥ 3% *via* thymidine kinase and C-reactive protein (15)), and presence of extramedullary disease (16).

Multiple Myeloma Precursor Stages

The presence of a precursor state is not known for most NDMM patients as most diagnoses occur at symptomatic stages. However, studies in 2009 from Drs. Michael Kuehl and Ola Landgren used molecular and biological markers to show that myeloma is preceded in virtually all cases by a premalignant state (17, 18). The following two subsections will refer to these precursor states.

Monoclonal Gammopathy of Undetermined Significance

MGUS was first described in 1961 by Dr. Jan Waldenström who identified a subset of patients with elevated serum and urine immunoglobulin levels without displaying symptoms of malignancy (19). Waldenström labelled this phenomenon a gammopathy, and the term, MGUS, was later coined in 1978 by Dr. Robert Kyle and colleagues (20). The IMWG now defines MGUS as the presence of a serum monoclonal (M) protein or M-protein at <3 g/dL concentration and <10% BMPC with the absence of CRAB criteria (6).

MGUS is found in 3% of Caucasians over the age of 50 and occurs at a 2 to 3-fold higher rate in African Americans (21, 22). Patients diagnosed with MGUS have a 1% risk per year of progressing to symptomatic myeloma, and therefore the standard of care is surveillance without intervention (23). Risk of patient progression can be further stratified using three risk factors: presence of a non-IgG M protein (IgA or IgG), M-protein >1.5 g/dL, and abnormal serum free light-chain (FLC) ratio (24) (**Table 1**). Recently, advancement of technology allowed for detection of precursor cells to MGUS, labelled pre-MGUS (3, 25). As many genomic alterations in MGUS originate in the germinal center, an aberrant clonal population of plasma cells can be formed prior to migration into the bone marrow (26, 27). Furthermore, microenvironment changes present in MGUS have shown to be key regulators in progression to symptomatic stages, and can be targeted in these early stages (3, 28).

Smoldering Multiple Myeloma

SMM is an intermediate clinical stage in progression between MGUS and multiple myeloma initially described in 1980 after observing a series of six patients with BMPC >10% that continued to have stable disease without treatment for >5 years (29). SMM is defined as the presence of an M-protein at ≥3 g/dL, and/or BMPC percentage of >10% with no evidence of end organ damage defined by the CRAB criteria (hypercalcemia, renal failure, anemia, bone lesions) (30). After the IMWG revised the diagnostic criteria of myeloma, a subset of patients previously classified as having SMM were now reclassified as having symptomatic myeloma. However, this reclassification ultimately only affected a small proportion of SMM patients, and the challenge still remained how to appropriately risk-stratify the remaining patients. SMM is a very heterogeneous disorder encompassing patients that will progress in the first two years and patients with stable low-level disease more than ten years after diagnosis. How then, do we identify which patients are at the highest risk of progression, and how do we safely manage them?

The Mayo 2018 model, also known as the 20/2/20 model, uses three independent risk factors of progression to myeloma: (1) a serum FLC ratio >20, (2) M-protein >2 g/dL, and (3) BMPC >20%. Depending on whether the patient has either 0, 1, or 2–3 of these factors, they are categorized as having either low, intermediate, or high risk SMM corresponding to a 5%, 17%, or 46% risk of progression at 2 years (31). The IMWG validated this model using a retrospective cohort, but added the high-risk cytogenetic features t(4,14), gain(1q), del(17p), and del(13q). Interestingly hyperdiploidy has been shown to be an adverse prognosticator in SMM despite its opposite meaning in MM (32). In this model, SMM patients were grouped into four risk categories (low risk, low-intermediate risk, intermediate risk, high risk) associated with a 2-year progression rate of 3.7%, 25%, 49%, and 72%, respectively (33) (**Table 1**).

Historically, observation was also the standard of care for SMM as with MGUS. However, recently published data has shown the benefit of early intervention with the immunomodulatory agent (IMiD) lenalidomide in high-risk SMM in terms of delaying progression to myeloma (34). The efficacy of using IMiDs in SMM illustrates the role that the microenvironment has in facilitating MM progression. Ongoing clinical trials continue to investigate different therapeutic strategies in SMM, as this continues to be an evolving area of research.

Extramedullary Multiple Myeloma

Extramedullary multiple myeloma (EMM) refers to hematogenous spread of clonal plasma cell tumors leading to soft tissue tumors at anatomic sites outside the bone marrow (35).

This is a separate diagnosis from solitary plasmacytomas which originate from the underlying bone marrow and grow through the cortical bone (36, 37). EMM can present in the liver, skin, central nervous system, pleura, kidneys, lymph nodes, and pancreas and is present in 6%–8% of NDMM cases and 10-30% of relapsed myeloma patients (38, 39). EMM may also present as plasma cell leukemia (PCL), an aggressive variant of the disease with >20% or ≥ 2*10 (9) circulating plasma cells in the blood (40). PCL can either present *de novo*, known as primary PCL, or more commonly as a progression from already diagnosed myeloma, known as secondary PCL.

Extramedullary disease and PCL are considered high risk entities and associated with a poor prognosis with a median OS of less than 6 months (37). Profiling of extramedullary tumors reveals differences from malignant bone marrow plasma cells. Cytogenetics that indicate standard risk myeloma such as hyperdiploidy and t(11,14) are mainly found in BMPC and rarely found in extramedullary plasmacytomas whereas t(4,14) is more commonly seen in EMM (35, 41). However, PCL, while heterogeneous, does have a higher incidence of t(11,14) translocations (40, 42). In relapsed patients, EMM cells undergo a shift from secretion of intact IgG to light chain, and most HMCL secrete only light chain, demonstrating its correlation with myeloma progression (43). The changes in molecular and protein expression that allow myeloma cells to survive and spread outside of the microenvironment will be addressed in a subsequent section of this review.

THE ROLE OF THE BONE MARROW MICROENVIRONMENT

In 1889, Stephen Paget introduced his "seed and soil" hypothesis which postulated that tumor cells (seed) grow preferentially in selective microenvironments (soil) (44, 45). We have seen that plasma cells undergo genomic alterations in the germinal center prior to MGUS (26, 27). Once this clonal population arrives in the bone marrow, it gains access to a wide array of microenvironment signals that facilitate plasma cell survival. Recent studies have found little difference between the microenvironments of MGUS and myeloma, demonstrating that the "soil" has a role in shaping the malignant progression (3, 46). The bone marrow microenvironment produces pro-survival signals for non-malignant long-lived plasma cells, which can live throughout the lifetime of the host, and secrete antibody titers as part of the adaptive immune response (2). Myeloma cells, the aggressive counterparts, use the supportive surrounding stromal cells, osteocytes, and endothelial cells to further their growth. Myeloma precursor states have been shown to mediate progressive growth *in vivo* in humanized mouse models supporting a dominant role for the microenvironment or tumor-extrinsic signals in regulating tumor growth (46). Initial small changes in the microenvironment or molecular changes to myeloma cells themselves cause an expansion of the plasma cell niche throughout the bone marrow.

Molecular Changes Driving Myeloma Growth

Myeloma cells undergo numerous molecular changes and genetic events which allow proliferation and induce further changes in the bone marrow microenvironment. One family of proteins commonly dysregulated in myeloma are D-type cyclins (47). D-type cyclins are cell cycle proteins that activate cyclin dependent kinase 4 (CDK4) and CDK6, which phosphorylate and inactivate Rb allowing for E2F activation and cell cycle progression (48). Primary genetic translocations such as t(11,14) and t(6,14) directly drive constitutive expression of cyclin D1 and D3 respectively (47, 49, 50). Another translocation t(4,14) which increases the expression of the histone methyltransferase MMSET (NSD2) also indirectly drives activation of cyclin D2 (47, 51). Cyclin D2 can also be dysregulated through t(14,16) and t(14,20) translocations which drive transcription factors that target Cyclin D2 (47). Although infrequent, biallelic inactivation of Rb itself is a subclonal mutation that occurs in 3% of tumors (52). Rb is found on chromosome 13q, and this deletion of this region is the most common mutation in myeloma, frequently accompanying t(4,14), t(14,16), and t (14,20) translocations (53, 54). Recently it was shown that monoallelic deletion of two other genes on 13q which code for Mir15A and Mir16-1 resulted in development of MGUS in wild type C57BL/6 mice and progression of myeloma in the Vk*Myc multiple myeloma mouse model (55).

Myeloma upregulates oncogenes that are typically associated with proliferation in cancer. One such gene is MYC, and its deregulation typically leads to a more aggressive disease phase (56). MYC translocations are found in 15% of human myeloma tumors (57) and include both IgH-MYC translocations [t(8,14)] and IgL-MYC translocations [t(8,22)]. The MYC locus is the most common source of light chain translocations accounting for 40% of these anomalies, and lambda light chain translocations portend a particularly poor outcome compared to kappa light chain translocations (58). Another pathway that is involved in myeloma proliferation is RAS signaling. A secondary mutation that is uncommon in MGUS, KRAS, and NRAS mutations are each found in ~20% of NDMM patients (27, 59). KRAS and NRAS mutations appear to not uniformly activate MAPK signaling pathways and actually lead to distinct downstream transcriptional signatures (60). Interestingly, FGFR3 mutations, which are mutually exclusive with RAS mutations appear to induce MAPK signaling more effectively (60, 61). Finally, the MAPK pathway can be activated by BRAF mutations. BRAF is mutated in 4% of patients with the V600E mutation being the most common (62). Additionally, recent studies have shown a role for cytidine deaminases such as AID and APOBEC in mediating genomic instability in MM cells (63). The expression of these genes, however, is also dependent on interactions with the microenvironment (64).

Extracellular Matrix

The bone marrow microenvironment provides a layered structure called the extracellular matrix (ECM) which acts as the "home base" for myeloma cells. Homing to the bone marrow is mediated by interaction of myeloma receptor CXCR4 with the chemokine SDF1α (65). This causes a subsequent migration to the stromal compartment of bone marrow. There, it will interact with ECM proteins or other native bone marrow cells.

The ECM consists of proteins such as fibronectin, collagen, osteopontin, hyaluronan, and laminin. Adhesion of myeloma cells has been shown to be important for survival and drug resistance (66, 67). A method of cell-ECM adhesion is activation of integrins, and myeloma cells have shown preference toward very large antigen-4 (VLA-4) aka integrin α4ß1 and integrin ß7 (ITGB7) (68–70). Binding of VLA-4 to fibronectin of the ECM induces activation of nuclear factor κB (NFκB) leading to cell adhesion-mediated drug resistance (CAM-DR) and pro-survival signaling (71). ITGB7 can be regulated by the MAF gene, and as a result, patients with t(14,16) have elevated levels of ITGB7 (51). ITGB7 is necessary for myeloma cell survival and CAM-DR, and has been shown to be constitutively active in myeloma cells (70, 72). Additional integrins such as VLA5 and the beta 5 integrin CD56 play a smaller but active role in myeloma progression (68, 73) (**Figure 1**).

Syndecan-1 or CD138 is a heparan sulfate proteoglycan and a surface marker of myeloma cells. It binds to type I collagen and induces expression of matrix metalloproteinase 1 (MMP1) to promote tumor invasion, bone resorption, and angiogenesis (74, 75). Additionally, syndecan-1 levels on cells correlate with cell survival and growth (76). Heparanase has an intricate interplay with syndecan-1, either causing its clustering and increased adhesion to the ECM or inducing its shedding (77, 78). Soluble syndecan-1 has been shown to promote myeloma tumor growth

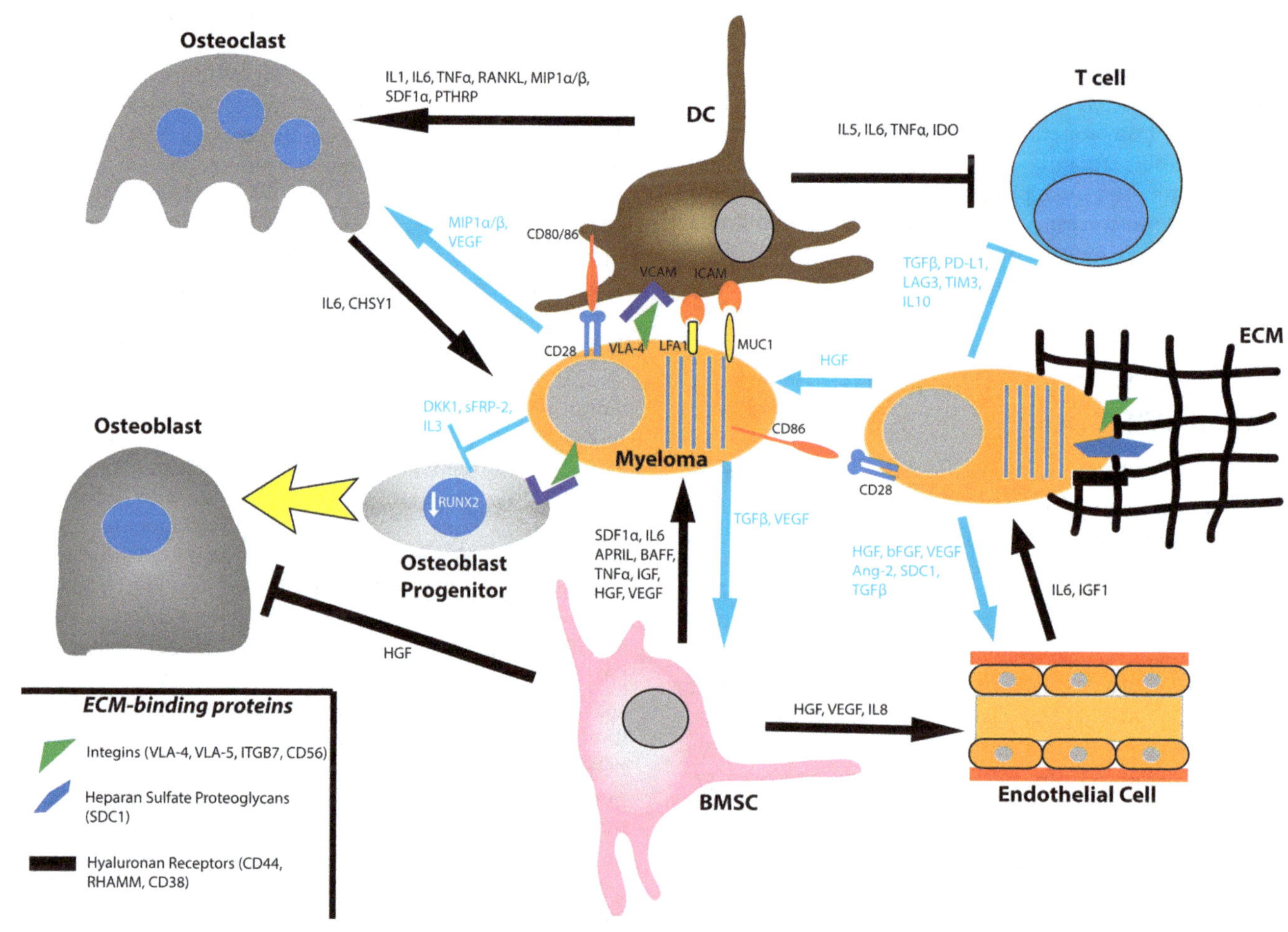

FIGURE 1 | Bone marrow interactions that promote myeloma growth and survival. Myeloma cells bind to the extracellular matrix (ECM) *via* integrins, proteoglycans, and hyaluronan receptors. They also directly bind to bone marrow stromal cell (BMSC) such as dendritic cells (DC) *via* the VCAM-VLA4, ICAM-LFA1, ICAM-MUC1, and CD80/86-CD28 axes. BMSC will produce the cytokines SDF1α, IL6, APRIL, BAFF, TNFα, IGF, HGF, and VEGF. In turn, myeloma cells secrete TGFβ and VEGF for BMSC. Myeloma cells promote osteoclast activation by secreting MIP1α/β and VEGF and by promoting BMSC secretion of IL1, IL6, TNFα, RANKL, MIP1α/β, SDF1, and PTHRP. They also prevent osteoblast differentiation by downregulating RUNX2 *via* direct binding of the VLA-VCAM axis and secretion of DKK1 and IL3. They also secrete sFRP-2 which also suppresses osteoblast differentiation. Osteoclasts produce IL6 and CHSY1 to promote myeloma cell survival. Myeloma cells induce angiogenesis in the bone marrow by secreting HGF, bFGF, VEGF, Ang-2, cleaved syndecan-1 (SDC1), and TGFβ. They also promote BMSC secretion of HGF, VEGF, and IL8. Endothelial cells produce IL6 and IGF1 to influence myeloma cell survival. Myeloma cells promote an immunosuppressive environment by inhibiting T cell function through production of TGFβ, PD-L1, LAG3, TIM3, and IL10. They also signal to BMSC to produce IL5, IL6, TNFα, and IDO.

in vivo (79). Finally, CD44, RHAMM, and CD38 are hyaluronan receptors (67). Hyaluronan is a secreted scaffold protein in the bone marrow. While certain splice variants of CD44 and RHAMM are active in the bone marrow as receptors for hyaluronan and osteopontin, they are generally more involved in extramedullary myeloma. Both proteins regulate the SDF1α/CXCR4 axis, and cell-ECM adhesion with RHAMM is more involved in cell motility (67). CD38 is another hyaluronic acid interacting partner that is expressed in high levels in plasma cells but low levels in other lymphoid and myeloid cells making it an effective target for antibody therapies like daratumumab and isatuximab (80)

Myeloma–Stroma Cell–Cell Contact

Binding of VLA-4 of a myeloma cell to VCAM of an adjacent stromal cell promotes downstream signaling pathways that activate NFκB and cause cellular survival and proliferation (74). Another myeloma receptor, lymphocyte function-associated antigen 1 (LFA1), will bind to ICAM-1 of an adjacent bone marrow stromal cell (BMSC). LFA1 is an integrin composed of αL and ß2 subunits and is associated with poor prognosis and disease progression in patients as well as increased proliferation in mice (81, 82). Mucin 1 (MUC1) is another transmembrane binding partner of ICAM-1 that has been shown to drive myeloma progression (**Figure 1**). MUC1 will induce proliferation in multiple myeloma by signaling *via* a ß-catenin/TCF4 mechanism to drive MYC gene expression (83).

Plasma and myeloma cells also express CD28, a transmembrane protein classically known for its role in T cell co-stimulation. During this process, MHC of an antigen presenting cell (APC) will first bind to the T cell receptor. The T cell is not fully activated unless CD80/86 of an APC binds to CD28 of a T cell, inducing survival, proliferation, and effector function in T cells (84). Plasma cells retain this CD28 pro-survival signaling capacity, and binding with CD80/86 of a BMSC, e.g., dendritic cell confers survival throughout the lifetime of the host (85, 86). Plasma and myeloma cells are dependent on CD28 signaling through both the PI3K and Vav signaling pathways (87, 88). Knockout of CD28 leads to decreased antibody titers of long-lived plasma cells in mice, and knockdown of CD28 or CD86 with short hairpin RNA leads to myeloma cell death in HMCL (86, 88, 89) (**Figure 1**).

Myeloma-Bone Marrow Stromal Cell Pro-Survival Cytokines

Multiple myeloma cells also pave the way for their own survival and proliferation by inducing cytokine secretion in BMSC. Direct binding of plasma and myeloma cells to BMSC leads to downstream pathways such as MAPK, NOTCH, and PI3K and cause subsequent transcription and secretion of numerous cytokines. One such cytokine is interleukin-6 (IL6), which has roles in myeloma growth, survival, migration, and drug resistance. IL6 binds to its cognate IL6-receptor (IL6R) and signals through MEK/MAPK, JAK/STAT, and PI3K/Akt pathways (90–92). It also increases dependence on Mcl-1, an anti-apoptotic Bcl-2 protein that is essential for plasma and myeloma cell survival. IL6 upregulates Mcl-1 in a STAT3 dependent manner and induces phosphorylation of Bim, thus increasing affinity of Bim for Mcl-1 over Bcl-2/Bcl-x. This increased binding of the two proteins ultimately leads to stabilization of Mcl-1 (93, 94).

In the absence of IL6, two other cytokines, B-cell activating factor (BAFF) and a proliferation inducing ligand (APRIL) have been shown to have a protective effect on myeloma cells particularly from treatment with corticosteroid (95). BAFF is a member of the tumor necrosis factor (TNF) family and is expressed on the surface of BMSC as well as in a cleaved soluble form. It has been shown to stimulate B cell growth, and, additionally, ligation of its receptors BAFF-R and TACI leads to increased proliferation and survival in myeloma cells (96, 97). APRIL is a secreted protein that will bind to TACI and B-cell maturation antigen (BCMA), a protein which has recently become a target for myeloma CAR-T cell therapy with an 88% response rate (98, 99). BAFF and APRIL-mediated signals also impact survival and growth signals to MM from surrounding dendritic cells (100). They are overexpressed in myeloma cells compared to normal plasma cells illustrating the importance of these cytokines (95). APRIL and BCMA promote cell growth (*via* MAPK and NFκB) and immunosuppression (*via* PD-L1, TGF-ß, and IL10) in myeloma cells (98).

Another member of the TNF family involved in myeloma growth and survival in the bone marrow microenvironment is TNFα. TNFα is a mediator of inflammation and has been found to be significantly higher in supernatants of patients with bone disease than those without (101). While TNFα signaling itself causes a modest increase in proliferation, it induces expression of adhesion molecules resulting in a 2–4 fold increase in binding of myeloma cells to BMSC. It also results in a significant increase in IL6 secretion. Interestingly, TNFα levels decrease with thalidomide treatment which may be a result of downstream effects of the drug's immunomodulatory effects on bone marrow myeloma cells (102).

Myeloma cells induce BMSC to secrete numerous growth factors. Among them, insulin-like growth factor (IGF) appears to have a sustained and pronounced effect on myeloma proliferation and antiapoptotic signaling. IGF binds to the tyrosine kinase receptor IGF-1R, and additionally influences proteasome and telomerase activities in myeloma cells. IGF is also implicated in drug resistance to cytotoxic chemotherapy, dexamethasone, and proteasome inhibitors (103). It primes myeloma cells to respond to other cytokines and to produce pro-angiogenic cytokines. BMSCs also produce other growth factors such as hepatocyte growth factor (HGF), basic fibroblast growth factor (bFGF) and vascular endothelial growth factor (VEGF) which influence osteoclast activation and angiogenesis (74) (**Figure 1**).

Osteoclast Interactions

Bone lesions result from osteoclast activation to enable further space for myeloma proliferation in the bone marrow. To directly activate osteoclasts, myeloma cells secrete macrophage inflammatory protein-1α (MIP1α) and MIP1ß. MIP1α binds to C-chemokine receptor 1 (CCR1) and CCR5 while MIP1ß binds to CCR5 and CCR8 to induce osteoclast formation and activity (104–106). MIP1α has been shown to lead to bone destruction, BMSC adhesion, and tumor burden in SCID mice with multiple myeloma (104). In turn, osteoclasts secrete IL6 to stimulate proliferation and growth of not only myeloma cells but other osteoclasts as well (107). Myeloma-osteoclast interaction also upregulates Chondroitin synthase 1 (CHSY1), which induces Notch signaling promoting the survival of myeloma cells (108). Notch signaling, particularly Notch3 and Notch4 stimulation leads to recruitment of osteoclast precursors and increased bone resorption (109, 110).

Interactions between myeloma cells and BMSCs also leads to production of cytokines that stimulate osteoclastogenesis. Binding of VLA4 with VCAM promotes secretion of cytokines such as IL1, IL6, TNFα, and parathyroid hormone related peptide (PTHRP) which promote osteoclast growth (111). Binding of VLA4 and VCAM also lead BMSC to produce receptor activator of NFκB ligand (RANKL). RANKL will bind to its receptor RANK to stimulate osteoclast activation and differentiation and bone lysis (111, 112). RANKL, MIP1α, and IL11 are upregulated by p38 MAPK in BMSCs, and inhibiting p38 MAPK decreases osteoclastogenesis and bone resorption (113) (**Figure 1**). The bone matrix glycoprotein, osteopontin, and the pro-inflammatory cytokine IL17 have also been implicated in osteoclastogenesis and bone resorption. They have been shown to be associated with poor prognosis and osteolytic lesions in patients (114–116).

Osteoblast Interactions

Myeloma cells also disrupt bone homeostasis by inhibiting osteoblast production and activation. Osteoblasts and BMSC produce osteoprotegerin (OPG) which inhibits the development of bone disease by competing for binding of RANK with RANKL (117). Binding of OPG with RANK prevents osteoclast maturation and activation (118). The ratio between RANKL and OPG is important prognostic indicator in patients and can be influenced in numerous ways (119–121). One way is binding of VLA4 on myeloma cells to VCAM of BMSCs which decreases secretion of OPG and increases secretion of RANKL, thereby tipping the balance in favor of osteoclasts (111, 112). Other factors which augment the RANKL/OPG ratio are activin A and sclerostin (122, 123). Sclerostin is cysteine knot protein which induces apoptosis in osteoblasts and inhibits bone formation (124). Activin A, a member of the TGF-ß superfamily, signals through numerous pathways to promote osteoclast differentiation and is a marker of poor prognosis (122, 125). Interestingly, IL3 can increase osteoclastogenesis by regulating activin A levels (126).

Myeloma cells can also prevent the maturation of osteoblast progenitor cells. Binding of VLA4 of myeloma cells to VCAM of osteoblast progenitors downregulates the activity of RUNX2, a transcription factor that is necessary for the differentiation of osteoblastic cells (127). In addition to increasing the RANKL/OPG ratio, IL7 secretion by BMSC also decreases RUNX2 activity and osteoblast differentiation (119, 127, 128). Recent studies from the Croucher lab have shown that MM-osteoblast interactions may also be important for maintaining dormancy of tumor cells (124)

Secretion of the cytokines Dickkopf 1 (DKK1) and Frizzled related protein 2 (sFRP-2) by myeloma cells contributes to bone resorption as well. DKK1 and sFRP-2 inhibit the canonical Wnt pathway which is responsible for the differentiation of osteoblast progenitor cells (127, 128). DKK1 and sFRP-2 are expressed in multiple myeloma cells of patients with bone lesions. Recombinant DKK1 and sFRP-2 or conditioned media containing either of the two cytokines inhibit differentiation of osteoblast precursor cells *in vitro* and suppress *in vitro* bone mineralization (129, 130). Interestingly, immunodepletion of sFRP-2 led to increased bone restoration suggesting it is necessary for bone resorption. Osteoblast differentiation may take place *via* the bone morphogenic protein 2 (BMP2) pathway. sFRP-2 as well as IL3 inhibit this pathway, thereby stunting osteoblast activation. Additionally, secretion of the cytokines TGF- ß and HGF by BMSC promote osteoclast generation while limiting osteoblast activity (74, 131) (**Figure 1**).

Endothelial Cell Interactions

Angiogenesis is the creation of new blood vessels through the use of endothelial cells. Patients with progressive myeloma disease show increased level of microvessel density (MVD), a measure of angiogenesis, when compared to those with inactive MGUS (132). This is because myeloma cells crowd the bone marrow microenvironment and generate hypoxic tumors, so they upregulate angiogenesis to deliver oxygen and nutrients while removing catabolites. In the presence of hypoxic conditions, myeloma cells upregulate hypoxia induced factor 1α (HIF1α), which regulates transcription of pro-angiogenic cytokines including HGF, bFGF, VEGF, and Angiopoietin-2 (Ang-2). Myeloma cells may also constitutively produce these cytokines due to genetic mutations or oncogene activation (133).

Adhesion of myeloma to the ECM increases angiogenesis. Expression of adhesion molecules VLA4, LFA1, and CD44 have been shown to correlate with increased angiogenesis in active myeloma (134). Syndecan-1 has been shown to have a prominent role in bone marrow angiogenesis as well. Syndecan-1 is correlated with MVD and facilitates binding of growth factors, particularly HGF, to cells. Not only can syndecan-1 potentiate the surface binding of HGF to cells, but it can also be shed in a soluble form that complexes with HGF to increase potency (135, 136). Myeloma cells also facilitate degradation of the ECM using matrix metalloproteinases (MMP) and heparanase to allow migration of endothelial cells into the surrounding tissue (137, 138).

Myeloma cells stimulate BMSCs to secrete HGF, VEGF, and IL8 to induce neovascularization (139). In turn, endothelial cells will produce IGF1 and IL6 to promote myeloma cell growth. This process can induce an autocrine loop in endothelial cells as they produce VEGF, platelet-derived growth factor (PDGF), Ang-1, HGF, and IL1 to further promote angiogenesis (140) (**Figure 1**).

Immune Cells

While the previous subsections have addressed allies that myeloma uses to advance itself in the Game of Bones, myeloma cells have an antagonist in the form of antitumor cells in the bone marrow. To overcome this, MM and its precursor MGUS are associated with several alterations in both innate and adaptive immunity. Immune cells increased in MM include regulatory T cells, IL-17-producing T cells, and terminally differentiated effector T cells, however, immunosuppression and exhaustion of these cells was present as early as the MGUS stage (3, 141). The bone marrow increases CD4(+) regulatory T cells and decreases CD4(-)CD8(-) regulatory T cells, and this correlates with increased disease burden (142). Myeloma cells produce proteins such as TGF- ß, PD-L1, LAG3, TIM3, and IL10 that contribute to the immunosuppressive phenotype and T cell anergy (**Figure 1**). Interestingly, these proteins are upregulated in myeloma cells by binding of APRIL to BCMA (98). CD28 ligation with CD80/86 has also been shown to cause BMSC secretion of IL6 and IDO. This occurs *via* "back signaling" of CD80/86 to activate the PI3K pathway. While IL6 normally activates T cells, IDO catabolizes tryptophan in the microenvironment into the toxic metabolite kynurenine. This results in T cell anergy *via* GCN2 kinase-mediated sensing of depleted intracellular tryptophan pools (143, 144). Interestingly, a subset of endothelial cells express low levels of CD80/86 as well as CD40 and ICOS-L in myeloma patients which can trap a population of T cells and stimulate them to induce immunosuppressive proteins (145). Autologous dendritic cells stimulated with tumor antigen can be used to activate T cells *ex vivo* to expand and attack the tumor. Emerging treatments such as targeted antibodies, checkpoint inhibitors and CAR-T cell therapy have aimed to increase the potency of the immune response (28, 141). Currently, advances in mass cytometry and RNA sequencing single cell analyses are being used to identify the immune checkpoint signature of the microenvironment (25). These methods have identified immunosuppressive phenotypes such as regulatory T-cell suppression, secretion of suppressive cytokines and interferons, and increased expression of PD-1 on CD8(+) T and NK cells as early as MGUS (146).

Myeloid derived suppressor cells (MDSC) have been shown to promote immune suppression and angiogenesis in multiple myeloma. They induce myeloma cell survival and proliferation by causing AMPK phosphorylation in myeloma cells. This increases levels of the anti-apoptotic proteins MCL-1 and BCL-2 and the autophagy marker LC3II (147). Myeloma cells in turn will cause an increase of MCL-1 expression and survival in MDSC (148). Another cell type, plasmacytoid dendritic cells (pDC), contribute to immunosuppression of the microenvironment when in direct contact with myeloma cells. While pDC can normally be activated to cause apoptosis of myeloma cells, pDC-myeloma binding *via* E-cadherin can convert pDC into tumor promoting cells (149). Myeloma cells use cell-cell contact to court the pDC to their advantage and signal downstream to inhibit pDC secretion of interferon-α (IFN- α) (149).

Natural killer (NK) cells induce cell death in myeloma cells *via* granzyme and perforin release and other proapoptotic ligands (150). Myeloma cells express CD1d and are also highly sensitive to lysis by NK cells. PD-L1 of a myeloma cell can bind PD-1 of NK cells to suppress their cytotoxic effect of myeloma cells. NK cells are a target of numerous therapies aimed at the immunosuppressive microenvironment. Lenalidomide can be added to checkpoint inhibitors to abrogate this effect and stimulate NK to target myeloma cells (151). The anti-SLAMF7 antibody elotuzumab can also be used to activate NK cells and mediate their activity in myeloma (152). In addition to targeting myeloma cells, the anti-CD38 antibody, daratumumab, also depletes CD38(+) regulatory cells in the bone marrow thus promoting an immune response (153). Recently, daratumumab has been shown to specifically stimulate NK cell activity in myeloma by selectively targeting CD38(+) NK cell populations (154). NK cells and other bone marrow resident immune cells are avenues for immunotherapy and have yielded some initial success in treating myeloma patients at precursor stages (28, 155–158).

MYELOMA TAKEOVER BEYOND THE MICROENVIRONMENT

While myeloma cells can be seen circulating in peripheral blood in advanced stages, most EMM is characterized by plasmacytomas in adjacent tissues and organs. Myeloma cells must develop the capacity to extravasate through stroma and ECM into the blood and navigate challenges such as building their own microenvironment in sites outside of the bone marrow. As the disease advances, cells undergo molecular and genomic alterations to promote autocrine loops that facilitate survival and proliferation away from its bone marrow sanctuary. It is notable that although extramedullary growth is a feature of advanced MM, circulating tumor cells can be detected even in early stages of MM (159). This section will explore a new landscape for the Game of Bones and how myeloma cells can undergo changes to survive and expand their niche independently of bone marrow signals.

Extravasation Model

While little is known about myeloma extravasation from the bone marrow, we can follow an adaptation of the leukocyte multistep model of extravasation and homing (**Figure 2**). In the standard model, cells first home to an environment as a result of chemoattractants. This is followed by adhesion of the cell to vascular endothelial cells and reorganization of the cytoskeleton to migrate through gaps between these endothelial cells. During this process, the cell degrades basement membrane and extracellular matrix to allow passage until its penetration through (160) (**Figure 2A**). We can reverse this first step for the myeloma cell extravasation model as they must first shed homing signals which tether them to the bone marrow. They must also reduce their affinity to ECM and cells that are specific to the bone marrow and upregulate migratory proteins. Finally, myeloma cells must also degrade the basement membrane to allow passage through gaps created in the bone marrow structure (**Figure 2B**). Once the myeloma cells are in circulation, they may re-enter the vasculature in other marrow compartments *via* the standard leukocyte model of extravasation. They may also form tumors in organs or remain circulating in the blood in the case of PCL.

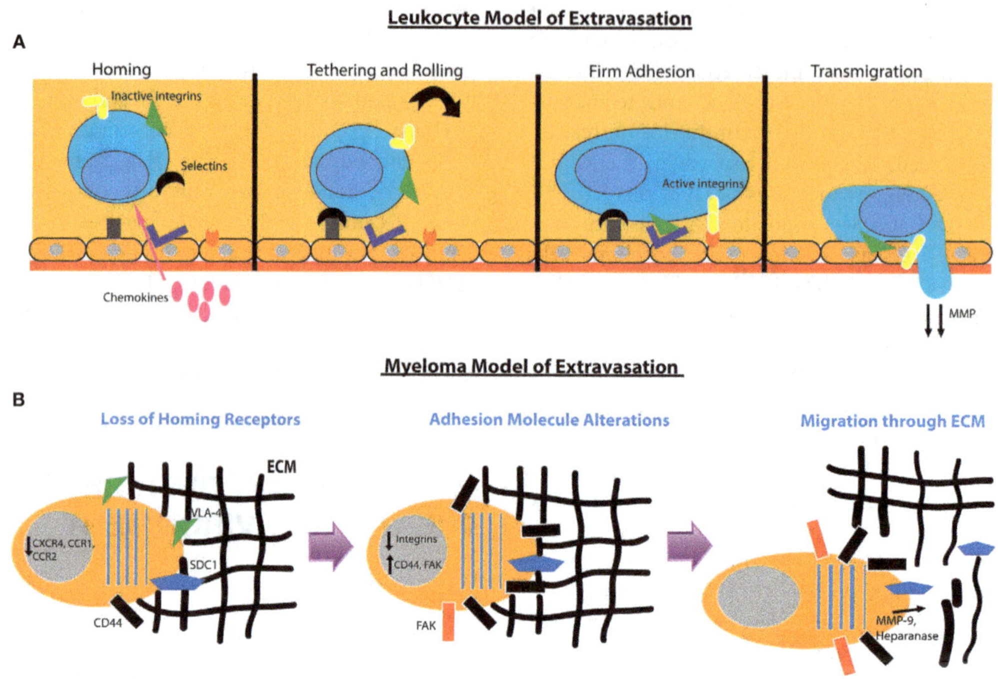

FIGURE 2 | Models for leukocyte and myeloma cell extravasation. **(A)** *Standard leukocyte multistep model of extravasation.* The leukocyte in the bloodstream receives homing signals from chemokines. This is followed by weak adhesion to the endothelium and rolling along the surface. Integrins such as VLA4 and LFA1 are activated to form tight adhesion to the endothelium. The leukocyte then reorganizes its cytoskeleton and degrades the basement membrane to transmigrate through. **(B)** *Model of myeloma extravasation out of the bone marrow.* Myeloma cells downregulate receptors used for homing to the bone marrow. They alter adhesion molecules by downregulating integrins and increasing hyaluronan receptors such as CD44 and RHAMM and expression of focal adhesion kinase (FAK). The myeloma cell will secrete MMP-9 and heparanase as well as induce production of MMP-9 *via* endothelial cells to degrade the extracellular matrix (ECM). Heparanase secretion can cause shedding of SDC1 which also contributes to cell motility. The myeloma cell will then reorganize its cytoskeleton and migrate through the ECM.

In order to home to the bone marrow, myeloma cells depend on chemokine signaling. The SDF1α/CXCR4 axis is the myeloma homing pathway most extensively characterized, and impairment of signaling between these molecules is associated with extramedullary transformation (39). Myeloma also depends on CCR1 and CCR2 signaling to regulate migration. Patients with active disease express significantly lower amounts of CXCR4, CCR1, and CCR2 than those with non-active disease, and expression of at least one of these receptors portends favorable clinical outcome (161). Additional chemokine receptors such as CXCR5 and CCR7 are downregulated to promote cell motility and decrease sensitivity to B and T cell cytokines (162).

Myeloma cells alter their adhesion properties to extravasate and migrate through the ECM. EMM plasma cells decrease expression of CD56 while increasing expression of certain CD44 isoforms that are important for proliferation and motility (163). In murine models, decreased expression of P-selectin and VLA4 are associated with increased extramedullary disease (164). Extramedullary myeloma cells also favor focal adhesion kinase (FAK), a protein that mediates an invasive and migratory phenotype. Patients with EMM have significantly increased expression of FAK mRNA compared with patients without extramedullary disease (165). The tetraspanin family of proteins is another family that modulates myeloma adhesion and migration. Two such proteins, CD81 and CD82, are downregulated in HMCL, and exogenous overexpression of these proteins reduces cell motility, invasion, and secretion of MMP-9 (166).

Finally, myeloma cells must degrade the ECM to allow passage through. MMP-9 will degrade basement membrane, and its secretion leads to increased invasion of tumor cells. HMCL have been shown to constitutively secrete MMP-9, and its expression is enhanced by HGF secretion by endothelial cells. Moreover, some HMCL can produce HGF, thus sustaining a loop of increased MMP-9 degradation. Interestingly, SDF1α stimulates MMP-9 production in mouse myeloma model suggesting that SDF1α may have pleiotropic effects in both myeloma cell homing and invasion (167). Myeloma cells also produce heparanase, an enzyme that cleaves heparanase sulfate chains of adhesive proteoglycans such as syndecan-1. Production of heparanase increases motility of myeloma cells and induces a migratory phenotype (168). In part, heparanase and syndecan appear to regulate one another throughout the progression of myeloma and EMM (**Figure 2B**).

Extramedullary Multiple Myeloma Molecular Changes

Comparison of myeloma cells at extramedullary sites with bone marrow myeloma cells revealed increased subclonal mutations in the extramedullary sites. Morgan et al. proposed a model of myeloma progression that follows the Darwinian mechanism of species evolution. In this model, myeloma cells undergo primary mutations that underlie their growth and expansion. When a bottleneck is applied, subsequent mutations of cells are selected for, thus resulting in surviving subclonal genetic populations (169). In addition to drug treatment, bottlenecks may refer to hypoxia, cell-competition in the microenvironment, and other novel environmental differences in extramedullary sites. Myeloma cells can migrate to other less populated marrow compartments or soft tissue sites and extravasate into these sites or form adjacent plasmacytomas to bone (167).

EMM cells upregulate the adhesion molecules platelet/endothelial cell adhesion molecule-1 (PECAM-1), secreted protein and rich in cysteine (SPARC), and endoglin (ENG), illustrating the shift in adhesion specificity in EMM (170). EMM cells also upregulate nestin, an intermediate filament implicated in metastasis and invasion (171).

A mechanism for myeloma autocrine pro-survival loop lies in the co-expression of CD28 and its ligand CD86. Ligation of CD28 promotes cellular survival and drug resistance in HMCL, and silencing of CD28 and CD86 leads to respective increases in cell death (88, 89). Recent work from our lab has shown that CD86 can signal to confer survival and drug resistance in HMCL. CD86 overexpression induces molecular changes such as increased expression of integrin ß1 and ß7 and interferon regulatory factor 4 (IRF4), a transcription factor necessary for myeloma survival which directly targets MYC (89, 172). Another autocrine loop involved in myeloma survival is secretion of HGF. HMCL and primary myeloma express the tyrosine kinase HGF receptor, c-Met, and produce HGF at variable levels. By this means, EMM cells can signal to stimulate c-Met thus preventing apoptosis and inducing proliferation through autocrine cytokine production (173, 174). Advances in screening technology using CRISPR offer new tools for future elucidation of genes necessary for HMCL survival and proliferation.

Extramedullary Multiple Myeloma Angiogenesis Signaling

One of the processes highly relied upon in the bone marrow microenvironment, angiogenesis, also has an important role in EMM. Hypoxia in the bone marrow causes myeloma cell upregulation of HIF1α which regulates secretion of proangiogenic cytokines. HIF1α is also upregulated in circulating plasma cells and is associated with myeloma EMT (175). Additional angiogenic factors are upregulated in EMM including VEGF, MMP-9, PECAM-1, and Ang-1. Other angiogenesis related genes such as PDGF, SPARC, NOTCH3, thrombospondin 2, TIMP3, and fibronectin 1 are overexpressed (162). Increased expression of these proteins indicates an important role for angiogenesis in EMM. Although current standard therapies for EMM such as lenalidomide (176) and bortezomib (140) are antiangiogenic, the role of angiogenesis in EMM remains largely unknown.

Plasma Cell Leukemia Molecular Alterations

PCL is an aggressive variant of EMM marked by rapidly proliferating circulating plasma cells and poor prognosis of patients. Primary immunoglobulin translocations are common in PCL with MAF translocations [t(14,16) and t(14,20)] being the most common followed by t(11,14) and t(4,14). Other common mutations in PCL are MYC translocations which can be found on IgH (5%), IgK(10%), and IgL (10%) loci, respectively (177).

PCL also overexpresses certain genes compared to plasmacytomas including RPL17, CD14, TRAF2, TRAF3, and CCL2. Other affected cancer driver genes include those involved in cell-matrix adhesion and membrane organization (SPTB, CELA1), cell cycle and apoptosis (CIDEC), genome stability (KIF2B), and protein folding (CMYA5). PCL cells are also enriched in functional pathways including Cadherin/Wnt signaling, ECM-receptor, and G2/M cell cycle checkpoint. As PCL are circulating in the blood, there is a downregulation of integrins (CD11a, CD11c, CD29, CD49, CD49e) and other adhesion molecules (CD33, CD117, CD138, CD81) in comparison to EMM. PCL also expresses decreased markers of plasma cells (CD28, CD38) and increased markers of B cells (CD19, CD20, CD45) due to their high prevalence of t(11,14) translocations (177, 178).

CONCLUSION

In the Game of Bones, myeloma cells are manipulators that identify allies within the bone marrow microenvironment to exploit and thereby enable their neutralization and evasion of their opposition, the host's immune defenses. Data that show microenvironment changes as early as MGUS propose that the microenvironment is susceptible to myeloma growth in precursor stages. Mutations in precursor stages beckon a "chicken or the egg" conundrum between myeloma cells and the microenvironment in assessing the advancement of this malignancy. By the time symptomatic myeloma develops, the Game of Bones has already tipped in favor of the cancer. This is because the disease is already quite evolved with numerous means of drug resistance and proliferation in its arsenal, and the cancer has a substantial advantage against innate defenses and chemotherapeutic intervention. In advanced stages, myeloma can readily proliferate in the bone marrow and develop the capacity to transcend the bone marrow.

Recent studies have aimed to tip the advantage back to the side of the host's defense system, either by effectively targeting myeloma cells and the microenvironment or by strengthening the immune response. As technology and detection tools improve, myeloma cells can be combatted at their early stages before treatment of myeloma or EMM is necessary. Modern genomic approaches such as single cell genomics, mass cytometry, ATAC-seq, whole genome bisulfite sequencing, and integrated phosphoproteomics can elucidate properly tailored treatments for improved efficacy and decreased toxicity of patients. The rise of IMiDs and targeted antibody treatments represent our growing understanding of the therapeutic role of targeting the microenvironment.

Mobilizing the body's own immune system also improves its odds at winning the Game of Bones. IMiDs, as well as CAR-T cell therapy are of particular interest as they can be utilized to bolster the body's defenses against its adversary. IMiDs are a potent frontline treatment for MM, and have even been shown to improve patient outcome in the SMM stage (34). Overall, studies of the cancer biology in myeloma cells and their surrounding microenvironment using *ex vivo* patient studies, murine models, and HMCL provide insight to future treatment options and increased efficacy of therapy.

AUTHOR CONTRIBUTIONS

TK conceived and wrote the review. NJ, MD, and KL contributed to the writing and editing of manuscript. LB conceived, edited, and oversaw the writing. All authors contributed to the article and approved the submitted version.

REFERENCES

1. Myeloma - SEER Stat Fact Sheets. . http://seer.cancer.gov/statfacts/html/mulmy.html.
2. Slifka MK, Ahmed R. Long-lived plasma cells: a mechanism for maintaining persistent antibody production. *Curr Opin Immunol* (1998) 10:252–8. doi: 10.1016/S0952-7915(98)80162-3
3. Dhodapkar MV. MGUS to myeloma: a mysterious gammopathy of underexplored significance. *Blood* (2016) 128:2599–606. doi: 10.1182/blood-2016-09-692954
4. Bailur JK, McCachren SS, Doxie DB, Shrestha M, Pendleton KE, Nooka AK, et al. Early Alterations in Stem-Like/Resident T Cells, Innate and Myeloid Cells in the Bone Marrow in Preneoplastic Gammopathy. *JCI Insight* (2019) 5:1–10. doi: 10.1172/jci.insight.127807
5. Hedvat CV, Comenzo RL, Teruya-Feldstein J, Olshen AB, Ely SA, Osman K, et al. Insights into extramedullary tumour cell growth revealed by expression profiling of human plasmacytomas and multiple myeloma. *Br J Haematol* (2003) 122:728–44. doi: 10.1046/j.1365-2141.2003.04481.x
6. Rajkumar SV, Dimopoulos MA, Palumbo A, Blade J, Merlini G, Mateos MV, et al. International Myeloma Working Group updated criteria for the diagnosis of multiple myeloma. *Lancet Oncol* (2014) 15:e538–48. doi: 10.1016/S1470-2045(14)70442-5
7. Larsen JT, Kumar SK, Dispenzieri A, Kyle RA, Katzmann JA, Rajkumar SV. Serum free light chain ratio as a biomarker for high-risk smoldering multiple myeloma. *Leukemia* (2013) 27:941–6. doi: 10.1038/leu.2012.296
8. Kastritis E, Terpos E, Moulopoulos L, Spyropoulou-Vlachou M, Kanellias N, Eleftherakis-Papaiakovou E, et al. Extensive bone marrow infiltration and abnormal free light chain ratio identifies patients with asymptomatic myeloma at high risk for progression to symptomatic disease. *Leukemia* (2013) 27:947–53. doi: 10.1038/leu.2012.309
9. Kastritis E, Moulopoulos LA, Terpos E, Koutoulidis V, Dimopoulos MA. The prognostic importance of the presence of more than one focal lesion in spine MRI of patients with asymptomatic (smoldering) multiple myeloma. *Leukemia* (2014) 28:2402–3. doi: 10.1038/leu.2014.230
10. Greipp PR, San Miguel J, Durie BGM, Crowley JJ, Barlogie B, Blade J, et al. International staging system for multiple myeloma. *J Clin Oncol* (2005) 23:3412–20. doi: 10.1200/JCO.2005.04.242
11. Palumbo A, Avet-Loiseau H, Oliva S, Lokhorst HM, Goldschmidt H, Rosinol L, et al. Revised International Staging System for Multiple Myeloma: A Report From International Myeloma Working Group. *J Clin Oncol* (2015) 33:2863–9. doi: 10.1200/JCO.2015.61.2267
12. Joseph NS, Kaufman JL, Dhodapkar MV, Hofmeister CC, Almaula DK, Heffner LT, et al. Long-Term Follow-Up Results of Lenalidomide, Bortezomib, and Dexamethasone Induction Therapy and Risk-Adapted Maintenance Approach in Newly Diagnosed Multiple Myeloma. *J Clin Oncol* (2020) 38:1928–37. doi: 10.1200/JCO.19.02515
13. Rajkumar SV. Multiple myeloma: 2020 update on diagnosis, risk-stratification and management. *Am J Hematol* (2020) 95:548–67. doi: 10.1002/ajh.25791
14. Schmidt TM, Barwick BG, Joseph NS, Heffner LT, Hofmeister CC, Bernal L, et al. Gain of Chromosome 1q is associated with early progression in multiple myeloma patients treated with lenalidomide, bortezomib, and dexamethasone. *Blood Cancer J* (2019) 9:1–13. doi: 10.1038/s41408-019-0254-0
15. Greipp PR, Lust JA, O'Fallon WM, Katzmann JA, Witzig TE, Kyle RA. Plasma cell labeling index and beta 2-microglobulin predict survival independent of thymidine kinase and C-reactive protein in multiple myeloma [see comments]. *Blood* (1993) 81:3382–7. doi: 10.1182/blood.V81.12.3382.bloodjournal81123382
16. Lonial S, Boise LH, Kaufman J. How I treat high-risk myeloma. *Blood* (2015) 126:1536–43. doi: 10.1182/blood-2015-06-653261
17. Landgren O, Kyle RA, Pfeiffer RM, Katzmann JA, Caporaso NE, Hayes RB, et al. Monoclonal gammopathy of undetermined significance (MGUS) consistently precedes multiple myeloma: a prospective study. *Blood* (2009) 113:5412–7. doi: 10.1182/blood-2008-12-194241
18. Weiss BM, Abadie J, Verma P, Howard RS, Kuehl WM. A monoclonal gammopathy precedes multiple myeloma in most patients. *Blood* (2009) 113:5418–22. doi: 10.1182/blood-2008-12-195008
19. Waldenstrom J. Studies on conditions associated with disturbed gamma globulin formation (gammopathies). *Harvey Lect* (1960) 56:211–31.
20. Kyle RA. Monoclonal Gammopathy of Undetermined Significance. Natural History in 241 Cases. *Am J Med* (1978) 64:814–26. doi: 10.1016/0002-9343(78)90563-6
21. Landgren O, Gridley G, Ingemar T, Caporaso NE, Goldin LR, Baris D, et al. Risk of monoclonal gammopathy of undetermined significance (MGUS) and subsequent multiple myeloma among African American and white veterans in the United States. *Blood* (2006) 107:904–6. doi: 10.1182/blood-2005-08-3449
22. Landgren O, Kyle RA, Rajkumar SV. From Myeloma Precursor Disease to Multiple Myeloma: New Diagnostic Concepts and Opportunities for Early Intervention. *Clin Cancer Res* (2011) 17:1243–52. doi: 10.1158/1078-0432.CCR-10-1822
23. Kyle RA, Therneau TM, Rajkumar SV, Offord JR, Larson DR, Plevak MF, et al. A Long-Term Study of Prognosis in Monoclonal Gammopathy of Undetermined Significance. *N Engl J Med* (2002) 346:564–9. doi: 10.1056/NEJMoa01133202
24. Kyle RA, Larson DR, Therneau TM, Dispenzieri A, Kumar S, Cerhan JR, et al. Long-Term Follow-up of Monoclonal Gammopathy of Undetermined Significance. *N Engl J Med* (2018) 378:241–9o. doi: 10.1056/NEJMoa1709974
25. Mills JR, Kohlhagen MC, Dasari S, Vanderboom PM, Kyle RA, Katzmann JA, et al. Comprehensive Assessment of M-Proteins Using Nanobody Enrichment Coupled to MALDI-TOF Mass Spectrometry. *Clin Chem* (2016) 62:1334–44. doi: 10.1373/clinchem.2015.253740
26. Zojer N, Ludwig H, Fiegl M, Stevenson FK, Sahota SS. Patterns of somatic mutations in VH genes reveal pathways of clonal transformation from MGUS to multiple myeloma. *Blood* (2003) 101:4137–9. doi: 10.1182/blood-2002-09-2825
27. Barwick BG, Gupta VA, Vertino PM, Boise LH. Cell of Origin and Genetic Alterations in the Pathogenesis of Multiple Myeloma. *Front Immunol* (2019) 10:1121. doi: 10.3389/fimmu.2019.01121
28. Cohen AD, Raje N, Fowler JA, Mezzi K, Scott EC, Dhodapkar MV. How to Train Your T Cells: Overcoming Immune Dysfunction in Multiple Myeloma. *Clin Cancer Res* (2020) 26:1541–54. doi: 10.1158/1078-0432.CCR-19-2111
29. Kyle RA, Greipp PR. Smoldering multiple myeloma. *N Engl J Med* (1980) 302:1347–9. doi: 10.1056/NEJM198006123022405
30. Rajkumar SV, Landgren O, Mateos M-V. Smoldering multiple myeloma. *Blood* (2015) 125:3069–75. doi: 10.1182/blood-2014-09-568899
31. Lakshman A, Rajkumar SV, Buadi FK, Binder M, Gertz MA, Lacy MQ, et al. Risk stratification of smoldering multiple myeloma incorporating revised

IMWG diagnostic criteria. *Blood Cancer J* (2018) 8:1–10. doi: 10.1038/s41408-018-0077-4

32. Neben K, Jauch A, Hielscher T, Hillengass J, Lehners N, Seckinger A, et al. Progression in Smoldering Myeloma Is Independently Determined by the Chromosomal Abnormalities del(17p), t(4;14), Gain 1q, Hyperdiploidy, and Tumor Load. *J Clin Oncol* (2013) 31:4325–32. doi: 10.1200/JCO.2012.48.4923
33. San Miguel J, Mateos MV, Gonzalez V, Dimopoulos MA, Kastritis E, Hajek R, et al. Updated risk stratification model for smoldering multiple myeloma (SMM) incorporating the revised IMWG diagnostic criteria. *J Clin Oncol* (2019) 37:8000–0. doi: 10.1200/JCO.2019.37.15_suppl.8000
34. Lonial S, Jacobus S, Fonseca R, Weiss M, Kumar S, Orlowski RZ, et al. Randomized Trial of Lenalidomide Versus Observation in Smoldering Multiple Myeloma. *J Clin Oncol* (2020) 38:1126–37. doi: 10.1200/JCO.19.01740
35. Weinstock M, Ghobrial IM. Extramedullary multiple myeloma. *Leuk Lymphoma* (2013) 54:1135–41. doi: 10.3109/10428194.2012.740562
36. Tsang RW, Campbell BA, Goda JS, Kelsey CR, Kirova YM, Parikh RR, et al. Radiation Therapy for Solitary Plasmacytoma and Multiple Myeloma: Guidelines From the International Lymphoma Radiation Oncology Group. *Int J Radiat Oncol Biol Phys* (2018) 101:794–808. doi: 10.1016/j.ijrobp.2018.08.004
37. Touzeau C, Moreau P. How I treat extramedullary myeloma. *Blood* (2016) 127:971–6. doi: 10.1182/blood-2015-07-635383
38. Varettoni M, Corso A, Pica G, Mangiacavalli S, Pascutto C, Lazzarino M. Incidence, presenting features and outcome of extramedullary disease in multiple myeloma: a longitudinal study on 1003 consecutive patients. *Ann Oncol* (2010) 21:325–30. doi: 10.1093/annonc/mdp329
39. Bladé J, Fernandez de Larrea F, Rosinol L, Cibeira MT, Jimenez R, Powles R. Soft-tissue plasmacytomas in multiple myeloma: incidence, mechanisms of extramedullary spread, and treatment approach. *J Clin Oncol* (2011) 29:3805–12. doi: 10.1200/JCO.2011.34.9290
40. Fernández de Larrea C, Kyle RA, Durie BGM, Ludwig H, Usmani S, Vesole DH, et al. Plasma cell leukemia: consensus statement on diagnostic requirements, response criteria and treatment recommendations by the International Myeloma Working Group. *Leukemia* (2013) 27:780–91. doi: 10.1038/leu.2012.336
41. Bink K, Haralambieva E, Kremer M, Ott G, Beham-Schmid C, de Leval L, et al. Primary extramedullary plasmacytoma: similarities with and differences from multiple myeloma revealed by interphase cytogenetics. *Haematologica* (2008) 93:623–6. doi: 10.3324/haematol.12005
42. Besse L, Sedlarikova L, Greslikova H, Kupska R, Almasi M, Penka M, et al. Cytogenetics in multiple myeloma patients progressing into extramedullary disease. *Eur J Haematol* (2016) 97:93–100. doi: 10.1111/ejh.12688
43. Dawson MA, Patil S, Spencer A. Extramedullary relapse of multiple myeloma associated with a shift in secretion from intact immunoglobulin to light chains. *Haematologica* (2007) 92:143–4. doi: 10.3324/haematol.10297
44. Langley RR, Fidler IJ. The seed and soil hypothesis revisited - the role of tumor-stroma interactions in metastasis to different organs. *Int J Cancer J Int Cancer* (2011) 128:2527–35. doi: 10.1002/ijc.26031
45. Paget S. The Distribution of Secondary Growths in Cancer of the Breast. 1889. *Cancer Metastasis Rev* (1989) 8:98–101.
46. Das R, Strowig T, Verma R, Koduru S, Hafemann A, Hopf S, et al. Microenvironment-dependent growth of preneoplastic and malignant plasma cells in humanized mice. *Nat Med* (2016) 22:1351–7. doi: 10.1038/nm.4202
47. Bergsagel PL, Kuehl WM, Zhan F, Sawyer J, Barlogie B, Shaughnessy J. Cyclin D dysregulation: an early and unifying pathogenic event in multiple myeloma. *Blood* (2005) 106:296–303. doi: 10.1182/blood-2005-01-0034
48. Bergsagel PL, Kuehl WM. Molecular pathogenesis and a consequent classification of multiple myeloma. *J Clin Oncol* (2005) 23:6333–8. doi: 10.1200/JCO.2005.05.021
49. Avet.-Loiseau H, Li JY, Facon T, Brigaudeau C, Morineau N, Maloisel F, et al. High Incidence of Translocations t(11;14)(q13;q32) and t(4;14)(p16;q32) in Patients With Plasma Cell Malignancies. *Cancer Res* (1998) 58:5640–5.
50. Shaughnessy J, Gabrea A, Qi Y, Brents L, Zhan F, Tian E, et al. Cyclin D3 at 6p21 Is Dysregulated by Recurrent Chromosomal Translocations to Immunoglobulin Loci in Multiple Myeloma. *Blood* (2001) 98. doi: 10.1182/blood.V98.1.217
51. Hurt EM, Wiestner A, Rosenwald A, Shaffer AL, Campo E, Grogan T, et al. Overexpression of c-maf is a frequent oncogenic event in multiple myeloma that promotes proliferation and pathological interactions with bone marrow stroma. *Cancer Cell* (2004) 5:191–9. doi: 10.1016/S1535-6108(04)00019-4
52. Walker BA, Leone PE, Chiecchio L, Dickens NJ, Jenner MW, et al. A Compendium of Myeloma-Associated Chromosomal Copy Number Abnormalities and Their Prognostic Value. *Blood* (2010) 116:e56–65. doi: 10.1182/blood-2010-04-279596
53. Chiecchio L, Dagrada GP, Ibrahim AH, Cabanas ED, Protheroe RKM, Stockley DM, et al. Timing of Acquisition of Deletion 13 in Plasma Cell Dyscrasias Is Dependent on Genetic Context. *Haematologica* (2009) 94:1708–13. doi: 10.3324/haematol.2009.011064
54. Biner M, Rajkumar SV, Ketterling RP, Greipp PT, Dispenzieri A, Lacy MQ, et al. Prognostic Implications of Abnormalities of Chromosome 13 and the Presence of Multiple Cytogenetic High-Risk Abnormalities in Newly Diagnosed Multiple Myeloma. *Blood Cancer J* (2017) 7:e600. doi: 10.1038/bcj.2017.83
55. Chesi M, Stein CK, Garbitt VM, Sharik ME, Asmann YW, Bergsagel M, et al. Monosomic Loss of MIR15A/MIR16-1 Is a Driver of Multiple Myeloma Proliferation and Disease Progression. *Blood Cancer Discov* (2020) 1:1–14. doi: 10.1158/0008-5472.BCD-19-0068
56. Nobuyoshi M, Kawano M, Tanaka H, Ishikawa H, Tanabe O, Iwato K, et al. Increased Expression of the C-Myc Gene May Be Related to the Aggressive Transformation of Human Myeloma Cells. *Br J Haematol* (1991) 77:523–8. doi: 10.1111/j.1365-2141.1991.tb08620.x
57. Avet-Loiseau H, Gerson F, Magrangeas F, Minvielle S, Harousseau JL, Bataille R, et al. Rearrangements of the c-myc oncogene are present in 15% of primary human multiple myeloma tumors. *Blood* (2001) 98:3082–6. doi: 10.1182/blood.V98.10.3082
58. Barwick BG, Neri P, Bahlis NJ, Nooka AK, Dhodapkar MV, Jaye DL, et al. Multiple myeloma immunoglobulin lambda translocations portend poor prognosis. *Nat Commun* (2019) 10:1911. doi: 10.1038/s41467-019-09555-6
59. Liu P, Leong T, Quam L, Billadeau D, Kay NE, Greipp P, et al. Activating Mutations of N- And K-ras in Multiple Myeloma Show Different Clinical Associations: Analysis of the Eastern Cooperative Oncology Group Phase III Trial. *Blood* (1996) 88:2699–706. doi: 10.1182/blood.V88.7.2699.bloodjournal8872699
60. Lin Y-HT, Way GP, Barwick BG, Mariano MC, Marcoulis M, Ferguson ID, et al. Integrated phosphoproteomics and transcriptional classifiers reveal hidden RAS signaling dynamics in multiple myeloma. *Blood Adv* (2019) 3:3214–27. doi: 10.1182/bloodadvances.2019000303
61. Chesi M, Brents LA, Ely SA, Bais C, Robbiani DF, Mesri EA, et al. Activated Fibroblast Growth Factor Receptor 3 Is an Oncogene That Contributes to Tumor Progression in Multiple Myeloma. *Blood* (2001) 97:729–36. doi: 10.1182/blood.V97.3.729
62. Andrulis M, Lehners N, Capper D, Penzel R, Heining C, Huellein J, et al. Targeting the BRAF V600E Mutation in Multiple Myeloma. *Cancer Discov* (2013) 3:862–9. doi: 10.1158/2159-8290.CD-13-0014
63. Maura F, Rustad EH, Yellapantula V, Luksza M, Hoyos D, Maclachlan KH, et al. Role of AID in the temporal pattern of acquisition of driver mutations in multiple myeloma. *Leukemia* (2020) 34:1476–80. doi: 10.1038/s41375-019-0689-0
64. Koduru S, Wong E, Strowig T, Sundaram R, Zhang L, Strout MP, et al. Dendritic cell-mediated activation-induced cytidine deaminase (AID)-dependent induction of genomic instability in human myeloma. *Blood* (2012) 119:2302–9. doi: 10.1182/blood-2011-08-376236
65. Menu E, Asosingh K, Indraccolo S, De Raeve H, Van Riet I, Van Valckenborgh E, et al. The involvement of stromal derived factor 1alpha in homing and progression of multiple myeloma in the 5TMM model. *Haematologica* (2006) 91:605–12. doi: 10.3324/%25x
66. Damiano JS, Cress AE, Hazlehurst LA, Shtil AA, Dalton WS. Cell adhesion mediated drug resistance (CAM-DR): role of integrins and resistance to apoptosis in human myeloma cell lines. *Blood* (1999) 93:1658–67. doi: 10.1182/blood.V93.5.1658

67. Katz B-Z. Adhesion molecules–The lifelines of multiple myeloma cells. *Semin Cancer Biol* (2010) 20:186–95. doi: 10.1016/j.semcancer.2010.04.003
68. Hosen N. Integrins in multiple myeloma. *Inflamm Regen* (2020) 40:4. doi: 10.1186/s41232-020-00113-y
69. Damiano JS. & Dalton W.S. Integrin-mediated Drug Resistance in Multiple Myeloma. *Leuk Lymphoma* (2000) 38:1658–67. doi: 10.3109/10428190009060320
70. Neri P, Ren L, Azab AK, Brentnall M, Gratton K, Klimowicz AC, et al. Integrin β7-mediated regulation of multiple myeloma cell adhesion, migration, and invasion. *Blood* (2011) 117:6202–13. doi: 10.1182/blood-2010-06-292243
71. Landowski TH, Olashaw NE, Agrawal D, Dalton WS. Cell adhesion-mediated drug resistance (CAM-DR) is associated with activation of NF-kappa B (RelB/p50) in myeloma cells. *Oncogene* (2003) 22:2417–21. doi: 10.1038/sj.onc.1206315
72. Hosen N, Matsunaga Y, Hasegawa K, Matsuno H, Nakamura Y, Makita M, et al. The activated conformation of integrin β 7 is a novel multiple myeloma-specific target for CAR T cell therapy. *Nat Med* (2017) 23:1436–43. doi: 10.1038/nm.4431
73. Riet IV, Waele MD, Remels L, Lacor P, Schots R, Camp BV, et al. Expression of cytoadhesion molecules (CD56, CD54, CD18 and CD29) by myeloma plasma cells. *Br J Haematol* (1991) 79:421–7. doi: 10.1111/j.1365-2141.1991.tb08050.x
74. Hideshima T, Mitsiades C, Tonon G, Richardson PG, Anderson KC. Understanding multiple myeloma pathogenesis in the bone marrow to identify new therapeutic targets. *Nat Rev Cancer* (2007) 7:585–98. doi: 10.1038/nrc2189
75. Sanderson RD, Turnbull JE, Gallagher JT, Lander AD. Fine structure of heparan sulfate regulates syndecan-1 function and cell behavior. *J Biol Chem* (1994) 269:13100–6. doi: 10.1016/S0021-9258(17)36804-7
76. Reijmers RM, Groen RWJ, Rozemuller H, Kuil A, de Haan-Kramer A, Csikos T, et al. Targeting EXT1 Reveals a Crucial Role for Heparan Sulfate in the Growth of Multiple Myeloma. *Blood* (2010) 115:601–4. doi: 10.1182/blood-2009-02-204396
77. Levy-Adam F, Feld S, Suss-Toby E, Vlodavsky I, Ilan N. Heparanase Facilitates Cell Adhesion and Spreading by Clustering of Cell Surface Heparan Sulfate Proteoglycans. *PLoS One* (2008) 3:e2319. doi: 10.1371/journal.pone.0002319
78. Yang Y, Macleod V, Miao MQ, Theus A, Zhan F, Shaughnessy JD, et al. Heparanase enhances syndecan-1 shedding: a novel mechanism for stimulation of tumor growth and metastasis. *J Biol Chem* (2007) 282:13326–33. doi: 10.1074/jbc.M611259200
79. Yang Y, Yaccoboy S, Liu W, Langford JK, Pumphrey CY, Theus A, et al. Soluble syndecan-1 promotes growth of myeloma tumors in vivo. *Blood* (2002) 100:610–7. doi: 10.1182/blood.V100.2.610
80. van de Donk NWCJ, Usmani SZ. CD38 Antibodies in Multiple Myeloma: Mechanisms of Action and Modes of Resistance. *Front Immunol* (2018) 9:2134. doi: 10.3389/fimmu.2018.02134
81. Ahsmann EJ, Lokhorst HM, Dekker AW, Bloem AC. Lymphocyte function-associated antigen-1 expression on plasma cells correlates with tumor growth in multiple myeloma. *Blood* (1992) 79:2068–75. doi: 10.1182/blood.V79.8.2068.bloodjournal7982068
82. Asosingh K, Vankerkhove V, Van Riet I, Van Camp B, Vanderkerken K. Selective in vivo growth of lymphocyte function- associated antigen-1-positive murine myeloma cells. Involvement of function-associated antigen-1-mediated homotypic cell-cell adhesion. *Exp Hematol* (2003) 31:48–55. doi: 10.1016/S0301-472X(02)00970-0
83. Tagde A, Rajabi H, Bouillez A, Alam M, Gali R, Bailey S, et al. MUC1-C drives MYC in multiple myeloma. *Blood* (2016) 127:2587–97. doi: 10.1182/blood-2015-07-659151
84. Linsley PS, Brady W, Grosmaire L, Aruffo A, Damle NK, Ledbetter JA. Binding of the B cell activation antigen B7 to CD28 costimulates T cell proliferation and interleukin 2 mRNA accumulation. *J Exp Med* (1991) 173:721–30. doi: 10.1084/jem.173.3.721
85. Bahlis NJ, King AM, Kolonias D, Carlson LM, Liu HY, Hussein MA, et al. CD28-mediated regulation of multiple myeloma cell proliferation and survival. *Blood* (2007) 109:5002–10. doi: 10.1182/blood-2006-03-012542
86. Rozanski CH, Arens R, Carlson LM, Nair JR, Boise LH, Chanan-Khan AA, et al. Sustained antibody responses depend on CD28 function in bone marrow-resident plasma cells. *J Exp Med* (2011) 208:1435–46. doi: 10.1084/jem.20110040
87. Rozanski CH, Utley A, Carlson LM, Farren MR, Murray M, Russell LM, et al. CD28 Promotes Plasma Cell Survival, Sustained Antibody Responses, and BLIMP-1 Upregulation through Its Distal PYAP Proline Motif. *J Immunol Baltim Md 1950* (2015) 194:4717–28. doi: 10.4049/jimmunol.1402260
88. Murray ME, Gavile CM, Nair JR, Koorella C, Carlson LM, Buac D, et al. CD28-mediated pro-survival signaling induces chemotherapeutic resistance in multiple myeloma. *Blood* (2014) 123:3770–9. doi: 10.1182/blood-2013-10-530964
89. Gavile CM, Barwick BG, Newman S, Neri P, Nooka AK, Lonial S, et al. CD86 regulates myeloma cell survival. *Blood Adv* (2017) 1:2307–19. doi: 10.1182/bloodadvances.2017011601
90. Hideshima T, Nakamura N, Chauhan D, Anderson KC. Biologic sequelae of interleukin-6 induced PI3-K/Akt signaling in multiple myeloma. *Oncogene* (2001) 20:5991–6000. doi: 10.1038/sj.onc.1204833
91. Chauhan D, Uchiyama H, Akbarali Y, Urashima M, Yamamoto, Libermann TA, et al. Multiple myeloma cell adhesion-induced interleukin-6 expression in bone marrow stromal cells involves activation of NF-kappa B. *Blood* (1996) 87:1104–12. doi: 10.1182/blood.V87.3.1104.bloodjournal8731104
92. Uchiyama H, Barut BA, Mohrbacher AF, Chauhan D, Anderson KC. Adhesion of human myeloma-derived cell lines to bone marrow stromal cells stimulates interleukin-6 secretion. *Blood* (1993) 82:3712–20. doi: 10.1182/blood.V82.12.3712.bloodjournal82123712
93. Gupta VA, Matulis SM, Conage-Pough JE, Nooka AK, Kaufman JL, Lonial S, et al. Bone marrow microenvironment-derived signals induce Mcl-1 dependence in multiple myeloma. *Blood* (2017) 129:1969–79. doi: 10.1182/blood-2016-10-745059
94. Conage-Pough JE. & Boise L.H. Phosphorylation Alters Bim-mediated Mcl-1 Stabilization and Priming. *FEBS J* (2018) 285:2626–40. doi: 10.1111/febs.14505
95. Moreaux J, Legouffe E, Jourdan E, Quittet P, Reme T, Lugagne C, et al. BAFF and APRIL protect myeloma cells from apoptosis induced by interleukin 6 deprivation and dexamethasone. *Blood* (2004) 103:3148–57. doi: 10.1182/blood-2003-06-1984
96. Schneider P, MacKay F, Steiner V, Hofman K, Bodmer JL, Holler N, et al. BAFF, a novel ligand of the tumor necrosis factor family, stimulates B cell growth. *J Exp Med* (1999) 189:1747–56. doi: 10.1084/jem.189.11.1747
97. Novak AJ, Darce JR, Arendt BK, Harder B, Henderson K, Kindsvogel W, et al. Expression of BCMA, TACI, and BAFF-R in multiple myeloma: a mechanism for growth and survival. *Blood* (2004) 103:689–94. doi: 10.1182/blood-2003-06-2043
98. Tai Y-T, Acharya C, An G, Moschetta M, Zhong MY, Feng X, et al. APRIL and BCMA promote human multiple myeloma growth and immunosuppression in the bone marrow microenvironment. *Blood* (2016) 127:3225–36. doi: 10.1182/blood-2016-01-691162
99. Timmers M, Roex G, Wang Y, Campillo-Davo D, Van Tendeloo VFI, Chu Y, et al. Chimeric Antigen Receptor-Modified T Cell Therapy in Multiple Myeloma: Beyond B Cell Maturation Antigen. *Front Immunol* (2019) 10:1613. doi: 10.3389/fimmu.2019.01613
100. Kukreja A, Hutchinson A, Dhodapkar A, Mazumder A, Vesole D, Angitapalli R, et al. Enhancement of clonogenicity of human multiple myeloma by dendritic cells. *J Exp Med* (2006) 203:1859–65. doi: 10.1084/jem.20052136
101. Hideshima T, Chauhan D, Schlossman R, Richardson P, Anderson KC. The role of tumor necrosis factor alpha in the pathophysiology of human multiple myeloma: therapeutic applications. *Oncogene* (2001) 20:4519–27. doi: 10.1038/sj.onc.1204623
102. Singhal S, Mehta J, Desikan R, Ayers D, Roberson P, Munshi N, et al. Antitumor Activity of Thalidomide in Refractory Multiple Myeloma. *N Engl J Med* (1999) 341:1565–71. doi: 10.1056/NEJM199911183412102
103. Mitsiades CS, Mitsiades NS, McMullan CJ, Poulaki V, Shringarpur R, Akiyama M, et al. Inhibition of the insulin-like growth factor receptor-1 tyrosine kinase activity as a therapeutic strategy for multiple myeloma, other hematologic malignancies, and solid tumors. *Cancer Cell* (2004) 5:221–30. doi: 10.1016/S1535-6108(04)00050-9

104. Choi SJ, Oba Y, Gazitt Y, Alsina M, Cruz J, Anderson J, et al. Antisense inhibition of macrophage inflammatory protein 1-alpha blocks bone destruction in a model of myeloma bone disease. *J Clin Invest* (2001) 108:1833–41. doi: 10.1172/JCI200113116
105. Abe M, Hiura K, Wilde J, Moriyama K, Hashimoto T, Ozaki S, et al. Role for Macrophage Inflammatory Protein (MIP)-1alpha and MIP-1beta in the Development of Osteolytic Lesions in Multiple Myeloma. *Blood* (2002) 100:2195–202. doi: 10.1182/blood.V100.6.2195.h81802002195_2195_2202
106. Oba Y, Lee JW, Ehrlich LA, Chung HY, Jelinek DF, Callander NS, et al. MIP-1alpha Utilizes Both CCR1 and CCR5 to Induce Osteoclast Formation and Increase Adhesion of Myeloma Cells to Marrow Stromal Cells. *Exp Hematol* (2005) 33:272–8. doi: 10.1016/j.exphem.2004.11.015
107. Han JH, Choi SJ, Kurihara N, Koide M, Oba Y, Roodman GD. Macrophage Inflammatory protein-1alpha Is an Osteoclastogenic Factor in Myeloma That Is Independent of Receptor Activator of Nuclear Factor kappaB Ligand. *Blood* (2001) 97:3349–53. doi: 10.1182/blood.V97.11.3349
108. Yin L. Chondroitin synthase 1 is a key molecule in myeloma cell-osteoclast interactions. *J Biol Chem* (2005) 280:15666–72. doi: 10.1074/jbc.M409877200
109. Colombo M, Mirandola L, Platonova N, Apicella L, Basile A, Figueroa AJ, et al. Notch-directed microenvironment reprogramming in myeloma: a single path to multiple outcomes. *Leukemia* (2013) 27:1009–18. doi: 10.1038/leu.2013.6
110. Delgado-Calle J, Anderson J, Cregor MD, Hiasa M, Chirgwin JM, Carlesso N, et al. Bidirectional Notch Signaling and Osteocyte-Derived Factors in the Bone Marrow Microenvironment Promote Tumor Cell Proliferation and Bone Destruction in Multiple Myeloma. *Cancer Res* (2016) 76:1089–100. doi: 10.1158/0008-5472.CAN-15-1703
111. Michigami T, Shimizu M, Williams PJ, Niewolna M, Dallas SL, Mundy GR, et al. Cell-cell contact between marrow stromal cells and myeloma cells via VCAM-1 and alpha(4)beta(1)-integrin enhances production of osteoclast-stimulating activity. *Blood* (2000) 96:1953–60. doi: 10.1182/blood.V96.5.1953.h8001953_1953_1960
112. Pearse RN, Sordillo EM, Yaccoby S, Wong BR, Liau DF, Colman N, et al. Multiple Myeloma Disrupts the TRANCE/ Osteoprotegerin Cytokine Axis to Trigger Bone Destruction and Promote Tumor Progression. *Proc Natl Acad Sci U S A* (2001) 98:11581–6. doi: 10.1073/pnas.201394498
113. Nguyen AN, Stebbins EG, Henson M, O'Young G, Choi SJ, Quon D, et al. Normalizing the bone marrow microenvironment with p38 inhibitor reduces multiple myeloma cell proliferation and adhesion and suppresses osteoclast formation. *Exp Cell Res* (2006) 312:1909–23. doi: 10.1016/j.yexcr.2006.02.026
114. Terpos E, Ntanasis-Stathopoulos I, Gavriatopoulou M, Dimopoulos MA. Pathogenesis of bone disease in multiple myeloma: from bench to bedside. *Blood Cancer J* (2018) 8:1–12. doi: 10.1038/s41408-017-0037-4
115. Saeki Y, Mima T, Ishii T, Ogata A, Kobayashi H, Ohshima S, et al. Enhanced production of osteopontin in multiple myeloma: clinical and pathogenic implications. *Br J Haematol* (2003) 123:263–70. doi: 10.1046/j.1365-2141.2003.04589.x
116. Noonan K, Marchionni L, Anderson J, Pardoll D, Roodman GD, Borrello I. A novel role of IL-17–producing lymphocytes in mediating lytic bone disease in multiple myeloma. *Blood* (2010) 116:3554–63. doi: 10.1182/blood-2010-05-283895
117. Terpos E, Dimopoulos M-A. Myeloma bone disease: pathophysiology and management. *Ann Oncol* (2005) 16:1223–31. doi: 10.1093/annonc/mdi235
118. Croucher PII, Shiman CM, Lippitt J, Perry M, Asosingh K, Hijzen A, et al. Osteoprotegerin inhibits the development of osteolytic bone disease in multiple myeloma. *Blood* (2001) 98:3534–40. doi: 10.1182/blood.V98.13.3534
119. Boyle WJ, Simonet WS, Lacey DL. Osteoclast differentiation and activation. *Nature* (2003) 423:337–42. doi: 10.1038/nature01658
120. Terpos E, Szydlo R, Apperley JF, Hatjiharissi E, Politou M, Meletis J, et al. Soluble receptor activator of nuclear factor kappaB ligand-osteoprotegerin ratio predicts survival in multiple myeloma: proposal for a novel prognostic index. *Blood* (2003) 102:1064–9. doi: 10.1182/blood-2003-02-0380
121. Giuliani N, Bataille R, Mancini C, Lazzaretti M, Barillé S. Myeloma cells induce imbalance in the osteoprotegerin/osteoprotegerin ligand system in the human bone marrow environment. *Blood* (2001) 98:3527–33. doi: 10.1182/blood.V98.13.3527
122. Sugatani T, Alvarez UM, Hruska KA. Activin A stimulates IkappaB-alpha/NFkappaB and RANK expression for osteoclast differentiation, but not AKT survival pathway in osteoclast precursors. *J Cell Biochem* (2003) 90:59–67. doi: 10.1002/jcb.10613
123. Colucci S, Brunetti G, Oranger A, Mori G, Sardone F, Specchia G, et al. Myeloma cells suppress osteoblasts through sclerostin secretion. *Blood Cancer J* (2011) 1:e27–7. doi: 10.1038/bcj.2011.22
124. Khoo WH, Ledergor G, Weiner A, Roden DL, Terry RL, McDonald MM, et al. A niche-dependent myeloid transcriptome signature defines dormant myeloma cells. *Blood* (2019) 134:30–43. doi: 10.1182/blood.2018880930
125. Terpos E, Kastritis E, Christoulas D, Gkotzamanidou M, Eleutherakis-Papaiakovou E, Kanellias N, et al. Circulating activin-A is elevated in patients with advanced multiple myeloma and correlates with extensive bone involvement and inferior survival; no alterations post-lenalidomide and dexamethasone therapy. *Ann Oncol* (2012) 23:2681–86. doi: 10.1093/annonc/mds068
126. Lee JW, Chung HY, Ehrlich LA, Jelinek DF, Callander NS, Roodman GD, et al. IL-3 expression by myeloma cells increases both osteoclast formation and growth of myeloma cells. *Blood* (2004) 103:2308–15. doi: 10.1182/blood-2003-06-1992
127. Giuliani N, Colla S, Morandi F, Lazzaretti M, Sala R, Bonomini S, et al. Myeloma cells block RUNX2/CBFA1 activity in human bone marrow osteoblast progenitors and inhibit osteoblast formation and differentiation. *Blood* (2005) 106:2472–83. doi: 10.1182/blood-2004-12-4986
128. Terpos E, Dimopoulos MA. Interaction between the skeletal and immune systems in cancer: mechanisms and clinical implications. *Cancer Immunol Immunother CII* (2011) 60:305–17. doi: 10.1007/s00262-011-0974-x
129. Oshima T, Abe M, Asano J, Hara T, Kitazoe K, Sekimoto E, et al. Myeloma cells suppress bone formation by secreting a soluble Wnt inhibitor, sFRP-2. *Blood* (2005) 106:3160–5. doi: 10.1182/blood-2004-12-4940
130. Yaccoby S, Ling W, Zhan F, Walker R, Barlogie B, Shaughnessy JD. Antibody-based inhibition of DKK1 suppresses tumor-induced bone resorption and multiple myeloma growth in vivo. *Blood* (2007) 109:2106–11. doi: 10.1182/blood-2006-09-047712
131. Ehrlich LA, Chung HY, Ghobrial I, Choi SJ, Morandi F, Colla S, et al. IL-3 Is a Potential Inhibitor of Osteoblast Differentiation in Multiple Myeloma. *Blood* (2005) 106:1407–14. doi: 10.1182/blood-2005-03-1080
132. Rajkumar SV, Mesa RA, Fonseca R, Schroeder G, Plevak MF, Dispenzieri A, et al. Bone marrow angiogenesis in 400 patients with monoclonal gammopathy of undetermined significance, multiple myeloma, and primary amyloidosis. *Clin Cancer Res* (2002) 8:2210–6.
133. Bhaskar A, Tiwary BN. Hypoxia inducible factor-1 alpha and multiple myeloma. *Int J Adv Res* (2016) 4:706–15.
134. Vacca A, Di Loreto M, Ribatti D, Di Stefano R, Gadaleta-Caldarola G, Iodice G, et al. Bone marrow of patients with active multiple myeloma: angiogenesis and plasma cell adhesion molecules LFA-1, VLA-4, LAM-1, and CD44. *Am J Hematol* (1995) 50:9–14. doi: 10.1002/ajh.2830500103
135. Andersen NF, Standal T, Nielsen JL, Heickendorff L, Borset M, Sorensen FB, et al. Syndecan-1 and angiogenic cytokines in multiple myeloma: correlation with bone marrow angiogenesis and survival. *Br J Haematol* (2005) 128:210–7. doi: 10.1111/j.1365-2141.2004.05299.x
136. Derksen PWB, Keehnen RMJ, Evers LM, van Oers MHL, Spaargaren M, Pals ST. Cell surface proteoglycan syndecan-1 mediates hepatocyte growth factor binding and promotes Met signaling in multiple myeloma. *Blood* (2002) 99:1405–10. doi: 10.1182/blood.V99.4.1405
137. Vande Broek I, Asosingh K, Allegaert V, Leleu X, Facon T, Vanderkerken K, et al. Bone marrow endothelial cells increase the invasiveness of human multiple myeloma cells through upregulation of MMP-9: evidence for a role of hepatocyte growth factor. *Leukemia* (2004) 18:976–82. doi: 10.1038/sj.leu.2403331
138. Purushothaman A, Uyama T, Kobayashi F, Yamada S, Sugahara K, Rapraeger AC, et al. Heparanase-enhanced Shedding of syndecan-1 by Myeloma Cells Promotes Endothelial Invasion and Angiogenesis. *Blood* (2010) 115:2449–57. doi: 10.1182/blood-2009-07-234757
139. Vacca A, Ribatti D, Presta M, Iurlaro M, Ria R, Albini A, et al. Bone Marrow Neovascularization, Plasma Cell Angiogenic Potential, and Matrix metalloproteinase-2 Secretion Parallel Progression of Human Multiple Myeloma. *Blood* (1999) 93:3064–73. doi: 10.1182/blood.V93.9.3064.409k07_3064_3073

140. Roccaro AM, Hideshima T, Raje N, Kumar S, Ishitsuka K, Yasui H, et al. Bortezomib Mediates Antiangiogenesis in Multiple Myeloma via Direct and Indirect Effects on Endothelial Cells. *Cancer Res* (2006) 66:184–91. doi: 10.1158/0008-5472.CAN-05-1195
141. Dhodapkar MV, Krasovsky J, Olson K. T cells from the tumor microenvironment of patients with progressive myeloma can generate strong, tumor-specific cytolytic responses to autologous, tumor-loaded dendritic cells. *Proc Natl Acad Sci* (2002) 99:13009–13. doi: 10.1073/pnas.202491499
142. Feyler S, von Lilienfeld-Toal M, Jarmin S, Marles L, Rawstron A, Ashcroft AJ, et al. CD4(+)CD25(+)FoxP3(+) regulatory T cells are increased whilst CD3 (+)CD4(-)CD8(-)alphabetaTCR(+) Double Negative T cells are decreased in the peripheral blood of patients with multiple myeloma which correlates with disease burden. *Br J Haematol* (2009) 144:686–95. doi: 10.1111/j.1365-2141.2008.07530.x
143. Nair JR, Carlson LM, Koorella C, Rozanski CH, Byrne GE, Bergsagel LP, et al. CD28 expressed on malignant plasma cells induces a prosurvival and immunosuppressive microenvironment. *J Immunol Baltim Md 1950* (2011) 187:1243–53. doi: 10.4049/jimmunol.1100016
144. Koorella C, Nair JR, Murray ME, Carlson LM, Watkins SK, Lee KP. Novel regulation of CD80/CD86-induced phosphatidylinositol 3-kinase signaling by NOTCH1 protein in interleukin-6 and indoleamine 2,3-dioxygenase production by dendritic cells. *J Biol Chem* (2014) 289:7747–62. doi: 10.1074/jbc.M113.519686
145. Leone P, Di Lernia G, Solimando AG, Cicco S, Saltarella I, Lamanuzzi A, et al. Bone marrow endothelial cells sustain a tumor-specific CD8+ T cell subset with suppressive function in myeloma patients. *Oncoimmunology* (2019) 8:e1486949. doi: 10.1080/2162402X.2018.1486949
146. Mouhieddine TH, Weeks LD, Ghobrial IM. Monoclonal gammopathy of undetermined significance. *Blood* (2019) 133:2484–94. doi: 10.1182/blood.2019846782
147. De Veirman K, Menu E, Maes K, De Beule N, De Smedt E, Maes A, et al. Myeloid-derived suppressor cells induce multiple myeloma cell survival by activating the AMPK pathway. *Cancer Lett* (2019) 442:233–41. doi: 10.1016/j.canlet.2018.11.002
148. De Veirman K, Van Ginderachter JA, Lub S, De Beule N, Thielemans K, Bautmans I, et al. Multiple myeloma induces Mcl-1 expression and survival of myeloid-derived suppressor cells. *Oncotarget* (2015) 6:10532–47. doi: 10.18632/oncotarget.3300
149. Bi E, Li R, Bover LC, Li H, Su P, Ma X, et al. E-cadherin expression on multiple myeloma cells activates tumor-promoting properties in plasmacytoid DCs. *J Clin Invest* (2018) 128:4821–31. doi: 10.1172/JCI121421
150. El-Sherbiny YM, Meade JL, Holmes TD, McGonagle D, Mackie SL, Morgan AW, et al. The Requirement for DNAM-1, NKG2D, and NKp46 in the Natural Killer Cell-Mediated Killing of Myeloma Cells. *Cancer Res* (2007) 67:8444–9. doi: 10.1158/0008-5472.CAN-06-4230
151. Görgün G, Samur MK, Cowens KB, Paula S, Bianchi G, Anderson JE, et al. Lenalidomide Enhances Immune Checkpoint Blockade-Induced Immune Response in Multiple Myeloma. *Clin Cancer Res* (2015) 21:4607–18. doi: 10.1158/1078-0432.CCR-15-0200
152. Pazina T, James AM, MacFarlane AW, Bezman NA, Henning KA, Bee C, et al. The anti-SLAMF7 antibody elotuzumab mediates NK cell activation through both CD16-dependent and -independent mechanisms. *Oncoimmunology* (2017) 6:e1339853. doi: 10.1080/2162402X.2017.1339853
153. Krejcik J, Casneuf T, Nijhof IS, Verbist B, Bald J, Plesner T, et al. Daratumumab depletes CD38+ immune regulatory cells, promotes T-cell expansion, and skews T-cell repertoire in multiple myeloma. *Blood* (2016) 128:384–94. doi: 10.1182/blood-2015-12-687749
154. Viola D, Dona A, Caserta E, Troadec E, Besi F, McDonald T, et al. Daratumumab induces mechanisms of immune activation through CD38+ NKcell targeting. *Leukemia* (2020) 35:1–12. doi: 10.1038/s41375-020-0810-4
155. Witzig TE, Laumann KM, Lacy MQ, Hayman SR, Dispenzieri A, Kumar S, et al. A Phase III Randomized Trial of Thalidomide Plus Zoledronic Acid Versus Zoledronic Acid Alone in Patients With Asymptomatic Multiple Myeloma. *Leukemia* (2013) 27:220–5. doi: 10.1038/leu.2012.236
156. Mateos MV, Hernandez MT, Giraldo P, de la Rubia J, de Arriba F, Corral LL, et al. Lenalidomide Plus Dexamethasone for High-Risk Smoldering Multiple Myeloma. *N Engl J Med* (2013) 369:438–47. doi: 10.1056/NEJMoa1300439
157. Korde N, Zingone A, Kwok M, Manasanch EE, Bhutani M, Costello R, et al. Phase II clinical and correlative study of carfilzomib, lenalidomide, and dexamethasone (CRd) in newly diagnosed multiple myeloma (MM) patients. *J Clin Oncol* (2012) 30:e18568–8. doi: 10.1200/jco.2012.30.15_suppl.e18568
158. Lonial S, Jacobus SJ, Weiss M, Kumar S, Orlowski RZ, Kaufman JL, et al. E3A06: Randomized phase III trial of lenalidomide versus observation alone in patients with asymptomatic high-risk smoldering multiple myeloma. *J Clin Oncol* (2019) 37:8001–1. doi: 10.1200/JCO.2019.37.15_suppl.8001
159. Kumar S, Rajkumar SV, Kyle RA, Lacy MQ, Dispenzieri A, Fonseca R, et al. Prognostic value of circulating plasma cells in monoclonal gammopathy of undetermined significance. *J Clin Oncol* (2005) 23:5668–74. doi: 10.1200/JCO.2005.03.159
160. Butcher EC, Picker LJ. Lymphocyte homing and homeostasis. *Science* (1996) 272:60–6. doi: 10.1126/science.272.5258.60
161. Vande Broek I, Leleu X, Schots R, Facon T, Vanderkerken K, Van Camp B, et al. Clinical significance of chemokine receptor (CCR1, CCR2 and CXCR4) expression in human myeloma cells: the association with disease activity and survival. *Haematologica* (2006) 91:200–6.
162. Bhutani M, Foureau DM, Atrash S, Voorhees PM, Usmani SZ. Extramedullary multiple myeloma. *Leukemia* (2020) 34:1–20. doi: 10.1038/s41375-019-0660-0
163. Dahl IMS, Rasmussen T, Kauric G, Husebekk A. Differential expression of CD56 and CD44 in the evolution of extramedullary myeloma. *Br J Haematol* (2002) 116:273–7. doi: 10.1046/j.1365-2141.2002.03258.x
164. Azab AK, Quang P, Azab F, Pitsillides C, Thompson B, Chonghaile T, et al. P-selectin glycoprotein ligand regulates the interaction of multiple myeloma cells with the bone marrow microenvironment. *Blood* (2012) 119:1468–78. doi: 10.1182/blood-2011-07-368050
165. Wang S-Y, Hao HL, Deng K, Li Y, Cheng ZY, Chao LV, et al. Expression levels of phosphatase and tensin homolog deleted on chromosome 10 (PTEN) and focal adhesion kinase in patients with multiple myeloma and their relationship to clinical stage and extramedullary infiltration. *Leuk Lymphoma* (2012) 53:1162–8. doi: 10.3109/10428194.2011.647311
166. Tohami T, Drucker L, Shapiro H, Radnay J, Lishner M. Overexpression of Tetraspanins Affects Multiple Myeloma Cell Survival and Invasive Potential. *FASEB J* (2007) 21:691–9. doi: 10.1096/fj.06-6610com
167. Broek IV, Vanderkerken K, Camp BV, Riet IV. Extravasation and homing mechanisms in multiple myeloma. *Clin Exp Metastasis* (2008) 25:325–34. doi: 10.1007/s10585-007-9108-4
168. Li J, Pan Q, Rowan PD, Trotter TN, Peker D, Regal KM, et al. Heparanase promotes myeloma progression by inducing mesenchymal features and motility of myeloma cells. *Oncotarget* (2016) 7:11299–309. doi: 10.18632/oncotarget.7170
169. Morgan GJ, Walker BA, Davies FE. The genetic architecture of multiple myeloma. *Nat Rev Cancer* (2012) 12:335–48. doi: 10.1038/nrc3257
170. Jelinek T, Bezdekova R, Zatopkova M, Burgos L, Simicek M, Sevcikova T, et al. Current applications of multiparameter flow cytometry in plasma cell disorders. *Blood Cancer J* (2017) 7:e617. doi: 10.1038/bcj.2017.90
171. Matsuda Y, Naito Z, Kawahara K, Nakazawa N, Korc M, Ishiwata T. Nestin is a novel target for suppressing pancreatic cancer cell migration, invasion and metastasis. *Cancer Biol Ther* (2011) 11:512–23. doi: 10.4161/cbt.11.5.14673
172. Shaffer AL, Emre NCT, Lamy L, Ngo VN, Wright G, Xiao W, et al. IRF4 addiction in multiple myeloma. *Nature* (2008) 454:226–31. doi: 10.1038/nature07064
173. Børset M, Lien E, Espevik T, Helseth E, Waage A, Sundan A. Concomitant Expression of Hepatocyte Growth Factor/Scatter Factor and the Receptor c-MET in Human Myeloma Cell Lines. *J Biol Chem* (1996) 271:24655–61. doi: 10.1074/jbc.271.40.24655
174. Derksen PWB, de Gorter DJJ, Meijer HP, Bende RJ, van Dijk M, Lokhorst HM, et al. The hepatocyte growth factor/Met pathway controls proliferation and apoptosis in multiple myeloma. *Leukemia* (2003) 17:764–74. doi: 10.1038/sj.leu.2402875
175. Azab AK, Hu J, Quang P, Azab F, Pitsillides C, Awwad R, et al. Hypoxia promotes dissemination of multiple myeloma through acquisition of epithelial to mesenchymal transition-like features. *Blood* (2012) 119:5782–94. doi: 10.1182/blood-2011-09-380410

176. Dimopoulos M, Spencer A, Attal M, Prince HM, Harousseau JL, Dmoszynska A, et al. Lenalidomide plus dexamethasone for relapsed or refractory multiple myeloma. *N Engl J Med* (2007) 357:2123–32. doi: 10.1056/NEJMoa070594
177. Schinke CD, Ashby C, Wang Y, Tytarenko RG, Boyle E, Wardell C, et al. The Mutational Landscape of Primary Plasma Cell Leukemia. *Blood* (2018) 132:114–4. doi: 10.1182/blood-2018-99-116758
178. Cifola I, Lionetti M, Pinatel E, Todoerti K, Mangano E, Pietrelli A, et al. Whole-exome sequencing of primary plasma cell leukemia discloses heterogeneous mutational patterns. *Oncotarget* (2015) 6:17543–58. doi: 10.18632/oncotarget.4028

6

Durable Response to Sintilimab and Chidamide in a Patient with Pegaspargase- and Immunotherapy-Resistant NK/T-Cell Lymphoma

*Zheng Yan[1], Shuna Yao[1], Yanyan Liu[1], Jianbo Zhang[2], Peng Li[3], Haiying Wang[1], Junfeng Chu[1], Shuang Zhao[1] and Zhihua Yao[1]**

[1] Department of Internal Medicine, Affiliated Cancer Hospital of Zhengzhou University and Henan Cancer Hospital, Zhengzhou, China, [2] Department of Pathology, Affiliated Cancer Hospital of Zhengzhou University and Henan Cancer Hospital, Zhengzhou, China, [3] The PET-CT Center of Henan Province, Affiliated Cancer Hospital of Zhengzhou University and Henan Cancer Hospital, Zhengzhou, China

***Correspondence:**
Zhihua Yao
zlyyyaozhihua1260@zzu.edu.cn

The prognosis of patients with relapsed/refractory NK/T-cell lymphoma (NKTCL) is dismal. Immunotherapy has showed encouraging anti-tumor activity in patients with asparaginase-resistant NKTCL; however, only a portion of patients benefit and the median response duration is rather short. Treatment strategies have not been identified for immunotherapy-resistant NKTCL. We describe a patient with primary cutaneous NKTCL experienced disease progression after pegaspargase-based chemotherapy and PD-1 inhibitor (sintilimab)-based immunotherapy. Following a combined treatment of sintilimab and the HDAC inhibitor chidamide, the patient achieved a durable complete molecular response with mild toxicity. This case indicates that the combination of PD-1 inhibitor and HDAC inhibitor might be a treatment choice for immunotherapy-resistant NKTCL.

Keywords: NK/T-cell lymphoma, immunotherapy, chidamide, immunotherapy resistance, sintilimab, case report

BACKGROUND

NK/T-cell lymphoma (NKTCL) is a rare and aggressive hematological malignancy. It mainly involves the upper aerodigestive tract, less commonly the skin, soft tissue, and gastrointestinal tract (1). Most patients with early-stage NKTCL can be cured with radiotherapy or combined radio-chemotherapy; however, patients with an advanced form of the disease have a dismal prognosis with a median survival of several months (2, 3). Historically, NKTCL responded poorly to conventional cytotoxic drugs probably because of inherent multidrug resistance; while it was sensitive to L-asparaginase (or pegaspargase) due to the unique anti-tumor mechanism for asparaginase and the fatal weakness of NKTCL cells. All normal body cells can produce asparagine by asparagine synthetase, while NKTCL cells are unable to synthesize the amino acid. Asparaginase therapy depletes serum asparagine. When the host serum asparagine is depleted by asparaginase, protein synthesis in NKTCL cells stops, leading to cancer cell death (4). Asparaginase alone or in combination with different cytotoxic drugs has showed good immediate efficacy in NKTCL treatment (5). However, disease relapse frequently occurs due to acquired drug resistance to asparaginase. Nowadays, there are limited treatment options for asparaginase-resistant NKTCL.

Recently, anti-PD-1/PD-L1 immunotherapy constitutes a new treatment option for relapsed/refractory (r/r) NKTCL. The PD-1 inhibitors pembrolizumab and sintilimab, as well as the PD-L1 inhibitor avelumab, have yielded encouraging effects in several case series reports and small sample-sized clinical trials (6); however, only a small portion of patients benefit, reflecting common primary and/or acquired resistance to immunotherapy and less durable response. Therefore, it is necessary to identify and evaluate novel treatment strategies for immunotherapy-resistant NKTCL. In this study, we reported a case with both pegaspargase- and immunotherapy-resistant NKTCL that achieved durable response to a combined treatment of sintilimab with the histone deacetylase inhibitor (HDACi) chidamide.

CASE PRESENTATION

At his first visit, a 24-year-old young man stated that two years ago his face, especially eyelids, was slightly red and swollen without any discomfort (**Figure 1A**). He had no notable past and family medical history. Since then, his facial swelling has persisted without obvious changes and medical intervention, but in recent two months the face swelling was rapidly aggravated with fever. He was admitted to our hospital in October 2019 with intermittent fever in the absence of weight loss and night sweat. The maximum body temperature was 38.3° C. Physical examination revealed that his whole face was red and swollen with a mucosal ulcer in the inner lower lip (**Figures 1B, C**). Laboratory examination revealed an elevated lactate dehydrogenase level of 319 U/L and erythrocyte sedimentation rate of 39 mm/h. Plasma EBV-DNA titer was 2.11×10^4 copies/ml. Other laboratory parameters were normal. Biopsy from the oral ulcer showed acute and chronic mucosal inflammation with infiltration of medium-sized atypical lymphoid cells. The infiltrating lymphocytes were positive for CD3, CD56, TIA-1, and Granzyme B, negative for CD20 and

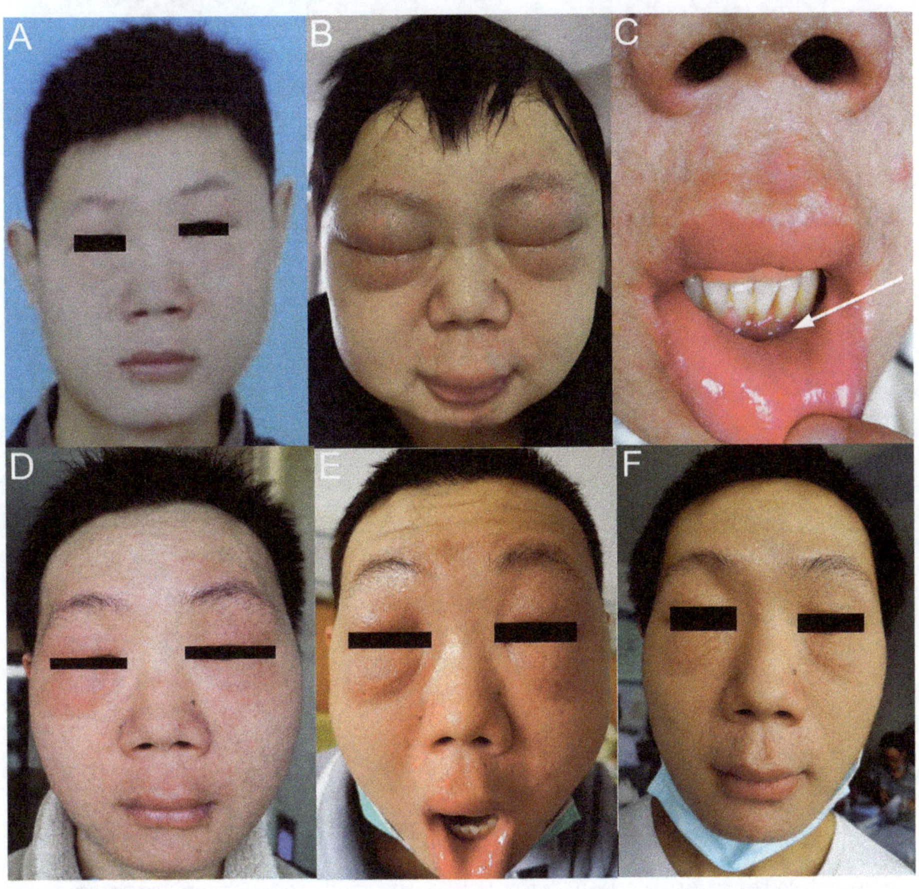

FIGURE 1 | Facial features of the patient with NKTCL. **(A)** Two years before diagnosis. **(B)** At the time of diagnosis of NKTCL. **(C)** Mucosal ulcer in the inner lower lip at diagnosis. **(D)** After completing 3 cycles of P-GemOx regimen chemotherapy. **(E)** After one cycle of sintilimab and decitabine combination treatment. **(F)** After four cycles of sintilimab and chidamide combination treatment.

CD30, and focally positive for CD8. Ki-67 was positive in 90% cancer cells. *In situ* hybridization revealed EBV infection in the majority of neoplastic cells (**Figure 2**). The diagnosis of NKTCL was made based on the morphology, immunohistochemistry, and EBV status. Positron emission tomography-computed tomography (PET/CT) (**Figures 3A–D**) and magnetic resonance imaging (MRI) (**Figures 3E, F**) showed that the facial soft tissues, eyelids, and lips were swollen with hypermetabolic activity (SUVmax 10.3). Bone marrow smear and flow cytometry analysis were negative.

From November 13, 2019 to December 27, 2019, the patient was given three cycles of P-GemOx regimen (pegaspargase, gemcitabine, and oxaliplatin) chemotherapy. After two cycles of treatment, his facial swelling alleviated, fever disappeared, and the plasma EBV-DNA titer reduced to an undetectable level. However, there was no further improvement for the facial swelling following the third cycle of chemotherapy (**Figure 1D**) and the plasma EBV-DNA titer came back and was increased to 1.15×10^3 copies/ml, indicating the development of acquired resistance to pegaspargase-based chemotherapy.

On January 15, 2020, the patient was treated with sintilimab (200 mg) as second-line treatment. In a prior study, decitabine, a DNA methyltransferase inhibitor, was showed to increase the efficacy of PD-1 blockade immunotherapy in patients with Hodgkin lymphoma (7). Considering only a short progression-free survival (PFS) in the trials of immunotherapy in r/r NKTCL patients (**Table 1**), a priming treatment with decitabine was administered to the patient in addition to sintilimab. Unexpectedly, the patient's facial swelling was slightly aggravated (**Figure 1E**), accompanied by the reappearance of fever, and the plasma EBV-DNA titer was increased to 7.02×10^3 copies/ml. Though the face swelling was not a definite indicator of drug efficacy, the reappearing fever and elevated plasma EBV-DNA titer strongly indicate the disease out of control.

We gave the patient an oral treatment of HDACi chidamide (30 mg every three days) beginning February 5, 2020.

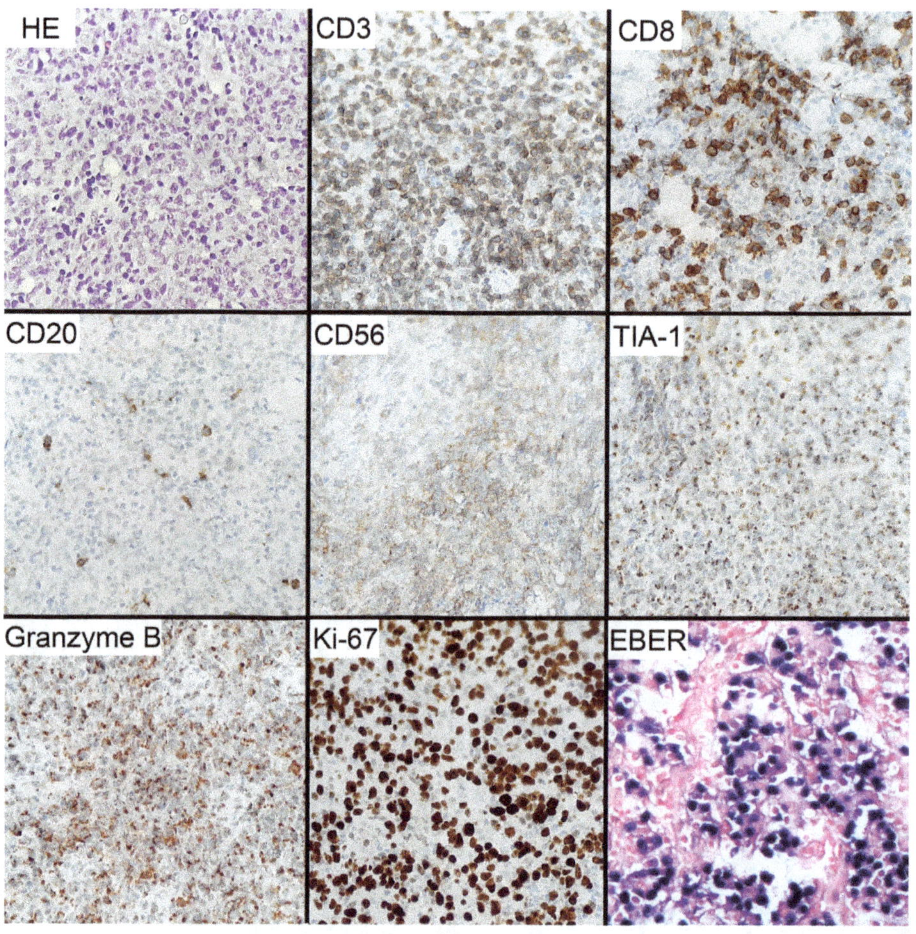

FIGURE 2 | Microscopic and immunohistochemical features of NKTCL tumor. Histological examination of H&E-stained tissues shows infiltration of medium-sized cells with irregular nuclei and inconspicuous nucleoli. Immunohistochemical staining shows positive CD3, CD56, TIA-1, and granzyme B, focally positive CD8, and negative CD20. Ki-67 proliferation index was about 90%. In situ hybridization for EBV-encoded RNA (EBER) reveals positive reaction. Original manifestation 400×.

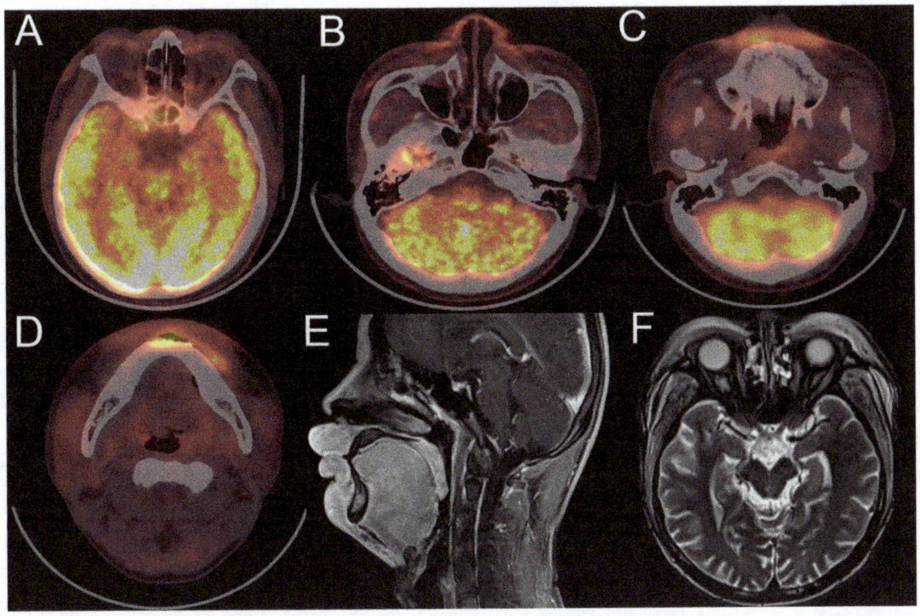

FIGURE 3 | Face imaging features of the patient at diagnosis. **(A–D)** PET/CT shows thickened and FDG-avid midline facial skin. **(E, F)** MRI sagittal plane and horizontal views show thickened facial skin and hyperintensity on T2-weighted imaging.

TABLE 1 | Reports of r/r NKTCL treated with immunotherapy.

Author	Study	No.	Treatment	Response	PFS
Tao et al. (8)	Phase 2	28	Sintilimab	19 (CR + PR)	–
Kim et al. (9)	Phase 2	21	Avelumab	5 CR, 3 PR	2.7 m (median)
Kim et al. (10)	Retrospective	14	Pembrolizumab	5 CR, 1 PR	–
Kwong et al. (11)	Case series	7	Pembrolizumab	5 CR, 2 PR	–
Li et al. (12)	Case series	7	pembrolizumab	2 CR, 2 PR	4.8 m (median)
Chan et al. (13)	Case series	3	Nivolumab	1 CR	–
Klee et al. (14)	Case report[a]	1	Pembrolizumab + radiotherapy	CR	>2 y
Kim et al. (15)	Case report	1	Pembrolizumab + haploidentical HSCT	CR	>6 m
Asif et al. (16)	Case report	1	Pembrolizumab + radiotherapy	CR	4 m
Lai et al. (17)	Case report	1	Pembrolizumab	CR[b]	>8 m

CR, complete response; PR, partial response; m, month; y, year. [a]This case had an early-stage disease; [b]This was a radiological complete response. The plasma EBV-DNA was persistent positive.

Meanwhile, the immunotherapy with sintilimab was administered continuously. The fever disappeared after several days of the combined treatment; the plasma EBV-DNA titer was quickly reduced to undetectable level at the end of the first cycle of the combined treatment and kept at this level thereafter, indicating a molecular complete response (CR) was achieved. A grade 1 thrombocytopenia and anemia occurred during the course of the combined treatment. After four cycles of the combined treatment, the patient's facial swelling had subsided, and he looked totally normal (**Figure 1F**). The dose of chidamide was reduced to 20 mg every three days thereafter and both thrombocytopenia and anemia were resolved. The patient was very satisfied with the treatment. He went to his work after six cycles of treatment. Hematopoietic stem cell transplantation was recommended in order to improve long-term outcome, but the patient refused. He has received nine cycles of treatment by the submission date of this article. A detailed treatment process and the changes of plasma EBV-DNA titers are shown in **Figure 4**.

DISCUSSION AND LITERATURE REVIEW

According to primary tumor location, NKTCL can be classified into two subtypes (1): nasal NKTCL involving the upper aerodigestive tract, including nasal cavity, nasopharynx, oral cavity, oropharynx, and hypopharynx; and (2) extranasal NKTCL involving any other organ or tissue such as skin, gastrointestinal tract, bone, and lung (18, 19). Extranasal NKTCL accounts for approximately 20% of newly diagnosed cases (20, 21). Generally, the prognosis of extranasal NKTCL is poorer than that of nasal NKTCL. The median overall survival

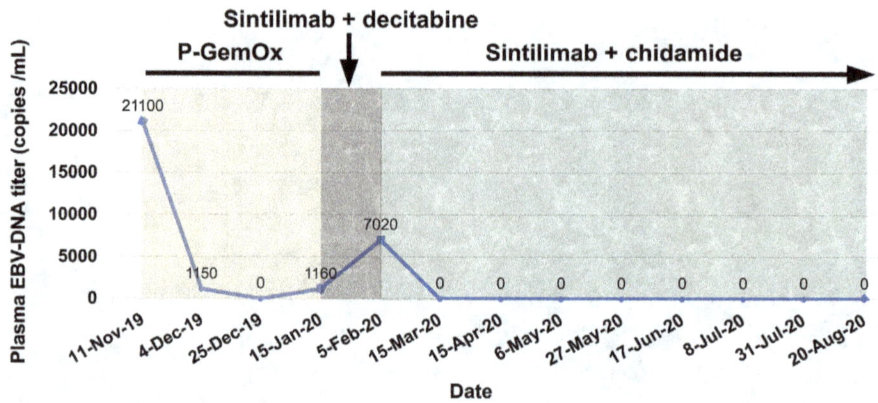

FIGURE 4 | Treatment process and the changes of plasma EBV-DNA titers.

time is only 3.4 months in patients with advanced extranasal NKTCL (19).

Over the past decade, significant progress has been made in the treatment of NKTCL. On the one hand, radiotherapy has been used as a curative option for early-stage NKTCL (22, 23). About 80% early-stage NKTCL patients were cured by radiotherapy alone or in combination with chemotherapy (2). One the other hand, the importance of L-asparaginase has been widely recognized in the treatment of NKTCL. The CR rate generally exceeded 50% in NKTCL patients treated with asparaginase (or pegaspargase)-containing chemotherapy. However, these progresses largely benefited those patients with early-stage disease. Relatively, patients with advanced disease had a dismal outcome, with a median survival of only several months even asparaginase-based chemotherapy was used (3, 21). Besides, asparaginase-based chemotherapy did not seem to improve the survival of patients with extranasal NKTCL (24, 25). Thus, novel treatment strategies are urgently needed for NKTCL patients with advanced disease, especially asparaginase-resistant disease.

NKTCL is universally associated with EBV infection in the lymphoma cells. EBV-DNA levels in peripheral blood are a surrogate biomarker of tumor loads, which are useful for prognostic assessment and treatment response evaluation. High plasma EBV-DNA levels, both pre- and post-treatment, correlate with worse clinical outcomes (26, 27). On the other hand, EBV infection is associated with higher PD-L1 expression in lymphoma cells and better response to immunotherapy (9, 10, 28, 29). Several case reports, case series, and small sample-sized phase 2 trials have demonstrated the anticancer activity of PD-1/PD-L1 blockade immunotherapy in NKTCL patients (**Table 1**). Based on these practices, the PD-1 inhibitors pembrolizumab and nivolumab were recently recommended by the NCCN guidelines as an alternative treatment option for r/r NKTCL. It seems that immunotherapy has convincing short-term efficacy in r/r NKTCL, but the long-term outcomes of immunotherapy-treated patients are still disappointing. Until now, the largest prospective clinical trial involving immunotherapy in r/r NKTCL patients has been conducted in China, in which 28 patients were treated with sintilimab. Of them, 19 patients achieved an objective response (8). In another phase 2 trial enrolling 21 patients in Korea, avelumab achieved CR in five patients and PR in three patients, with a median PFS of 2.7 months (9). Kim et al. reported five out of 14 patients treated with pembrolizumab achieved CR (10). Two retrospective case series studies reported five CR and one CR in seven and three patients, respectively (11, 13). In another case series study with seven patients with pembrolizumab treatment, two patients achieved CR, and the median PFS was 4.8 months (12). Klee et al. reported one patient who had survived more than 2 years following a combined treatment of pembrolizumab and radiotherapy, but it should be noted that this case had an early-stage disease (14). With the emergence of various new anti-tumor drugs, immunotherapy-based treatment for NKTCL is continuously evolving to improve patient outcomes. Clinical trials evaluating the combination of immunotherapy with various cancer therapies are currently under investigation, including cytotoxic drugs, PI3K inhibitor, HDACi, CAR-T cell therapy, and antiangiogenic agent (**Table 2**).

Chidamide, a subtype-selective HDACi, was approved in China for patients with relapsed or refractory peripheral T-cell lymphoma. It is also used to treat r/r NKTCL. In a phase 2 trial including various types of T- and NK-cell lymphomas, the ORR was 19% in 16 NKTCL patients and the median PFS was 2.1 months (30). In addition to its direct anticancer activity, HDACi has pleiotropic immunomodulatory effects (31–33). HDACi can enhance the intratumoral infiltration of CD8+ T cells and macrophages, decrease the intratumoral infiltration of T-regulatory cells, myeloid-derived suppressor cells, and pro-tumorigenic M2 macrophages, induce the intratumoral expression of multiple chemokines, upregulate the expression of MHC and co-stimulatory molecules, enhance immune recognition, promote tumor-specific T cell-mediated killing of cancer cells, and sensitize tumor cells to NK cell lysis (32, 34–42). Preclinical studies have demonstrated that HDACi can enhance the anticancer activity of immunotherapy in several types of cancers (36, 37, 43–45). Currently, there are dozens of clinical trials evaluating the feasibility of combining HDACi and immunotherapy across multiple cancer types (32, 34).

TABLE 2 | Ongoing clinical trials utilizing immune checkpoint blockade in NKTCL (by 10-Aug-2020).

Phase	Trial Intervention	Status; Estimated completion date	NCT ID
1	MEDI-570 (anti-ICOS antibody)	Recruiting; December 2020	02520791
1	Pembrolizumab + modified SMILE and ASCT	Recruiting; December 2023	03719105
1/2	Pembrolizumab Pembrolizumab + copanlisib	Recruiting; December 2022	02535247
1/2	Sintilimab + chidamide	Recruiting; February 2025	03820596
1/2	Pembrolizumab + romidepsin	Active, not recruiting; November 2020	03278782
1/2	Pembrolizumab + pralatrexate	Recruiting; April 2021	03598998
2	Nivolumab + talimogene laherparepvec	Recruiting; June 2021	02978625
2	Pembrolizumab + radiotherapy	Recruiting; November 2020	03210662
NA	Cemrelizumab + pegaspargase + apatinib	Recruiting; December 2023	04366128

ICOS, Inducible T-cell co-stimulator; SMILE, Dexamethasone, methotrexate, ifosfamide, pegaspargase, and etoposide; ASCT, Allogeneic stem cell transplantation; NA, not availabe.

In this study, the primary cutaneous NKTCL acquired resistance after a short response to pegaspargase-based chemotherapy. It was known that a transient increase of tumor volume, called pseudoprogression, in immunotherapy-treated patients. Nevertheless, it was unlikely a pseudogprogression in this case after one cycle of sintilimab and decitabine combination therapy, as together with tumor regrowth, the lymphoma-related fever reappeared and the plasma EBV-DNA titer, a sensitive indicator of NKTCL load, was increased following the combined treatment. Therefore, we believe that this case was primarily resistant to sintilimab. Based on the aforementioned immunomodulatory effects of HDACi, chidamide was used in combination with sintilimab as third-line treatment for this patient. An excellent response was observed: the fever and plasma EBV-DNA disappeared very quickly after the first cycle of the combined regimen treatment, and the response has lasted for over 6 months so far. The result of this study should be interpreted with caution, because chidamide alone has anti-cancer activity. It is not sure whether the excellent response in this patient was attributed to the synergistic action of sintilimab and chidamide or to chidamide alone. Currently, there is an ongoing phase 1/2 trial assessing the efficacy and safety of sintilimab plus chidamide in patients with r/r NKTCL (NCT 03820596). It may take time to get the results but it is worth the wait.

CONCLUSION

There are limited treatment options for patients with r/r NKTCL, especially those resistant to asparaginase and immunotherapy. We reported herein that a pegaspargase- and immunotherapy-resistant patient achieved durable response from the combined treatment of sintilimab and chidamide with mild toxicity. This combination regimen of immunotherapy and HDACi is a promising treatment choice for patients with r/r NKTCL.

ETHICS STATEMENT

The studies involving human participants were reviewed and approved by Institutional Review Board of Affiliated Cancer Hospital of Zhengzhou University. The patients/participants provided their written informed consent to participate in this study. Written informed consent was obtained from the individuals for the publication of any potentially identifiable images or data included in this article.

AUTHOR CONTRIBUTIONS

ZheY and ZhiY: designed the study. ZheY, SY, YL, HW, JC, SZ, and ZhiY: treated the patient and collected the data. ZheY, JZ, and PL: collected and analyzed the data. ZheY and ZhiY: wrote the original draft. All authors contributed to the article and approved the submitted version.

REFERENCES

1. Aozasa K, Zaki MA. Epidemiology and pathogenesis of nasal NK/T-cell lymphoma: a mini-review. *ScientificWorldJournal* (2011) 11:422–8. doi: 10.1100/tsw.2011.41
2. Qi SN, Yang Y, Zhang YJ, Huang HQ, Wang Y, He X, et al. Risk-based, response-adapted therapy for early-stage extranodal nasal-type NK/T-cell lymphoma in the modern chemotherapy era: A China Lymphoma Collaborative Group study. *Am J Hematol* (2020). doi: 10.1002/ajh.25878
3. Kim SJ, Park S, Kang ES, Choi JY, Lim DH, Ko YH, et al. Induction treatment with SMILE and consolidation with autologous stem cell transplantation for newly diagnosed stage IV extranodal natural killer/T-cell lymphoma patients. *Ann Hematol* (2015) 94(1):71–8. doi: 10.1007/s00277-014-2171-4
4. Ando M, Sugimoto K, Kitoh T, Sasaki M, Mukai K, Ando J, et al. Selective apoptosis of natural killer-cell tumours by l-asparaginase. *Br J Haematol* (2005) 130(6):860–8. doi: 10.1111/j.1365-2141.2005.05694.x
5. Pokrovsky VS, Vinnikov D. L-Asparaginase for newly diagnosed extra-nodal NK/T-cell lymphoma: systematic review and meta-analysis. *Expert Rev Anticancer Ther* (2017) 17(8):759–68. doi: 10.1080/14737140.2017.1344100
6. Wang L, Li LR, Zhang L, Wang JW. The landscape of new drugs in extranodal NK/T-cell lymphoma. *Cancer Treat Rev* (2020) 89:102065. doi: 10.1016/j.ctrv.2020.102065

7. Nie J, Wang C, Liu Y, Yang Q, Mei Q, Dong L, et al. Addition of Low-Dose Decitabine to Anti-PD-1 Antibody Camrelizumab in Relapsed/Refractory Classical Hodgkin Lymphoma. *J Clin Oncol* (2019) 37: (17):1479–89. doi: 10.1200/JCO.18.02151
8. Tao R. *Sintilimab for relapsed/refractory (r/r) extranodal NK/T cell lymphoma (ENKTL): A multicenter s-a, phase 2 trial (ORIENT-4).* Chicago, IL: John Wiley and Sons (2019) p. 102–3.
9. Kim SJ, Lim JQ, Laurensia Y, Cho J, Yoon SE, Lee JY, et al. Avelumab for the treatment of relapsed or refractory extranodal NK/T-cell lymphoma: an open-label phase 2 study. *Blood* (2020) 113:3931–7. doi: 10.1182/blood.2020007247
10. Kim SJ, Hyeon J, Cho I, Ko YH, Kim WS. Comparison of Efficacy of Pembrolizumab between Epstein-Barr VirusPositive and Negative Relapsed or Refractory Non-Hodgkin Lymphomas. *Cancer Res Treat* (2019) 51(2):611–22. doi: 10.4143/crt.2018.191
11. Kwong YL, Chan TSY, Tan D, Kim SJ, Poon LM, Mow B, et al. PD1 blockade with pembrolizumab is highly effective in relapsed or refractory NK/T-cell lymphoma failing l-asparaginase. *Blood* (2017) 129(17):2437–42. doi: 10.1182/blood-2016-12-756841
12. Li X, Cheng Y, Zhang M, Yan J, Li L, Fu X, et al. Activity of pembrolizumab in relapsed/refractory NK/T-cell lymphoma. *J Hematol Oncol* (2018) 11(1):15. doi: 10.1186/s13045-018-0559-7
13. Chan TSY, Li J, Loong F, Khong PL, Tse E, Kwong YL. PD1 blockade with low-dose nivolumab in NK/T cell lymphoma failing L-asparaginase: efficacy and safety. *Ann Hematol* (2018) 97(1):193–6. doi: 10.1007/s00277-017-3127-2
14. Klee G, von Ducker L, Terheyden P. Sustained complete remission of extranodal NK/T-cell lymphoma, nasal type, following pembrolizumab and radiation therapy. *J Dtsch Dermatol Ges* (2020) 98:1647–55. doi: 10.1111/ddg.14142
15. Kim YE, Kim H, Shin J, Min SY, Kang SH, Suh JK, et al. Stage IV natural killer/T-cell lymphoma with chronic active Epstein-Barr virus, treated with pembrolizumab and TCRalphabeta-depleted haploidentical hematopoietic stem cell transplantation. *Leuk Lymphoma* (2020) 1-4:106284. doi: 10.1080/10428194.2020.1757666
16. Asif S, Begemann M, Bennett J, Fatima R, Masood A, Raza S. Pembrolizumab in newly diagnosed EBV-negative extranodal natural killer/T-cell lymphoma: A case report. *Mol Clin Oncol* (2019) 10(3):397–400. doi: 10.3892/mco.2019.1805
17. Lai J, Xu P, Jiang X, Zhou S, Liu A. Successful treatment with anti-programmed-death-1 antibody in a relapsed natural killer/T-cell lymphoma patient with multi-line resistance: a case report. *BMC Cancer* (2017) 17 (1):507. doi: 10.1186/s12885-017-3501-4
18. Jo JC, Yoon DH, Kim S, Lee BJ, Jang YJ, Park CS, et al. Clinical features and prognostic model for extranasal NK/T-cell lymphoma. *Eur J Haematol* (2012) 89(2):103–10. doi: 10.1111/j.1600-0609.2012.01796.x
19. Au WY, Weisenburger DD, Intragumtornchai T, Nakamura S, Kim WS, Sng I, et al. Clinical differences between nasal and extranasal natural killer/T-cell lymphoma: a study of 136 cases from the International Peripheral T-Cell Lymphoma Project. *Blood* (2009) 113(17):3931–7. doi: 10.1182/blood-2008-10-185256
20. Suzuki R, Suzumiya J, Yamaguchi M, Nakamura S, Kameoka J, Kojima H, et al. Prognostic factors for mature natural killer (NK) cell neoplasms: aggressive NK cell leukemia and extranodal NK cell lymphoma, nasal type. *Ann Oncol* (2010) 21(5):1032–40. doi: 10.1093/annonc/mdp418
21. Yan Z, Huang HQ, Wang XX, Gao Y, Zhang YJ, Bai B, et al. A TNM Staging System for Nasal NK/T-Cell Lymphoma. *PLoS One* (2015) 10(6):e0130984. doi: 10.1371/journal.pone.0130984
22. Deng XW, Wu JX, Wu T, Zhu SY, Shi M, Su H, et al. Radiotherapy is essential after complete response to asparaginase-containing chemotherapy in early-stage extranodal nasal-type NK/T-cell lymphoma: A multicenter study from the China Lymphoma Collaborative Group (CLCG). *Radiother Oncol* (2018) 129(1):3–9. doi: 10.1016/j.radonc.2018.04.026
23. Vargo JA, Patel A, Glaser SM, Balasubramani GK, Farah RJ, Marks SM, et al. The impact of the omission or inadequate dosing of radiotherapy in extranodal natural killer T-cell lymphoma, nasal type, in the United States. *Cancer* (2017) 123(16):3176–85. doi: 10.1002/cncr.30697
24. Yamaguchi M, Suzuki R, Miyazaki K, Amaki J, Takizawa J, Sekiguchi N, et al. Improved prognosis of extranodal NK/T cell lymphoma, nasal type of nasal origin but not extranasal origin. *Ann Hematol* (2019) 98(7):1647–55. doi: 10.1007/s00277-019-03689-9
25. Jiang L, Li P, Quan Q, Chen P, Qiu H, Zhang B. Cutaneous extranodal natural killer (NK) / T - cell lymphoma: A comprehensive clinical features and outcomes analysis of 71 cases. *Leuk Res* (2020) 88:106284. doi: 10.1016/j.leukres.2019.106284
26. Suzuki R, Yamaguchi M, Izutsu K, Yamamoto G, Takada K, Harabuchi Y, et al. Prospective measurement of Epstein-Barr virus-DNA in plasma and peripheral blood mononuclear cells of extranodal NK/T-cell lymphoma, nasal type. *Blood* (2011) 118(23):6018–22. doi: 10.1182/blood-2011-05-354142
27. Kimura H, Kwong YL. EBV Viral Loads in Diagnosis, Monitoring, and Response Assessment. *Front Oncol* (2019) 9:62. doi: 10.3389/fonc.2019.00062
28. Bi XW, Wang H, Zhang WW, Wang JH, Liu WJ, Xia ZJ, et al. PD-L1 is upregulated by EBV-driven LMP1 through NF-kappaB pathway and correlates with poor prognosis in natural killer/T-cell lymphoma. *J Hematol Oncol* (2016) 9(1):109. doi: 10.1186/s13045-016-0341-7
29. Chen BJ, Chapuy B, Ouyang J, Sun HH, Roemer MG, Xu ML, et al. PD-L1 expression is characteristic of a subset of aggressive B-cell lymphomas and virus-associated malignancies. *Clin Cancer Res* (2013) 19(13):3462–73. doi: 10.1158/1078-0432.CCR-13-0855
30. Shi Y, Dong M, Hong X, Zhang W, Feng J, Zhu J, et al. Results from a multicenter, open-label, pivotal phase II study of chidamide in relapsed or refractory peripheral T-cell lymphoma. *Ann Oncol* (2015) 26(8):1766–71. doi: 10.1093/annonc/mdv237
31. Zhao LM, Zhang JH. Histone Deacetylase Inhibitors in Tumor Immunotherapy. *Curr Med Chem* (2019) 26(17):2990–3008. doi: 10.2174/0929867324666170801102124
32. Mazzone R, Zwergel C, Mai A, Valente S. Epi-drugs in combination with immunotherapy: a new avenue to improve anticancer efficacy. *Clin Epigenet* (2017) 9:59. doi: 10.1186/s13148-017-0358-y
33. Conte M, De Palma R, Altucci L. HDAC inhibitors as epigenetic regulators for cancer immunotherapy. *Int J Biochem Cell Biol* (2018) 98:65–74. doi: 10.1016/j.biocel.2018.03.004
34. Briere D, Sudhakar N, Woods DM, Hallin J, Engstrom LD, Aranda R, et al. The class I/IV HDAC inhibitor mocetinostat increases tumor antigen presentation, decreases immune suppressive cell types and augments checkpoint inhibitor therapy. *Cancer Immunol Immunother* (2018) 67 (3):381–92. doi: 10.1007/s00262-017-2091-y
35. Hicks KC, Fantini M, Donahue RN, Schwab A, Knudson KM, Tritsch SR, et al. Epigenetic priming of both tumor and NK cells augments antibody-dependent cellular cytotoxicity elicited by the anti-PD-L1 antibody avelumab against multiple carcinoma cell types. *Oncoimmunology* (2018) 7 (11):e1466018. doi: 10.1080/2162402X.2018.1466018
36. Bretz AC, Parnitzke U, Kronthaler K, Dreker T, Bartz R, Hermann F, et al. Domatinostat favors the immunotherapy response by modulating the tumor immune microenvironment (TIME). *J Immunother Cancer* (2019) 7(1):294. doi: 10.1186/s40425-019-0745-3
37. Knox T, Sahakian E, Banik D, Hadley M, Palmer E, Noonepalle S, et al. Selective HDAC6 inhibitors improve anti-PD-1 immune checkpoint blockade therapy by decreasing the anti-inflammatory phenotype of macrophages and down-regulation of immunosuppressive proteins in tumor cells. *Sci Rep* (2019) 9(1):6136. doi: 10.1038/s41598-019-42237-3
38. Ugurel S, Spassova I, Wohlfarth J, Drusio C, Cherouny A, Melior A, et al. MHC class-I downregulation in PD-1/PD-L1 inhibitor refractory Merkel cell carcinoma and its potential reversal by histone deacetylase inhibition: a case series. *Cancer Immunol Immunother* (2019) 68(6):983–90. doi: 10.1007/s00262-019-02341-9
39. Adeshakin AO, Yan D, Zhang M, Wang L, Adeshakin FO, Liu W, et al. Blockade of myeloid-derived suppressor cell function by valproic acid enhanced anti-PD-L1 tumor immunotherapy. *Biochem Biophys Res Commun* (2020) 522(3):604–11. doi: 10.1016/j.bbrc.2019.11.155
40. Kim YD, Park SM, Ha HC, Lee AR, Won H, Cha H, et al. HDAC Inhibitor, CG-745, Enhances the Anti-Cancer Effect of Anti-PD-1 Immune Checkpoint Inhibitor by Modulation of the Immune Microenvironment. *J Cancer* (2020) 11(14):4059–72. doi: 10.7150/jca.44622
41. Wang X, Waschke BC, Woolaver RA, Chen SMY, Chen Z, Wang JH. HDAC inhibitors overcome immunotherapy resistance in B-cell lymphoma. *Protein Cell* (2020) 11(7):472–82. doi: 10.1007/s13238-020-00694-x
42. Yeon M, Kim Y, Jung HS, Jeoung D. Histone Deacetylase Inhibitors to Overcome Resistance to Targeted and Immuno Therapy in Metastatic Melanoma. *Front Cell Dev Biol* (2020) 8:486. doi: 10.3389/fcell.2020.00486

43. Terranova-Barberio M, Thomas S, Ali N, Pawlowska N, Park J, Krings G, et al. HDAC inhibition potentiates immunotherapy in triple negative breast cancer. *Oncotarget* (2017) 8(69):114156–72. doi: 10.18632/oncotarget.23169
44. Llopiz D, Ruiz M, Villanueva L, Iglesias T, Silva L, Egea J, et al. Enhanced anti-tumor efficacy of checkpoint inhibitors in combination with the histone deacetylase inhibitor Belinostat in a murine hepatocellular carcinoma model. *Cancer Immunol Immunother* (2019) 68(3):379–93. doi: 10.1007/s00262-018-2283-0
45. Burke B, Eden C, Perez C, Belshoff A, Hart S, Plaza-Rojas L, et al. Inhibition of Histone Deacetylase (HDAC) Enhances Checkpoint Blockade Efficacy by Rendering Bladder Cancer Cells Visible for T Cell-Mediated Destruction. *Front Oncol* (2020) 10:699. doi: 10.3389/fonc.2020.00699

7

Harnessing the Immune System against Multiple Myeloma: Challenges and Opportunities

Leona Yamamoto[1], *Nicola Amodio*[2], *Annamaria Gulla*[1*†] *and Kenneth Carl Anderson*[1*†]

[1] *Division of Hematologic Malignancy, Department of Medical Oncology, Jerome Lipper Multiple Myeloma Center, Dana-Farber Cancer Institute, Harvard Medical School, Boston, MA, United States,* [2] *Department of Experimental and Clinical Medicine, Magna Graecia University of Catanzaro, Catanzaro, Italy*

Correspondence:
Kenneth Carl Anderson
kenneth_anderson@dfci.harvard.edu
Annamaria Gulla
annamaria_gulla@dfci.harvard.edu

†These authors have contributed equally to this work

Multiple myeloma (MM) is an incurable malignancy of plasma cells that grow within a permissive bone marrow microenvironment (BMM). The bone marrow milieu supports the malignant transformation both by promoting uncontrolled proliferation and resistance to cell death in MM cells, and by hampering the immune response against the tumor clone. Hence, it is expected that restoring host anti-MM immunity may provide therapeutic benefit for MM patients. Already several immunotherapeutic approaches have shown promising results in the clinical setting. In this review, we outline recent findings demonstrating the potential advantages of targeting the immunosuppressive bone marrow niche to restore effective anti-MM immunity. We discuss different approaches aiming to boost the effector function of T cells and/or exploit innate or adaptive immunity, and highlight novel therapeutic opportunities to increase the immunogenicity of the MM clone. We also discuss the main challenges that hamper the efficacy of immune-based approaches, including intrinsic resistance of MM cells to activated immune-effectors, as well as the protective role of the immune-suppressive and inflammatory bone marrow milieu. Targeting mechanisms to convert the immunologically "cold" to "hot" MM BMM may induce durable immune responses, which in turn may result in long-lasting clinical benefit, even in patient subgroups with high-risk features and poor survival.

Keywords: myeloma, immunotherapy, microenvironment, immune system, challanges

INTRODUCTION

Multiple myeloma (MM) is a plasma cell (PC) malignancy that accounts for approximately 1.5% of all cancers, and 10% of hematological malignancies (1). Abnormal proliferation of malignant PCs in the bone marrow (BM) in most cases leads to excessive secretion of immunoglobulin in the blood and urine, associated with organ dysfunction including hypercalcemia, renal dysfunction, anemia and/or bone disease (CRAB) (2). MM onset follows a multistep development process: tumor immune escape and accumulation of genomic aberrations in the malignant clone(s) drives the progression from precursor stages, namely monoclonal gammopathy of undetermined significance (MGUS) and smoldering multiple myeloma (SMM), to overt MM (1, 3). Current therapy consists of combination of novel agents with remarkable efficacy in MM. Specifically, combination proteasome inhibitor (PIs), immunomodulatory drugs (IMiDs), and dexamethasone used alone or integrated into high dose melphalan and autologous stem cell transplantation (ASCT) paradigm, increased rate, extent, and duration of response (4)..

Immunotherapy has recently demonstrated remarkable activity in many human solid tumors and is also transforming MM treatment as well. Recent approval of monoclonal antibodies (moAb) for the treatment of both newly diagnosed (NDMM) and relapsed/refractory (RRMM) MM patients highlights the fundamental role of therapies targeting the immunosuppressive microenvironment. The success of these approaches underlies the potential benefit of combination of immune- and targeted-therapies to overcome inter- and intra-patient heterogeneity characteristic of MM. In this review, we will discuss the role of the immunosuppressive BM microenvironment in MM, and outline novel immunotherapeutic approaches to effectively restore anti-MM immunity.

IMMUNE DYSFUNCTION AND TUMOR IMMUNE EVASION MECHANISMS

BM-mediated immune dysfunction and tumor immune evasion represent the main challenges for immunotherapy in MM (5). However, although qualitative and/or quantitative alterations of cellular and non-cellular components of the BM *niche* in MM confer immunosuppression, they similarly represent ideal targets for novel therapeutics. Immune dysfunction not only confers MM cell growth and resistance to therapy, but also is associated with higher susceptibility to infections and impaired cellular immunity, evidenced by lack of a strong immune response to vaccinations (6–9). Alterations in accessory and immune cells in the BM including regulatory T cells, myeloid-derived suppressor cells (4, 10), Th17 cells, tumor-associated macrophages, mesenchymal stromal cells, and osteoclasts contribute to immune suppression and immune exhaustion (5, 11). Interaction of MM cells with plasmacytoid dendritic cells further promotes MM cell survival and therapy resistance, providing the rationale for targeting this interaction in novel therapeutic approaches (12, 13). Recent reports show a stepwise immune dysregulation in MM which occurs as early as in SMM stage, and the potential role of immune-based therapeutic interventions in premalignant precursor stages to delay or prevent progression to active MM in under active investigation in ongoing clinical trials (14–17).

During progression of disease, MM cells acquire the ability to evade the immune system and subvert cancer immunoediting, a dynamic process encompassing multiple aspects of tumor cell-immune system interactions (10, 18). Immunoediting, a process that is well described for solid tumors, shapes cancer cell immunogenicity in three phases: elimination, equilibrium, and escape. In the first phase, both innate and adaptive immunity recognize and eliminate early tumor cells (elimination). However, a state of dormancy next occurs in which a functional immune system maintains the survival of tumor cells under constant immune pressure (equilibrium). In this phase, resistant tumor cells acquire genetic and epigenetic alterations that eventually lead to escape the immune recognition, allowing for uncontrolled proliferation and clinical progression (escape) (19–21). A potential application of this model in MM identifies in the MGUS/SMM precursor stages a phase of immune equilibrium (22). In this context, marked heterogeneity of MM cells, along with constitutive and ongoing genomic instability, and modulations occurring in the composition of the BM *milieu* may underlie immune escape and disruption of the immune equilibrium during disease progression (22). Specifically, the strict and symbiotic interaction between MM cells and the BM microenvironment facilitate tumor immune escape *via* several mechanisms: immunosuppressive cells in the BM; disruption of antigen presentation by downregulating major histocompatibility complex and/or costimulatory molecules; loss or mutation of cancer-specific antigens; and upregulation of decoy receptors or complement inhibitory receptors (5, 23). Moreover, secretion of immunoregulatory soluble factors from both MM and BM microenvironment cells including transforming growth factor TGF-β, interleukin IL-10, IL-6, prostaglandin E2, and APRIL; as well as adhesion of MM cells to extracellular matrix proteins and accessory cells further promotes immune evasion and inhibition of apoptosis (5). Lastly, immune evasion also results from increased expression of immune checkpoints, i.e. PD-1/PD-L1, in T cells and MM cells, which has been associated with progression from precursor stages to clinically active MM, as well as with progression from NDMM to RRMM. As will be discussed later, clinically active agents blocking PD-1/PDL-1 axis have been associated with adverse events and are not approved for MM treatment; and ongoing studies are exploring the role of other potential immune checkpoint or agonist molecules including LAG 3 or TIGIT and OX40, respectively (24).

IMMUNOTHERAPY IN MM

The potential benefit of immunotherapeutic approaches in MM was first demonstrated by the curative effect achieved in some MM patients by the graft-*versus*-myeloma effect induced by allogeneic stem cell transplantation (23). Importantly, several moAbs and an immunotoxin have been FDA approved to treat MM and already improved patient outcome. Here, we review these therapies, as well as novel approaches under investigation in preclinical and clinical studies to further boost anti-MM immune response (**Figure 1**).

Direct Targeting of MM Cell Tumor Antigens

Monoclonal Antibody Therapy

Monoclonal antibody (moAb) therapy is a successful strategy for both solid tumors and hematological malignancies; and recently has also transformed MM treatment (25). A key determinant for an optimal moAb efficacy is identification of a target uniquely or selectively and highly expressed by MM cells (26). To date, the targeting of two MM surface antigens, CD-38 and SLAMF7, has led to the Food and Drug Administration (FDA) approval of

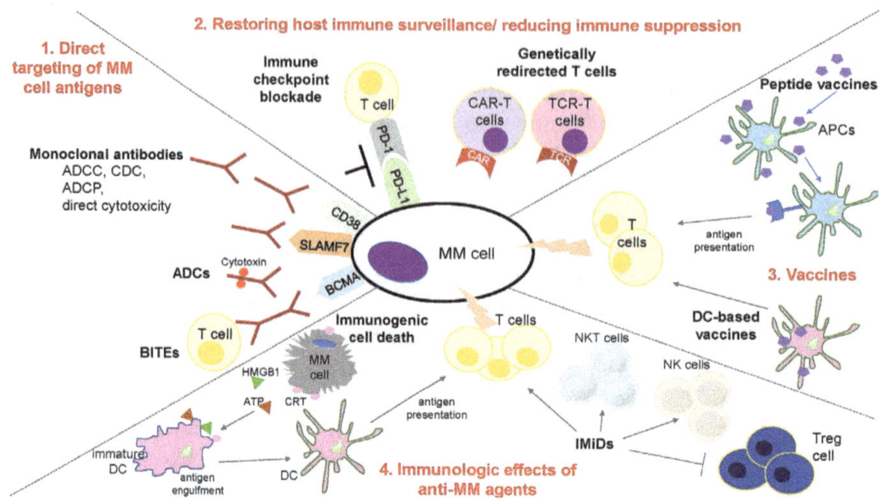

FIGURE 1 | Schematic overview of immune therapies in MM. 1. Strategies for the direct targeting of MM cell antigens includes: (a) moAbs: anti-CD38 and -SLAMF7 antibodies induce ADCC, CDC, ADCP, and direct cytotoxic effect on MM cells; (b) ADCs: conjugation of moAbs and cytotoxic compounds provides direct and selective tumor killing; (c) BiTEs: dual interaction with surface antigen of tumor cells and the TCR complex enables T cell activation and tumor lysis of MM cells. 2. Restoration of host immune surveillance and decrease of immune suppression can be achieved by the blockade of immune-checkpoint, such as PD-1/PD-L1 axis, that are responsible for inactivation and loss of proliferative capacity of T cells; or by the use of genetically redirected T cells including CAR-T and TCR-T cells. CAR-T cells mediate MHC-unrestricted tumor cell killing *via* recognition of tumor antigen. TCR-T cells mediate MHC-restricted tumor cell killing by recognizing the intracellular antigen fragment presented by MHC molecules. 3. Peptide- or DC-based vaccination represents an additional strategy to increase a MM specific anti-tumor immunity. Peptide vaccines binds to restricted MHC molecule in APCs and after intracellular processing, peptide/MHC complex is transported to the cell surface for antigen presentation and activation of T cells. In DC-based vaccines, DCs are generated to present tumor associated antigens to T cells. 4. Anti-MM agents such as IMiDs and PIs may affect the immune compartment composition and increase anti-MM immune response. IMiDs increase and stimulate T, NK, and NKT cells, along with a decrease of immunosuppressive Treg cells. Novel reports also show the ability of anti-MM agents, such as bortezomib to induce immunogenic cell death (ICD) and stimulate an immune response against MM cells. Specifically, dying tumor cells expose specific damage associated molecular patterns (DAMPs) that induce the functional maturation of DCs, and the efficient presentation of tumor antigens to the T cells. *ADCC*, Antibody-dependent cellular cytotoxicity; *ADCP*, Antibody-dependent cellular phagocytosis; *CDC*, Complement-dependent cytotoxicity; *ADC*, Antibody drug conjugate; *BiTE*, Bi-specific T cell engager; *CAR*, Chimeric antigen receptor; *TCR*, T cell receptor; *APC*, Antigen presenting cell; *NK*, Natural Killer; *Treg*, regulatory T cells; *DC*, dendritic cell; *CRT*, Calreticulin.

moAbs Daratumumab or Isatuximab and Elotuzumab, respectively, for MM treatment. Anti-MM immune effects of these moAbs include antibody-dependent cellular cytotoxicity (ADCC), antibody-dependent cellular phagocytosis (ADCP), complement activation, and direct effects on MM cells. Specifically, Elotuzumab is a humanized IgG1 monoclonal antibody that targets SLAMF7, which is highly expressed on PCs, natural killer (NK) cells, and activated monocytes (27). It induces ADCC while also activating NK cells and inhibiting MM cell adhesion to BMSCs (28, 29). Although no single agent activity has been reported in a phase I study (30), increased overall response (ORR) and median progression free survival (PFS) in the phase III Eloquent-2 trial provided the basis for its FDA approval in combination with lenalidomide and dexamethasone (Rd) in RRMM (31). More recently, the Eloquent-3 trial led to its approval in combination with pomalidomide and low dose dexamethasone (PomDex) in RRMM (32).

Daratumumab is an IgG1 kappa fully human moAb that targets CD38, which is highly expressed on malignant MM cells, but is also expressed on lymphoid and myeloid cells, hematopoietic progenitor cells, as well as non-hematopoietic tissues (18, 33). Anti-MM effects of daratumumab include: Fc fragment-dependent complement-dependent cytotoxicity (CDC), where the Fc fragment binds C1q, initiates complement cascade, and induces the formation of the membrane attack complex (MAC) that leads to MM cell lysis; ADCC, where Fc fragment binds an FcR-bearing effector cells such as natural killer (NK) cells, thus stimulating MM cytotoxicity; ADCP, where Fc fragment binds an Fc-bearing macrophage, thus stimulating MM cells phagocytosis; tumor cell apoptosis upon FcγR cross-linking (34–38); and immunomodulatory effects due to killing of CD-38-positive immune suppressor cells including regulatory T and B cells (Treg and Breg) and MDSCs (35), associated with an increase in T cell number, clonality, activation, and killing capacity due to higher levels of granzyme B (35). All these effects both induce MM cytotoxicity and increase host-anti MM response, associated with durable responses (**Table 1**). In the phase I/II GEN501 study and phase II SIRIUS study, Daratumumab monotherapy induced significant responses in heavily pretreated RRMM, leading to its FDA approval as monotherapy to treat RRMM in 2015 (39, 40). Combinations of daratumumab with Rd, PomDex, Bortezomib and dexamethasone (Vd), and carfilzomib dexamethasone are all

TABLE 1 | Daratumumab.

Treatment	Clinical trials	Patient population	ORR%	PFS	OS at 12 m	Date of approval
D monotherapy	**GEN501**	RRMM	36*	5.6 m	77%*	Nov 16, 2015
	SIRIUS	RRMM	29.2	3.7 m	64.8%	
	POLLUX	RRMM	92.9 *vs* 76.4	12 m: 83.2 *vs* 60.1%	92.1 *vs* 86.8%	Nov 21, 2016
D-Rd vs Rd						
	MAIA	NDMM transplant-ineligible	92.9 *vs* 81.3	30 m: 70.6 *vs* 55.6%		June 27, 2019
D-Vd vs Vd	**CASTOR**	RRMM	82.9 *vs* 63.2	12 m: 60.7 *vs* 26.9 %		Nov 21, 2016
D plus PomDex	**EQUULEUS**	RRMM	60	13.1 m: 8.8 m (median)	66% (median)	June 16, 2017
D-VMP vs VMP	**ALCYONE**	NDMM transplant-ineligible	90.9 *vs* 73.9	18 m: 71,6 *vs* 50.2%		May 7, 2018
D-VTd vs VTd	**CASSIOPEIA**	NDMM transplant-eligible	92.6 *vs* 89.9	18 m: 93 *vs* 85%		Sept 26, 2019
D-RVd vs RVd	**GRIFFIN**	NDMM transplant-eligible	99 *vs* 91.8	24 m: 95.8 *vs* 89.9 %		

**in the cohort of patients receiving 16 mg/kg dose.*
NDMM, newly diagnosed MM patients; RRMM, relapsed refractory MM patients; D, daratumumab; R, lenalidomide; Pom, pomalidomide; V, bortezomib; M, melphalan; T, thalidomide; P, prednisone; d, dexamethasone; ORR, overall response rate; PFS, progression free survival; OS, overall survival; m, months.

FDA approved to treat RRMM; moreover, recent studies led to the FDA approval of Daratumumab in combination with Rd, or bortezomib, melphalan, and prednisolone (VMP), or bortezomib, thalidomide, and dexamethasone (VTd) to treat NDMM (41–46) due increased frequency and extent of durable responses (**Table 1**). A co-formulated product of daratumumab and recombinant human hyaluronidase PH20 suitable for subcutaneous administration has recently shown non-inferiority in the COLUMBA and PLEIADES trials as compared to intravenous infusion (47); and subcutaneous Daratumumab is now FDA approved, thus reducing infusion time and rate of infusion-related reactions.

Isatuximab (SAR650984) is another humanized IgG1 chimeric moAb that targets CD38. Its mechanisms of actions include CDC, ADCC, ADCP, and direct cytotoxicity without crosslinking of the Fc receptors of the antibody (48, 49). Moreover, both Daratumumab and Isatuximab may induce the depletion of CD38+ immune suppressor cells such as Tregs and Bregs (21, 50, 51). In the phase III ICARIA-MM study, isatuximab combined with PomDex showed superiority in terms of ORR (60.4 *vs* 35.3%) and median PFS (11.5 months *vs* 6.5 months) (52). This result led the FDA to approve isatuximab as a combination therapy with PomDex to treat RRMM in March 2020.

Antibody Drug Conjugate (ADC) and Bi-Specific Antibody (BiTEs)

Monoclonal antibodies have been recently used to develop Ab drug conjugates (ADC) and bispecific T cell engagers (BiTEs). ADCs are moAbs conjugated to cytotoxic compounds (such as auristatin) *via* synthetic linkers (53, 54). This conjugation provides both selective targeting and direct tumor killing, along with immune-mediated cytotoxicity (54–58). Several ADCs are under investigation in pre-clinical and clinical settings; among them, B cell maturation antigen (BCMA)-directed ADCs are showing promising effect due to the high and unique expression of BCMA on MM and late memory B cells, and to the oncogenic role of BCMA/APRIL pathway in the disease (56, 58, 59). Specifically, BCMA is a member of the tumor necrosis factor receptor superfamily (TNF) with high affinity for B cell activating factor (BAFF) and a proliferation-inducing ligand (APRIL). BCMA is essential for long-lived bone marrow PCs survival and regulates B cell differentiation into PCs (60, 61), thus representing an ideal target for MM therapy. Importantly, we have carried out preclinical studies of belantamab mafodotin, a BCMA-aurostatin immunotoxin, which recently received FDA approval in RRMM (58, 62). Balantamab mafodotin specifically blocks cell growth *via* G2/M arrest, induces caspase-dependent apoptosis, and ADCC (58). These multiple cytotoxic mechanisms enable potent and selective anti-MM activity.

BiTEs are bispecific antibodies which bind to specific tumor antigens on one side, and to the CD3 epsilon chain of the T-cell receptor complex on the other (63, 64). This dual interaction enables T cells engagement with tumor cells, which leads to T cell activation, cytolytic synapses, and tumor cell lysis (65, 66). In MM CD19, CD38, CD138, BCMA, GPRC5D, and Fc receptor-like 5 antigens have been tested (67–69), with early promising responses from BCMA BiTEs treatment in RRMM (66, 69). Novel bispecific antibodies are under clinical development and have shown encouraging data in preclinical studies. Specifically, AMG 701 holds an extended half-life *in vivo* and mediates T-cell dependent cellular cytotoxicity (TDCC) of BCMA positive MM cells and is currently under clinical investigation (NCT03287908). We have also shown that MM cytotoxicity can be augmented at lower effector: tumor cell ratios when low doses of AMG 701 are combined with lenalidomide or pomalidomide, suggesting a favorable therapeutic index (70). Although early results look promising and both ADC and Bites approaches have the advantage for "off the shelf" availability, longer follow-up in larger studies is needed to assess their clinical efficacy and toxicity.

Restoring Host Immune Surveillance/Reducing Immune Suppression

Genetically Redirected T Cells

Cellular therapies represent an optimal strategy to restore host immune surveillance using either adoptive T-cell (ACT) or engineered T cell approaches (71–73). Expansion and activation of immunosuppressive T cells from the tumor microenvironment has shown best responses to date in solid tumors (72, 73). In MM, early experience showed that marrow-infiltrating lymphocytes (MILs) can be effectively used as a source of tumor specific T cells for ACT (74). Although these results are encouraging, ACT in MM has mainly utilized TCR and chimeric antigen receptor (CAR) T cell strategies, facilitated by recent progress in gene engineering technology (23). In the first approach, a TCR is cloned within patient T cells, thereby enabling specific recognition of patient's tumor antigens in an MHC-dependent manner (71). Promising results were obtained in a phase I/II trial in which MM patients received high dose melphalan, ASCT, and two days later infusion of T cells engineered to express an affinity-enhanced TCR recognizing a naturally processed peptide shared by two cancer/testis antigens NY-ESO-1 and LAGE-1 (NY-ESOc259) (75, 76). Responses were noted in 80% patients with RRMM, and severe adverse events were not observed. Long-term persistence of NY-ESOc259 targeting T cells was detected and correlated with clinical activity against antigen-expressing MM cells (75). Importantly, CAR-T cell technology overcomes potential limitations of TCR-T cells by allowing recognition of unprocessed tumor antigen in an MHC-independent manner; however TCR, but not CAR-T, cells can also recognize intracellular proteins (23, 24). CARs are chimeric proteins that couple the constant region of a TCR and the tumor-associated antigen binding domain of a variable fragment of a moAb (23, 24, 77). Second-generation CAR-T cells also include costimulatory molecules, thus enhancing T cell activation and tumor killing by mimicking a physiological T cell response (23, 24, 77, 78). Patient's T cells are engineered by means of electroporation, retroviral, or lentiviral transduction, expanded *ex vivo*, and then reinfused to the patient, leading to profound and rapid tumor killing (23, 24, 77). A major determinant of successful CAR-T therapy is the identification of the appropriate antigen, which is uniquely and highly expressed by MM cells, in order to avoid adverse events. Specifically, the main challenge of CAR-T therapy is the appropriate target selection, which is critical in the management of on-target, off-tumor toxicity to avoid excess cytokine release after target recognition on non-malignant cells (79). Similarly, the major on-target, on-tumor adverse events of CAR-T cells include cytokine release syndrome (CRS) characterized by fever, hypotension and/or renal failure, as well as neurotoxicity (80); and are mainly due to the CAR-T cell activation and expansion and uncontrolled cytokine release (79). Importantly, clinical experience has now shown that targeting interleukin-6 and use of dexamethasone can treat these toxicities (23, 24, 77, 81). Nonetheless, several strategies have been developed to overcome these toxicities and include either modifications of CAR-T cell activation kinetics to maintain activation and cytokine release under a controlled level, or approaches to restrict the recognition of normal cells by optimizing CAR-T/tumor cells interaction (79). Among several antigens including CD19, CD138 and SLAMF7, B-cell maturation antigen (BCMA) represents the most promising to date due to its high selective expression on normal plasma and MM cells (82, 83).

Several CAR-T products have been clinically evaluated in heavily pretreated (PIs-IMiDs-CD38 mAb) RRMM and demonstrated remarkable efficacy, including high rates of CR with minimal residual disease (MRD) negativity (77, 84). In the phase 1 study of bb2121, an anti-BCMA CAR-T, 85% of heavily pretreated RRMM patients had a clinical response lasting a median of 10.9 months without additional MM treatment (84). Encouraging results from the LEGEND-2 (NCT03090659) and CARTITUDE-1 (NCT03548207) clinical trials have been recently disclosed and show high overall response rate (ORR) with deep responses by using a different CAR-T product LCAR-B38M, also called JNJ 4528, which possesses a 4-1BB costimulatory domain and two BCMA-targeting domains (*Wang et al. ASH 2019; Madduri et al. ASH 2019*). Similarly, preliminary results from a phase 1 dose-escalating trial of a dual-target BM38 CAR recognizing both CD38 and BCMA are showing high ORR with a long duration of stringent CR and elimination of extramedullary lesions in RRMM patients (*Li et al., 2019 ASH*). However, relapse of disease occurs in most patients; and ongoing studies are evaluating mechanisms of CAR-T resistance in order to achieve durable responses. These include use of combination with immune approaches, treatment earlier in the disease course, and use of gamma secretase inhibitors to upregulate BCMA expression, among others.

Immune Checkpoint Blockade

Cancer cells may escape from T cell surveillance by altering the balance of costimulatory and coinhibitory molecular interactions. Stimulatory checkpoints and their ligands (CD27/CD70, CD40/CD40L, OX40/OX40L, GITR/GITL, CD137/CD137L, CD28/CD80 and CD86, ICOS/ICOSL) support T cell activation, whereas inhibitory checkpoints and their ligands (A2AR/adenosine, CTLA-4/CD80 and CD86, KIR/MHC class I, LAG3/MHC class II, PD-1/PD-L1 and PD-L2) lead to T cell suppression and induce their apoptosis (85). The PD-1/PD-L1 axis is the most studied pathway in MM. Programmed -death 1 (PD-1) receptor is a member of B7 family of costimulatory molecules and is expressed on antigen-activated and exhausted T, B, and NK cells (60, 86). PD-L1 expressing cells may evade T cell attack *via* several mechanisms, including induction of apoptosis, anergy or exhaustion of T cells, formation of a molecular shield to protect tumor cells from lysis, increased production of immunosuppressive IL-10, and stimulation of Treg cell-mediated suppression (87). Numerous studies have shown that PD-1 is overexpressed on CD4+ and CD8+ T cells of MM patients (88, 89), and that its expression is higher in patients with RRMM and MRD positive MM (90). Likewise, MM cells express PD-L1 at varying intensity (91–93), with a progressive increase in expression with progression from MGUS/SMM to NDMM to RRMM. Its oncogenic role in MM pathophysiology is also supported by the evidence that PD-L1 expressing MGUS or

SMM show a rapid progression to symptomatic disease (94). MM cells-microenvironment interaction and secretion of proinflammatory cytokines (such as IL-6) promote PD-L1 upregulation on MM cell surface, which both inhibits T cell-mediated anti-MM immunity (94) and promotes MM cell survival by inducing reverse signaling to MM cells and activating the PI3K/AKT pathway (94). Although preclinical data have demonstrated the potential utility of PD-1/PD-L1 blockade in MM therapy, early clinical trials have been discouraging (95). Pembrolizumab immunotherapy did not show any activity in MM (96), and its combination with IMiDs, lenalidomide, or pomalidomide in RRMM patients was associated with immune-related toxicities and mortality in two phase III studies (KEYNOTE-183 and KEYNOTE-185), leading to a FDA clinical hold (24, 97). The precise mechanisms that lead to immune-related toxicities are still unknown (98); however, immune checkpoints are regulators of immunological homeostasis, and their functional disruption may unbalance immune tolerance that can lead to uncontrolled immune response (98, 99). Clinically, patients experience autoimmune-like/inflammatory reactions that can cause organ and tissue damages (98, 99). Although the mechanisms underlying the severity of such adverse events in some patients is yet to be elucidated, some reports suggest an association with underlying germline genetic factors or patient microbiota (98, 100). To date, the mechanisms underlying higher toxicity observed in MM patients as compared to other tumors are unknown. Pembrolizumab and nivolumab monotherapy in RRMM patients displayed similar safety profile as in other cancers (99); however, combination of pembrolizumab with IMiDs resulted in higher toxicity, with severe and unanticipated adverse events (99). Future analysis of combinations with other agents, patient selection, and timing of treatment initiation may allow for optimal therapeutical application of PD-1/PD-L1 axis blockade in MM. Recent studies suggest the potential role of other immune checkpoint or agonist proteins (i.e. LAG 3 or TIGIT and OX40, respectively) as MM therapeutic targets, alone and in combination with MM targeted and immune therapies (101). These novel studies, along with the identification of patients who may most benefit of immune checkpoint therapy, may allow for their future clinical use.

Vaccine Strategies

Antigen-specific anti-tumor immunity can be primed by vaccination through several strategies including tumor cell-based vaccines (autologous or allogeneic), dendritic cell (DC)-based vaccines, protein/peptide-based vaccines, and genetic vaccines (DNA vaccines, RNA vaccine, viral based-vaccines) (102, 103). Among them, tumor cell-, protein/peptide-, and DC-based vaccines have been explored, although the main challenge to their efficacy has been represented by hallmark immunosuppression in MM (104, 105). GVAX (Aduro Biotech) is a vaccine platform that uses tumor cells which are genetically engineered to produce granulocyte-macrophage colony-stimulating factor GM-CSF (106), which can recruit and activate DCs and other APCs (107). This vaccine is now being tested in combination with lenalidomide in patients with CR and near CR (NCT03376477). Several antigens that are broadly expressed in MM cells, such as MAGE-A3, WT-1, SLAMF7, CD138, and XBP-1 have been examined alone or in combination in the context of peptide/protein-based vaccines (108–110). Although the clinical efficacy seems modest, new approaches using a multipeptide-based vaccine induced an effective and durable memory multipeptide-specific cytotoxic T lymphocytes response in patients with SMM, suggesting its potential utility to delay disease progression (111). Similarly, a novel engineered heteroclitic BCMA peptide can induce BCMA-specific memory immunity, providing the rationale for its clinical evaluation (112). Additionally, previous reports have also explored the idiotype (Id) vaccination in which early-stage MM patients are immunized with autologous tumor-derived clone-specific immunoglobulin, both as a peptide vaccine and a DNA vaccine (113–115). Id specific immunological responses were reported, although clinical responses were infrequent.

DC-based vaccines are also under investigation in MM. Two approaches can be used to augment presentation of tumor antigens in DC: to chemically fuse patient DCs with autologous MM cells (MM cells/DCs fusion vaccine); or to load DCs with tumor antigens in the form of peptides, proteins, tumor lysates, and mRNAs (106, 116). In the first phase I clinical trial, 16 patients were treated with MM cell/DC fusion vaccine with GM-CSF as an adjuvant. The majority of patients (11 of 15) showed disease stabilization, associated with expansion of circulating CD4+ and CD8+ lymphocytes reactive against autologous MM cells (116). In the phase II trial, patients received vaccination post-ASCT. In this setting, vaccination induced effective anti-MM immunity and increases the depth of response, with 78% of the patients showing CR/VGPR (117). Moreover, 24% patients converted from PR to CR/near CR after vaccination at more than 3 months post-ASCT, suggesting a vaccine-mediated effect targeting residual disease (117). To confirm these results, phase II trial in the same setting (NCT02728102) is ongoing. Another DC-based vaccine approach in which Langerhans-type DCs (LCs) are electroporated with mRNAs encoding MM antigens CT7, MAGE-A3, and WT-1 is now being evaluated in the post-ASCT setting in phase I clinical trial (NCT01995708). This trial is based on preclinical data showing that LCs induce a more potent T cell response than monocyte-derived DCs, and that the electroporation of mRNA stimulates their maturation and activation (118, 119).

Of note, due to the lack of an optimal response after vaccination in MM patients to date, an ongoing trial (NCT02728102) is exploring whether combination with IMiDs may increase a clinically significant immune response.

Immunologic Effects of Anti-MM Agents

Several studies have focused on the effects of anti-MM agents on cellular and non-cellular components of the bone marrow microenvironment, including immune cells. Immunomodulatory agents (IMiDs) thalidomide and its more potent derivatives lenalidomide and pomalidomide represent the best example of drugs with both direct cytotoxic activity on MM cells and immunomodulatory effects (24). Thalidomide is approved to treat both NDMM and RRMM in combination with bortezomib and dexamethasone (VTd), and the recent phase III CASSIOPEIA study granted its FDA approval in combination with daratumumab (D-VTd) in NDMM (46). However, occurrence of peripheral neuropathy and introduction of lenalidomide and pomalidomide in the MM armamentarium, has progressively decreased its clinical use. Lenalidomide is used in combination with bortezomib and dexamethasone (RVd) to treat transplant-eligible NDMM (120, 121); a dose modification (RVd-lite) has also shown a favorable therapeutic index in transplant-ineligible NDMM patients (121, 122). Lenalidomide is also FDA approved post-ASCT as maintenance therapy as it prolongs both PFS and OS (123); in RRMM setting, it is FDA approved in combination with daratumumab (41), elotuzumab (31), ixazomib (124), and carfilzomib (125). Pomalidomide is FDA approved to treat RRMM patients in combination with dexamethasone along with elotuzumab, bortezomib, daratumumab, and isatuximab (32, 44, 126), and its role in this setting has become more evident due to the broad use of lenalidomide in both NDMM and in maintenance and the development of lenalidomide resistance leading to relapse. Elegant mechanistic studies identified cereblon (CRBN) as a major target for IMiDs in MM cells, and showed that they induce growth arrest and caspase-8–mediated apoptosis, associated with CRBN-dependent degradation of Ikaros (IKZF1) and aiolos (IKZF3) transcription factors, followed by IRF4 downregulation (24, 127, 128). IMiDs treatment impacts the MM cell/microenvironment interaction by decreasing cell surface expression of adhesion molecules, modulating cytokine and growth factor secretion, and inhibiting angiogenesis (24). Immunomodulatory effects include activation of cytotoxic CD8+ T, NK, and NKT cells, along with a decrease of Treg (24). CRBN targeting is also responsible for the immune effects of IMiDs, as degradation of IKZF1/3 in T cells increases IL-2 secretion (129) and NK and NKT cell cytotoxicity (24). More recently, it has been shown that IMiDs can enhance NK and T cell cytotoxicity by triggering granzyme-B *via* either CRBN or ZAP-70 dependent mechanisms, thus providing the rationale for novel therapeutics to activate ZAP-70 in MM (130). Recent studies are also suggesting different mechanisms of action between pomalidomide and lenalidomide *in vivo*, consistent with clinical responses observed in patients with lenalidomide RRMM (131, 132).

Importantly, the identification of the mechanism of action of IMiDs has informed the development of a new class of drugs, CELMoD agents which are higher affinity CRBN E3-ligase modulators (24). Among them, Iberdomide and CC-92480 have shown significant preclinical activity and are currently under investigation in the RRMM clinical setting (133, 134).

Proteasome Inhibitors (PI) bortezomib, carfilzomib, and ixazomib represent the backbone of MM therapy in both NDMM and RRMM. MM cells are highly dependent on proteasome activity due to their high turnover of abnormal immunoglobulins (24, 135). Although PIs exert a primarily cytotoxic effect on MM cells, the biological outcome of proteasome inhibition also targets the MM microenvironment. PI treatment can disrupt MM cell/bone marrow cell adhesion by decreasing the expression of adhesion molecules, inhibit angiogenesis by modulating secretion of several cytokines, and modify osteoclast activity and bone turnover (136). However, the effect of this class of agents on the immune cells is still largely unknown, with preclinical data suggesting an immunosuppressive role (137). Interestingly, a more recent elegant study has instead shown an immunogenic potential role of bortezomib in eliciting an anti-MM immune response *in vitro* (138). Moreover, our recent studies using both syngeneic *in vivo* MM model and MM patient samples show that bortezomib treatment triggers immunogenic MM cell death, which in turn primes an effective anti-MM immune response and disease control *in vivo* models and in patients (*Gulla et al., ASH 2019*). A deep understanding of the immunomodulatory role of PIs will be instrumental to inform their clinical use in combination with immune therapies.

As shown in several types of cancers, histone deacetylase (HDAC) inhibitors are powerful epigenetic regulators with a wide range of effects, including immune modulation (139). For example, recent evidence has shown that an HDAC6 specific inhibitor ACY241 exerts its anti-MM activity, at least in part, by enhancing anti-tumor response of antigen-specific central memory cytotoxic T lymphocytes against MM (140). Future studies will better inform the therapeutic use of HDAC inhibitors as immune regulators in this disease.

DISCUSSIONS

Increasing knowledge of MM pathobiology and immune microenvironment dysfunction, along with the introduction of PIs and IMiDs-based regimens, has already transformed patient outcome in MM patients. The advent of immunotherapy in MM has already shown remarkable effects in terms of extent and frequency of response. Moreover, immune-based approaches, alone and in combination, have the potential to overcome not only immune dysfunction, but also constitutive and ongoing genomic heterogeneity of MM cells, and thereby improve patient long-term control of disease. However, several challenges remain for effective translation of novel immune strategies into clinical practice, as well as for optimal clinical use of drugs including moAbs that are already incorporated in the treatment regimens (141). Clinical challenges are associated with moAbs use, including infusion reactions, infection risk and blood typing interference that causes positive indirect Coombs test occurring with Daratumumab treatment. Moreover no clear data are available that identify alternative combinations besides their incorporation in triplet regimens, or the characteristic of the patient population in which Daratumumab may be preferably used as single drug (141).

Similarly, resistance to immune approaches hamper their long-term efficacy and may develop due to the loss of target antigen or immune suppression. To address this concern, novel approaches targeting multiple antigens are under investigation (24). Along with loss of surface expression of target protein, antigen in soluble form may potentially interfere with immune-targeted strategies. For example, soluble BCMA, which is cleaved by γ-secretase, inhibits CART cell recognition of surface BCMA (142, 143). High levels of soluble BCMA are present in RRMM, and a clinical trial is testing the combination of anti-BCMA

CAR-T therapy with γ-secretase inhibitor to block BCMA cleavage from the MM cell surface (NCT03502577). Although CAR-T therapies represent a very promising strategy, several challenges intrinsic to the technology may limit their efficacy; and ongoing efforts are optimizing their design to avoid antigen-independent tonic signaling, and to increase their expansion and persistence *in vivo*, by enriching for early memory T cell phenotype and/or intensifying lymphodepletion to promote CAR-T persistence (77). Moreover, the optimal timing for immune intervention during MM the disease course remains undefined. Early immune-based intervention in high-risk SMM patients to avoid development of active MM is promising strategy, but must be balanced against adverse events and therapeutic index. Finally, correlative studies using MM patient samples will delineate mechanisms of action and resistance and thereby inform clinical application of immune therapies in combination with other anti-MM agents. Restoring host anti-MM immunity along with MRD negativity will be required for the long-term control of disease and its potential cure.

AUTHOR CONTRIBUTIONS

AG and KA conceived the review. LY and AG collected the literature. LY, AG, and NA drafted the manuscript and prepared the table and figure. KA provided critical comments on the manuscript—review and editing. All authors contributed to the article and approved the submitted version.

REFERENCES

1. Kumar SK, Rajkumar V, Kyle RA, van Duin M, Sonneveld P, Mateos MV, et al. Multiple myeloma. *Nat Rev Dis Primers* (2017) 3:17046. doi: 10.1038/nrdp.2017.46
2. Palumbo A, Anderson K. Multiple myeloma. *N Engl J Med* (2011) 364 (11):1046–60. doi: 10.1056/NEJMra1011442
3. Landgren O, Kyle RA, Pfeiffer RM, Katzmann JA, Caporaso NE, Hayes RB, et al. Monoclonal gammopathy of undetermined significance (MGUS) consistently precedes multiple myeloma: a prospective study. *Blood* (2009) 113(22):5412–7. doi: 10.1182/blood-2008-12-194241
4. Guang MHZ, McCann A, Bianchi G, Zhang L, Dowling P, Bazou D, et al. Overcoming multiple myeloma drug resistance in the era of cancer 'omics'. *Leuk Lymphoma* (2018) 59(3):542–61. doi: 10.1080/10428194.2017.1337115
5. Holthof LC, Mutis T. Challenges for Immunotherapy in Multiple Myeloma: Bone Marrow Microenvironment-Mediated Immune Suppression and Immune Resistance. *Cancers (Basel)* (2020) 12(4). doi: 10.3390/cancers12040988
6. Blimark C, Holmberg E, Mellqvist UH, Landgren O, Bjorkholm M, Hultcrantz M, et al. Multiple myeloma and infections: a population-based study on 9253 multiple myeloma patients. *Haematologica* (2015) 100 (1):107–13. doi: 10.3324/haematol.2014.107714
7. Kristinsson SY, Tang M, Pfeiffer RM, Bjorkholm M, Goldin LR, Blimark C, et al. Monoclonal gammopathy of undetermined significance and risk of infections: a population-based study. *Haematologica* (2012) 97(6):854–8. doi: 10.3324/haematol.2011.054015
8. Robertson JD, Nagesh K, Jowitt SN, Dougal M, Anderson H, Mutton K, et al. Immunogenicity of vaccination against influenza, Streptococcus pneumoniae and Haemophilus influenzae type B in patients with multiple myeloma. *Br J Cancer* (2000) 82(7):1261–5. doi: 10.1054/bjoc.1999.1088
9. Ljungman P, Nahi H, Linde A. Vaccination of patients with haematological malignancies with one or two doses of influenza vaccine: a randomised study. *Br J Haematol* (2005) 130(1):96–8. doi: 10.1111/j.1365-2141.2005.05582.x
10. Gorgun GT, Whitehill G, Anderson JL, Hideshima T, Maguire C, Laubach J, et al. Tumor-promoting immune-suppressive myeloid-derived suppressor cells in the multiple myeloma microenvironment in humans. *Blood* (2013) 121(15):2975–87. doi: 10.1182/blood-2012-08-448548
11. Tamura H. Immunopathogenesis and immunotherapy of multiple myeloma. *Int J Hematol* (2018) 107(3):278–85. doi: 10.1007/s12185-018-2405-7
12. Chauhan D, Singh AV, Brahmandam M, Carrasco R, Bandi M, Hideshima T, et al. Functional interaction of plasmacytoid dendritic cells with multiple myeloma cells: a therapeutic target. *Cancer Cell* (2009) 16(4):309–23. doi: 10.1016/j.ccr.2009.08.019
13. Ray A, Song Y, Chauhan D, Anderson KC. Blockade of ubiquitin receptor Rpn13 in plasmacytoid dendritic cells triggers anti-myeloma immunity. *Blood Cancer J* (2019) 9(8):64. doi: 10.1038/s41408-019-0224-6
14. Das R, Strowig T, Verma R, Koduru S, Hafemann A, Hopf S, et al. Microenvironment-dependent growth of preneoplastic and malignant plasma cells in humanized mice. *Nat Med* (2016) 22(11):1351–7. doi: 10.1038/nm.4202
15. Glavey SV, Naba A, Manier S, Clauser K, Tahri S, Park J, et al. Proteomic characterization of human multiple myeloma bone marrow extracellular matrix. *Leukemia* (2017) 31(11):2426–34. doi: 10.1038/leu.2017.102
16. Paiva B, Mateos MV, Sanchez-Abarca LI, Puig N, Vidriales MB, Lopez-Corral L, et al. Immune status of high-risk smoldering multiple myeloma patients and its therapeutic modulation under LenDex: a longitudinal analysis. *Blood* (2016) 127(9):1151–62. doi: 10.1182/blood-2015-10-662320
17. Mateos MV, Hernandez MT, Giraldo P, de la Rubia J, de Arriba F, Lopez Corral L, et al. Lenalidomide plus dexamethasone for high-risk smoldering multiple myeloma. *N Engl J Med* (2013) 369(5):438–47. doi: 10.1056/NEJMoa1300439
18. Malavasi F, Deaglio S, Funaro A, Ferrero E, Horenstein AL, Ortolan E, et al. Evolution and function of the ADP ribosyl cyclase/CD38 gene family in physiology and pathology. *Physiol Rev* (2008) 88(3):841–86. doi: 10.1152/physrev.00035.2007
19. Dunn GP, Bruce AT, Ikeda H, Old LJ, Schreiber RD. Cancer immunoediting: from immunosurveillance to tumor escape. *Nat Immunol* (2002) 3(11):991–8. doi: 10.1038/ni1102-991
20. Mittal D, Gubin MM, Schreiber RD, Smyth MJ. New insights into cancer immunoediting and its three component phases–elimination, equilibrium and escape. *Curr Opin Immunol* (2014) 27:16–25. doi: 10.1016/j.coi.2014.01.004
21. Ho M, Goh CY, Patel A, Staunton S, O'Connor R, Godeau M, et al. Role of the Bone Marrow Milieu in Multiple Myeloma Progression and Therapeutic Resistance. *Clin Lymphoma Myeloma Leuk* (2020) 20(10):e752–68. doi: 10.1016/j.clml.2020.05.026
22. Minnie SA, Hill GR. Immunotherapy of multiple myeloma. *J Clin Invest* (2020) 130(4):1565–75. doi: 10.1172/JCI129205
23. Rodriguez-Otero P, Paiva B, Engelhardt M, Prosper F, San Miguel JF. Is immunotherapy here to stay in multiple myeloma? *Haematologica* (2017) 102(3):423–32. doi: 10.3324/haematol.2016.152504
24. Gulla A, Anderson KC. Multiple myeloma: the (r)evolution of current therapy and a glance into future. *Haematologica* (2020) 105(10):2358–67. doi: 10.3324/haematol.2020.247015

25. Scott AM, Allison JP, Wolchok JD. Monoclonal antibodies in cancer therapy. *Cancer Immun* (2012) 12:14.
26. Scott AM, Wolchok JD, Old LJ. Antibody therapy of cancer. *Nat Rev Cancer* (2012) 12(4):278–87. doi: 10.1038/nrc3236
27. Hsi ED, Steinle R, Balasa B, Szmania S, Draksharapu A, Shum BP, et al. CS1, a potential new therapeutic antibody target for the treatment of multiple myeloma. *Clin Cancer Res* (2008) 14(9):2775–84. doi: 10.1158/1078-0432.CCR-07-4246
28. Tai YT, Dillon M, Song W, Leiba M, Li XF, Burger P, et al. Anti-CS1 humanized monoclonal antibody HuLuc63 inhibits myeloma cell adhesion and induces antibody-dependent cellular cytotoxicity in the bone marrow milieu. *Blood* (2008) 112(4):1329–37. doi: 10.1182/blood-2007-08-107292
29. Collins SM, Bakan CE, Swartzel GD, Hofmeister CC, Efebera YA, Kwon H, et al. Elotuzumab directly enhances NK cell cytotoxicity against myeloma via CS1 ligation: evidence for augmented NK cell function complementing ADCC. *Cancer Immunol Immunother* (2013) 62(12):1841–9. doi: 10.1007/s00262-013-1493-8
30. Zonder JA, Mohrbacher AF, Singhal S, van Rhee F, Bensinger WI, Ding H, et al. A phase 1, multicenter, open-label, dose escalation study of elotuzumab in patients with advanced multiple myeloma. *Blood* (2012) 120(3):552–9. doi: 10.1182/blood-2011-06-360552
31. Lonial S, Dimopoulos M, Palumbo A, White D, Grosicki S, Spicka I, et al. Elotuzumab Therapy for Relapsed or Refractory Multiple Myeloma. *N Engl J Med* (2015) 373p(7):621–31. doi: 10.1056/NEJMoa1505654
32. Dimopoulos MA, Dytfeld D, Grosicki S, Moreau P, Takezako N, Hori M, et al. Elotuzumab plus Pomalidomide and Dexamethasone for Multiple Myeloma. *N Engl J Med* (2018) 379(19):1811–22. doi: 10.1056/NEJMoa1805762
33. Lin P, Owens R, Tricot G, Wilson CS. Flow cytometric immunophenotypic analysis of 306 cases of multiple myeloma. *Am J Clin Pathol* (2004) 121 (4):482–8. doi: 10.1309/74R4TB90BUWH27JX
34. Moreno L, Perez C, Zabaleta A, Manrique I, Alignani D, Ajona D, et al. The Mechanism of Action of the Anti-CD38 Monoclonal Antibody Isatuximab in Multiple Myeloma. *Clin Cancer Res* (2019) 25(10):3176–87. doi: 10.1158/1078-0432.CCR-18-1597
35. van de Donk N, Usmani SZ. CD38 Antibodies in Multiple Myeloma: Mechanisms of Action and Modes of Resistance. *Front Immunol* (2018) 9:2134. doi: 10.3389/fimmu.2018.02134
36. Sanchez L, Wang Y, Siegel DS, Wang ML. Daratumumab: a first-in-class CD38 monoclonal antibody for the treatment of multiple myeloma. *J Hematol Oncol* (2016) 9(1):51. doi: 10.1186/s13045-016-0283-0
37. de Weers M, Tai YT, van der Veer MS, Bakker JM, Vink T, Jacobs DC, et al. Daratumumab, a novel therapeutic human CD38 monoclonal antibody, induces killing of multiple myeloma and other hematological tumors. *J Immunol* (2011) 186(3):1840–8. doi: 10.4049/jimmunol.1003032
38. Overdijk MB, Verploegen S, Bogels M, van Egmond M, Lammerts van Bueren JJ, Mutis T, et al. Antibody-mediated phagocytosis contributes to the anti-tumor activity of the therapeutic antibody daratumumab in lymphoma and multiple myeloma. *MAbs* (2015) 7(2):311–21. doi: 10.1080/19420862.2015.1007813
39. Lokhorst HM, Plesner T, Laubach JP, Nahi H, Gimsing P, Hansson M, et al. Targeting CD38 with Daratumumab Monotherapy in Multiple Myeloma. *N Engl J Med* (2015) 373(13):1207–19. doi: 10.1056/NEJMoa1506348
40. Lonial S, Weiss BM, Usmani SZ, Singhal S, Chari A, Bahlis NJ, et al. Daratumumab monotherapy in patients with treatment-refractory multiple myeloma (SIRIUS): an open-label, randomised, phase 2 trial. *Lancet* (2016) 387(10027):1551–60. doi: 10.1016/S0140-6736(15)01120-4
41. Dimopoulos MA, Oriol A, Nahi H, San-Miguel J, Bahlis NJ, Usmani SZ, et al. Daratumumab, Lenalidomide, and Dexamethasone for Multiple Myeloma. *N Engl J Med* (2016) 375(14):1319–31. doi: 10.1056/NEJMoa1607751
42. Facon T, Kumar S, Plesner T, Orlowski RZ, Moreau P, Bahlis N, et al. Daratumumab plus Lenalidomide and Dexamethasone for Untreated Myeloma. *N Engl J Med* (2019) 380(22):2104–15. doi: 10.1056/NEJMoa1817249
43. Palumbo A, Chanan-Khan A, Weisel K, Nooka AK, Masszi T, Beksac M, et al. Daratumumab, Bortezomib, and Dexamethasone for Multiple Myeloma. *N Engl J Med* (2016) 375(8):754–66. doi: 10.1056/NEJMoa1606038
44. Chari A, Suvannasankha A, Fay JW, Arnulf B, Kaufman JL, Ifthikharuddin JJ, et al. Daratumumab plus pomalidomide and dexamethasone in relapsed and/or refractory multiple myeloma. *Blood* (2017) 130(8):974–81. doi: 10.1182/blood-2017-05-785246
45. Mateos MV, Dimopoulos MA, Cavo M, Suzuki K, Jakubowiak A, Knop S, et al. Daratumumab plus Bortezomib, Melphalan, and Prednisone for Untreated Myeloma. *N Engl J Med* (2018) 378(6):518–28. doi: 10.1056/NEJMoa1714678
46. Moreau P, Attal M, Hulin C, Arnulf B, Belhadj K, Benboubker L, et al. Bortezomib, thalidomide, and dexamethasone with or without daratumumab before and after autologous stem-cell transplantation for newly diagnosed multiple myeloma (CASSIOPEIA): a randomised, open-label, phase 3 study. *Lancet* (2019) 394(10192):29–38. doi: 10.1016/S0140-6736(19)31240-1
47. Mateos MV, Nahi H, Legiec W, Grosicki S, Vorobyev V, Spicka I, et al. Subcutaneous versus intravenous daratumumab in patients with relapsed or refractory multiple myeloma (COLUMBA): a multicentre, open-label, non-inferiority, randomised, phase 3 trial. *Lancet Haematol* (2020) 7(5):e370–80. doi: 10.1016/S2352-3026(20)30070-3
48. Jiang H, Acharya C, An G, Zhong M, Feng X, Wang L, et al. SAR650984 directly induces multiple myeloma cell death via lysosomal-associated and apoptotic pathways, which is further enhanced by pomalidomide. *Leukemia* (2016) 30(2):399–408. doi: 10.1038/leu.2015.240
49. Deckert J, Wetzel MC, Bartle LM, Skaletskaya A, Goldmacher VS, Vallee F, et al. SAR650984, a novel humanized CD38-targeting antibody, demonstrates potent antitumor activity in models of multiple myeloma and other CD38+ hematologic malignancies. *Clin Cancer Res* (2014) 20 (17):4574–83. doi: 10.1158/1078-0432.CCR-14-0695
50. Krejcik J, Casneuf T, Nijhof IS, Verbist B, Bald J, Plesner T, et al. Daratumumab depletes CD38+ immune regulatory cells, promotes T-cell expansion, and skews T-cell repertoire in multiple myeloma. *Blood* (2016) 128(3):384–94. doi: 10.1182/blood-2015-12-687749
51. Feng X, Zhang L, Acharya C, An G, Wen K, Qiu L, et al. Targeting CD38 Suppresses Induction and Function of T Regulatory Cells to Mitigate Immunosuppression in Multiple Myeloma. *Clin Cancer Res* (2017) 23 (15):4290–300. doi: 10.1158/1078-0432.CCR-16-3192
52. Attal M, Richardson PG, Rajkumar SV, San-Miguel J, Beksac M, Spicka I, et al. Isatuximab plus pomalidomide and low-dose dexamethasone versus pomalidomide and low-dose dexamethasone in patients with relapsed and refractory multiple myeloma (ICARIA-MM): a randomised, multicentre, open-label, phase 3 study. *Lancet* (2019) 394(10214):2096–107. doi: 10.1016/S0140-6736(19)32556-5
53. McCombs JR, Owen SC. Antibody drug conjugates: design and selection of linker, payload and conjugation chemistry. *AAPS J* (2015) 17(2):339–51. doi: 10.1208/s12248-014-9710-8
54. Cho SF, Anderson KC, Tai YT. Targeting B Cell Maturation Antigen (BCMA) in Multiple Myeloma: Potential Uses of BCMA-Based Immunotherapy. *Front Immunol* (2018) 9:1821. doi: 10.3389/fimmu.2018.01821
55. Xing L, Lin L, Yu T, Li Y, Cho SF, Liu J, et al. A novel BCMA PBD-ADC with ATM/ATR/WEE1 inhibitors or bortezomib induce synergistic lethality in multiple myeloma. *Leukemia* (2020) 34(8):2150–62. doi: 10.1038/s41375-020-0745-9
56. Trudel S, Lendvai N, Popat R, Voorhees PM, Reeves B, Libby EN, et al. Targeting B-cell maturation antigen with GSK2857916 antibody-drug conjugate in relapsed or refractory multiple myeloma (BMA117159): a dose escalation and expansion phase 1 trial. *Lancet Oncol* (2018) 19 (12):1641–53. doi: 10.1016/S1470-2045(18)30576-X
57. Kinneer K, Meekin J, Tiberghien AC, Tai YT, Phipps S, Kiefer CM, et al. SLC46A3 as a Potential Predictive Biomarker for Antibody-Drug Conjugates Bearing Noncleavable Linked Maytansinoid and Pyrrolobenzodiazepine Warheads. *Clin Cancer Res* (2018) 24(24):6570–82. doi: 10.1158/1078-0432.CCR-18-1300
58. Tai YT, Mayes PA, Acharya C, Zhong MY, Cea M, Cagnetta A, et al. Novel anti-B-cell maturation antigen antibody-drug conjugate (GSK2857916) selectively induces killing of multiple myeloma. *Blood* (2014) 123 (20):3128–38. doi: 10.1182/blood-2013-10-535088
59. Trudel S, Lendvai N, Popat R, Voorhees PM, Reeves B, Libby EN, et al. Antibody-drug conjugate, GSK2857916, in relapsed/refractory multiple

myeloma: an update on safety and efficacy from dose expansion phase I study. *Blood Cancer J* (2019) 9(4):37. doi: 10.1038/s41408-019-0196-6

60. Benson DM Jr, Bakan CE, Mishra A, Hofmeister CC, Efebera Y, Becknell B, et al. The PD-1/PD-L1 axis modulates the natural killer cell versus multiple myeloma effect: a therapeutic target for CT-011, a novel monoclonal anti-PD-1 antibody. *Blood* (2010) 116(13):2286–94. doi: 10.1182/blood-2010-02-271874
61. Yu B, Jiang T, Liu D. BCMA-targeted immunotherapy for multiple myeloma. *J Hematol Oncol* (2020) 13(1):125. doi: 10.1186/s13045-020-00962-7
62. Lonial S, Lee HC, Badros A, Trudel S, Nooka AK, Chari A, et al. Belantamab mafodotin for relapsed or refractory multiple myeloma (DREAMM-2): a two-arm, randomised, open-label, phase 2 study. *Lancet Oncol* (2020) 21 (2):207–21. doi: 10.1016/S1470-2045(19)30788-0
63. Smits NC, Sentman CL. Bispecific T-Cell Engagers (BiTEs) as Treatment of B-Cell Lymphoma. *J Clin Oncol* (2016) 34(10):1131–3. doi: 10.1200/JCO.2015.64.9970
64. Fu M, He Q, Guo Z, Zhou X, Li H, Zhao L, et al. Therapeutic Bispecific T-Cell Engager Antibody Targeting the Transferrin Receptor. *Front Immunol* (2019) 10:1396. doi: 10.3389/fimmu.2019.01396
65. Seckinger A, Delgado JA, Moser S, Moreno L, Neuber B, Grab A, et al. Target Expression, Generation, Preclinical Activity, and Pharmacokinetics of the BCMA-T Cell Bispecific Antibody EM801 for Multiple Myeloma Treatment. *Cancer Cell* (2017) 31(3):396–410. doi: 10.1016/j.ccell.2017.02.002
66. Hipp S, Tai YT, Blanset D, Deegen P, Wahl J, Thomas O, et al. A novel BCMA/CD3 bispecific T-cell engager for the treatment of multiple myeloma induces selective lysis in vitro and in vivo. *Leukemia* (2017) 31(8):1743–51. doi: 10.1038/leu.2016.388
67. Zou J, Chen D, Zong Y, Ye S, Tang J, Meng H, et al. Immunotherapy based on bispecific T-cell engager with hIgG1 Fc sequence as a new therapeutic strategy in multiple myeloma. *Cancer Sci* (2015) 106(5):512–21. doi: 10.1111/cas.12631
68. Lejeune M, Kose MC, Duray E, Einsele H, Beguin Y, Caers J. Bispecific, T-Cell-Recruiting Antibodies in B-Cell Malignancies. *Front Immunol* (2020) 11:762. doi: 10.3389/fimmu.2020.00762
69. Topp MS, Duell J, Zugmaier G, Attal M, Moreau P, Langer C, et al. Anti-B-Cell Maturation Antigen BiTE Molecule AMG 420 Induces Responses in Multiple Myeloma. *J Clin Oncol* (2020) 38(8):775–83. doi: 10.1200/JCO.19.02657
70. Cho SF, Lin L, Xing L, Li Y, Wen K, Yu T, et al. The immunomodulatory drugs lenalidomide and pomalidomide enhance the potency of AMG 701 in multiple myeloma preclinical models. *Blood Adv* (2020) 4(17):4195–207. doi: 10.1182/bloodadvances.2020002524
71. Morgan RA, Dudley ME, Wunderlich JR, Hughes MS, Yang JC, Sherry RM, et al. Cancer regression in patients after transfer of genetically engineered lymphocytes. *Science* (2006) 314(5796):126–9. doi: 10.1126/science.1129003
72. Rosenberg SA, Packard BS, Aebersold PM, Solomon D, Topalian SL, Toy ST, et al. Use of tumor-infiltrating lymphocytes and interleukin-2 in the immunotherapy of patients with metastatic melanoma. *A Prelim Rep N Engl J Med* (1988) 319(25):1676–80. doi: 10.1056/NEJM198812223192527
73. Rosenberg SA, Restifo NP. Adoptive cell transfer as personalized immunotherapy for human cancer. *Science* (2015) 348(6230):62–8. doi: 10.1126/science.aaa4967
74. Noonan KA, Huff CA, Davis J, Lemas MV, Fiorino S, Bitzan J, et al. Adoptive transfer of activated marrow-infiltrating lymphocytes induces measurable antitumor immunity in the bone marrow in multiple myeloma. *Sci Transl Med* (2015) 7(288):288ra78. doi: 10.1126/scitranslmed.aaa7014
75. Rapoport AP, Stadtmauer EA, Binder-Scholl GK, Goloubeva O, Vogl DT, Lacey SF, et al. NY-ESO-1-specific TCR-engineered T cells mediate sustained antigen-specific antitumor effects in myeloma. *Nat Med* (2015) 21(8):914–21. doi: 10.1038/nm.3910
76. Thomas R, Al-Khadairi G, Roelands J, Hendrickx W, Dermime S, Bedognetti D, et al. NY-ESO-1 Based Immunotherapy of Cancer: Current Perspectives. *Front Immunol* (2018) 9:947. doi: 10.3389/fimmu.2018.00947
77. D'Agostino M, Raje N. Anti-BCMA CAR T-cell therapy in multiple myeloma: can we do better? *Leukemia* (2020) 34(1):21–34. doi: 10.1038/s41375-019-0669-4
78. Eshhar Z, Waks T, Gross G, Schindler DG. Specific activation and targeting of cytotoxic lymphocytes through chimeric single chains consisting of antibody-binding domains and the gamma or zeta subunits of the immunoglobulin and T-cell receptors. *Proc Natl Acad Sci U.S.A.* (1993) 90 (2):720–4. doi: 10.1073/pnas.90.2.720
79. Garcia-Guerrero E, Sierro-Martinez B, Perez-Simon JA. Overcoming Chimeric Antigen Receptor (CAR) Modified T-Cell Therapy Limitations in Multiple Myeloma. *Front Immunol* (2020) 11:1128. doi: 10.3389/fimmu.2020.01128
80. Lee DW, Gardner R, Porter DL, Louis CU, Ahmed N, Jensen M, et al. Current concepts in the diagnosis and management of cytokine release syndrome. *Blood* (2014) 124(2):188–95. doi: 10.1182/blood-2014-05-552729
81. Barrett DM, Teachey DT, Grupp SA. Toxicity management for patients receiving novel T-cell engaging therapies. *Curr Opin Pediatr* (2014) 26 (1):43–9. doi: 10.1097/MOP.0000000000000043
82. Ali SA, Shi V, Maric I, Wang M, Stroncek DF, Rose JJ, et al. T cells expressing an anti-B-cell maturation antigen chimeric antigen receptor cause remissions of multiple myeloma. *Blood* (2016) 128(13):1688–700. doi: 10.1182/blood-2016-04-711903
83. Garfall AL, Maus MV, Hwang WT, Lacey SF, Mahnke YD, Melenhorst JJ, et al. Chimeric Antigen Receptor T Cells against CD19 for Multiple Myeloma. *N Engl J Med* (2015) 373(11):1040–7. doi: 10.1056/NEJMoa1504542
84. Raje N, Berdeja J, Lin Y, Siegel D, Jagannath S, Madduri D, et al. Anti-BCMA CAR T-Cell Therapy bb2121 in Relapsed or Refractory Multiple Myeloma. *N Engl J Med* (2019) 380(18):1726–37. doi: 10.1056/NEJMoa1817226
85. Jelinek T, Mihalyova J, Kascak M, Duras J, Hajek R. PD-1/PD-L1 inhibitors in haematological malignancies: update 2017. *Immunology* (2017) 152 (3):357–71. doi: 10.1111/imm.12788
86. Ishida Y, Agata Y, Shibahara K, Honjo T. Induced expression of PD-1, a novel member of the immunoglobulin gene superfamily, upon programmed cell death. *EMBO J* (1992) 11(11):3887–95. doi: 10.1002/j.1460-2075.1992.tb05481.x
87. Zou W, Chen L. Inhibitory B7-family molecules in the tumour microenvironment. *Nat Rev Immunol* (2008) 8(6):467–77. doi: 10.1038/nri2326
88. Gorgun G, Samur MK, Cowens KB, Paula S, Bianchi G, Anderson JE, et al. Lenalidomide Enhances Immune Checkpoint Blockade-Induced Immune Response in Multiple Myeloma. *Clin Cancer Res* (2015) 21(20):4607–18. doi: 10.1158/1078-0432.CCR-15-0200
89. Hallett WH, Jing W, Drobyski WR, Johnson BD. Immunosuppressive effects of multiple myeloma are overcome by PD-L1 blockade. *Biol Blood Marrow Transplant* (2011) 17(8):1133–45. doi: 10.1016/j.bbmt.2011.03.011
90. Paiva B, Azpilikueta A, Puig N, Ocio EM, Sharma R, Oyajobi BO, et al. PD-L1/PD-1 presence in the tumor microenvironment and activity of PD-1 blockade in multiple myeloma. *Leukemia* (2015) 29(10):2110–3. doi: 10.1038/leu.2015.79
91. Liu J, Hamrouni A, Wolowiec D, Coiteux V, Kuliczkowski K, Hetuin D, et al. Plasma cells from multiple myeloma patients express B7-H1 (PD-L1) and increase expression after stimulation with IFN-{gamma} and TLR ligands via a MyD88-, TRAF6-, and MEK-dependent pathway. *Blood* (2007) 110 (1):296–304. doi: 10.1182/blood-2006-10-051482
92. Tamura H, Ishibashi M, Yamashita T, Tanosaki S, Okuyama N, Kondo A, et al. Marrow stromal cells induce B7-H1 expression on myeloma cells, generating aggressive characteristics in multiple myeloma. *Leukemia* (2013) 27(2):464–72. doi: 10.1038/leu.2012.213
93. Ray A, Das DS, Song Y, Richardson P, Munshi NC, Chauhan D, et al. Targeting PD1-PDL1 immune checkpoint in plasmacytoid dendritic cell interactions with T cells, natural killer cells and multiple myeloma cells. *Leukemia* (2015) 29(6):1441–4. doi: 10.1038/leu.2015.11
94. Tamura H, Ishibashi M, Sunakawa-Kii M, Inokuchi K. PD-L1-PD-1 Pathway in the Pathophysiology of Multiple Myeloma. *Cancers (Basel)* (2020) 12(4):924. doi: 10.3390/cancers12040924
95. Lesokhin AM, Ansell SM, Armand P, Scott EC, Halwani A, Gutierrez M, et al. Nivolumab in Patients With Relapsed or Refractory Hematologic Malignancy: Preliminary Results of a Phase Ib Study. *J Clin Oncol* (2016) 34 (23):2698–704. doi: 10.1200/JCO.2015.65.9789

96. Ribrag V, Avigan DE, Green DJ, Wise-Draper T, Posada JG, Vij R, et al. Phase 1b trial of pembrolizumab monotherapy for relapsed/refractory multiple myeloma: KEYNOTE-013. *Br J Haematol* (2019) 186(3):e41–4. doi: 10.1111/bjh.15888
97. Costello C. The future of checkpoint inhibition in multiple myeloma? *Lancet Haematol* (2019) 6(9):e439–40. doi: 10.1016/S2352-3026(19)30149-8
98. Postow MA, Sidlow R, Hellmann MD. Immune-Related Adverse Events Associated with Immune Checkpoint Blockade. *N Engl J Med* (2018) 378 (2):158–68. doi: 10.1056/NEJMra1703481
99. Jelinek T, Paiva B, Hajek R. Update on PD-1/PD-L1 Inhibitors in Multiple Myeloma. *Front Immunol* (2018) 9:2431. doi: 10.3389/fimmu.2018.02431
100. Oliva S, Troia R, D'Agostino M, Boccadoro M, Gay F. Promises and Pitfalls in the Use of PD-1/PD-L1 Inhibitors in Multiple Myeloma. *Front Immunol* (2018) 9:2749. doi: 10.3389/fimmu.2018.02749
101. Costa F, Das R, Kini Bailur J, Dhodapkar K, Dhodapkar MV. Checkpoint Inhibition in Myeloma: Opportunities and Challenges. *Front Immunol* (2018) 9:2204. doi: 10.3389/fimmu.2018.02204
102. Guo C, Manjili MH, Subjeck JR, Sarkar D, Fisher PB, Wang XY. Therapeutic cancer vaccines: past, present, and future. *Adv Cancer Res* (2013) 119:421–75. doi: 10.1016/B978-0-12-407190-2.00007-1
103. Maurer DM, Butterfield LH, Vujanovic L. Melanoma vaccines: clinical status and immune endpoints. *Melanoma Res* (2019) 29(2):109–18. doi: 10.1097/CMR.0000000000000535
104. Garfall AL, Stadtmauer EA. Cellular and vaccine immunotherapy for multiple myeloma. *Hematol Am Soc Hematol Educ Program* (2016) 2016 (1):521–7. doi: 10.1182/asheducation-2016.1.521
105. Cohen AD, Raje N, Fowler JA, Mezzi K, Scott EC, Dhodapkar MV. How to Train Your T Cells: Overcoming Immune Dysfunction in Multiple Myeloma. *Clin Cancer Res* (2020) 26(7):1541–54. doi: 10.1158/1078-0432.CCR-19-2111
106. Le DT, Pardoll DM, Jaffee EM. Cellular vaccine approaches. *Cancer J* (2010) 16(4):304–10. doi: 10.1097/PPO.0b013e3181eb33d7
107. Dranoff G. GM-CSF-based cancer vaccines. *Immunol Rev* (2002) 188:147–54. doi: 10.1034/j.1600-065X.2002.18813.x
108. Rapoport AP, Aqui NA, Stadtmauer EA, Vogl DT, Xu YY, Kalos M, et al. Combination immunotherapy after ASCT for multiple myeloma using MAGE-A3/Poly-ICLC immunizations followed by adoptive transfer of vaccine-primed and costimulated autologous T cells. *Clin Cancer Res* (2014) 20(5):1355–65. doi: 10.1158/1078-0432.CCR-13-2817
109. Tsuboi A, Oka Y, Nakajima H, Fukuda Y, Elisseeva OA, Yoshihara S, et al. Wilms tumor gene WT1 peptide-based immunotherapy induced a minimal response in a patient with advanced therapy-resistant multiple myeloma. *Int J Hematol* (2007) 86(5):414–7. doi: 10.1007/BF02983998
110. Bae J, Smith R, Daley J, Mimura N, Tai YT, Anderson KC, et al. Myeloma-specific multiple peptides able to generate cytotoxic T lymphocytes: a potential therapeutic application in multiple myeloma and other plasma cell disorders. *Clin Cancer Res* (2012) 18(17):4850–60. doi: 10.1158/1078-0432.CCR-11-2776
111. Bae J, Prabhala R, Voskertchian A, Brown A, Maguire C, Richardson P, et al. A multiepitope of XBP1, CD138 and CS1 peptides induces myeloma-specific cytotoxic T lymphocytes in T cells of smoldering myeloma patients. *Leukemia* (2015) 29(1):218–29. doi: 10.1038/leu.2014.159
112. Bae J, Samur M, Richardson P, Munshi NC, Anderson KC. Selective targeting of multiple myeloma by B cell maturation antigen (BCMA)-specific central memory CD8(+) cytotoxic T lymphocytes: immunotherapeutic application in vaccination and adoptive immunotherapy. *Leukemia* (2019) 33(9):2208–26. doi: 10.1038/s41375-019-0414-z
113. Hansson L, Abdalla AO, Moshfegh A, Choudhury A, Rabbani H, Nilsson B, et al. Long-term idiotype vaccination combined with interleukin-12 (IL-12), or IL-12 and granulocyte macrophage colony-stimulating factor, in early-stage multiple myeloma patients. *Clin Cancer Res* (2007) 13(5):1503–10. doi: 10.1158/1078-0432.CCR-06-1603
114. McCann KJ, Godeseth R, Chudley L, Mander A, Di Genova G, Lloyd-Evans P, et al. Idiotypic DNA vaccination for the treatment of multiple myeloma: safety and immunogenicity in a phase I clinical study. *Cancer Immunol Immunother* (2015) 64(8):1021–32. doi: 10.1007/s00262-015-1703-7
115. Coscia M, Mariani S, Battaglio S, Di Bello C, Fiore F, Foglietta M, et al. Long-term follow-up of idiotype vaccination in human myeloma as a maintenance therapy after high-dose chemotherapy. *Leukemia* (2004) 18(1):139–45. doi: 10.1038/sj.leu.2403181
116. Rosenblatt J, Vasir B, Uhl L, Blotta S, Macnamara C, Somaiya P, et al. Vaccination with dendritic cell/tumor fusion cells results in cellular and humoral antitumor immune responses in patients with multiple myeloma. *Blood* (2011) 117(2):393–402. doi: 10.1182/blood-2010-04-277137
117. Rosenblatt J, Avivi I, Vasir B, Uhl L, Munshi NC, Katz T, et al. Vaccination with dendritic cell/tumor fusions following autologous stem cell transplant induces immunologic and clinical responses in multiple myeloma patients. *Clin Cancer Res* (2013) 19(13):3640–8. doi: 10.1158/1078-0432.CCR-13-0282
118. Romano E, Cotari JW, Barreira da Silva R, Betts BC, Chung DJ, Avogadri F, et al. Human Langerhans cells use an IL-15R-alpha/IL-15/pSTAT5-dependent mechanism to break T-cell tolerance against the self-differentiation tumor antigen WT1. *Blood* (2012) 119(22):5182–90. doi: 10.1182/blood-2011-09-382200
119. Chung DJ, Romano E, Pronschinske KB, Shyer JA, Mennecozzi M, St Angelo ET, et al. Langerhans-type and monocyte-derived human dendritic cells have different susceptibilities to mRNA electroporation with distinct effects on maturation and activation: implications for immunogenicity in dendritic cell-based immunotherapy. *J Transl Med* (2013) 11:166. doi: 10.1186/1479-5876-11-166
120. Benboubker L, Dimopoulos MA, Dispenzieri A, Catalano J, Belch AR, Cavo M, et al. Lenalidomide and dexamethasone in transplant-ineligible patients with myeloma. *N Engl J Med* (2014) 371(10):906–17. doi: 10.1056/NEJMoa1402551
121. Durie BGM, Hoering A, Abidi MH, Rajkumar SV, Epstein J, Kahanic SP, et al. Bortezomib with lenalidomide and dexamethasone versus lenalidomide and dexamethasone alone in patients with newly diagnosed myeloma without intent for immediate autologous stem-cell transplant (SWOG S0777): a randomised, open-label, phase 3 trial. *Lancet* (2017) 389 (10068):519–27. doi: 10.1016/S0140-6736(16)31594-X
122. O'Donnell EK, Laubach JP, Yee AJ, Chen T, Huff CA, Basile FG, et al. A phase 2 study of modified lenalidomide, bortezomib and dexamethasone in transplant-ineligible multiple myeloma. *Br J Haematol* (2018) 182(2):222–30. doi: 10.1111/bjh.15261
123. Joseph NS, Kaufman JL, Dhodapkar MV, Hofmeister CC, Almaula DK, Heffner LT, et al. Long-Term Follow-Up Results of Lenalidomide, Bortezomib, and Dexamethasone Induction Therapy and Risk-Adapted Maintenance Approach in Newly Diagnosed Multiple Myeloma. *J Clin Oncol* (2020) 38(17):1928–37. doi: 10.1200/JCO.19.02515
124. Moreau P, Masszi T, Grzasko N, Bahlis NJ, Hansson M, Pour L, et al. Oral Ixazomib, Lenalidomide, and Dexamethasone for Multiple Myeloma. *N Engl J Med* (2016) 374(17):1621–34. doi: 10.1056/NEJMoa1516282
125. Stewart AK, Rajkumar SV, Dimopoulos MA, Masszi T, Spicka I, Oriol A, et al. Carfilzomib, lenalidomide, and dexamethasone for relapsed multiple myeloma. *N Engl J Med* (2015) 372(2):142–52. doi: 10.1056/NEJMoa1411321
126. Richardson PG, Oriol A, Beksac M, Liberati AM, Galli M, Schjesvold F, et al. Pomalidomide, bortezomib, and dexamethasone for patients with relapsed or refractory multiple myeloma previously treated with lenalidomide (OPTIMISMM): a randomised, open-label, phase 3 trial. *Lancet Oncol* (2019) 20(6):781–94. doi: 10.1016/S1470-2045(19)30152-4
127. Kronke J, Udeshi ND, Narla A, Grauman P, Hurst SN, McConkey M, et al. Lenalidomide causes selective degradation of IKZF1 and IKZF3 in multiple myeloma cells. *Science* (2014) 343(6168):301–5. doi: 10.1126/science.1244851
128. Lu G, Middleton RE, Sun H, Naniong M, Ott CJ, Mitsiades CS, et al. The myeloma drug lenalidomide promotes the cereblon-dependent destruction of Ikaros proteins. *Science* (2014) 343(6168):305–9. doi: 10.1126/science.1244917
129. Gandhi AK, Kang J, Havens CG, Conklin T, Ning Y, Wu L, et al. Immunomodulatory agents lenalidomide and pomalidomide co-stimulate T cells by inducing degradation of T cell repressors Ikaros and Aiolos via modulation of the E3 ubiquitin ligase complex CRL4(CRBN.). *Br J Haematol* (2014) 164(6):811–21. doi: 10.1111/bjh.12708
130. Hideshima T, Ogiya D, Liu J, Harada T, Kurata K, Bae J, et al. Immunomodulatory drugs activate NK cells via both Zap-70 and cereblon-dependent pathways. *Leukemia* (2020) 35(1):177–88. doi: 10.1038/s41375-020-0809-x

131. Ocio EM, Fernandez-Lazaro D, San-Segundo L, Lopez-Corral L, Corchete LA, Gutierrez NC, et al. In vivo murine model of acquired resistance in myeloma reveals differential mechanisms for lenalidomide and pomalidomide in combination with dexamethasone. *Leukemia* (2015) 29 (3):705–14. doi: 10.1038/leu.2014.238

132. Sehgal K, Das R, Zhang L, Verma R, Deng Y, Kocoglu M, et al. Clinical and pharmacodynamic analysis of pomalidomide dosing strategies in myeloma: impact of immune activation and cereblon targets. *Blood* (2015) 125 (26):4042–51. doi: 10.1182/blood-2014-11-611426

133. Bjorklund CC, Kang J, Amatangelo M, Polonskaia A, Katz M, Chiu H, et al. Iberdomide (CC-220) is a potent cereblon E3 ligase modulator with antitumor and immunostimulatory activities in lenalidomide- and pomalidomide-resistant multiple myeloma cells with dysregulated CRBN. *Leukemia* (2020) 34(4):1197–201. doi: 10.1038/s41375-019-0620-8

134. Hansen JD, Correa M, Nagy MA, Alexander M, Plantevin V, Grant V, et al. Discovery of CRBN E3 Ligase Modulator CC-92480 for the Treatment of Relapsed and Refractory Multiple Myeloma. *J Med Chem* (2020) 63 (13):6648–76. doi: 10.1021/acs.jmedchem.9b01928

135. Bianchi G, Oliva L, Cascio P, Pengo N, Fontana F, Cerruti F, et al. The proteasome load versus capacity balance determines apoptotic sensitivity of multiple myeloma cells to proteasome inhibition. *Blood* (2009) 113 (13):3040–9. doi: 10.1182/blood-2008-08-172734

136. Gandolfi S, Laubach JP, Hideshima T, Chauhan D, Anderson KC, Richardson PG. The proteasome and proteasome inhibitors in multiple myeloma. *Cancer Metastasis Rev* (2017) 36(4):561–84. doi: 10.1007/s10555-017-9707-8

137. Ettari R, Zappala M, Grasso S, Musolino C, Innao V, Allegra A. Immunoproteasome-selective and non-selective inhibitors: A promising approach for the treatment of multiple myeloma. *Pharmacol Ther* (2018) 182:176–92. doi: 10.1016/j.pharmthera.2017.09.001

138. Spisek R, Charalambous A, Mazumder A, Vesole DH, Jagannath S, Dhodapkar MV. Bortezomib enhances dendritic cell (DC)-mediated induction of immunity to human myeloma via exposure of cell surface heat shock protein 90 on dying tumor cells: therapeutic implications. *Blood* (2007) 109(11):4839–45. doi: 10.1182/blood-2006-10-054221

139. Hull EE, Montgomery MR, Leyva KJ. HDAC Inhibitors as Epigenetic Regulators of the Immune System: Impacts on Cancer Therapy and Inflammatory Diseases. *BioMed Res Int* (2016) 2016:8797206. doi: 10.1155/2016/8797206

140. Bae J, Hideshima T, Tai YT, Song Y, Richardson P, Raje N, et al. Histone deacetylase (HDAC) inhibitor ACY241 enhances anti-tumor activities of antigen-specific central memory cytotoxic T lymphocytes against multiple myeloma and solid tumors. *Leukemia* (2018) 32(9):1932–47. doi: 10.1038/s41375-018-0062-8

141. Laubach JP, van de Donk N, Davies FE, Mikhael J. Practical Considerations for Antibodies in Myeloma. *Am Soc Clin Oncol Educ Book* (2018) 38:667–74. doi: 10.1200/EDBK_205443

142. Laurent SA, Hoffmann FS, Kuhn PH, Cheng Q, Chu Y, Schmidt-Supprian M, et al. gamma-Secretase directly sheds the survival receptor BCMA from plasma cells. *Nat Commun* (2015) 6:7333. doi: 10.1038/ncomms8333

143. Pont MJ, Hill T, Cole GO, Abbott JJ, Kelliher J, Salter AI, et al. gamma-Secretase inhibition increases efficacy of BCMA-specific chimeric antigen receptor T cells in multiple myeloma. *Blood* (2019) 134(19):1585–97. doi: 10.1182/blood.2019000050

8

CDC27 Promotes Tumor Progression and Affects PD-L1 Expression in T-Cell Lymphoblastic Lymphoma

Yue Song[1,2,3†], *Wei Song*[4†], *Zhaoming Li*[1,3], *Wenting Song*[1,2,3], *Yibo Wen*[2], *Jiwei Li*[1,3], *Qingxin Xia*[4*] *and Mingzhi Zhang*[1,3*]

[1] Department of Oncology, The First Affiliated Hospital of Zhengzhou University, Zhengzhou, China, [2] The Academy of Medical Science of Zhengzhou University, Zhengzhou, China, [3] Lymphoma Diagnosis and Treatment Center of Henan Province, Zhengzhou, China, [4] Department of Pathology, The Affiliated Cancer Hospital of Zhengzhou University, Henan Cancer Hospital, Zhengzhou, China

***Correspondence:**
Qingxin Xia
tudou414135404@163.com
Mingzhi Zhang
mingzhi_zhang1@163.com

† These authors have contributed equally to this work

T-lymphoblastic lymphoma (T-LBL) is a rare hematological malignancy with highly aggressive, unique clinical manifestations, and poor prognosis. Cell division cycle 27 (CDC27) was previously reported to be a significant subunit of the anaphase-promoting complex/cyclosome. However, the specific functions and relevant mechanisms of CDC27 in T-LBL remain unknown. Through immunohistochemistry staining, we identified that CDC27 was overexpressed in T-LBL tissues and related to tumor progression and poor survival. Functional experiments demonstrated that CDC27 promoted proliferation *in vivo* and *in vitro*. Further experiment suggested the role of CDC27 in facilitating G1/S transition and promoting the expression of Cyclin D1 and CDK4. Then the effect of CDC27 in inhibiting apoptosis was also identified. Furthermore, we found a positive correlation between the expression of CDC27 and Programmed death ligand-1 (PD-L1) by immunohistochemistry staining. The interaction between CDC27 and PD-L1 was also proved by western blot, luciferase gene reporter assay and immunofluorescence. Taken together, our results showed that CDC27 contributes to T-LBL progression and there is a positive correlation between PD-L1 and CDC27, which offers novel perspectives for future studies on targeting CDC27 in T-LBL.

Keywords: CDC27, T-cell lymphoblastic lymphoma, PD-L1, cell cycle, APC/C

INTRODUCTION

Lymphoblastic lymphoma is a rare type of non-Hodgkin lymphoma (NHL) with biological characteristics similar to acute lymphoblastic leukemia (ALL). On the basis of the origin of tumor cells, it is primarily classified into B-cell lymphoblastic lymphoma and T-cell lymphoblastic lymphoma (T-LBL) (1). Because of the progressive improvements in therapeutic strategies, especially the wide application of targeted therapies, the prognosis of B-cell lymphoma has improved obviously. However, the clinical progression of T-LBL is rapid and the prognosis is poor. The standard NHL-like treatment plan is less effective with higher probability of recurrence and metastasis. Because of the rarity of the disease and limited materials for research, there is also a lack of knowledge about the molecular genetics and effective targeted therapies for T-LBL (2). Therefore, the molecular mechanisms related to tumor formation and progression of T-LBL should be studied to provide effective therapies for its prevention.

The anaphase-promoting complex/cyclosome (APC/C) plays an important role in the process of protein degradation during mitosis (3). APC/C is significant in a variety of cellular events, including mitotic progression, controlling differentiation, etc. (4). Moreover, the aberrant expression of APC/C is relevant to cancer occurrence (5). Cell division cycle 27 (CDC27) is a critical subunit of APC/C that is in charge of binding to two coactivators: CDH1 and cell division cycle 20 (CDC20) (6). CDH1 and CDC20 have tumor suppressor function and oncogenic function, respectively (7–9). Although many studies have shown that CDC27 mutations are detected in various cancer specimens, the role of CDC27 in cancer is uncertain, especially in lymphoma (10).

Programmed death ligand-1 (PD-L1), as the ligand of programmed cell death protein 1 (PD-1), is a key immune checkpoint molecule that is frequently overexpressed in various tumors and correlates with tumor cells evading immune surveillance (11). Therefore, blocking the PD-1/PD-L1 axis is critical for cancer immunotherapy. However, the response rates to PD-1/PD-L1 immune checkpoint blockade therapy are likely to vary widely, ~10–20% across whole tumor types (12, 13). It is urgent to find predictive molecules and relevant pathways for PD-1/PD-L1 checkpoint blockade immunotherapy to develop innovative treatments.

In our previous studies, we found some prognostic clinical indicators in T-LBL (14, 15). We also found that the novel mutation in CDC27, which ranked highly in the samples (16). However, the function of relative targeted gene or therapy, such as CDC27, is not completely clear. In the present study, we aimed to determine whether CDC27 can be used as a target for T-LBL patients by analyzing 46 cases of T-LBL tissues and the T-LBL cells. The results offer new insights into the mechanisms of T-LBL tumorigenesis and suggest that the CDC27-PD-L1 axis could be used as a target in T-LBL treatment.

MATERIALS AND METHODS

Cell Lines and Culture

Sup-T1 cells were purchased from American Type Culture Collection (Manassas, VA, USA). Jurkat and 293T cells were purchased From the Cell Bank of Type Culture Collection of the Chinese Academy of Sciences (Shanghai, China). 293T cell line was cultured in high glucose DMEM medium (Thermo Fisher Scientific), and the other cell lines were cultured in RPMI 1640 medium (Thermo Fisher Scientific). The cells were cultured in corresponding medium supplemented with 10% fetal bovine serum (Sigma-Aldrich, St. Louis, MO, USA), 100 U/mL penicillin, and 100 mg/mL streptomycin (Invitrogen, California, USA) in an incubator maintained at 37°C in a humidified atmosphere containing 5% CO_2 and 95% air.

Abbreviations: T-LBL, T-lymphoblastic lymphoma; CDC27, Cell division cycle 27; PD-L1, Programmed death ligand-1; NHL, non-Hodgkin lymphoma; ALL, acute lymphoblastic leukemia; APC/C, anaphase-promoting complex/cyclosome; CDC20, cell division cycle 20; PD-1, programmed cell death protein 1; PBS, phosphate buffer saline; IHC, Immunohistochemistry; OD, optic density; SD, standard deviation; OS, overall survival; PFS, progression free survival.

Patient Tissue Samples and Clinicopathological Characteristics

Forty-six T-LBL tissues and 30 reactive hyperplasia of the lymph node tissues were collected in this study. All patients were histologically and clinically diagnosed between 2014 and 2019 in the First Affiliated Hospital of Zhengzhou University (Henan, China) and signed informed consent for the collection of tissues. The protocols were confirmed by the Institutional Research Ethics Committee of the First Affiliated Hospital of Zhengzhou University (Henan, China).

Immunohistochemistry (IHC)

The detailed method has been described in a previous study (17). Sections were incubated with the primary antibodies overnight at 4°C, including CDC27 (Santa Cruz, CA, USA, sc-9972, 1:50), Ki67 (Abcam, MA, USA, ab15580, 1:100), and PD-L1 (Proteintech, Wuhan, China, 17952-1-AP, 1:100). The protein expression levels were evaluated semi-quantitatively according to the intensity and the percentage of staining area (18). The score criterion of intensity is as follows: <5%, - (negative = 0); 6–20%, + (weakly positive = 1); 21–50%, ++ (moderately positive = 2); >50%, + + + (strongly positive = 3). The scores were assessed by pathologists without prior knowledge of the patients' and the xenograft tumors' information. H-score that ranged from 0 (no staining) to 300 (maximum staining) were calculated with the following formula: 1 × (% light staining) + 2 × (% moderate staining) + 3 × (% strong staining).

Stable Cell Line Construction

To overexpress CDC27, 12 μg purified pCDH- CMV-MCS-EF1- copGFP- T2A- puro- vector or pCDH- CMV- MCS-EF1- copGFP- T2A- puro- CDC27 plasmid was cotransfected with 6 μg pMDL-G/P-RRE, 6 μg pCMV-VSVG, and 7.5 μg pRSV-REV using Lipofectamine 6000 (Introgen, Carlsbad, CA, USA) according to the manufacturer's protocol. After 72 h, the viruses were harvested and used for transduction with 8 mg/ml polybrene. Stable CDC27 knockdown cell lines were generated using lentiviral constructs expressing short hairpin RNA (shRNA) of CDC27 (target sequence: shCDC27 #1 CAAGTACCTAATCATAGTTTA; shCDC27 #2 GAGCCAATAACCCAAGAAGAA) and negative control (target sequence: TTCTCCGAACGTGTCACGT), which were synthesized by Shanghai GeneChem (Shanghai, China). Cells were infected with lentivirus (multiplicity of infection = 50) by using polybrene (5 μg/ml) for 16 h.

Cell Viability Assay

Cell proliferation was assayed by using the Cell Counting Kit-8 (CCK-8; Dojindo Laboratories, Tokyo, Japan) according to the manufacturer's protocol. First, T-LBL cells were seeded into 96-well-plates in triplicate (2 × 10^3 cells per well) and totally cultured for 5 days. Then, the cells were incubated with a CCK-8 solution for 2 h at 37°C in an atmosphere containing 5% CO_2. Absorbance was determined at OD 450 nm using a Multiskan FC microplate reader (Thermo Scientific, Waltham, MA, USA).

Colony Formation Assays

In the colony formation assay (GENMED, SCIENTIFICS INC, USA), cells were seeded into 6-well-culture plates (1,000 cells per well) with Reagent A and incubated at 37°C for 14 days. Then, the cells were fixed and stained with 0.1% crystal violet solution (Amresco: C3886). The number of colonies containing more than 50 cells was counted.

EdU-647 Labeling

1×10^6 cells were seeded in 24-well-plates and labeled with 10 μM EdU (Click-iT™ Plus EdU Alexa Fluor™ 647 Flow Cytometry Assay Kit, lot: C10634) in 37°C for 2 h. After staining, fixation, and membrane permeability, cells were treated with 1 × Click-iT staining reaction solution for 30 min in darkness. After three washes, samples were added with 5 μl 7-AAD and analysis was performed on a flow cytometer (FACSCanto II, BD Bioscience, San Jose, CA, USA).

Cell Cycle Analysis

Cells were harvested, washed, and fixed in precooled 75% ethanol mixed with phosphate buffer saline (PBS) at 4°C overnight. The next day, the cells were washed and resuspended in 500 μl RNase and propidium Iodide (PI) mixed solution from a cell cycle detection kit (KeyGen Biotech, KGA512), and the cells were incubated at 37°C for 30 min for staining. All cell samples were harvested and analyzed on a flow cytometer.

Apoptosis Detection

Cell apoptosis was analyzed with an APC-annexin V Kit (BD Pharmingen). After 48 h of serum-starved culture, cells in each group were fully harvested and resuspended in annexin-V binding buffer. Next, cells were stained with APC-annexin V and 7-AAD Viability Staining Solution and incubated in the dark for 30 min at room temperature before being detected by a flow cytometer.

Luciferase Gene Reporter Assay

The pGL3 plasmid containing the PD-L1 promoter region and luciferase reporter gene was purchased from GeneChem (Shanghai, China). The detailed procedures of the luciferase gene reporter assay were performed as previously described (19). According to the manufacturer's instructions, 24-well-plates were used to seed a total of 1×10^5 293T cells which were co-transfected with the corresponding plasmids, including the pGL3-luciferase plasmids (control vector or containing PD-L1 promoter), the indicated silencing transfection plasmids (shNC or shCDC27#1), and pRL-TK-Renilla vector. After 48 h, firefly and Renilla luciferase activities were measured and normalized by the Dual Luciferase Assay Kit (Promega, lot: 0000322867) according to the manufacturer's recommendations.

Immunofluorescence Staining

The cells were fixed with 4% formaldehyde in PBS for 30 min at room temperature. After three washes with PBS, the cells were incubated in 0.25% Triton X-100 for 10 min to penetrate the membranes. To block the samples, the cells were treated with 5% bovine serum albumin in PBS for 1 h at room temperature. Then, the cells were incubated with the corresponding primary antibodies overnight at 4°C. Then the cells were washed and stained with a mixture of fluorescent secondary antibodies (Alexa Fluor 488 goat anti-mouse IgG, 1:100: Alexa Fluor 568 goat anti-rabbit IgG, 1:100, Life Technologies) and incubated for 1 h at room temperature in the dark. After three washes with PBS, the cells were stained with DAPI (sc-24941, Santa Cruz Biotechnology). Images were captured using a fluorescence microscope (DMI400B, Leica Company, Germany).

Western Blotting Analysis

The detailed procedures of protein extraction and western blot analyses were previously described (20). Cells were washed and lysed in RIPA buffer with protease and phosphatase inhibitor cocktail (Thermo Scientific, Waltham, MA, USA). Protein samples were loaded and separated by 10% SDS-PAGE and then transferred to PVDF membranes. The membranes were then blocked with 5% non-fat milk in TBS/Tween (0.05% Tween-20 in TBS) for 2 h. Membranes were incubated with primary antibodies including CDC27 (Santa Cruz, sc-9972; 1:200), CDK4 (Proteintech, 11026-1-AP, 1:1,000), cyclin D1 (Proteintech, 26939-1-AP, 1:1,000), cleaved PARP (Cell Signaling Technology, #5625, 1:1,000), cleaved caspase 3 (Cell Signaling Technology, #9664, 1:1,000), PD-L1 (Abcam, ab205921, 1:1,000), and GAPDH (Proteintech, 60004-1-lg, 1:10,000) overnight at 4°C and then with secondary antibodies (anti-rabbit or anti-mouse; Proteintech) for 1 h at room temperature. To quantify the relative protein levels, the band images were gathered by using a ChemiDoc™ XRS+ system (Bio-Rad Laboratories, Hercules, CA, USA).

Animal Experiment

Female BALB/c nude mice (4–5 weeks old, 15–18 g) were purchased from the GemPharmatech Company (Jiangsu, China). The nude mice were housed five per cage and fed a standard sterile laboratory diet under humidity and temperature-controlled conditions. Human tumor xenograft models were created by subcutaneous injection of 1.0×10^7 Jurkat cells (sh-NC/sh-CDC27, $n = 5$) in 0.1 ml of PBS/Matrigel (1:1 mixture, BD Biosciences, CA, USA) into the flank regions of the mice; tumors were allowed to form for 5 weeks. During the experiments, the tumor burden, general conditions and weight of nude mice were monitored twice daily. After 35 days, the nude mice were euthanized. The tumor volumes and tumor weights were measured. Balb/c nude mice were handled and treated under animal laboratory conditions according to the approved guidelines of the Institutional Animal Care and Use Committee of the First Affiliated Hospital of Zhengzhou University (Henan, China).

Statistical Analysis

Statistical analyses were performed using SPSS software version 19.0 (IBM Corp., Armonk, NY, USA) or GraphPad Prism version 7.01 (GraphPad Software, Inc., La Jolla, CA, USA). Data were expressed as the mean ± Standard Deviation (SD). Comparisons between two groups and among three groups were performed by using Student's t-test and one-way ANOVA, respectively. Pearson's correlation was used for correlation analysis. Protein expression and clinicopathological indicators were assessed using χ^2-test. The Kaplan-Meier estimator method and log-rank test were used to analyze survival data. A value of $p < 0.05$ was considered statistically significant.

RESULTS

CDC27 Is Overexpressed and Correlated With Progression in T-LBL

Firstly, we used immunohistochemistry to evaluate CDC27 expression in tumor tissues from 46 T-LBL patients and 30 cases of reactive hyperplasia of the lymph node tissues. The results showed that CDC27 was mainly expressed in the nucleus. Compared with the reactive hyperplasia of the lymph node tissues, the tumor tissues had stronger staining intensity (**Figures 1A,B**). To analyze the relationship between CDC27 expression and the clinicopathological characteristics, we summarized the clinical information of the 46 cases of T-LBL in **Table 1**. There were 29 cases of tumor samples (63.1%) that were highly positive (**Figure 1C**). Further study showed that the expression of CDC27 had a significant correlation with the stage of disease ($p = 0.014$), which revealed that CDC27 expression may be associated with T-LBL progression. Then we investigated the correlation between CDC27 and the survival of T-LBL patients. The results of Kaplan-Meier survival analysis and log-rank tests in **Figure 1D** showed that T-LBL patients with high CDC27 expression exhibited significantly shorter overall survival (OS) than patients with low CDC27 expression ($p < 0.01$, hazard ratio = 5.182, CI = 1.871–14.35). And the correlation between CDC27 expression and progression free survival (PFS) was not statistically significant ($p = 0.064$, hazard ratio = 2.681, CI = 1.032–6.968; **Figure 1E**). The results demonstrated that high expression of CDC27 in T-LBL may be associated with poor prognosis to some extent.

CDC27 Promotes Cell Growth in T-LBL Cell Lines

To test whether CDC27 alterations could affect the proliferation of T-LBL, we first examined the expression of CDC27 in five T cell lymphoma cell lines and primary normal T cells extracted from peripheral blood mononuclear cells using western blotting (**Figure 2A**). According to the results, we constructed stable CDC27-downregulated Jurkat cell lines that were transfected with shRNAs targeting CDC27 (sh1-CDC27, sh2-CDC27) or negative control shRNA (shNC-CDC27). In addition, we constructed a control Sup-T1 cell lines (control) and

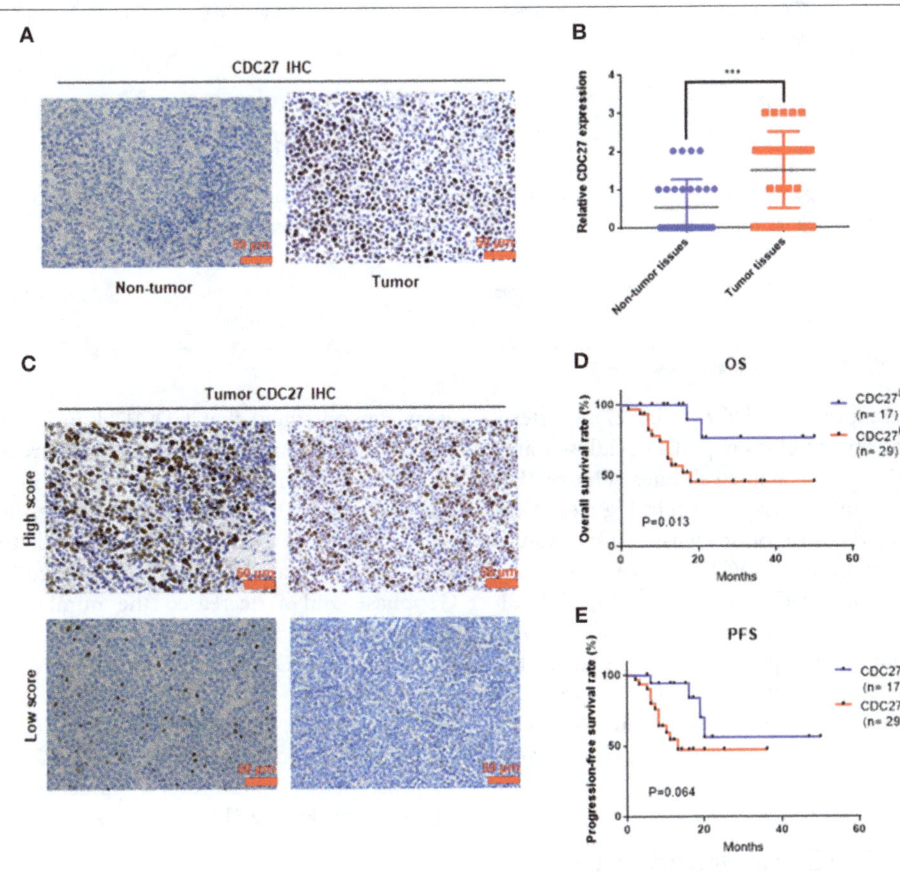

FIGURE 1 | CDC27 is overexpressed in patient tumor samples and predicts decreased survival in T-LBL. **(A)** Representative images of CDC27 expression in T-LBL tissues ($n = 46$) and reactive hyperplasia ($n = 30$) of the lymph node tissues by IHC (×400 magnification). **(B)** Relative immunohistochemistry analysis for CDC27 expression T-LBL tissues and reactive hyperplasia of the lymph node tissues.-20 ***$P < 0.001$. **(C)** Representative images by IHC (×400 magnification) of T-LBL tissues which were divided into high score group (score = 2 or 3) or low score group (score = 0 or 1). **(D,E)** Kaplan-Meier analysis of OS and PFS in T-LBL patients.

TABLE 1 | Clinicopathological findings and correlation with CDC27 expression in T-LBL.

Variables	N (%)	CDC27-low (%)	CDC27-high (%)	χ^2	*P* value
Total cases	46 (100%)	17 (36.9%)	29 (63.1%)		
Gender					
Male	34 (73.9%)	13 (28.3%)	21 (45.6%)	0.091	0.762
Female	12 (26.1%)	4 (8.7%)	8 (17.4%)		
Age (years)					
<60	35(76.1%)	15 (32.6%)	20 (43.5%)	2.187	0.139
≥60	11(23.9%)	2 (4.3%)	9 (19.6%)		
Stage					
I-II	8 (17.4%)	6 (13.1%)	2 (4.3%)	6.016	**0.014***
III-IV	38 (82.6%)	11 (23.9%)	27 (58.7%)		
LDH increased					
Y	13 (28.3%)	4 (8.7%)	9 (19.6%)	0.298	0.585
N	33 (71.7%)	13 (28.2%)	20 (43.5%)		
Intrathoracic effusions					
Y	31 (67.4%)	9 (19.6%)	22 (47.8%)	2.562	0.109
N	15 (32.6%)	8 (17.4%)	7 (15.2%)		
Bone marrow					
Y	28 (60.9%)	11 (23.9%)	17 (37.0%)	0.167	0.686
N	18 (39.1%)	6 (13.0%)	12 (26.1%)		
ECOG					
0–2	37 (80.4%)	16 (34.8%)	21 (45.6%)	3.208	0.073
3–5	9 (19.6%)	1 (2.2%)	8 (17.4%)		
B symptoms					
Y	17 (37%)	7 (15.2%)	10 (21.8%)	0.206	0.650
N	29 (63%)	10 (21.7%)	19 (41.3%)		
Ki67					
<80%	24 (52.2%)	10 (21.8%)	14 (30.4%)	0.478	0.489
≥80%	22 (47.8%)	7 (15.2%)	15 (32.6%)		
IPI score					
0-2	31 (67.4%)	11 (23.9%)	20 (43.5%)	0.088	0.766
3-5	15 (32.6%)	6 (13.0%)	9 (19.6%)		

*T-LBL T-cell lymphoblastic lymphoma; LDH, lactate dehydrogenase; *P < 0.05.*

stable Sup-T1 cell line overexpressing CDC27 (CDC27). Western blotting was used to confirm the efficiency of knockdown and overexpression of CDC27 in these stable cell lines (**Figure 2B**). The results of the cell proliferation assay shown in **Figures 2C,D** indicated that the cell survival, or optic density (OD) value, was significantly decreased in the CDC27 shRNA-expressing Jurkat cells and increased in CDC27-overexpressing SUP-T1 cells. In addition, the sh-CDC27 group had weaker colony formation ability than the shNC group of Jurkat cells (**Figure 2E**). Furthermore, exogenous CDC27 expression also increased the colony formation capacity in Sup-T1 cells (**Figure 2F**). The results above indicated that CDC27 promotes cell growth in T-LBL.

CDC27 Promotes G1/S Transition in the Cell Cycle

EdU cell staining and cell cycle detection assays were performed to verify whether the cell proliferation induced by CDC27 was related to cell cycle progression. The results of the EdU assay demonstrated that CDC27 knockdown decreased the S-phase proportion of Jurkat cells (**Figure 3A**). Overexpression of CDC27 promoted EdU synthesis in S-phase in Sup-T1 cells (**Figure 3B**). Furthermore, the results of the cell cycle assay showed that compared with Jurkat-shNC cells, Jurkat-shCDC27 had a significantly increased number of cells in G1 phase and a decreased the number of cells in S phase (**Figure 3C**). In stable Sup-T1 cells, CDC27 overexpression facilitated the G1/S transition (**Figure 3D**). Next, the level of G1/S-related cyclin D1 and CDK4 protein were detected by western blot. CDC27 knockdown decreased CyclinD1 and CDK4 expression (**Figure 3E**). In CDC27 overexpressing Sup-T1 cells, the expression level of CDK4 and cyclin D1 increased significantly (**Figure 3F**).

CDC27-Knockdown Facilitates T-LBL Cell Apoptosis

To clarify whether CDC27 knockdown influenced the apoptosis of T-LBL cell lines, Jurkat and Sup-T1 cells were starved for

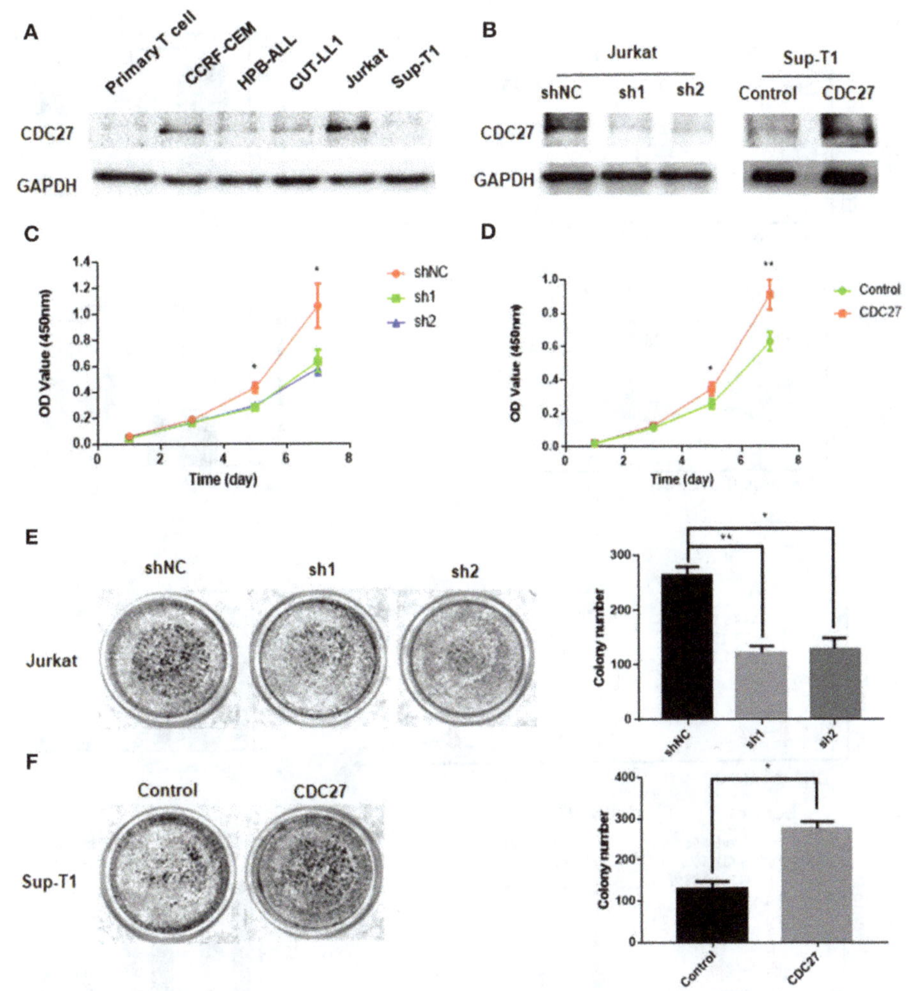

FIGURE 2 | CDC27 promotes proliferation of CRC cells. **(A)** Protein expression was identified by western blotting analysis in T cell lymphoma cell lines. **(B)** The efficient overexpression or suppression of CDC27 was detected by western blotting. **(C,D)** Effects of CDC27 knockdown and over-expression on the proliferation of T-LBL cells (Jurkat and Sup-T1) *in vitro* by CCK-8 assay. $^*P < 0.05$, $^{**}P < 0.01$. **(E)** Colony formation number decreased under CDC27 knockdown in Jurkat cells. $^*P < 0.05$, $^{**}P < 0.01$. **(F)** CDC27 overexpression promoted cell growth in colony formation assays. $^*P < 0.05$.

48 h and subjected to Annexin V/7-AAD staining analysis. The percentage of apoptotic cells were counted as the sum of early apoptotic cells (quadrants Q4) and late apoptotic cells (quadrants Q2). The results showed that the proportion of apoptotic cells was significantly higher in CDC27 shRNA-expressing Jurkat and lower in CDC27 overexpressing SUP-T1 cells than in control cells (**Figures 4A,B**). We next verified the effect of CDC27 on several apoptosis-related proteins (**Figures 4C,D**). Given that PARP (poly ADP-ribose polymerase) is a kind of DNA repair enzyme that plays a significant role in DNA damage repair and apoptosis, the overexpression of CDC27 induced an obvious decrease in the levels of cleaved PARP. In addition, the expression of cleaved PARP remarkably increased in the shCDC27 group compared with the shNC group. The same trend in the expression of cleaved caspase 3 was also identified. These results suggested that CDC27 may influence the progression of T-LBL by regulating apoptosis.

The Effect of CDC27 on PD-L1 Expression

Given that APC/C^{Cdh1} can influence the expression of PD-L1 via degradation of SPOP, we wondered whether CDC27 can regulate PD-L1 in T-LBL cells (21). Firstly, we found a positive correlation between CDC27 and PD-L1 expression in human T-LBL tissues by IHC. The results showed that tissues with a higher score for CDC27 also had a higher level of PD-L1 expression (**Figures 5A,B**). There was an obvious positive correlation between CDC27 expression and PD-L1 expression in T-LBL tissues. In addition, the protein expression level of PD-L1 was significantly decreased in shCDC27 Jurkat cells compared with the control cells (**Figure 5C**). And in CDC27-overexpressing cells, the expression level of PD-L1 increased (**Figure 5D**). Moreover, 293T cells were transfected with luciferase reporter plasmids driven by the PD-L1 promoter (**Figures 5E,F**). Western blotting was used to confirm the efficiency of knockdown of CDC27 in 293T cells (**Figure 5E**).

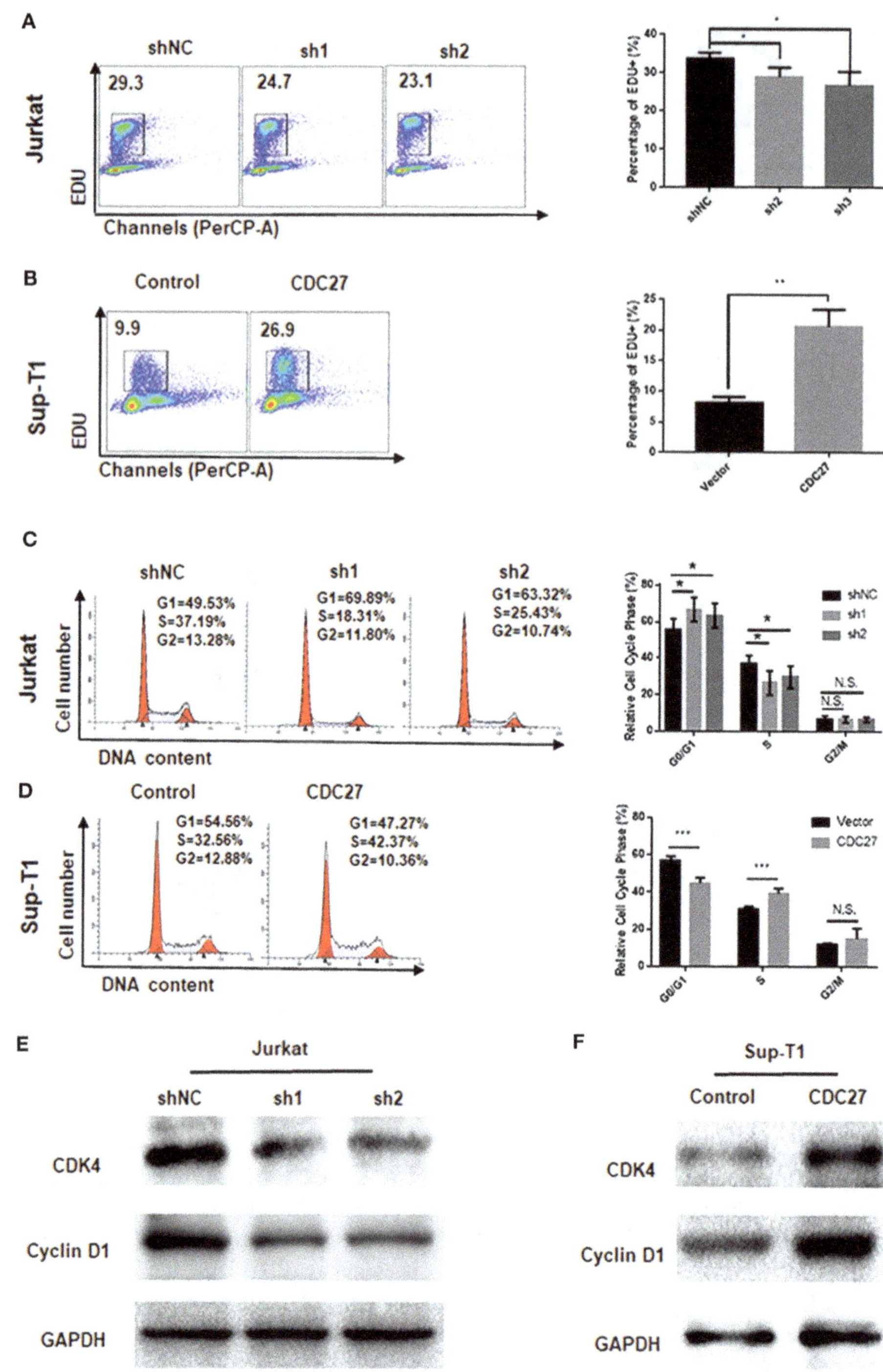

FIGURE 3 | CDC27 influence the G1/S phase transition. **(A,B)** Cell proliferation were assessed by EdU incorporation assay. Data are representative of at least three independent experiments. $^{**}P < 0.01$, $^{*}P < 0.05$. **(C,D)** Flow cytometry was used to examine the cell cycle by PI staining of both Jurkat and Sup-T1 cells. Images and qualification of the cell cycle distribution in three independent experiments are shown. $^{*}P < 0.05$, $^{***}P < 0.001$. N.S., not significant. **(E,F)** Western blot was performed to detect the expression levels of cell cycle related proteins in both Jurkat and Sup-T1 cells, respectively.

The results indicated that silencing CDC27 inhibited the activity of the PD-L1 promoter which demonstrated that CDC27 can regulate PD-L1 expression at transcriptional level at least in part (**Figure 5F**). We also found that PD-L1 protein expression was increased in high-CDC27 expression areas of the tumor cells by an immunofluorescence assay (**Figures 5G,H**). All the results

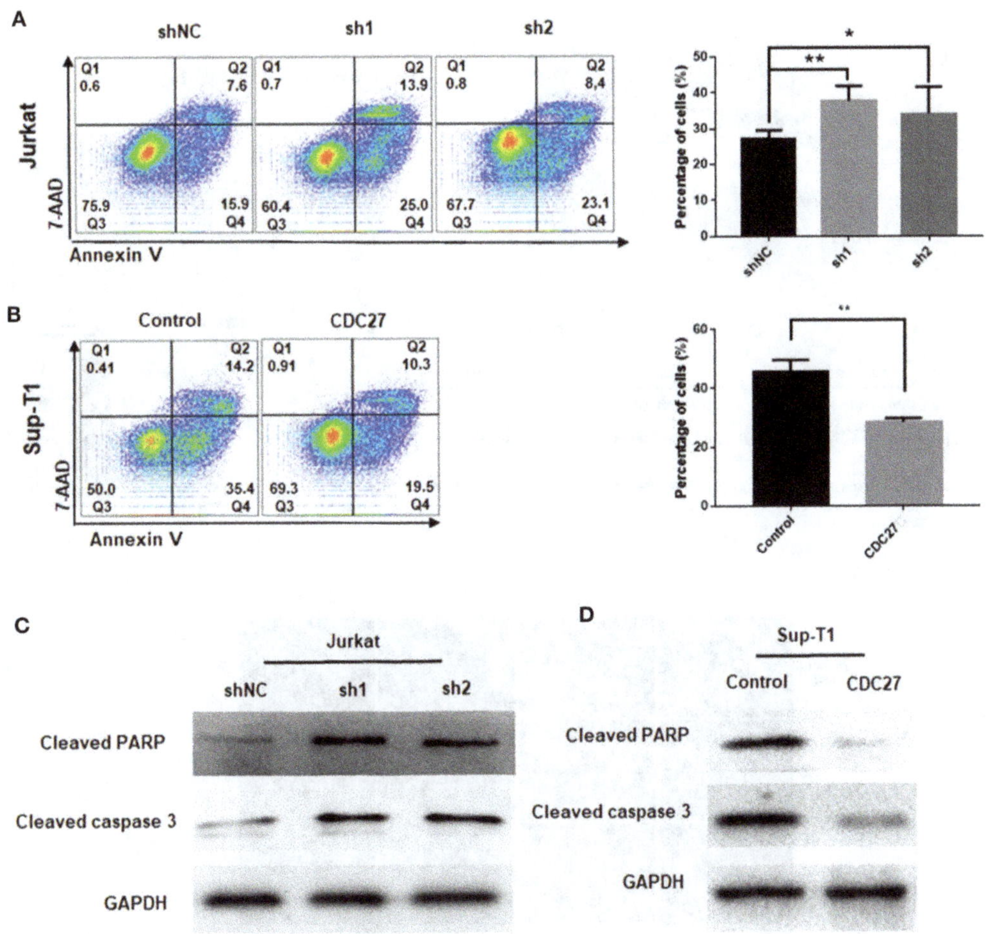

FIGURE 4 | CDC27 inhibits cell apoptosis in T-LBL cells. **(A,B)** Flow cytometry was used to examine the apoptosis as the sum of both Q2 and Q4 quadrants (early + late apoptosis) by Annexin V/7-AAD staining of both Jurkat and Sup-T1 cells. Apoptosis rates were expressed as the mean (Q2 + Q4) ± SD of values from experiments performed in triplicate by using Student's *t*-test. *$P < 0.05$, **$P < 0.01$. **(C,D)** Western blot was performed to detect the expression levels of apoptotic related proteins in both Jurkat and Sup-T1 cells, respectively.

suggested a positive correlation between CDC27 and PD-L1 in T-LBL.

CDC27 Promotes Tumor growth in a Xenograft Mouse Model

Then, we used stable Jurkat cell lines to establish a BALB/c nude mouse xenograft model. ShNC or shCDC27 Jurkat cells were injected subcutaneously into female nude mice. Tumor volume was calculated according to the measured tumor size. After 5 weeks, the mice were killed and then the tumors were collected and weighed. The results showed that compared with the control group, knockdown of CDC27 in stable Jurkat cell contributed to a marked decrease in both tumor weight and volume ($n = 5$, **Figures 6A–C**). Next, we detected the expression of Ki67, which is a marker of nuclear cell proliferation, in excised mouse tumors by IHC. The staining intensity of Ki67 in the Jurkat-shCDC27 group was weaker than that in the control group (**Figure 6D**). In addition, the results of IHC also showed that the expression of PD-L1 had a positive correlation with CDC27 expression in tumors (**Figures 6D,E**). The results demonstrated that CDC27 is not only related to tumor proliferation but also affects PD-L1 expression in T-LBL.

DISCUSSION

The deregulation of APC/C has been reported to be connected with the genomic instability of tumor cells (22). As a core subunit of APC/C, CDC27 can bind CDH1 or CDC20, playing a key role in the process of recognizing and degrading target substrates. In recent years, several studies have reported that CDC27 can facilitate cell proliferation, migration and invasion in some types of cancers (23–25). Nevertheless, few studies indicated the opposite influence of CDC27 on cell functions and patients' survival analysis (26, 27). The expression and effect of CDC27 in lymphoma has not been reported or clarified. In our present study, CDC27 regulated the proliferation, apoptosis, and

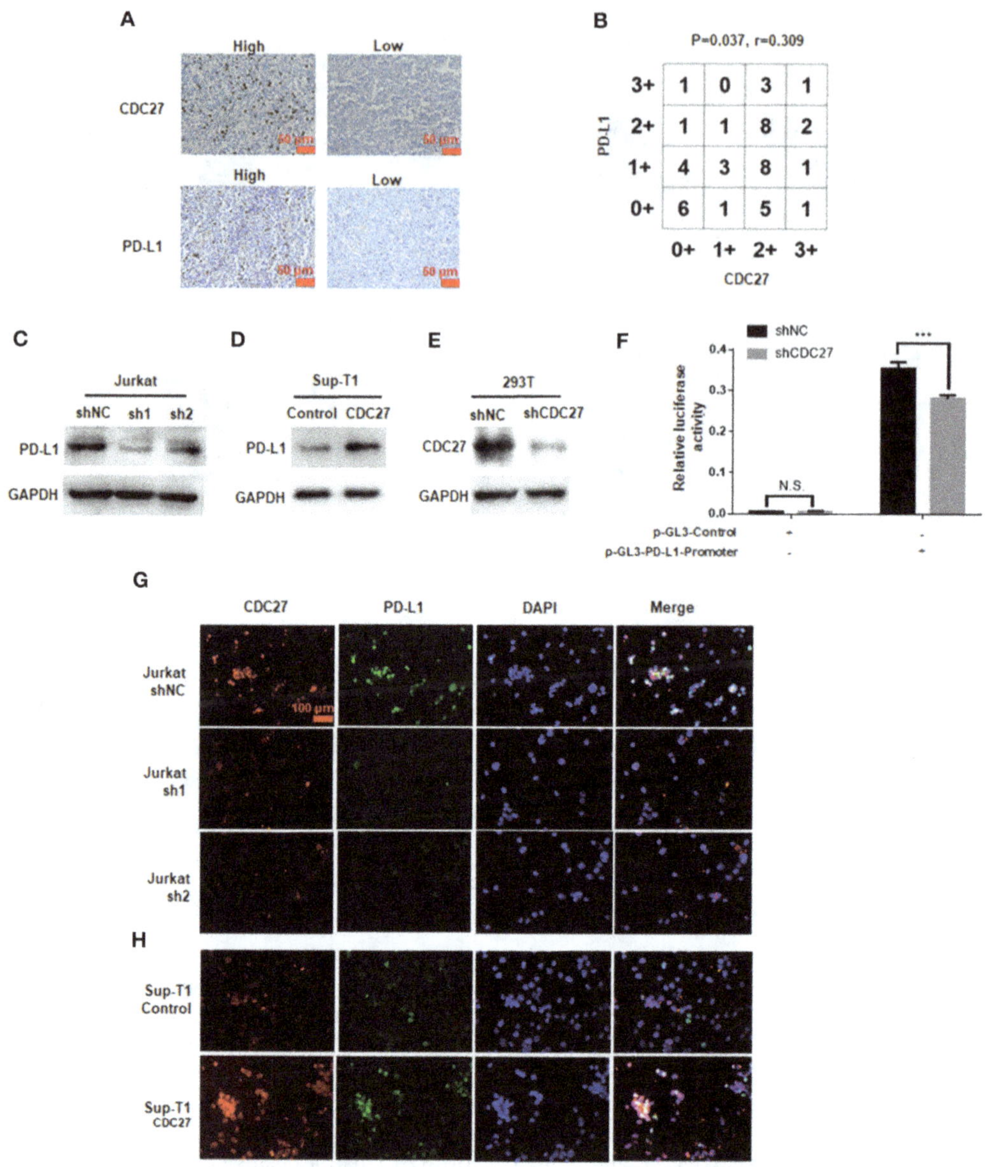

FIGURE 5 | The effect of CDC27 on PD-L1 expression. **(A,B)** Representative IHC images and interaction plots of serial sections derived from patients with T-LBL ($n = 46$) were stained for CDC27 and PD-L1. **(C)** The protein expression of PD-L1 in shCDC27 Jurkat cells compared to control. **(D)** The protein expression of PD-L1 in CDC27 overexpression Sup-T1 cells compared to control. **(E)** The reduction of CDC27 protein levels in shCDC27-transfected 293T cells was detected by western blotting. **(F)** Luciferase reporter assays were performed to detect PD-L1 expression in the indicated cells with CDC27 suppressed. $^{***}P < 0.001$. N.S., not significant. **(G,H)** Immunofluorescence analysis of CDC27 and PD-L1 expression in Jurkat and Sup-T1 cells, respectively.

the cell cycle. By means of *in vitro* and *in vivo* experiments as well as clinical information analysis, we claimed that targeting CDC27 might offer new thoughts to the treatment of T-LBL.

Our study found that the expression of CDC27 was significantly unregulated in T-LBL tissues compared with the control tissues, which suggested that CDC27 may facilitate tumorigenesis of T-LBL and laid a foundation for further study. First, the proliferative effect of CDC27 was proven by cell viability assay and *in vivo* study. EdU-647 labeling assays and cell cycle assays revealed that the cancer-promoting function of CDC27 may be primarily because of the promotion of the G1/S phase transition. In addition, through the apoptosis detection test and western blotting experiments, we found that CDC27 could inhibit the apoptosis of T-LBL cells, which might be connected with the upregulation of related proteins in the apoptosis pathway. All of our functional studies in T-LBL cells demonstrated that CDC27 could promote tumor progression in various aspects. Intriguingly, Qiu et al. did not find evidence to prove that CDC27 is associated with apoptosis in colorectal cancer cells (23). This may be due to the tumor

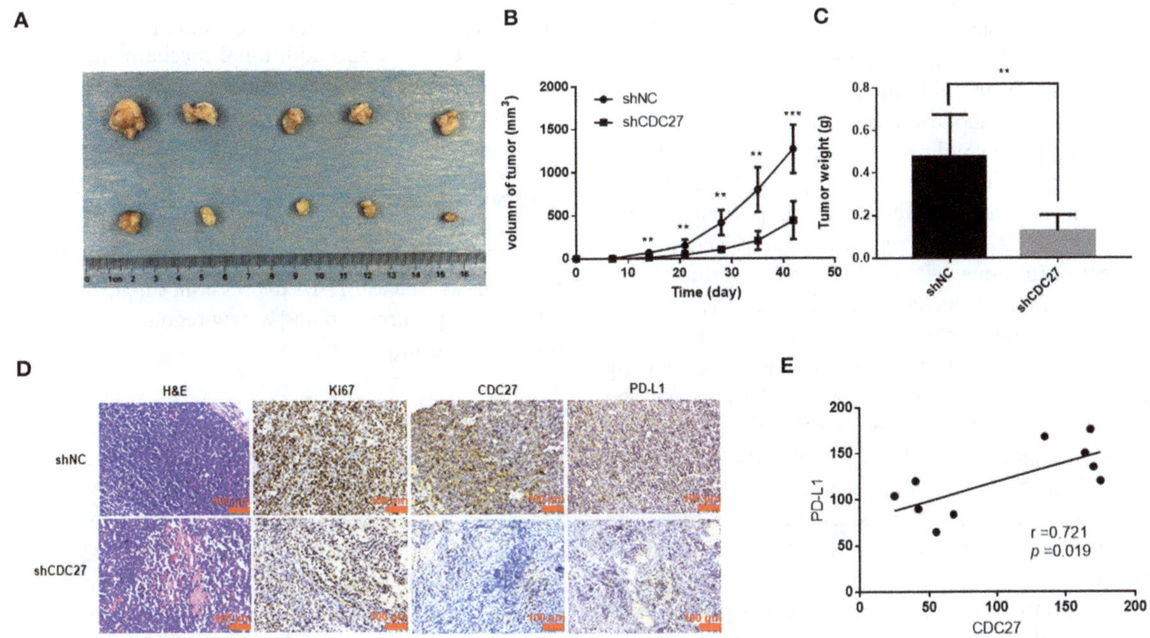

FIGURE 6 | CDC27 promotes tumor growth *in vivo*. **(A)** Representative images of xenograft tumors Jukat cells with expression of shNC and shCDC27 ($n = 5$ in each group). **(B,C)** Tumor volume and tumor weight were analyzed. $^{**}P < 0.01$, $^{***}P < 0.001$. **(D)** Representative H&E staining and immunohistochemistry staining of Ki67, CDC27, and PD-L1 in the xenograft tumor tissues (×200 magnification). **(E)** Correlations between CDC27 and PD-L1 expression in the xenograft tumor tissues were analyzed by Pearson's test.

heterogeneity and more experiments are needed to confirm this point.

Although intensive chemotherapy has been applied in treating T-LBL patients, the 5-year OS is <67%, and the recurrence rate is over 30% (28). In this study, majority of T-LBL patients received regimens including dose-adjusted BFM-90 (prednisone, Vincristine, daunorubicin, L-Asaraginase, cyclophosphamide, cytarabine, bleomycin) or Hyper CVAD (cyclophosphamide, vincristine, doxorubicin, and dexamethasone, alternating with methotrexate and cytarabine). No research reported that the drugs mentioned above targeted CDC27. Our study revealed that CDC27 was overexpressed in T-LBL tumor tissues and correlated with OS. As for the negative results of PFS, it may be due to the limited number of cases that could be included in this study. Collectively, the detection of CDC27 expression could help to evaluate tumor staging and prognosis in T-LBL to a certain extent.

In recent years, immune checkpoint inhibition has been considered as a novel treatment method (29). PD-1 is one of the immune checkpoints responsible for regulating the immune response. Its ligand on tumor cells, PD-L1, can bind PD-1 and transmit suppression signals to T cells (30). Therefore, it is important to reverse immune escape by inhibiting the interaction between PD-1 and PD-L1. Nevertheless, most of patients fail to respond to PD-1/PD-L1 axis inhibitors. The abnormal expression of PD-L1 can be used as a predictive or prognostic marker of PD-1/PD-L1 inhibition therapy for patients (31–33). However, few studies have studied the expression and regulatory mechanisms of PD-1 or PD-L1 expression in T- LBL (34, 35). In this study, we first found a prominent positive relationship between tumor CDC27 and PD-L1 expression by IHC staining of T-LBL tissues. To further investigate and prove this connection, we also performed the western blotting, luciferase gene reporter assays and immunofluorescence staining, the results of which also proved our assumption that the expression of CDC27 is indirectly associated with PD-L1 in T-LBL tumor cells. However, the regulatory mechanisms between CDC27 and PD-L1 is uncertain, which may consist of a meshwork of proteins and pathways. A study of Zhang et al. showed that the activation of APC/C^{Cdh1} can promote the degradation of SPOP, which reduces ubiquitination-mediated PD-L1 degradation, resulting in increased PD-L1 levels (21). This study provided strong support that CDC27, as the most notable APC/C subunit, may participate in the regulation of PD-L1. Furthermore, Zhang et al. also indicated that CDK inhibitor plays a key facilitating role in the whole process (21). Recently, several studies indicated that CDK family had a close correlation with PD-L1 expression and immune escape (36–38). It gave clues that CDC27 may influence PD-L1 expression via modulating certain potential CDKs and their cell cycle or apoptosis related downstream molecules in the tumor microenvironment. Besides, previous studies have proved that TGF-β signaling can facilitate the activation of APC/C via CDC27, which allowing the transcription of genes necessary for growth inhibition and in turn leads to the transactivation of TGF-β-responsive genes for cell cycle arrest or apoptosis (39). Notably, the activation of TGF-β pathway can also induce the expression of

PD-L1 and promote the occurrence of immunosuppression (33, 40, 41). Collectively, crosstalk among TGF-β signaling pathway may play a significant role in the regulation network of CDC27-PD-L1, which needs to be tested in the future.

The research findings above indicated that CDC27 may be involved in the progression and prognosis of T-LBL patients and is expected to become a promising novel target for the treatment. Based on current experimental basis, we hope that special inhibitors against CDC27 or its regulators can reactivate the anti-cancer effect of immune cells in T-LBL by reducing PD-L1 expression. And the CDC27 blockades can be designed and tested in conjunction with immune checkpoint inhibitors to overcome the therapeutic resistance. With the development of sequencing technologies, the personalized combination therapy will be feasible in the near future. A study showed that the pre-therapy tumor clone with mutations in CDC27 could not be detected after anti-PD-1 treatment in patients with hyperprogressive disease (42). In addition, CDC27 was also reported to be the most frequently mutated gene of resistant clones in a patient with exceptional response to immune checkpoint inhibitor (43). Therefore, it is worth to investigate whether the newly discovered "partner molecule" of PD-L1 can be served as a biomarker to predict the response of T-LBL patients to immunotherapy.

However, this study also has some limitations. Firstly, in recent years, CDC27 mutations have been found in some cancers (44–46). A study has identified mutated CDC27 as a tumor antigen which leaded to massive changes of chromosomal number (47). The mutated CDC27, which has not been investigated thoroughly by a conventional approach, may play an important role in cancer development. We tried to investigate the presence of alleles related to T-LBL. However, we have not found the key mutations of CDC27 that can influence the tumor progression or tumorigenesis until now. This need to be confirmed by rigorous experiments and larger cohort studies in the future. Secondly, because of the low incidence of T-LBL, the number of patients included in the study was limited. Some intriguing molecular genetics of T-LBL patients are not well-characterized, mainly due to the scarcity of samples. Hence, more researches with larger sample sizes are needed to verify our conclusions and explore novel fields. Thirdly, there may be various mediators and additional mechanisms involved in PD-L1 regulation by CDC27. Further studies are required to identify more target proteins in CDC27-PD-L1 axis.

CONCLUSION

CDC27 is overexpressed in T-LBL tissues and influences the cell functions as well as PD-L1 expression, suggesting a novel insight into tumor progression and a new regulatory axis with potential therapeutic utility.

ETHICS STATEMENT

The studies involving human participants were reviewed and approved by Institutional Research Ethics Committee of the First Affiliated Hospital of Zhengzhou University (Henan, China). Written informed consent to participate in this study was provided by the participants' legal guardian/next of kin. This animal study was reviewed and approved by Institutional Animal Care and Use Committee of the First Affiliated Hospital of Zhengzhou University (Henan, China). Written informed consent was obtained from the individual(s), and minor(s)' legal guardian/next of kin, for the publication of any potentially identifiable images or data included in this article.

AUTHOR CONTRIBUTIONS

MZ, YS, and ZL conceived the project. YS, WenS, and YW performed most of the experiments. QX and WeiS provided help for data analysis and curation. YS wrote the manuscript. ZL, JL, and MZ improved and revised this manuscript. All authors have read and agreed to the published version of the manuscript.

REFERENCES

1. You MJ, Medeiros LJ, Hsi ED. T-lymphoblastic leukemia/lymphoma. *Am J Clin Pathol.* (2015) 144:411–22. doi: 10.1309/AJCPMF03LVSBLHPJ
2. Jain N, Lamb AV, O'Brien S, Ravandi F, Konopleva M, Jabbour E, et al. Early T-cell precursor acute lymphoblastic leukemia/lymphoma (ETP-ALL/LBL) in adolescents and adults: a high-risk subtype. *Blood.* (2016) 127:1863–9. doi: 10.1182/blood-2015-08-661702
3. Morgan DO. Regulation of the APC and the exit from mitosis. *Nat Cell Biol.* (1999) 1:E47. doi: 10.1038/10039
4. Peters JM. The anaphase promoting complex/cyclosome: a machine designed to destroy. *Nat Rev Mol Cell Biol.* (2006) 7:644–656. doi: 10.1038/nrm1988
5. Penas C, Ramachandran V, Ayad NG. The APC/C ubiquitin ligase: from cell biology to tumorigenesis. *Front Oncol.* (2011) 1:60. doi: 10.3389/fonc.2011.00060
6. Kim HS, Vassilopoulos A, Wang RH, Lahusen T, Xiao Z, Xu X, et al. SIRT2 maintains genome integrity and suppresses tumorigenesis through regulating APC/C activity. *Cancer Cell.* (2011) 20:487–99. doi: 10.1016/j.ccr.2011.09.004
7. Chang DZ, Ma Y, Ji B, Liu Y, Hwu P, Abbruzzese JL, et al. Increased CDC20 expression is associated with pancreatic ductal adenocarcinoma differentiation and progression. *J Hematol Oncol.* (2012) 5:15. doi: 10.1186/1756-8722-5-15

8. Kato T, Daigo Y, Aragaki M, Ishikawa K, Sato M, Kaji M. Overexpression of CDC20 predicts poor prognosis in primary non-small cell lung cancer patients. *J Surg Oncol.* (2012) 106:423–30. doi: 10.1002/jso.23109
9. Wu WJ, Hu KS, Wang DS, Zeng ZL, Zhang DS, Chen DL, et al. CDC20 overexpression predicts a poor prognosis for patients with colorectal cancer. *J Transl Med.* (2013) 11:142. doi: 10.1186/1479-5876-11-142
10. Melloy PG. The anaphase-promoting complex: a key mitotic regulator associated with somatic mutations occurring in cancer. *Genes Chromos Cancer.* (2020) 59:189–202. doi: 10.1002/gcc.22820
11. Pardoll D. The blockade of immune checkpoints in cancer immunotherapy. *Nat Rev Cancer.* (2012) 12:252–64. doi: 10.1038/nrc3239
12. Song Y, Li Z, Xue W, Zhang M. Predictive biomarkers for PD-1 and PD-L1 immune checkpoint blockade therapy. *Immunotherapy.* (2019) 11:515–29. doi: 10.2217/imt-2018-0173
13. Liu L, Ruiz J, O'Neill S, Grant S, Petty W, Yang M, et al. Favorable outcome of patients with lung adenocarcinoma harboring POLE mutations and expressing high PD-L1. *Mol Cancer.* (2018) 17:81. doi: 10.1186/s12943-018-0832-y
14. Feng X, Li L, Wu J, Zhang L, Sun Z, Li X, et al. Complete blood count score model integrating reduced lymphocyte-monocyte ratio, elevated neutrophil-lymphocyte ratio, and elevated platelet-lymphocyte ratio predicts inferior clinical outcomes in adult T-lymphoblastic lymphoma. *Oncologist.* (2019) 24:e1123–31 doi: 10.1634/theoncologist.2018-0789
15. Dong M, Zhang X, Yang Z, Wu S, Ma M, Li Z, et al. Patients over 40 years old with precursor T-cell lymphoblastic lymphoma have different prognostic factors comparing to the youngers. *Sci Rep.* (2018) 8:1088. doi: 10.1038/s41598-018-19565-x
16. Li Z, Song Y, Zhang Y, Li C, Wang Y, Xue W, et al. Genomic and outcome analysis of adult T-cell lymphoblastic lymphoma. *Haematologica.* (2020) 105:e107–10. doi: 10.3324/haematol.2019.220863
17. Li Z, Lu L, Zhou Z, Xue W, Wang Y, Jin M, et al. Recurrent mutations in epigenetic modifiers and the PI3K/AKT/mTOR pathway in subcutaneous panniculitis-like T-cell lymphoma. *Br J Haematol.* (2018) 181:406–10. doi: 10.1111/bjh.14611
18. McCarty KS Jr., Miller LS, Cox EB, Konrath J, McCarty KS Sr. Estrogen receptor analyses. Correlation of biochemical and immunohistochemical methods using monoclonal antireceptor antibodies. *Archiv Pathol Lab Med.* (1985) 109:716–21.
19. Yu Y, Chen L, Zhao G, Li H, Guo Q, Zhu S, et al. RBBP8/CtIP suppresses P21 expression by interacting with CtBP and BRCA1 in gastric cancer. *Oncogene.* (2019):39:1273–89. doi: 10.1038/s41388-019-1060-7
20. Li Z, Zhang X, Xue W, Zhang Y, Li C, Song Y, et al. Recurrent GNAQ mutation encoding T96S in natural killer/T cell lymphoma. *Nat Commun.* (2019) 10:4209. doi: 10.1038/s41467-019-12032-9
21. Zhang J, Bu X, Wang H, Zhu Y, Geng Y, Nihira NT, et al. Cyclin D-CDK4 kinase destabilizes PD-L1 via cullin 3-SPOP to control cancer immune surveillance. *Nature.* (2018) 553:91–5. doi: 10.1038/nature25015
22. Wasch R, Engelbert D. Anaphase-promoting complex-dependent proteolysis of cell cycle regulators and genomic instability of cancer cells. *Oncogene.* (2005) 24:1–10. doi: 10.1038/sj.onc.1208017
23. Qiu L, Wu J, Pan C, Tan X, Lin J, Liu R, et al. Downregulation of CDC27 inhibits the proliferation of colorectal cancer cells via the accumulation of p21Cip1/Waf1. *Cell Death Dis.* (2016) 7:e2074. doi: 10.1038/cddis.2015.402
24. Qiu L, Tan X, Lin J, Liu RY, Chen S, Geng R, et al. CDC27 induces metastasis and invasion in colorectal cancer via the promotion of epithelial-to-mesenchymal transition. *J Cancer.* (2017) 8:2626–35. doi: 10.7150/jca.19381
25. Xin Y, Ning S, Zhang L, Cui M. CDC27 facilitates gastric cancer cell proliferation, invasion and metastasis via twist-induced epithelial-mesenchymal transition. *Cell Physiol Biochem.* (2018) 50:501–11. doi: 10.1159/000494164
26. Talvinen K, Karra H, Pitkänen R, Ahonen I, Nykänen M, Lintunen M, et al. Low cdc27 and high securin expression predict short survival for breast cancer patients. *Apmis.* (2013) 121:945–53. doi: 10.1111/apm.12110
27. Feng Z, Zhang L, Zhou J, Zhou S. mir-218-2 promotes glioblastomas growth, invasion and drug resistance by targeting CDC27. *Oncotarget.* (2017) 8:6304–6318. doi: 10.18632/oncotarget.13850
28. Liu Y, Rao J, Li J, Wen Q, Wang S, Lou S, et al. Tandem autologous hematopoietic stem cell transplantation for treatment of adult T-cell lymphoblastic lymphoma: a multiple center prospective study in China. *Haematologica* (2019). haematol.2019.226985. doi: 10.3324/haematol.2019.226985
29. Wakabayashi G, Lee YC, Luh F, Kuo CN, Chang WC, Yen Y. Development and clinical applications of cancer immunotherapy against PD-1 signaling pathway. *J Biomed Sci.* (2019) 26:96. doi: 10.1186/s12929-019-0588-8
30. Chen L, Flies DB. Molecular mechanisms of T cell co-stimulation and co-inhibition. *Nat Rev Immunol.* (2013) 13:227–42. doi: 10.1038/nri3405
31. Kloten V, Lampignano R, Krahn T, Schlange T. Circulating tumor cell pd-l1 expression as biomarker for therapeutic efficacy of immune checkpoint inhibition in NSCLC. *Cells.* (2019) 8:809. doi: 10.3390/cells8080809
32. Sun Y, Yu W, Guan W, Cai L, Qiao M, Zheng L, et al. Integrated assessment of PD-L1 expression and molecular classification facilitates therapy selection and prognosis prediction in gastric cancer. *Cancer Manag Res.* (2019) 11:6397–410. doi: 10.2147/CMAR.S206189
33. Shen X, Zhang L, Li J, Li Y, Wang Y, Xu ZX. Recent findings in the regulation of programmed death ligand 1 expression. *Front Immunol.* (2019) 10:1337. doi: 10.3389/fimmu.2019.01337
34. Kim S-J, Hyeon J, Cho I, Ko YH, Kim WS. Comparison of efficacy of pembrolizumab between epstein-barr virus–positive and –negative relapsed or refractory non-hodgkin lymphomas. *Cancer Res Treat.* (2019) 51:611–22. doi: 10.4143/crt.2018.191
35. Santos J, Gonzalez-Sanchez L, Villa-Morales M, Ors I, Lopez-Nieva P, Vaquero C, et al. The stromal gene encoding the CD274 antigen as a genetic modifier controlling survival of mice with γ-radiation-induced T-cell lymphoblastic lymphomas. *Oncogene.* (2010) 29:5265–73. doi: 10.1038/onc.2010.280
36. Mok MT, Zhou J, Tang W, Zeng X, Oliver AW, Ward SE, et al. CCRK is a novel signalling hub exploitable in cancer immunotherapy. *Pharmacol Ther.* (2018) 186:138–51. doi: 10.1016/j.pharmthera.2018.01.008
37. Dorand RD, Nthale J, Myers JT, Barkauskas DS, Avril S, Chirieleison SM, et al. Cdk5 disruption attenuates tumor PD-L1 expression and promotes antitumor immunity. *Science.* (2016) 353:399–403. doi: 10.1126/science.aae0477
38. Zhao L, Li P, Zhao L, Wang M, Tong D, Meng Z, et al. Expression and clinical value of PD-L1 which is regulated by BRD4 in tongue squamous cell carcinoma. *J Cell Biochem.* (2020) 121:1855–69. doi: 10.1002/jcb.29420
39. Zhang L, Fujita T, Wu G, Xiao X, Wan Y. Phosphorylation of the anaphase-promoting complex/Cdc27 is involved in TGF-beta signaling. *J Biol Chem.* (2011) 286:10041–50. doi: 10.1074/jbc.M110.205518
40. Jiang X, Wang J, Deng X, Xiong F, Ge J, Xiang B, et al. Role of the tumor microenvironment in PD-L1/PD-1-mediated tumor immune escape. *Molecular Cancer.* (2019) 18:10. doi: 10.1186/s12943-018-0928-4
41. Ni XY, Sui HX, Liu Y, Ke SZ, Wang YN, Gao FG. TGF-β of lung cancer microenvironment upregulates B7H1 and GITRL expression in dendritic cells and is associated with regulatory T cell generation. *Oncol Rep.* (2012) 28:615–21. doi: 10.3892/or.2012.1822
42. Xiong D, Wang Y, Singavi AK, Mackinnon AC, George B, You M. Immunogenomic landscape contributes to hyperprogressive disease after anti-PD-1 immunotherapy for cancer. *iScience.* (2018) 9:258–77. doi: 10.1016/j.isci.2018.10.021
43. Boilève A, Carlo MI, Barthélémy P, Oudard S, Borchiellini D, Voss MH, et al. Immune checkpoint inhibitors in *MITF* family translocation renal cell carcinomas and genetic correlates of exceptional responders. *J Immuno Ther Cancer.* (2018) 6:159. doi: 10.1186/s40425-018-0482-z
44. Guo J, Huang J, Zhou Y, Zhou Y, Yu L, Li H, et al. Germline and somatic variations influence the somatic mutational signatures of esophageal squamous cell carcinomas in a Chinese population. *BMC Genomics.* (2018) 19:538. doi: 10.1186/s12864-018-4906-4

45. Chen C, Shi C, Huang X, Zheng J, Zhu Z, Li Q, et al. Molecular profiles and metastasis markers in chinese patients with gastric carcinoma. *Sci Rep.* (2019) 9:13995. doi: 10.1038/s41598-019-50171-7
46. Yu M, Hong W, Ruan S, Guan R, Tu L, Huang B, et al. Genome-wide profiling of prognostic alternative splicing pattern in pancreatic cancer. *Front Oncol.* (2019) 9:773. doi: 10.3389/fonc.2019.00773
47. Wang R-F, Wang X, Atwood AC, Topalian SL, Rosenberg SA. Cloning genes encoding MHC class II-restricted antigens: mutated CDC27 as a tumor antigen. *Science.* (1999) 284:1351–4. doi: 10.1126/science.284.5418.1351

9

Multiple Myeloma Cells Alter Adipogenesis, Increase Senescence-Related and Inflammatory Gene Transcript Expression and Alter Metabolism in Preadipocytes

Heather Fairfield[1,2,3], *Samantha Costa*[1,2,3], *Carolyne Falank*[1,2,3], *Mariah Farrell*[1,2,4], *Connor S. Murphy*[1,2,3], *Anastasia D'Amico*[1,2,4], *Heather Driscoll*[5] *and Michaela R. Reagan*[1,2,3,4*]

[1] *Center for Molecular Medicine, Maine Medical Center Research Institute, Scarborough, ME, United States,* [2] *School of Medicine, Tufts University, Boston, MA, United States,* [3] *Graduate School of Biomedical Science and Engineering, University of Maine, Orono, ME, United States,* [4] *Biology Department, University of Southern Maine, Portland, ME, United States,* [5] *Biology Department, Norwich University, Northfield, VT, United States*

Correspondence:
Michaela R. Reagan
Mreagan@mmc.org

Within the bone marrow microenvironment, mesenchymal stromal cells (MSCs) are an essential precursor to bone marrow adipocytes and osteoblasts. The balance between this progenitor pool and mature cells (adipocytes and osteoblasts) is often skewed by disease and aging. In multiple myeloma (MM), a cancer of the plasma cell that predominantly grows within the bone marrow, as well as other cancers, MSCs, preadipocytes, and adipocytes have been shown to directly support tumor cell survival and proliferation. Increasing evidence supports the idea that MM-associated MSCs are distinct from healthy MSCs, and their gene expression profiles may be predictive of myeloma patient outcomes. Here we directly investigate how MM cells affect the differentiation capacity and gene expression profiles of preadipocytes and bone marrow MSCs. Our studies reveal that MM.1S cells cause a marked decrease in lipid accumulation in differentiating 3T3-L1 cells. Also, MM.1S cells or MM.1S-conditioned media altered gene expression profiles of both 3T3-L1 and mouse bone marrow MSCs. 3T3-L1 cells exposed to MM.1S cells before adipogenic differentiation displayed gene expression changes leading to significantly altered pathways involved in steroid biosynthesis, the cell cycle, and metabolism (oxidative phosphorylation and glycolysis) after adipogenesis. MM.1S cells induced a marked increase in 3T3-L1 expression of MM-supportive genes including *Il-6* and *Cxcl12* (SDF1), which was confirmed in mouse MSCs by qRT-PCR, suggesting a forward-feedback mechanism. *In vitro* experiments revealed that indirect MM exposure prior to differentiation drives a senescent-like phenotype in differentiating MSCs, and this trend was confirmed in MM-associated MSCs compared to MSCs from normal donors. In direct co-culture, human mesenchymal stem cells (hMSCs) exposed to MM.1S, RPMI-8226, and OPM-2 prior to and during differentiation, exhibited different levels of lipid accumulation as well as secreted cytokines. Combined, our results suggest that MM cells can inhibit adipogenic differentiation while stimulating expression of the senescence associated secretory phenotype (SASP) and other pro-myeloma molecules. This study provides insight into a novel way in which MM cells manipulate their microenvironment by altering the expression of supportive cytokines and skewing the cellular diversity of the marrow.

Keywords: myeloma, bone marrow, adipocytes, senescence, microarray, mesenchymal stromal cells (MSCs), preadipocytes

INTRODUCTION

The pathogenesis of multiple myeloma (MM) involves bidirectional interactions of MM cells with bone marrow (BM) resident cells. MM cells often depend on these host cells to provide factors that aid in drug resistance and proliferation. Specifically, MM cells interact with osteoblasts (1–3), osteoclasts (4, 5), osteocytes (6), BM mesenchymal stem cells (MSCs) (7), and bone marrow adipocytes (BMAds) (8, 9), each playing a unique type of supportive role for MM cells. MSCs are a common progenitor for pericytes, osteoblasts, osteocytes, and adipocytes. The differentiation capacity of MSCs is influenced and regulated by many growth factors, canonical WNT signaling (10), and metabolic programming (11). Indeed, high fat diet in mice (11) and obesity in humans (12) have recently been shown to modulate the number of adipocyte progenitors in the marrow, skewing the delicate balance between MSCs, osteoblasts, and BMAds. Interestingly, obesity is also a risk factor for MM development and progression, with obese patients being 20% more likely than non-obese patients to transition from a premalignant stage, monoclonal gammopathy of undetermined significance (MGUS), to overt MM (13, 14). Obesity likely contributes to MM in many ways; for example, Bullwinkle et al. found that conditioned media from white adipocytes from obese patients contained increased IL-6, and when cultured with MM cells, led to increased MM cell survival and adhesion *via* increased STAT-3 (15). Lwin et al. found that diet-induced obesity increased IGF1 levels in mice and created a permissive BM microenvironment for the progression of MM from MGUS (16). Increased levels of BMAds have also been correlated with obesity in human patients (17), suggesting that obesity-associated levels of increased BMAds, likely contribute to an optimal MM microenvironment. Moreover, MM incidence increases with age, and BMAds make up 0% of BM cells in infancy and almost 70% in the elderly (18), again demonstrating a correlation between increased BMAds and MM. Thus, understanding the role of BMAds in MM, and how MM influences BMAds and their progenitors, is crucial for fully understanding MM disease progression and incidence.

The bidirectional relationship between myeloma cells and BMAds is yet to be fully elucidated; however, the data suggest that BMAds typically support myeloma cells. BMAds were previously believed to be inert bystanders, but in recent years, they were found to be intricate and responsive players in the BM microenvironment. BMAds contribute to systemic metabolism (19), bone remodeling (20), and hematopoiesis (21). Several studies have shown that BMAds influence MM cell proliferation, apoptosis, migration, and homing to the marrow (18, 22). Adipocyte-derived factors such as MCP-1/*CCL2* and SDF1α/*CXCL12* are chemotactic factors for myeloma cells (8, 15), while other adipokines promote myeloma proliferation (e.g., leptin/LEP) (18) and resistance to chemotherapies (e.g., leptin/LEP, adipsin/CFD) (9, 23). Recent studies have demonstrated that BMAds are modulated by MM cells (22, 24–26) and that MM-reprogrammed BMAds contribute to myeloma-induced bone disease (27). Myeloma patient-derived MSCs (MM-MSCs) also have alterations in the expression of transcripts involved in MM disease pathogenesis (IL-6) (28) as well as impaired osteogenic capabilities (7, 28–30). Evidence suggests that MM-MSCs have senescent characteristics accompanied by an aberrant secretory profile that may impair bone formation (7, 28, 30). Here we further investigate the adipogenic capacity of patient-derived MM-MSCs and model MM-induced changes in adipogenic progenitors with a co-culture system.

MATERIAL AND METHODS

Cell Culture

3T3-L1, human BM MSCs from normal, non-malignant bone marrow (NBM-MSCs), or myeloma patient bone marrow (MM-MSCs) (7), and naïve mouse BM MSCs (mMSCs) were cultured and differentiated as previously described (6). mMSCs were extracted from wild-type mice of C57BL6/J background of approximately 2–3 months of age. All experimental studies and procedures involving mice were performed in accordance with approved protocols from the Maine Medical Center Research Institute (Scarborough, ME, USA) Institutional Animal Care and Use Committee (IACUC), Reagan Laboratory protocol #1812. NBM-MSCs were isolated and utilized for experiments as previously described (31). 5TGM1, MM.1S, RPMI-8226, and OPM-2 cells were cultured as previously described (22, 31). For transwell co-culture experiments, stromal cells were seeded into the bottom of 6- or 24-well plates prior to adipogenic differentiation, allowed to adhere, and grown to 80–100% confluence depending on the cell type. Myeloma cells were then seeded either directly, or into the top of 0.4 μm transwell membranes (Corning; Corning, NY) and cultured for 48 h for indirect co-culture experiments, or allowed to remain in direct co-culture throughout adipogenic differentiation. Lipid droplets from adipocytes *in vitro* were labeled with Oil Red O alone, or in combination with DAPI (Thermo Fisher Scientific, Waltham,

MA) and AF488-phalloidin (Invitrogen, Carlsbad, CA) and analyzed as previously described (6). All cell culture reagents were acquired from VWR unless stated.

Total mRNA Extraction and Quantitative Reverse Transcriptase Polymerase Chain Reaction

Total RNA was harvested in QIAzol and prepared *via* Qiagen miRNEASY Kit with DNase On-column digestion (Qiagen; Hilden, Germany) according to the manufacturer's protocol. Ribolock (1U/μl; Thermo Fisher Scientific) was added to inhibit RNA degradation in samples processed for microarray. mRNA was quantified and tested for quality and contamination using a Nanodrop 2000 (Thermo Fisher Scientific) and subjected to quality control minimum standards of 260/230 > 2 and 260/280 > 1.8 prior to downstream applications. qRT-PCR experiments were carried out as previously described (6). Ranges of Cq values utilized for qPCR experiments include human mesenchymal stem cells (hMSCs): *ACTB* (22.08–30.84), *PPARG* (25.80–34.45), *CEBPA* (27.62–35.03), *FABP4* (22.30–39.51); mBMSCs: *Actb* (17.56–19.25), *Pparg* (23.48–25.71), *Cebpa* (24.44–27.8), *Fabp4* (18.30–28.81), *Cxcl1* (27.50–34.40), *Cxcl2* (25.03–34.79), *Il6* (32.46–37.57); 3T3L1: *Actb* (18.37–38.15), *Pparg* (22.39–39.05), *Adipoq* (21.09–38.30), *Cxcl12* (19.45–37.30), *Cxcl1* (27.79–39.36), *Il6* (30.09–39.04).

3T3-L1 Gene Expression Assessed by Microarray

Total RNA (100 ng) was used for cRNA synthesis, prepared, and purified as previously described (22); 5.5 μg of fragmented single-strand cDNA (GeneChip ® WT PLUS reagent Kit) was purified, labeled, and hybridized prior to injection into Mouse Clariom S arrays, also as previously described (22). Arrays were placed in the Affymetrix® GeneChip® Hybridization Oven 645 and stained with the Affymetrix GeneChip® Fluidics Station 450 prior to scanning (7G Affymetrix GeneChip Scanner 3000). Raw data (Affymetrix CEL files) were imported into the Gene Expression Workflow (Partek Genomics Suite v. 6.17.0918, Partek, St Louis, MO) (GSE143269) and normalized prior to log2 transformation, and differential expression (DE) analysis, as previously described (22), except here a one-way ANOVA was utilized in the DE analysis and DE genes were defined based on an absolute fold change > 1.5 in combination with an unadjusted p-value of 0.05 or less.

Differential expression of functional groups was assessed through Pathway-ANOVA and GO-ANOVA analyses in Partek Genomic Suite, which utilized Kyoto Encyclopedia of Genes and Genomes (KEGG) Pathway and GO term databases, respectively. Both Pathway- and GO-ANOVA were performed on normalized expression data without filtering using the method of moments algorithm. Parameters for the Pathway- and GO-ANOVA analyses were configured such that only pathways with more than two and fewer than 500 genes are considered and only GO-terms with more than two and fewer than 100 genes were considered.

Normalized gene expression values were also subjected to a gene set enrichment analysis (GSEA) using the Java implementation from the Broad Institute (32). Array probe sets were collapsed into gene symbols for the analysis and the chip platform used for annotation was Clariom_S_Mouse.r1.chip available from the annotation directory within the GSEA software. Phenotype labels for treatment (the factor of interest) were "MM.1S" and "Control." "Diff_of_Classes" was used as the gene ranking metric. Several Molecular Signatures Database Collections (MSigDB v6.1, Dec 2, 2017) were used to identify gene sets significantly enriched in MM.1S vs control cultures for both the preadipocyte and mature adipocyte experiments, including H (Hallmark), C2 (curated gene sets), and C5 (Gene Ontology, GO, gene sets), which contained 50, 3,689, and 4,429 gene sets respectively, when gene set size filters min=15 and max=500 were applied (33). Only those gene sets with a false discovery rate (FDR) < 25% were considered significantly enriched.

Analysis of External Multiple Myeloma-Mesenchymal Stromal Cells and Normal Bone Marrow-Mesenchymal Stromal Cells Dataset

Microarray gene expression data from Corre et al. (28) was accessed for MSCs derived from non-malignant, normal bone marrow (NBM; n=7) or multiple myeloma (MM; n=6) patient bone marrow. Differentially expressed (DE) genes were determined *via* unpaired, two-tailed t-test for each transcript ($p<0.05$). Gene relatedness was assessed with a tool for recurring instances of neighboring genes (STRING v11.0), input was limited to significant DE genes with a fold-change ≥|2| (34). Heatmaps were generated using the publicly available Morpheus data visualization tool through the Broad Institute (https://software.broadinstitute.org/morpheus/).

Analysis of p16 and p21 in Adipogenic Precursors and Adipocytes

Protein from cell lysates was extracted using RIPA buffer (Santa Cruz, 24948) and quantified using DC protein assay kit II (Bio-Rad, 5000112). Each sample was denatured in 4x laemmli buffer (Bio-Rad, 1610747) for 5 minutes at 95°C. Samples were run on 12% polyacrylamide gels (Bio-Rad, 5671043) and transferred onto PVDF membranes (Bio-Rad, 1704156). Primary antibodies anti-p16 (Abcam, ab108349; 5% milk in TBS-T, 3 days), p21 Waf1/Cip1 (Cell Signaling Technology, #2947; 5% BSA in TBS-T, 1 day) and β-tubulin (Cell Signaling Technology, #2146; 5% BSA in TBS-T, 1 day) were used at a 1:1,000 dilution with incubation at 4°C. HRP-linked anti-rabbit IgG (Cell signaling technology, #7074; 5% BSA in TBS-T) was used as the secondary antibody at a 1:5,000 dilution with incubation at 4°C for 24 h.

Analysis of Secreted Cytokines Following Exposure to Multiple Myeloma Cells

Cell culture conditioned media (CM) was collected from mature naïve adipocytes or MM-adipocytes in culture after 48 (mouse) or 72 (human) hours of incubation and frozen at −20°C. Secreted cytokines in the CM were quantified with either the Mouse Cytokine Array A (R&D; Minneapolis, MN) or the Human Cytokine Array (R&D) per the manufacturer's instructions.

In Vitro Myeloma Cell Functional Characterization

Myeloma cell number was assessed using bioluminescence (MM.1S, OPM-2) or CellTiter-Glo (5TGM1, RPMI-8226; Promega, City, State). Cells were collected and stained with APC-Annexin V (BioLegend, San Diego, CA) and DAPI (Thermo Fisher Scientific, Waltham, MA) for apoptosis. For proliferation, cells were fixed in fixation buffer (BioLegend) prior to washing and staining with Alexa Fluor 647 anti-human Ki-67 antibody (BioLegend) prior to flow cytometry *via* MACSQuant Analyzer (Miltenyi Biotec, Bergisch Gladbach, Germany). A minimum of 10,000 events were captured and analyzed using FlowJo v.10.1 (Becton, Dickinson & Company, Ashland, OR).

Statistical Analysis

All graphs were created with GraphPad Prism (version 7); statistical significance was determined by using two-way ANOVA (multiple groups) or Student's T-test (two groups) unless otherwise stated. For these tests, we made the assumptions that the data had a Gaussian distribution and that they meet the qualifications for a parametric test (normality, equal variance, and independence). All data are expressed as mean ± SEM. For more information, please reference *Supplemental Methods.* Statistical analyses for the microarray data were completed as outlined above.

RESULTS

Multiple Myeloma Patient-Derived Mesenchymal Stromal Cells Exhibit Changes in Key Metabolic Genes

We began with a thorough analysis of the publicly available data from Corre et al. (28), investigating relative differences in the gene expression profiles in MSCs from normal bone marrow (NBM) and multiple myeloma (MM) patient bone marrow. We found 224 downregulated genes in MM-MSCs compared to NBM-MSC controls, and 183 of these genes were connected nodes in our gene network analysis (STRINGv11.0, **Supplementary Figure 1A**). In the significantly downregulated genes, we observed significant enrichment of transcripts encoding genes in the cellular differentiation pathway (GO:0030154; FDR<0.05) including the transcription factors forkhead box transcription factors A1 and M1 (*FOXA1, FOXM1*), pioneering transcription factors that can enhance or suppress the expression of differentiation and/or proliferation factors (35, 36) as well as lim homeobox 8 (*LHX8*), which is involved in the pro-osteogenic BMP signaling cascade (37). Nine genes specifically involved in osteogenesis were also significantly downregulated including collagen type XI alpha 1 chain (*COL11A1*), the BMP4 antagonist chordin like 1 (*CHRDL1*), insulin like growth factor 1 (*IGF1*), and asporin (*ASPN*) which binds collagen and calcium in cartilage, inducing cartilage mineralization. The leptin receptor (*LEPR*), a known regulator of osteogenic and adipogenic progenitors (38), was also significantly decreased in MM-MSCs compared to controls, suggesting that in addition to impaired osteogenic capacity, as previously described (28), adipogenic capacity may also be impaired in MM-MSCs.

We next created two clusters of transcripts involved in both the KEGG PPAR signaling pathway (**Figure 1A**) and the Hallmark adipogenesis gene set (**Figure 2**) to begin to specifically investigate the effects of MM exposure on lipid metabolism and metabolic homeostasis. Within the PPAR signaling pathway, we observed significantly altered expression of 14 transcripts (associated with nine genes) within this cluster (**Table 1**). Seven out of nine genes were downregulated, including fatty acid desaturase 1 (*FADS1*; **Figure 1B, Supplementary Figure 1A**) and fatty acid desaturase 2 (*FADS2*; **Figure 1C**), potentially representing a modulation of the processing of long-chain polyunsaturated fatty acids in MM-MSCs. MM-MSCs exhibited slight but significant increases in acetyl-coA acyltransferase 1 (*ACAA1*), acyl-CoA oxidase 1 (*ACOX1*), and acyl-CoA oxidase 2 (*ACOX2*), which are involved in fatty acid oxidation. These findings led us to hypothesize that MM cells modulate the metabolism of MSCs and may alter their adipogenic differentiation. As previously reported by Corre *et al.*, we also confirmed >2 fold increases in two transcripts for angiopoietin like 4 (*ANGPTL4*; **Figure 1D, Supplementary Figure 1B**), the expression of which is responsive to peroxisome proliferation activators (28).

By further examining genes that were significantly different (p<0.05) between MM and NBM-MSCs in the Corre dataset, we observed differential expression of 68 genes that are specifically upregulated during adipogenesis (**Figure 2**). The cluster of genes upregulated in MM-MSCs included acyl-CoA dehydrogenase long chain (*ACADL*)—a mitochondrial enzyme involved in fatty acid metabolism, as well as aldolase fructose-bisphosphate A (*ALDOA*), a glycolytic enzyme, suggesting that MM-MSCs burn rather than store more fatty acids than normal MSCs. ATP binding cassette subfamily A member 1 (*ABCA1*), a membrane-associated protein involved in cellular lipid removal, was also upregulated in MM-MSCs. The cluster of transcripts downregulated in MM-MSCs included metabolic enzymes 1-acylglycerol-3-phosphate O-acyltransferase 3 (*AGPAT3*), ectonucleotide pyrophosphatase/phosphodiesterase 2 (*ENPP2*), and dihydrolipoamide S-acetyltransferase (*DLAT*). Signal transducer and activator of transcription 5A (*STAT5A*), a key molecule involved in the signaling cascades triggered by many ligands including interleukins and growth hormones, was also downregulated in MM-MSCs compared to controls. Interestingly, key regulators of cell cycle and apoptosis were downregulated in MM-MSCs, including cyclin dependent kinase inhibitor 2C (*CDKN2C*), a cell cycle regulator that controls G1 progression, and programmed cell death 4 (*PDCD4*), which regulates proliferation by inducing cell cycle arrest at G1 (39). Overall, these data suggest that MM patient derived MSCs exhibit changes in key metabolic genes that may inhibit their ability to differentiate into adipocytes.

In a second study utilizing mesenchymal cells isolated from patient bone marrow biopsies (40), MM-MSCs exhibited differential expression profiles compared to ND-MSCs. The authors identified seventy-eight differentially expressed genes

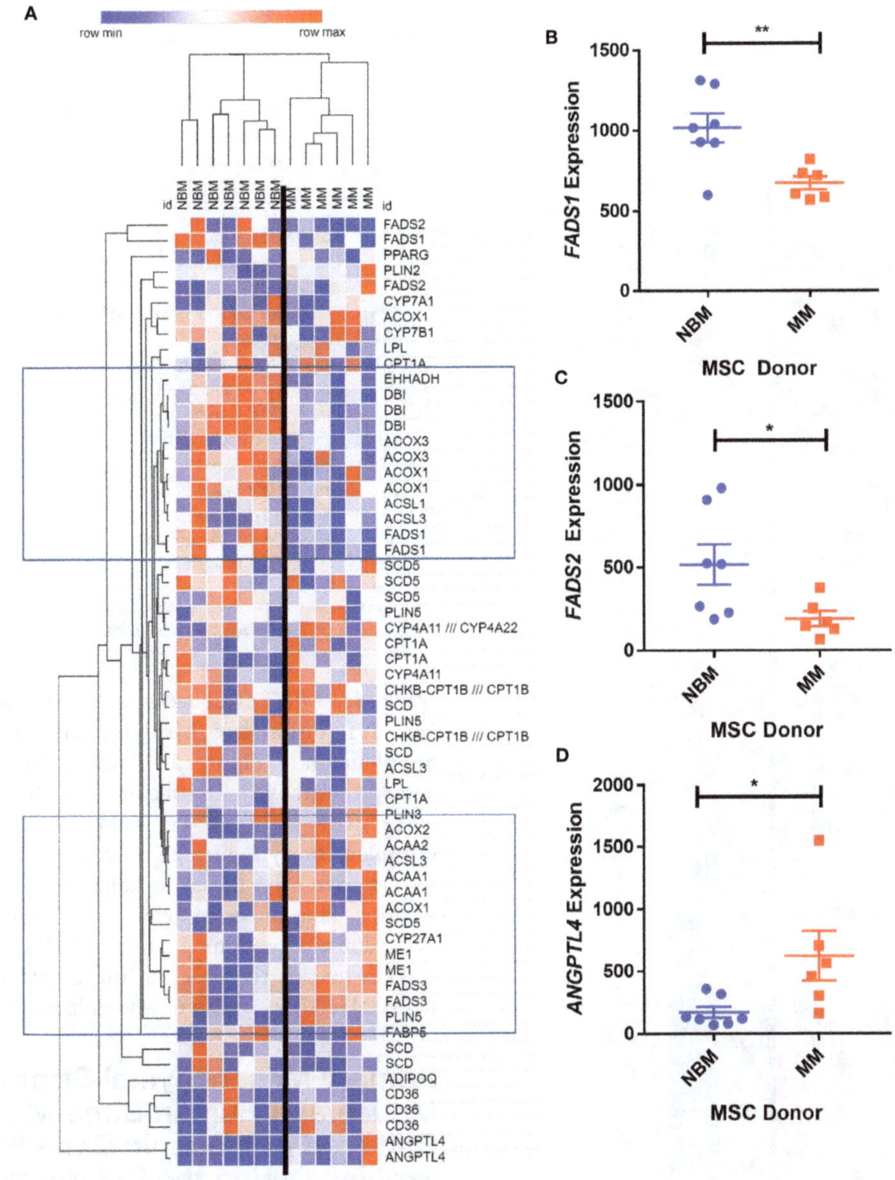

FIGURE 1 | Expression of genes encoding key metabolic proteins in myeloma patient mesenchymal stromal cells (MSCs). Expression of transcripts involved in PPAR signaling Kyoto Encyclopedia of Genes and Genomes (KEGG) pathway **(A)**, in MSCs derived from normal patient bone marrow (NBM) or myeloma patients (MM), graphically demonstrated using Morpheus software (The Broad Institute). Groups of down and upregulated genes can roughly be seen in the top and bottom boxed regions. Reduced gene expression of *FADS1* **(B)** and *FADS2* **(C)** and increased expression of *ANGPTL4* **(D)**. Analysis of publicly available data from Corre *et al.* 2007, *Leukemia*.

between MM- and ND-MSCs, with transcripts representing processes such as cell adhesion, cell cycle and proliferation, and transcriptional regulation. We utilized the data from this study to investigate functional enrichments and connectedness of the DE genes (**Supplementary Figure 2**). Our analysis revealed that 31 of the 78 genes (approximately 40% of the differentially expressed genes) were involved in the regulation of cellular metabolic process (GO:0031325), including a number of transcription factors (**Supplementary Figure 2A**) including nuclear receptor subfamily 1, group D, member2 (NR1D2), SRY-box transcription factor 9 (SOX9), nuclear receptor subfamily 2 group F member 1 (NR2F1), paired like homeodomain 2 (PITX2), and YY1 transcription factor (*YY1*). *ENPP1* was also significantly decreased in MM-MSCs compared to controls (**Supplementary Figure 2B**), as we have highlighted above in the dataset from Corre et al. In addition, in this second

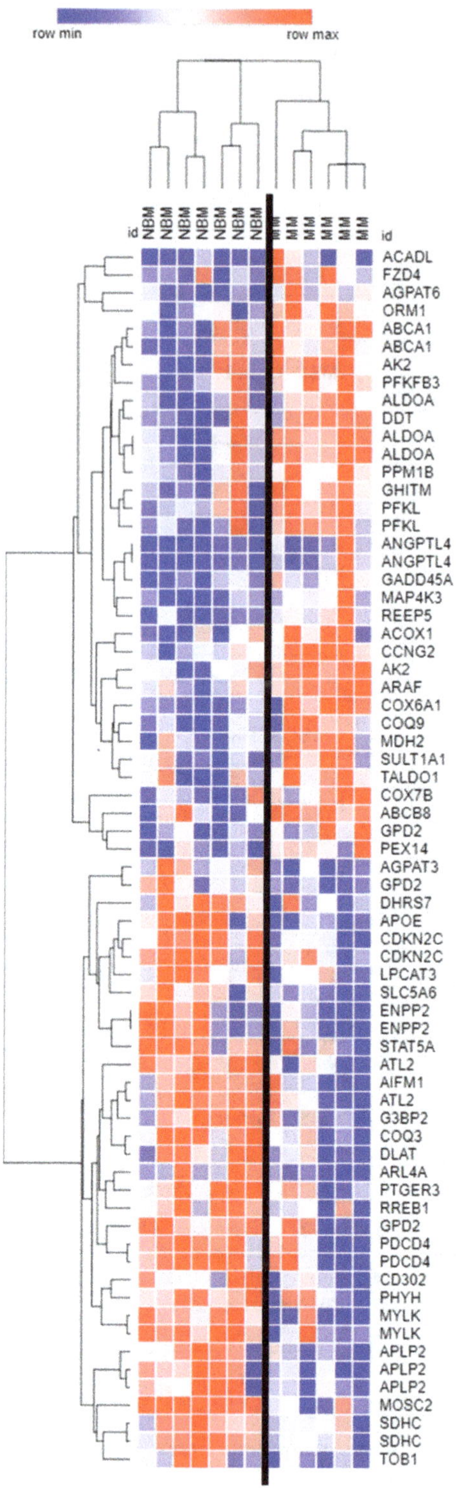

FIGURE 2 | Expression of genes encoding key adipogenic proteins in myeloma patient mesenchymal stromal cells (MSCs). Expression of transcripts included in the Hallmark Adipogenesis Gene Set, in MSCs derived from normal patient bone marrow (NBM) or myeloma patients (MM). Graphically demonstrated using Morpheus software (The Broad Institute). Analysis of publicly available data from Corre *et al.* 2007, *Leukemia*.

TABLE 1 | 14 Metabolic genes significantly altered in myeloma patient-derived mesenchymal stem cells (MM-MSCs).

Gene symbol	Gene name	P-value	Relative expression (MM/NBM)
EHHADH	Enoyl-CoA hydratase and 3-hydroxyacyl CoA dehydrogenase	0.0024	0.64
DBI	Diazepam binding inhibitor, acyl-CoA binding protein	0.0028	0.80
FADS1	Fatty acid desaturase 1	0.0030	0.57
DBI	Diazepam binding inhibitor, acyl-CoA binding protein	0.0037	0.81
DBI	Diazepam binding inhibitor, acyl-CoA binding protein	0.0045	0.78
ACOX2	Acyl-CoA oxidase 2	0.0046	1.17
FADS1	Fatty acid desaturase 1	0.0083	0.66
FADS1	Fatty acid desaturase 1	0.0143	0.48
ACOX3	Acyl-CoA oxidase 3, pristanoyl	0.0300	0.75
ANGPTL4	Angiopoietin like 4	0.0355	2.68
ANGPTL4	Angiopoietin like 4	0.0365	3.63
FADS2	Fatty acid desaturase 2	0.0384	0.37
ACAA1	Acetyl-CoA acyltransferase 1	0.0447	1.17
ACOX1	Acyl-CoA oxidase 1	0.0452	1.35

Analysis of publicly available data from Corre et al. 2007, Leukemia; p<0.05. Blue text indicates downregulated; red indicates upregulated.

study MM-MSCs exhibited significantly decreased expression of CCAAT enhancer binding protein alpha (*CEBPA*; **Supplementary Figure 2B**), which functions as a key early adipogenic transcription factor. In addition, *SOX9* and *MEIS1* were upregulated in MM-MSCs vs. NBM-MSCs (**Supplementary Figure 2C**), but the inactivation of these two factors have been linked to adipogenic differentiation (41). In addition, zinc finger protein 36 (*ZFP36*) and Salvador family WW domain containing protein 1 (*SAV1*), which have been linked to positive regulation of fat cell differentiation (GO:0045600) were also downregulated in MM-MSCs.

Primary Mesenchymal Stromal Cells From Mouse and Human Bone Marrow Exhibit Reduced Adipogenic Gene Expression Profiles During the Differentiation Process

To determine if the gene expression changes above translated to functional effects, we next tested our hypothesis that adipogenesis is inhibited in MM-MSCs by comparing the *in vitro* differentiation capacity of normal bone marrow (NBM) and myeloma donor (MM) MSCs (**Figure 3A**). While NBM-MSCs readily differentiated into adipocytes (**Figure 3B**), MM-MSCs exhibited diminished differentiation capacity (**Figure 3C**; **Supplementary Figure 2A**). Having observed phenotypic differences in differentiated MM-MSCs, we next tested their relative gene expression of key adipogenic transcripts by qRT-PCR and observed suppression of *PPARG* (**Figure 3D**), *CEBPA* (**Figure 3E**), and *FABP4* (**Figure 3F**). These findings demonstrate significantly reduced adipogenic capacity of MM-MSCs compared to NBM-MSCs using patient stromal cells.

This led to us to ask if MM cells themselves directly cause these alterations in MSCs, thus, we next tested the hypothesis that MM

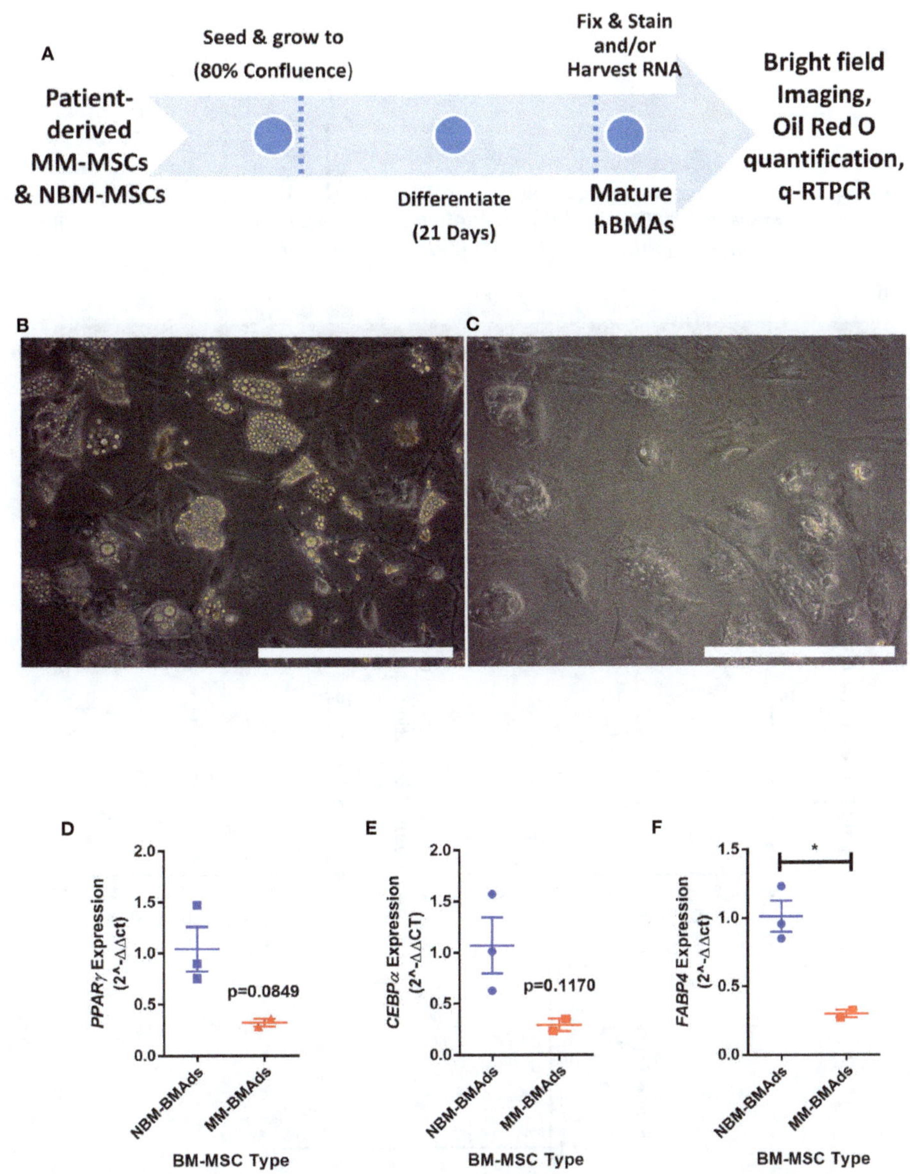

FIGURE 3 | Mesenchymal stromal cells (MSCs) derived from myeloma patients exhibit impaired adipogenic differentiation. Experimental design of MSC differentiation experiment **(A)**. MSCs differentiated into adipocytes for 21 days from normal donor bone marrow (NBM-BMAds), **(B)**, or myeloma patient bone marrow (MM-BMAds, **(C)** for 21 days; images taken at 20X, scale bars = 250 μm. *PPARG* **(D)**, *CEBPA* **(E)**, and *FABP4* **(F)** expression are decreased at the end of the adipogenic differentiation period in adipocytes derived from myeloma patient MSCs (MM-BMAds), relative to normal donor controls (NBM-BMAds) (n=3); *p < 0.05.

cells can directly induce changes in primary BM stromal cells with *in vitro* co-culture. Primary BM stromal cells from naïve mice (**Supplementary Figure 2B**) were exposed to MM.1S myeloma cells *via* transwell co-culture for 72 h prior to adipogenic differentiation (**Figure 4A**). Imaging after differentiation revealed significantly fewer lipid-containing adipocytes in cultures with MM pre-exposure, compared to controls (**Figure 4B**). Immediately after MM exposure (day 3), and 2 days later (day 5), mouse MSCs exhibited suppression of the key adipogenic transcription factor *Pparg* (**Figure 4C**) with slight, but non-significant suppression of both *Cebpa* (**Figure 4D**) and the mature adipocyte marker *Fabp4* (**Figure 4E**). While expression levels of these adipogenic transcripts were reduced, the overall pattern of induction mirrored that of the control cells, suggesting that adipogenic differentiation was occurring at some capacity. These experiments support the hypothesis that MM cells induce rapid and long-lasting effects on adipocyte precursors, and that these effects are at least in part mediated through soluble molecules.

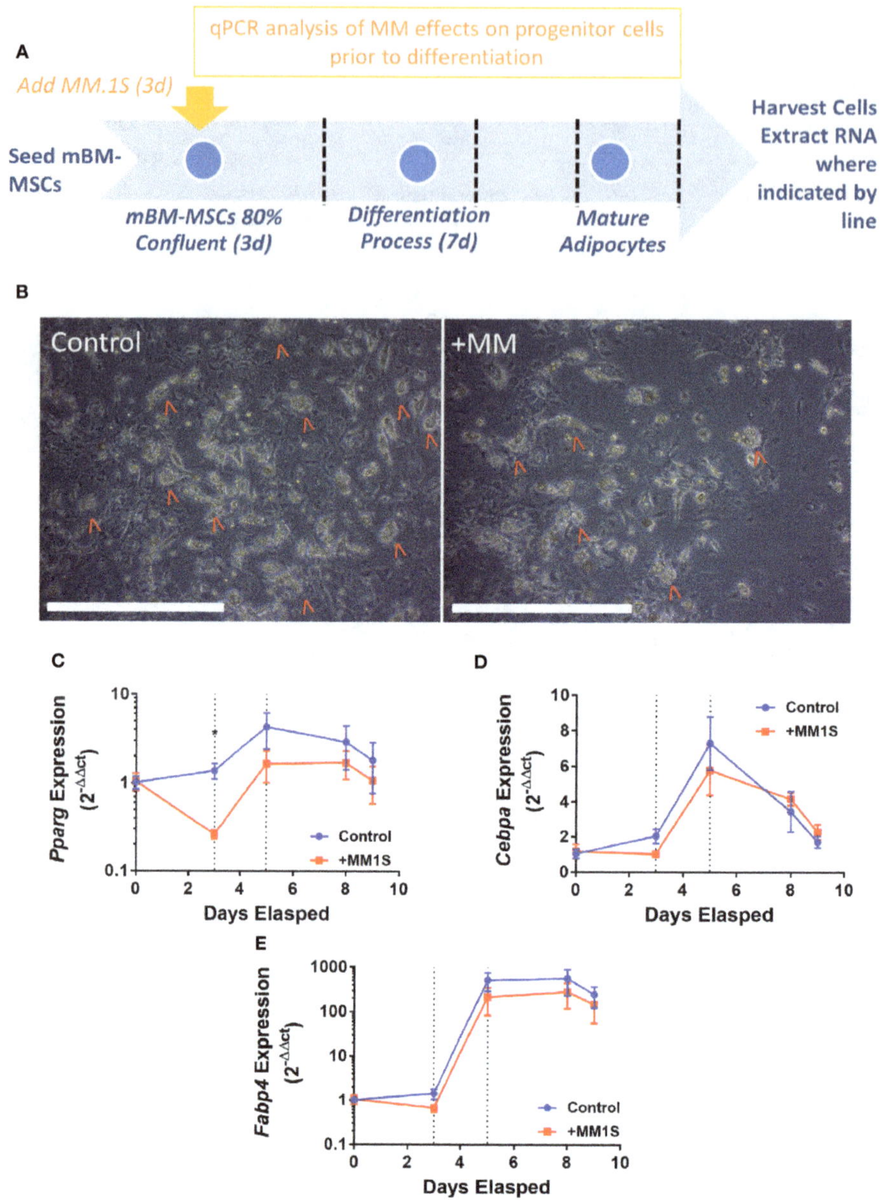

FIGURE 4 | Mouse bone marrow mesenchymal stem cells (BM-MSCs) exposed to multiple myeloma (MM) cells *via* indirect co-culture *in vitro* exhibit reduced adipogenesis. Experimental design of co-culture experiment **(A)**. Images taken with 10X objective (scale bars = 500 µm) at terminal differentiation following pre-exposure (day 9; **B**). *Pparg* **(C)**, *Cebpa* **(D)**, and *Fabp4* **(E)** expression as assessed by qRT-PCR is suppressed in mouse MSCs "pre-exposed" to myeloma cells *in vitro* for 72-h *prior to differentiation* (first dotted line indicates the end of pre-exposure and start of differentiation), and levels are slightly suppressed throughout differentiation (second dotted line represents day 2 of adipogenic differentiation) (n=3); $^{*}p \leq 0.05$.

Indirect Co-Culture with Myeloma Cells Results in Reduced Lipid Accumulation and Inhibition of Adipogenic Transcripts in Differentiating Mouse Preadipocytes

Having observed similar effects in primary human samples and *in vitro* with co-cultures, we next investigated MM-induced changes in adipogenic precursors using the 3T3-L1 murine preadipocyte cell line, to eliminate donor variability. We utilized multiple different experimental designs to characterize the effects of MM cells on 3T3-L1 cells (MM-3T3-L1s): pre-exposure of 3T3-L1 cells to MM cells for 2 days *prior to* differentiation (using direct or indirect co-cultures; **Supplementary Figure 4A**), and co-culture of 3T3-L1 cells with MM cells *during* differentiation (through exposure to MM conditioned media (MM-CM) during differentiation; **Supplementary Figure 4B**). 3T3-L1 preadipocytes exposed to MM.1S cells during differentiation exhibited significantly reduced lipid content in direct co-culture and this trend also

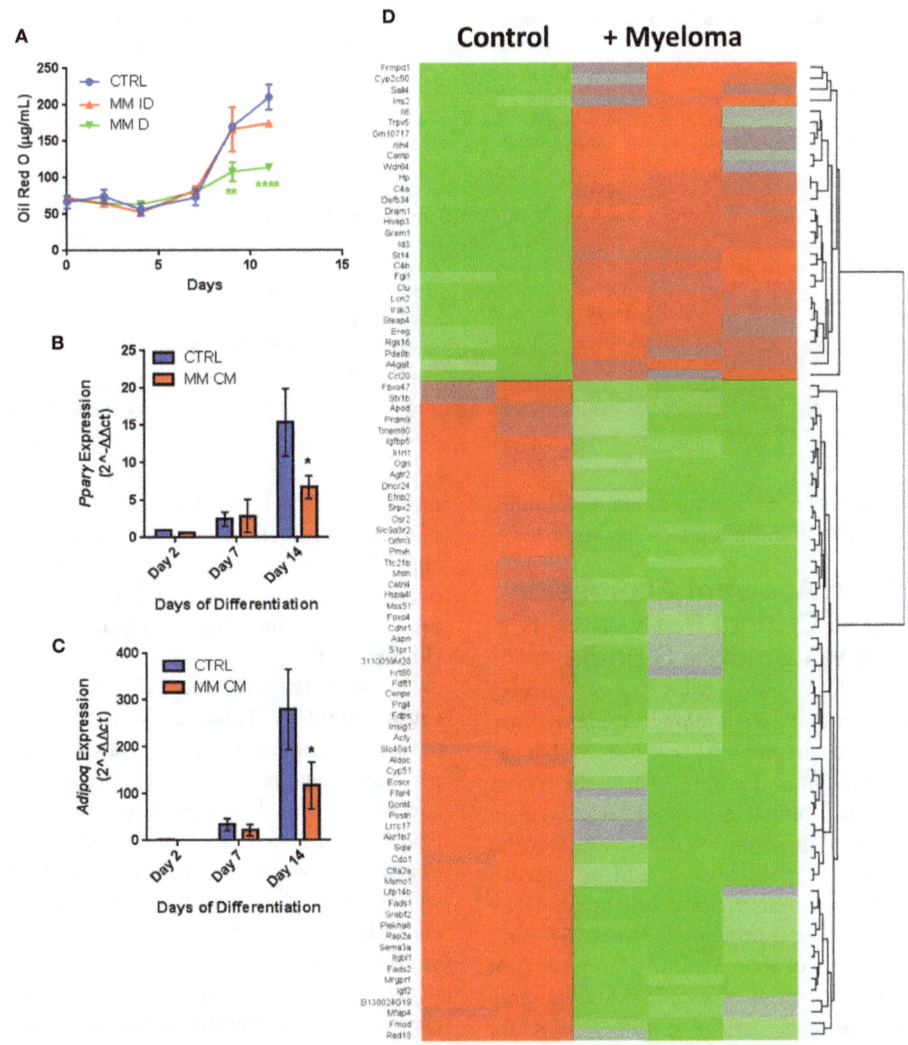

FIGURE 5 | Adipogenic differentiation of 3T3-L1 preadipocytes is inhibited by MM.1S myeloma cells. 3T3-L1 adipocytes were assessed for Oil Red-O content either alone (control) or with exposure to MM.1S cells prior to differentiation process *via* indirect (+MM ID) or direct (+ MM D) co-culture (day 11). Lipid content is significantly reduced by MM.1S co-culture (indirect, MM ID; direct, MM D) *during* differentiation compared to 3T3-L1 cells on their own (CTRL); quantification of Oil Red-O staining **(A)**. Expression of adipogenic transcripts *Pparg* **(B)** and *Adipoq* **(C)** are suppressed *during* differentiation in the presence of conditioned media from MM.1S cells; n=4. Significant differences in gene expression ($p \leq 0.05$, FC |1.8|, red is upregulated, green is downregulated) in 3T3-L1 adipocytes exposed to myeloma cells for 48-h *prior* to differentiation as measured by microarray **(D)**; control n=2, MM.1S n=3; *$p < 0.05$, **$p < 0.01$, ****$p < 0.0001$.

seen in indirect co-culture (**Figure 5A**). Similarly, 3T3-L1 cells exposed to MM-CM during differentiation exhibited significantly reduced *Pparg* gene expression (**Figure 5B**), and adiponectin, *Adipoq* (**Figure 5C**) at day 14. Although we observed these reductions with MM co-culture, lipid accumulation did increase over the course of differentiation, and the expression of adipogenic transcripts was also turned on, suggesting that MM cells inhibit, but do not completely block adipogenesis.

Indirect exposure of 3T3-L1 preadipocytes to MM.1S cells *via* transwell for 48 h prior to differentiation (**Supplementary Figure 4A**), revealed significant differences in the expression of 1287 total genes as assessed by microarray (**Figure 5D**). Of these, 105 transcripts were significantly upregulated (>1.5-fold, p<0.05; **Supplementary Table 1**) and 179 were significantly downregulated (<1.5-fold, p<0.05; **Supplementary Table 2**). Among them, we observed increased expression of interleukin-1-receptor- associated kinase 3 (*Irak3*) and lipocalin 2 (*Lcn2*) (**Table 2**; **Supplementary Table 1**), a small transport protein involved in the shuttling of small hydrophobic molecules. We also detected decreased expression of insulin growth factor (*Igf2;* **Table 2**; **Supplementary Table 2**), a growth factor which promotes subcutaneous preadipocyte differentiation (42). Also, of note, we detected significantly reduced expression of odd-skipped related 2 (*Osr2*), which has been linked to the control of BMP and semaphorin 3A (SEMA3A) signaling. Interestingly, *Sema3a* was also suppressed in MM-3T3-L1s (**Table 2**; **Supplementary Table 2**), and its expression is known to inhibit MM progression in mouse models (43). Overall, we

TABLE 2 | Altered expression of transcripts in 3T3-L1 adipocytes with exposure to MM.1S cells.

Increased in adipocytes w/pre-exposure to MM cells	p-value	Fold change (MM/CTRL)	Decreased in adipocytes w/pre-exposure to MM cells	P-value	Fold change (MM/CTRL)
Cathelicidin antimicrobial peptide *(Camp)*	0.046908	*3.725*	Angiotensin II receptor, type 2 *(Agtr2)*	0.002039	−9.069
Interleukin-1 receptor associated kinase 3 *(Irak3)*	0.011152	*3.644*	Aldolase C, fructose-bisphosphate *(Aldoc)*	0.012447	−4.186
CD4 antigen *(C4a)*	0.004946	*2.405*	Interleukin 1 receptor-like 1 *(Il1rl1)*	0.009467	−4.055
Lipocalin 2 *(Lcn2)*	0.012884	*2.346*	Apolipoprotein D *(Apod)*	0.02907	−3.747
Complement component 4 b *(C4b)*	0.000832	*2.300*	**Semaphorin 3a *(Sema3a)***	0.001421	−3.282
Fibrinogen-like protein 1 *(Fgl1)*	0.01909	*2.241*	UTP14B small subunit processome component *(Utp14b)*	0.025423	−3.246
Inhibitor of DNA binding 3 *(Id3)*	0.00221	*2.195*	**Odd-skipped related 2 *(Osr2)***	0.002808	−3.191
Alpha 1,4, galctosyltransferase *(A4galt)*	0.047703	*2.181*	Cytochrome P450, family 51 *(Cyp51)*	0.005149	−3.089
Haptoglobin *(Hp)*	0.004879	*2.170*	**Insulin-like growth factor 2 *(Igf2)***	0.000666	−2.955
STEAP family member 4 *(Steap4)*	0.014702	*2.125*	Integrin, beta-like 1 *(Itgbl1)*	0.000345	−2.891

Top 10 most significant gene expression changes in 3T3-L1 adipocytes with exposure to MM.1S cells prior to differentiation derived from microarray data. Bold indicates discussed in text. Blue text indicates downregulated and red text indicates upregulated.

have seen that MM cells reduce lipid accumulation and inhibit adipogenic transcripts in differentiating mouse preadipocytes.

Myeloma Cells Drive Aberrant Expression of Genes Involved in Critical Pathways in Mouse Adipocytes via Soluble Signals

Utilizing our indirect co-culture system with pre-exposure of 3T3-L1 cells to MM cells prior to differentiation (**Supplementary Figure 4A**), we next examined whether MM cells induce changes in major pathways when co-cultured with 3T3-L1 cells within the microarray data. The differential expression results from Pathway-ANOVA analysis of microarray data show several significantly enriched KEGG pathways including steroid biosynthesis and oxidative phosphorylation, cell cycle, DNA replication, and ubiquitin-mediated proteolysis (**Table 3**). Both the oxidative phosphorylation (**Table 3**) and glycolysis (not shown) KEGG pathways were enriched in 3T3-L1 adipocytes with pre-exposure to MM cells prior to differentiation, suggesting that exposure to MM-derived factors leads to metabolic dysfunction in preadipocytes and mature adipocytes. In addition to KEGG pathway analysis, we utilized normalized microarray data to perform gene set enrichment analysis (GSEA). While many signatures were not significant, GSEA analysis indicated significant enrichment (FDR<25%) in 14 out of 50 Hallmark gene sets (**Table 4**) including glycolysis (**Figure 6A**), fatty acid metabolism (**Figure 6B**), and mTORC signaling (**Figure 6C**).

Within the 179 significantly downregulated genes (**Supplementary Table 2**) in MM-3T3-L1s (**Figure 6D**), we observed enrichment in sterol, lipid, and cholesterol metabolic processes by gene network analysis- including 27 genes specifically linked to lipid metabolic processes. Like our data from analysis of normal donor versus myeloma patient MSCs (**Table 1**), we again found that *Fads1* and *Fads2* were significantly downregulated in MM-3T3-L1s compared to controls. Additionally, the expression of the key enzymes fatty acid synthase (*Fasn*) and carnitine palmitoyltransferase 1a (*Cpt1a*) were both suppressed in adipocytes with MM pre-exposure demonstrating altered metabolic activity, with specific implications for fatty acid synthesis and β-oxidation.

TABLE 3 | Microarray data reveal key cellular Kyoto Encyclopedia of Genes and Genomes (KEGG) pathways altered in response to multiple myeloma (MM) cell exposure.

KEGG pathway (pretreat)	P-value	FC
Steroid biosynthesis	5.84E−16	−1.41136
Cell cycle	1.67E−12	−1.08717
Terpenoid backbone biosynthesis	1.22E−08	−1.2398
DNA replication	1.23E−07	−1.13989
Rheumatoid arthritis	4.03E−07	1.08281
Ubiquitin mediated proteolysis	5.50E−07	−1.0509
Protein processing in endoplasmic reticulum	1.02E−06	−1.04289
Oxidative phosphorylation	1.46E−06	1.03672
Phagosome	2.37E−06	1.04667
Systemic lupus erythematosus	4.97E−06	1.05049

KEGG Pathways significantly altered in 3T3-L1 adipocytes with exposure to MM.1S cells prior to differentiation derived from microarray data. Pathway analyses incorporate all robust multi-array average (RMA)-normalized genes. Bold indicates discussed in text. Blue text indicates downregulated and red text indicates upregulated.

TABLE 4 | Key gene sets revealed as altered in response to multiple myeloma (MM) cell exposure.

Hallmark gene set enriched	FDR (<0.25)
Androgen response	0.091
Mitotic spindle	0.091
mTORC1 signaling	0.091
Cholesterol signaling	0.091
G2M checkpoint	0.118
Protein secretion	0.122
Myogenesis	0.129
E2F targets	0.142
Glycolysis	0.148
Hypoxia	0.155
UV response DNA	0.155
Fatty acid metabolism	0.157
Apical junction	0.198
PI3K-AKT-MTOR signaling	0.206

Significant gene set enrichment analysis (GSEA) results in 3T3-L1 adipocytes with exposure to MM.1S cells prior to differentiation compared to controls. Derived from microarray data; analyses incorporate all robust multi-array average (RMA)-normalized genes. Bold indicates discussed in text.

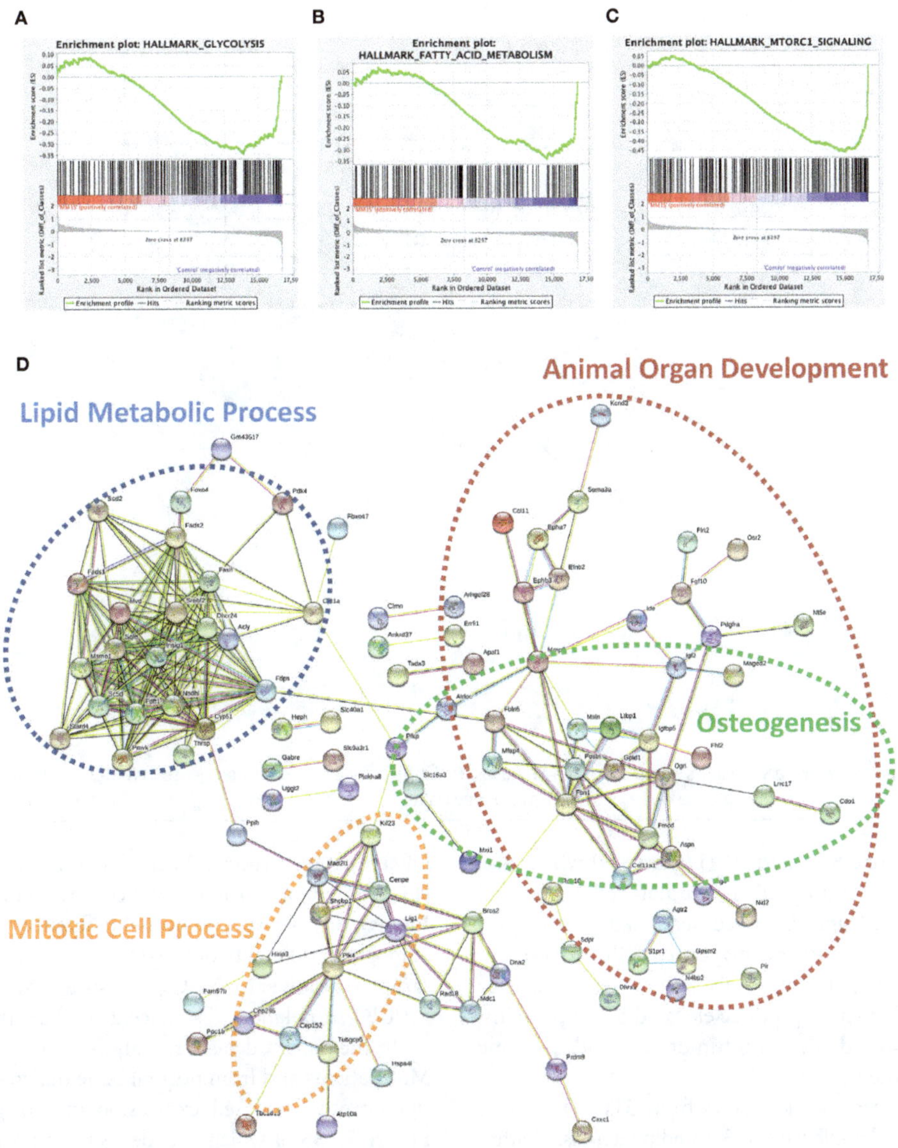

FIGURE 6 | Cellular metabolism and key signaling pathways are altered in myeloma-associated mouse adipocytes. 3T3-L1 adipocytes exposed to MM.1S prior to differentiation have altered expression of genes involved with glycolysis **(A)**, fatty acid metabolism **(B)**, and mTORC signaling **(C)** as determined *via* gene set enrichment analysis (GSEA) analysis of 3T3-L1 microarray data. Expression of genes involved in lipid metabolism and encoding essential growth factors are downregulated in MM-3T3-L1 adipocytes **(D)** as visualized by string-db analysis of 3T3-L1 microarray data ($p < 0.05$, FC<–1.5).

By specifically examining the 103 significantly upregulated genes in 3T3-L1 adipocytes with prior exposure to MM cells, we further identified a network of genes with *Il6* as a central node (**Figure 7**). Collectively, these genes are enriched for GO terms such as "cellular response to interleukin-1" (GO:0071347), "inflammatory response" (GO:0006954), and "response to tumor necrosis factor" (GO:0034612). These results suggest that 3T3-L1 adipocytes exposed to MM cells in their progenitor stage increase the expression of genes that produce inflammatory proteins known to modulate the bone marrow microenvironment, and many of these are known members of the senescence-associated secretory phenotype (SASP).

Multiple Myeloma Induces Expression of Key Transcripts Involved in the Senescence Associated Secretory Phenotype in Adipocyte Lineage Cells

Having obtained evidence that MM-3T3-L1s express genes encoding SASP proteins, we wanted to verify this in each of our cell types. We confirmed that *Cxcl12* and two traditional SASP genes, *Cxcl1*, and *Il6*, were elevated in MM-3T3-L1s *versus* control 3T3-L1s by qRT-PCR (**Figure 8A**). To confirm the presence of elevated SASP transcripts in primary cells, we first utilized mouse MSCs pre-exposed to MM.1S cells. After 24 h of MM exposure, we observed extremely high expression of *Cxcl1*

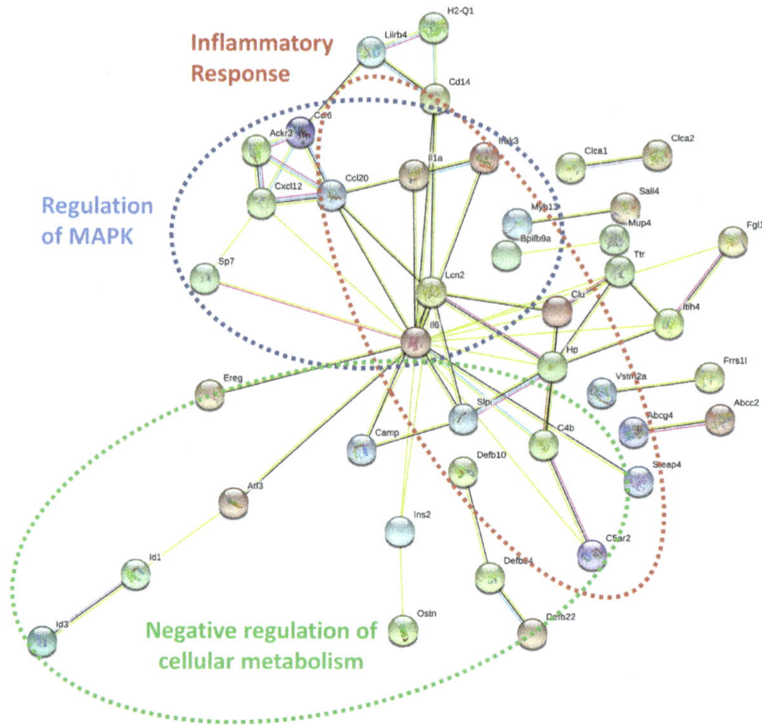

FIGURE 7 | Key signaling pathways are altered in myeloma-associated mouse 3T3-L1 adipocytes. Upregulated genes in MM-3T3-L1s are connected *via* the central node of Il6 as demonstrated graphically by string-db analysis of 3T3-L1 microarray data.

(**Figure 8B**), *Cxcl2* (**Figure 8C**), and *Il6* (**Figure 8D**) which was not basally expressed in mouse BM stromal cells. Elevated expression of both *Cxcl2* and *Il6* were sustained in the pre-exposure group throughout adipogenic differentiation. Combined these data suggest that mouse adipocytes with prior exposure to MM soluble factors produce elevated SASP proteins, which would have profound effects on tumor cells and the bone marrow microenvironment.

We next tested whether soluble factors from 5TGM1 murine myeloma cells have a similar effect on 3T3-L1 adipogenesis. Neither indirect pre-exposure to 5TGM1 cells prior to differentiation, or exposure to 5TGM1 soluble factors (conditioned media, CM) during differentiation resulted in phenotypic changes in 3T3-L1 adipocytes at terminal differentiation (**Supplementary Figure 5A**). Lipid content, as assessed *via* Oil Red-O staining and quantification, also was not significantly different (**Supplementary Figures 5B, C**). Exposure to 5TGM1 soluble factors CM (Supplementary **Figure 5D**), or with transwell indirect co-culture (**Supplementary Figure 5E**), also had no significant effects on in the secretion of over 40 cytokines, (including IL-6, CXCL1, and CXCL2), assessed *via* cytokine array; suggesting a differential effect of either myeloma cell line, or between species. To explore whether indirect co-culture with myeloma cells increases p16 or p21, commonly implicated in cellular senescence, NBM-MSCs were exposed to MM.1S and RPMI-8226 myeloma cells *via* transwell co-culture for 48 h prior to adipogenic differentiation (21 days). MSCs were harvested for total protein either immediately after co-culture, or at the end of the differentiation process. MM co-culture seemingly had very little effect on p16 or p21 in hMSCs compared to naïve (**Supplementary Figures 6A, B**), with no overall differences at the end of 21 days of adipogenic differentiation. p21 and p16 also increased in BMAT samples relative to MSCs, consistent with previous reports of PPARG stimulation of senescent markers (p16) expression (44).

In the patient dataset reanalysis (28), we compared MSCs from MM patients and from normal bone marrow (NBM), and observed significantly increased expression of 267 genes (**Supplementary Figure 7**), 36 of which encode secreted proteins (KW-0964; **Table 5**). These include key signaling molecules known to modulate the BM microenvironment including: C-C motif chemokine ligand 5 (*CCL5*), C-X-C motif chemokine ligand 8 (*CXCL8/IL-8*), platelet derived growth factor B (*PDGFB*), as well as transforming growth factors A and B (*TGFA*, *TGFB*). Secreted phosphoprotein 1 (*SPP1*) was also increased in MM-MSCs relative to NBM-MSCs, suggesting that myeloma MSCs may be similar to other types of cancer-associated stromal cells and adipocytes (45–47). In the DE genes reported by Todoerti et al. (40), only 21 genes were significantly upregulated in MM- *vs.* NBM-MSCs, which were predominantly enriched for factors involved in transcription, including *YY1* which may regulate p16 expression (48) (**Supplementary Figure 2**).

We further examined the expression of senescence-associated genes and observed a general trend for increased SASP gene expression (including *CXCL1*, *CXCL2*, and *IL6*) in MM-MSCs when compared to NBM-MSCs (**Figure 8E**) (28). Elevated expression of *IL6* in MM-MSCs relative to normal donor

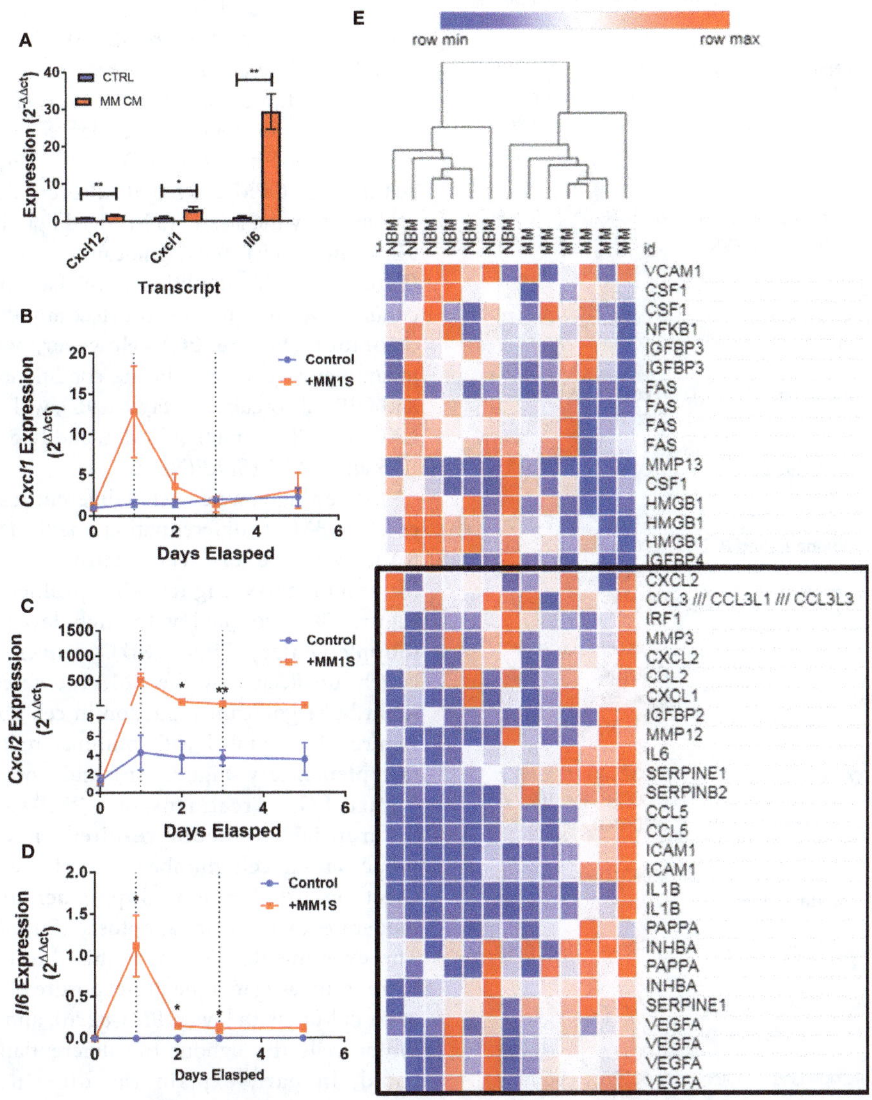

FIGURE 8 | Exposure to myeloma cells prior to adipogenic differentiation induces SASP production in adipocyte precursors. 3T3-L1 cells exposed to MM.1S soluble factors during differentiation exhibit increased expression of: *Il6*, *Cxcl1*, and *Cxcl12* after terminal differentiation **(A)**. Mouse bone marrow MSCs were exposed to MM.1S cells *in vitro* for up to 72 h prior to adipogenic differentiation. Cells were harvested for RNA extraction after 24 (first dotted line), 48, and 72 (second dotted line; change to adipogenic media) hours of pre-exposure, and after the first treatment of adipogenic media (day 5). *Cxcl1* **(B)**, *Cxcl2* **(C)**, and *Il6* **(D)** gene expression was quantified in mMSCs at each time point; n=3 per group, $^*p < 0.05$, $^{**}p < 0.01$. Reanalysis of previously published MSC gene expression data comparing bone marrow from normal donors (NBM) and myeloma donors (MM) examining the SASP gene cluster **(E)** data from Corre *et al*. 2007, *Leukemia*.; heatmap generated *via* Morpheus.

MSCs was observed in an independent experiment utilizing nanostring gene expression data (~2.5-fold, data not shown), and has been previously reported (7, 30). Overexpression of SASP genes Interleukin 1 beta (*IL1B)* and serpin family E member 1 (*SERPINE1)* were also previously reported (28). Additionally, we found that cyclin dependent kinase inhibitor 2A (*CDKN2A*) and high mobility group AT-hook 2 (*HMGA2*) were significantly increased in MM-MSCs 2- and 2.4-fold respectively; these genes encode proteins involved in senescence-associated heterochromatin foci (GO:0035985; **Supplementary Figure 7**). In the Todoerti et al. dataset, MM-MSCs overexpressed NR2F1, a transcription factor that has been linked to increased expression of *CXCL12* (49), however none of the signaling molecules listed above were included in the list of significantly different genes. In addition, among the downregulated genes were those associated with response to cytokine stimulus (GO:0071345), and the interferon signaling pathway (HSA-913531), suggesting that these processes are aberrant in MM-MSCs compared to NBM-MSCs, although the specific relationships remain unclear.

TABLE 5 | Genes upregulated in myeloma patient-derived mesenchymal stem cells (MM-MSCs) compared to non-malignant bone marrow-MSCs (NBM-MSCs) that encode secreted proteins.

Gene Symbol	Gene Name	P-Value	Relative Expression (MM/NBM)
ADAM23	a disintegrin and metallopeptidase domain 23	0.00242	2.7021
ADAMTS12	a disintegrin-like and metallopeptidase (reprolysin type) with thrombospondin type 1 motif, 12	0.00848	2.2248
ANGPTL4	angiopoietin-like 4	0.03554	2.6803
ASAH1	N-acylsphingosine amidohydrolase 1	0.00302	2.4670
BAGE5	B melanoma antigen	0.00811	2.6112
CA6	carbonic anhydrase 6	0.00703	2.3897
CCL5	**chemokine (C-C motif) ligand 5**	0.00968	2.9745
CLEC3A	C-type lectin domain family 3, member a	0.03478	3.6175
CSHL1	chorionic somatomammotropin hormone like 1	0.00117	2.2147
CST2	cystatin SA	0.04382	2.2356
CXCL8	**C-X-C motif chemokine ligand 8**	0.00164	2.2690
DPP4	dipeptidylpeptidase 4	0.00266	2.4102
ENPP5	ectonucleotide pyrophosphatase/ phosphodiesterase 5	0.03128	3.0575
HPX	hemopexin	0.03025	2.3668
IL17D	interleukin 17D	0.00164	2.3558
IL1A	interleukin 1 alpha	0.04260	3.1132
LRRC17	leucine rich repeat containing 17	0.01147	2.6269
LYZ	lysozyme	0.03481	2.5119
MSMB	beta-microseminoprotein	0.03234	2.1747
NPPB	natriuretic peptide type B	0.00038	3.9836
OLR1	oxidized low density lipoprotein (lectin-like) receptor 1	0.00918	3.3160
PAPPA2	pappalysin 2	0.04318	2.2153
PDGFB	**platelet derived growth factor, B polypeptide**	0.01085	2.7339
PDGFRL	platelet-derived growth factor receptor-like	0.04730	3.1235
PLAT	plasminogen activator, tissue	0.00253	2.2369
RSPO2	R-spondin 2	0.01459	2.3071
SEMG1	semenogelin 1	0.00777	3.0290
SERPINB2	serine (or cysteine) peptidase inhibitor, clade B, member 2	0.00028	3.7445
SPP1	**CXXC finger 1 (PHD domain)**	0.01160	5.0380
SPX	spexin hormone	0.03056	3.4733
TFPI	tissue factor pathway inhibitor	0.00222	2.0072
TGFA	**transforming growth factor alpha**	**0.03717**	2.6374
TGFB2	**transforming growth factor, beta 2**	**0.01007**	2.0666
THPO	thrombopoietin	0.00976	2.1998
VWA5B1	von Willebrand factor A domain containing 5B1	0.00672	4.1775
ZG16B	zymogen granule protein 16B	0.00238	2.4187

Reanalysis of Corre et al. 2007 Leukemia. Bold indicates discussed in text.

To specifically test whether MM cells can inhibit adipogenesis and promote expression of SASPs in hMSCs, we directly co-cultured NBM-MSCs with tumor cells prior to and during differentiation (**Figure 9A**). NBM-MSCs were exposed directly to MM.1S, RPMI-8226, and OPM-2 cells for 48-h prior to the initiation of differentiation. At day 0 of differentiation, the co-culture media was removed, and cells were washed gently prior to the addition of fresh adipogenic differentiation media which was changed 1–2 times weekly until day 18 at which time conditioned media was collected from the co-cultures and cells were fixed and stained for analysis (**Figure 9B**). We found that direct co-culture with MM.1S resulted in no net change in lipid content, while RPMI-8226 tumor cells a slight, non-significant decrease on lipid accumulation or content as evidenced by fluorescent microscopy and quantified by Oil Red-O elution (**Figure 9C**). However, co-culture with OPM-2 resulted in severe decreased adipogenesis as evidenced by the lack of full-fledged lipid laden adipocytes (**Figure 9B**, bottom left) and significantly reduced Oil Red-O content (**Figure 9C**). In conditioned media from MM.1S+BMAT co-cultures, we were unable to detect any differences in 36 different cytokines (**Figure 9C**). However, we observed increased inflammatory cytokines in the conditioned media of RPMI-8226 and OPM-2 co-cultures (**Figure 9C**), with significant differences in CXCL1 (OPM-2 only), ICAM-1, and IL-8 and trends for increased IL-6 and PAI-1 (*SERPINE1*).

Interestingly, we detected different responses of the myeloma cells to BMAT differentiation media (**Supplementary Figure 8A**), with severe reduction in MM.1S cell number (**Supplementary Figure 8B**), proliferation (**Supplementary Figure 8C**), coupled with high levels (~80%) of apoptosis (**Supplementary Figure 8D**). Conversely, OPM-2 cells were largely unaffected by the BMAT differentiation media, with a slight but significant reduction in cell number (**Supplementary Figure 8E**), coupled with minimal reductions in proliferation (**Supplementary Figure 8F**) and apoptosis (**Supplementary Figure 8G**). Treatment of RPMI-8226 cells with BMAT differentiation media resulted in an approximate 50% reduction in cell number (**Supplementary Figure 8H**), no effect on proliferation (**Supplementary Figure 8I**), with a moderate increase in apoptosis (**Supplementary Figure 8J**). The experimental design of this direct co-culture experiment therefor investigated the pre-exposure of MSCs (MM.1S), as well as co-culture with low (RPMI-8226), and high (OPM-2) levels of tumor cells throughout the differentiation process. This data could, in part, explain the differing levels of adipocyte differentiation and/or lipid accumulation, and its correlation with the production of SASPs, if these processes are tied to tumor cell presence, but cannot be teased apart from cell-line specific signals that might be involved in altering adipogenesis. Combined these results suggest that MM cells are likely inducing senescence in cells within the marrow niche including both adipocytes and their precursors (MSCs), which has implications for tumor cell proliferation and survival.

DISCUSSION

In this study, we demonstrate that exposure to myeloma cells modulates adipocyte progenitors by altering adipogenic differentiation capacity, skewing metabolism-related transcripts, and increasing the expression of inflammatory cytokines. Our data build on what is known in the field of myeloma, to demonstrate that preadipocytes that are exposed to soluble MM-derived factors are phenotypically altered. Overall,

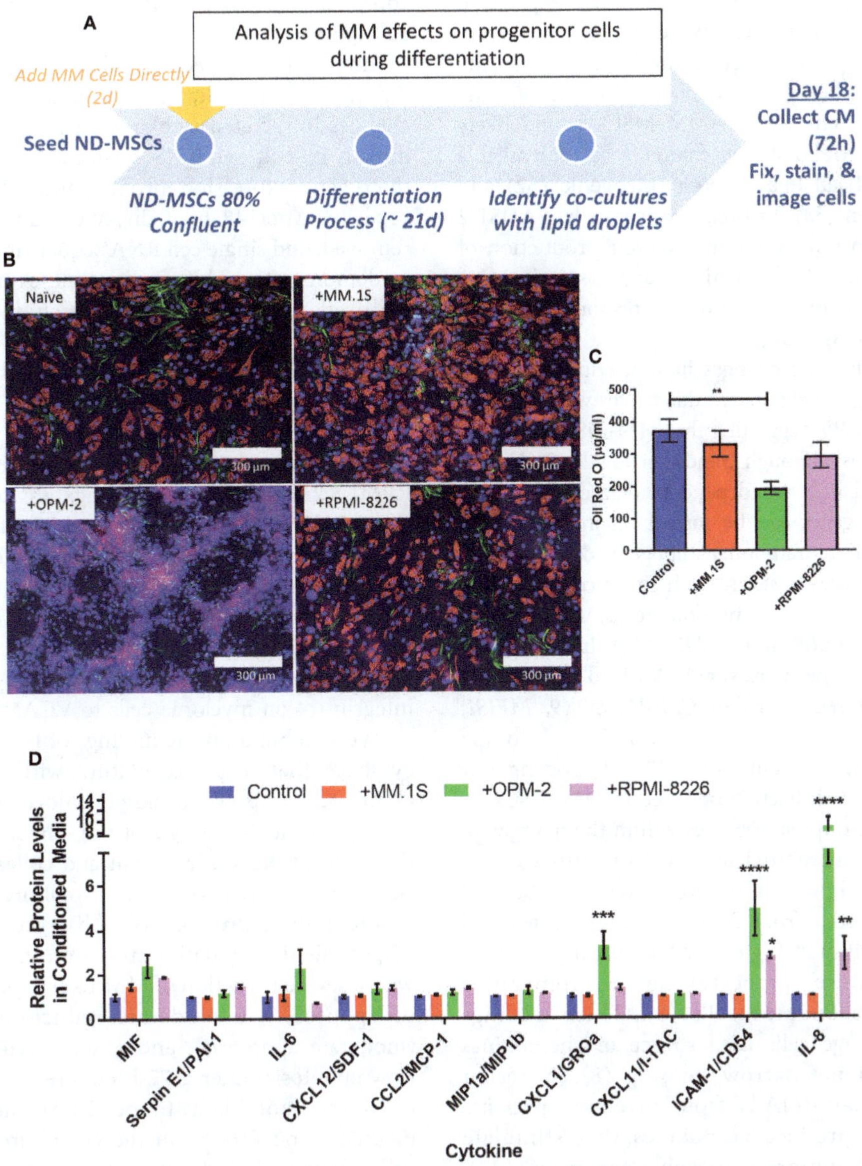

FIGURE 9 | Direct co-culture of human mesenchymal stem cells (hMSCs) with myeloma cells reveals cell-line specific effects on lipid accumulation and cytokine production. Experimental design of co-culture experiment **(A)** where multiple myeloma (MM) cells (MM.1S, RPMI-8226, OPM-2) were added 2 days prior to the start of differentiation. Myeloma cells were allowed to persist during differentiation with adipogenic media. Fresh adipogenic media was incubator for 72 h prior to the collection of conditioned media. Conditioned media was collected and cells were fixed and stained on day 18 of differentiation, a few days prior to terminal differentiation. Adipocytes were fixed, stained (phalloidin=green, Oil Red-O=red, DAPI=blue), and imaged with a 10X objective after differentiation and co-culture with or without myeloma cells **(B)**; images are from one hMSC donor, but are representative of n=3 donors. Lipid content was assessed by Oil Red-O staining, elution, and quantification **(C)**. Cytokines were assessed in conditioned media by human cytokine array (R&D) **(D)**; n=3 donors for each condition (control=naïve, +MM.1S, +OPM-2, +RPMI-8226). Significance was assessed *via* two-way ANOVA. $^{*}p < 0.05$, $^{**}p < 0.01$, $^{***}p < 0.001$, $^{****}p < 0.0001$.

these data support the interpretation that MM cells modulate adipocytes and their precursors by inducing senescence, and stimulating production of MM-supportive cytokines and other factors that likely contribute to "the vicious cycle" (2) of bone destruction and release of growth factors fueling myeloma cells in the bone marrow.

Corre and colleagues determined that MM-MSCs exhibit extremely different expression profiles from NBM-MSCs (28). Among the upregulated genes highlighted in these findings were factors that promote lipolysis, *ANGPTL4* (50), growth differentiation factor 15 (*GDF15*) (51), and known SASPs *IL1B* and *SERPINE1*. This study also detected downregulation of chemokine C-X-C motif ligand 12 (*CXCL12, SDF1*) and insulin-like growth factor 1 (*IGF1*), and aberrant expression of genes encoding molecules involved in WNT signaling Dickkopf homolog 1 (*DKK1*) and WNT1 inducible signaling protein 1

(*WISP1*) (28). By relaxing the stringency of our reanalysis, we were able to detect additional differences in gene expression ($p<0.05$; FC>|2|), confirm diminished expression of osteogenic-related transcripts and growth factors, and further identify *FADS1* and *FADS2* as being elevated in MM-MSCs. The downregulation of these enzymes in MM-MSCs would likely manifest in an altered portfolio of long-chain fatty acids available to the cell, which has been tied to both osteogenic (52) and adipogenic differentiation (53). In breast cancer cells, FADS1/2 have also been linked to inflammation *via* their production of arachidonic acid (54), suggesting that their suppression in MM-MSCs may be linked to an anti-inflammatory response linked to increased cytokine signaling (55).

While we did observe some changes in transcript expression related to PPAR signaling, no significant differences were detected in *PPARG* or *CEBPA/CEBPB*, suggesting that MM-MSCs were not committed to adipogenesis, although trends for low-level elevated expression were observed in two independent datasets. Our data suggest that while these genes can be turned on in MM-MSCs during *in vitro* differentiation, traditional adipogenic differentiation is inhibited. Our findings are consistent with single cell qRT-PCR analysis of normal MSCs exposed to myeloma cells, which exhibit trends for suppression of *LEPR* and *PPARG* (26). In addition, a second dataset comparing gene expression in MM- to NBM-MSCs demonstrated significant reductions in *CEBPA*, *SOX9*, *MEIS1*, *ZFP36*, and *SAV1*—all of which have been linked to the promotion of adipogenic differentiation (40), supporting our hypothesis that adipogenesis is likely suppressed in MM-MSCs.

An increased number of preadipocytes within the marrow of myeloma patients has been reported, as well as supportive effects of preadipocytes and adipocytes on MM cells (8). Studies utilizing conditioned media from 3T3-L1 preadipocytes and mature adipocytes specifically highlighted a recruitment/pro-migration role for mature adipocytes, and a proliferative effect of preadipocytes on MM cells (8). These findings implicate adipocyte-lineage cells as a source of chemokines that drive myeloma bone marrow homing (8). A recent study demonstrated that BMAds from myeloma patients are reprogrammed to produce adipokines that stimulate osteoclastogenesis and suppress osteoblastogenesis (27). Our studies build on these findings by highlighting both similar and new chemokines produced by uncommitted MSCs, differentiating MSCs, and committed adipocytes, and recapitulate their production after MM exposure. Within our reanalysis of the data from Corre et al., we uncovered significantly decreased expression of *FOXA1*, a transcription factor whose suppression in cancer stem cells has been tied to increased *IL6* expression (56). We hypothesize that a similar mechanism is controlling expression of *IL6* in MM-MSCs, and potentially other SASP proteins. We specifically highlight SASP-related transcripts encoding inflammatory cytokines in each of our adipocyte-lineage experiments and demonstrate that the induction of these transcripts is sustained after differentiation. In addition, we found that direct co-culture of hMSCs with two myeloma cell lines prior to and during adipogenic differentiation resulted in increased secretion of CXCL1/GRO, IL-8, and ICAM-1 in co-culture conditioned medium samples. We also observed complete inhibition of adipogenic differentiation with OPM-2 co-culture.

Interestingly, direct co-culture with MM.1S myeloma cells, did not inhibit adipogenesis and resulted in no significant changes in secreted cytokines. A recent study by Liu et al. (57) directly co-cultured hMSCs with MM.1S cells and characterized their gene expression profiles and adipogenic differentiation capacity. After 48 h of direct co-culture, myeloma cells were removed, and single cell RNA sequencing (scRNA-seq) was used to demonstrate a shift in the gene expression profile of MSCs cultured with MM.1S cells, including enrichment of the adipokine signaling pathway. They also demonstrated impaired mineralization with osteogenic differentiation (as assessed with alizarin red staining) and elevated Oil Red O staining in MSCs previously cultured with MM.1S cells compared to naïve MSCs (57). Similar findings were also observed with ARP-1, U266, and RPMI-8,226 cells. These findings are consistent with the data presented in our current study, which utilizes a slightly different experimental design, and demonstrates no negative effect in Oil Red O staining in adipocytes directly co-cultured with either MM.1S cells or RPMI-8226 cells. Liu et al. demonstrate that MM.1S and ARP-1 cells stimulate PPARG in MSCs *via* a protein kinase C-mediated mechanism that is triggered by the binding of integrin-α4 on myeloma cells to VCAM1 on MSCs (57).

We also build on the findings of Liu et al. (57), by providing evidence that direct co-culture with OPM-2 myeloma cells eliminates or prevents adipogenic differentiation of hMSCs. The experimental design of our direct co-culture experiments differs from the study by Liu and colleagues (57), as myeloma cells were allowed to persist in culture during the adipogenic differentiation process. We observed adverse effects of the adipogenic differentiation media on the tumor cells themselves, with a severe reduction of MM.1S cells (coupled with a high level of apoptosis), a moderate reduction of RPMI-8226 cells (moderate apoptosis), and a slight reduction of OPM-2 cells (low apoptosis) after a 72-h culture. This suggests that MM.1S cells were not likely to persist throughout the adipogenic differentiation process in the co-culture system, while OPM-2 cells remained and interacted with MSCs throughout the duration of the experiment. Indeed, we observed complete inhibition of the presence of lipid laden adipocytes in OPM-2 hMSC co-cultures, and significantly elevated levels of the SASPs, GROα (*CXCL1*), IL8, and CD54 (*ICAM-1*), in the culture media. Elevated levels of IL-6 and SDF-1 (*CXCL12*) protein were also detected, although these were not significant by two-way ANOVA. Interestingly, hMSCs differentiating with RPMI-8226 in direct co-culture were able to differentiate into lipid-laden adipocytes and expressed significantly more CD54 (ICAM-1) and IL-8, and slightly more PAI-1 (SERPINE1), SDF-1, MCP-1 (CCL2), and GROα. Further investigation is required to determine whether the differences observed in direct co-culture with these three cell lines is cell-line specific, or dependent on the absence/presence of MM cells during differentiation.

Our findings are consistent with previous reports of myeloma "primed" MSCs differentiated into adipocytes such as the

Mehdi et al. study that demonstrated MSC-MM co-culture for 3 days suppressed adipogenic differentiation and reduced the overall size and lipid content of those adipocytes (26). In patient samples, the authors suggest that production of small, immature IGFBP2+ adipocytes is negatively correlated with disease progression- suggesting that myeloma inhibits the formation of these cells, or that these cells are somehow utilized during MM progression (26). In 3T3-L1 adipocytes, we observed a slight, non-significant increase in *Igfbp2* expression after a two-day exposure to MM cells by indirect co-culture. The authors did report an increase in genes associated with senescence in MM patient MSCs, consistent with our findings, and adding strength to a potential role of SASPs in myeloma disease progression (31). Indeed, two key risk factors for myeloma—aging (58) and obesity (12)—have been shown to increase senescence in the bone marrow, suggesting that targeting senescent cells *via* senolytic therapies (59) may be beneficial in myeloma treatment.

We see a number of ways in which our work could translate to the clinic. First, as mentioned above, targeting senescent cells using senolytic treatment may remove senescent, myeloma-associated bone marrow adipocytes (31), or pre-adipocytes, as shown here, from the microenvironment. New ways to remove senescent cells are being developed in the field of aging, such as quercetin or dasatinib + quercetin, and the role of local senescent cells in tumor growth is becoming increasingly evident in a variety of cancers (60). The field of senotherapeutics is burgeoning and senolytics as well as senomorphics, which act to interfere with a specific senescence pathway in order to restore the appropriate cellular function, may prove useful in cancer treatment. Interestingly, dormant myeloma cells themselves (61), or MGUS (monoclonal gammopathy of undetermined) cells may also be removed through targeting senescent cells, as Weivoda et al. have recently suggested at the ASBMR, 2020 annual meeting. Others have also seen that other types of tumor cells can express senescent genes and are sensitive to senolysis (60). Overall, targeting senescence clinically may be a new means by which to target the tumor cells and the host microenvironment simultaneously.

Moreover, targeting SASPs and other factors from myeloma-associated adipocytes is another potential way to translate our findings to the bedside. For example, targeting IL6 (e.g., Johnson and Johnson's drug sirukumab), or the IL6 receptor (e.g., Regeneron's sarilumab) could be tailored perhaps by using BMAT biomarkers (62), knowing now that BMAds, especially myeloma-associated adipocyte lineage cells, are a source of IL6. Better alignment with patient populations for enhanced precision medicine could also be considered based on our data, for therapies targeting the CXCL12/CXCR4 axis, such as the CXCR4 inhibitor AMD3100 (plerixafor) (63), or the CXCL12 antagonist NOX-A12 (64). Our data may also help explain the ability of treatment with plerixafor to overcome bortezomib resistance and mobilize stem cells and immune cells, which was recently reported in a phase I/II trial (65), by providing new insight into the players in the bone marrow niche involved in this pathway. Interestingly, new data *in vitro* has shown that SDF-1α stimulation of CXCR4 on MM cells may up-regulate the expression of IL-6 through the activation of the PI3K/AKT, suggesting that the IL6 and CXCR4/CXCL12 pathways overlap in MM cells (64). Overall, our study provides insight into the mechanism of action of drugs targeting the CXCL12/CXCR4 axis, the IL6/IL6R axis, or other SASP protein signaling pathways in MM, and suggests that targeting proteins identified herein may lead to new therapeutic avenues.

In conclusion, our studies demonstrate that adipocyte-lineage cells are dramatically altered by MM cells. MSCs exposed to myeloma-derived soluble factors exhibited reduced differentiation capacity, and elevated expression of senescence-related transcripts including MM-supportive *Il6/IL6*. Mouse preadipocytes exposed to MM.1S myeloma cells can differentiate, but accumulate less lipid and exhibit aberrant gene expression, including upregulation of key SASP genes; however this was not observed with exposure to 5TGM1 murine myeloma soluble factors. Direct co-culture of hMSCs with human myeloma cell lines revealed extreme differences in the effects of myeloma cells on adipogenic differentiation, with an increase in adipogenesis observed in response to MM.1S co-culture, and an inhibitory response observed in response to OPM-2 co-culture, which stimulated SASP production. The induction of SASP gene expression by MM cells in adipocyte lineage cells underlines the importance of future studies to examine whether SASPs promote MM tumor initiation, disease stage transition, or resistance to traditional chemotherapies. Moreover, the myeloma-derived factors that induce senescence and modulate adipogenesis and in pre-adipocytes should be explored in future experiments. Our studies indicate that myeloma cells induce senescence in adipocyte-lineage cells and add to the building knowledgebase that SASP proteins are involved in MM pathogenesis.

ETHICS STATEMENT

The animal study was reviewed and approved by The Maine Medical Center Research Institute (Scarborough, ME, USA) Institutional Animal Care and Use Committee (IACUC).

AUTHOR CONTRIBUTIONS

HF, CF, and MR conceptualized and designed the study. HF, CF, and MR developed the methodology. HF, CF, and SC acquired the data. HF, CF, SC, HD, and MR analyzed and interpreted the data. HF and MR wrote, reviewed, and/or revised the manuscript. All authors contributed to the review and revision of the manuscript. HF, HD, AD, and MR provided administrative support. HF, SC, and CF provided technical support. HF and MR supervised the study. All authors contributed to the article and approved the submitted version.

ACKNOWLEDGMENTS

We would like to thank Dr. Clifford Rosen for feedback on this research and Dr. Patricia Maiso for help in collating the Corre et al. dataset.

REFERENCES

1. Yaccoby S. Osteoblastogenesis and tumor growth in myeloma. *Leuk Lymphoma* (2010) 51:213–20. doi: 10.3109/10428190903503438
2. Guise TA, Mohammad KS, Clines G, Stebbins EG, Wong DH, Higgins LS, et al. Basic mechanisms responsible for osteolytic and osteoblastic bone metastases. *Clin Cancer Res* (2006) 12:6213s–6s. doi: 10.1158/1078-0432.CCR-06-1007
3. Roodman GD. Osteoblast function in myeloma. *Bone* (2011) 48:135–40. doi: 10.1016/j.bone.2010.06.016
4. Fu J, Li S, Feng R, Ma H, Sabeh F, Roodman GD, et al. Multiple myeloma-derived MMP-13 mediates osteoclast fusogenesis and osteolytic disease. *J Clin Invest* (2016) 126:1759–72. doi: 10.1172/JCI80276
5. Colombo M, Thümmler K, Mirandola L, Garavelli S, Todoerti K, Apicella L, et al. Notch signaling drives multiple myeloma induced osteoclastogenesis. *Oncotarget* (2014) 5:10393–406. doi: 10.18632/oncotarget.2084
6. Fairfield H, Falank C, Harris E, Demambro V, McDonald M, Pettitt JAJ, et al. The skeletal cell-derived molecule sclerostin drives bone marrow adipogenesis. *J Cell Physiol* (2017) 233:1156–67. doi: 10.1002/jcp.25976
7. Reagan MR, Mishima Y, Glavey SV, Zhang YY, Manier S, Lu ZN, et al. Investigating osteogenic differentiation in multiple myeloma using a novel 3D bone marrow niche model. *Blood* (2014) 124:3250–9. doi: 10.1182/blood-2014-02-558007
8. Trotter TN, Gibson JT, Sherpa TL, Gowda PS, Peker D, Yang Y. Adipocyte-Lineage Cells Support Growth and Dissemination of Multiple Myeloma in Bone. *Am J Pathol* (2016) 186:3054–63. doi: 10.1016/j.ajpath.2016.07.012
9. Liu Z, Xu J, He J, Liu H, Lin P, Wan X, et al. Mature adipocytes in bone marrow protect myeloma cells against chemotherapy through autophagy activation. *Oncotarget* (2015) 6:34329–41. doi: 10.18632/oncotarget.6020
10. Baron R, Rawadi G. Minireview: Targeting the Wnt/β-catenin pathway to regulate bone formation in the adult skeleton. *Endocrinology* (2007) 148:2635–43. doi: 10.1210/en.2007-0270
11. Tencerova M, Rendina-Ruedy E, Neess D, Færgeman N, Figeac F, Ali D, et al. Metabolic programming determines the lineage-differentiation fate of murine bone marrow stromal progenitor cells. *Bone Res* (2019) 7:1–14. doi: 10.1038/s41413-019-0076-5
12. Tencerova M, Frost M, Figeac F, Nielsen TK, Ali D, Lauterlein JL, et al. Obesity-Associated Hypermetabolism and Accelerated Senescence of Bone Marrow Stromal Stem Cells Suggest a Potential Mechanism for Bone Fragility. *Cell Rep* (2019) 27:2050–62.e6. doi: 10.1016/J.CELREP.2019.04.066
13. Marinac CR, Suppan CA, Giovannucci E, Song M, Kværner AS, Townsend MK, et al. Elucidating Under-Studied Aspects of the Link Between Obesity and Multiple Myeloma: Weight Pattern, Body Shape Trajectory, and Body Fat Distribution. *JNCI Cancer Spectr* (2019) 3:pkz044. doi: 10.1093/jncics/pkz044
14. Birmann BM, Andreotti G, De Roos AJ, Camp NJ, Chiu BCH, Spinelli JJ, et al. Young adult and usual adult body mass index and multiple myeloma risk: A pooled analysis in the international multiple myeloma consortium (IMMC). *Cancer Epidemiol Biomarkers Prev* (2017) 26:876–85. doi: 10.1158/1055-9965.EPI-16-0762-T
15. Bullwinkle EM, Parker MD, Bonan NF, Falkenberg LG, Davison SP, DeCicco-Skinner KL. Adipocytes contribute to the growth and progression of multiple myeloma: Unraveling obesity related differences in adipocyte signaling. *Cancer Lett* (2016) 380:114–21. doi: 10.1016/j.canlet.2016.06.010
16. Lwin ST, Olechnowicz SWZ, Fowler JA, Edwards CM. Diet-induced obesity promotes a myeloma-like condition in vivo. *Leukemia* (2015) 29:507–10. doi: 10.1038/leu.2014.295
17. Bredella MA, Torriani M, Ghomi RH, Thomas BJ, Brick DJ, Gerweck AV, et al. Vertebral bone marrow fat is positively associated with visceral fat and inversely associated with IGF-1 in obese women. *Obesity* (2011) 19:49–53. doi: 10.1038/oby.2010.106
18. Caers J, Deleu S, Belaid Z, De Raeve H, Van Valckenborgh E, De Bruyne E, et al. Neighboring adipocytes participate in the bone marrow microenvironment of multiple myeloma cells. *Leukemia* (2007) 21:1580–4. doi: 10.1038/sj.leu.2404658
19. Fowler JA, Lwin ST, Drake MT, Edwards JR, Kyle RA, Mundy GR, et al. Host-derived adiponectin is tumor-suppressive and a novel therapeutic target for multiple myeloma and the associated bone disease. *Blood* (2011) 118:5872–82. doi: 10.1182/blood-2011-01-330407
20. Fan Y, Hanai J, Le PT, Bi R, Maridas D, DeMambro V, et al. Parathyroid Hormone Directs Bone Marrow Mesenchymal Cell Fate. *Cell Metab* (2017) 25:661–72. doi: 10.1016/j.cmet.2017.01.001
21. Boyd AL, Reid JC, Salci KR, Aslostovar L, Benoit YD, Shapovalova Z, et al. Acute myeloid leukaemia disrupts endogenous myelo-erythropoiesis by compromising the adipocyte bone marrow niche. *Nat Cell Biol* (2017) 19:1336–47. doi: 10.1038/ncb3625
22. Fairfield H, Falank C, Farrell M, Vary C, Boucher JM, Driscoll H, et al. Development of a 3D bone marrow adipose tissue model. *Bone* (2018) 118:77–88. doi: 10.1016/j.bone.2018.01.023
23. Falank C, Fairfield H, Farrell M, Reagan MR. New Bone Cell Type Identified As Driver of Drug Resistance in Multiple Myeloma: The Bone Marrow Adipocyte. *Blood* (2017) 130:122. doi: 10.1182/blood.V130.Suppl_1.122.122
24. Fairfield H, Harris EJ, Falank C, Reagan MR. Myeloma-Associated Adipocytes Exhibit Reduced Adipogenic Gene Expression and Delipidation. *Blood* (2017) 130:1768. doi: 10.1182/blood.V130.Suppl_1.1768.1768
25. Morris EV, Suchacki KJ, Hocking J, Cartwright R, Sowman A, Gamez B, et al. Myeloma Cells Down-Regulate Adiponectin in Bone Marrow Adipocytes Via TNF-Alpha. *J Bone Miner Res* (2019) 53(5). doi: 10.1002/jbmr.3951
26. Mehdi SJ, Johnson SK, Epstein J, Zangari M, Qu P, Hoering A, et al. Mesenchymal stem cells gene signature in high-risk myeloma bone marrow linked to suppression of distinct IGFBP2-expressing small adipocytes. *Br J Haematol* (2018) 184(4):578–93. doi: 10.1111/bjh.15669
27. Liu H, He J, Koh SP, Zhong Y, Liu Z, Wang Z, et al. Reprogrammed marrow adipocytes contribute to myeloma-induced bone disease. *Sci Transl Med* (2019) 11:eaau9087. doi: 10.1126/scitranslmed.aau9087
28. Corre J, Mahtouk K, Attal M, Gadelorge M, Huynh A, Fleury-Cappellesso S, et al. Bone marrow mesenchymal stem cells are abnormal in multiple myeloma. *Leukemia* (2007) 21:1079–88. doi: 10.1038/sj.leu.2404621
29. Garcia-Gomez A. Multiple myeloma mesenchymal stromal cells: Contribution to myeloma bone disease and therapeutics. *World J Stem Cells* (2014) 6:322. doi: 10.4252/wjsc.v6.i3.322
30. André T, Meuleman N, Stamatopoulos B, De Bruyn C, Pieters K, Bron D, et al. Evidences of Early Senescence in Multiple Myeloma Bone Marrow Mesenchymal Stromal Cells. *PLoS One* (2013) 8:e59756. doi: 10.1371/journal.pone.0059756
31. Fairfield H, Dudakovic A, Khatib CM, Farrell M, Costa S, Falank C, et al. Myeloma-modified adipocytes exhibit metabolic dysfunction and a senescence-associated secretory phenotype (SASP). *Cancer Res* (2020) 82:634–47. doi: 10.1158/0008-5472.CAN-20-1088

32. Subramanian A, Tamayo P, Mootha VK, Mukherjee S, Ebert BL, Gillette MA, et al. Gene set enrichment analysis: a knowledge-based approach for interpreting genome-wide expression profiles. *Proc Natl Acad Sci U S A* (2005) 102:15545–50. doi: 10.1073/pnas.0506580102
33. Liberzon A, Birger C, Thorvaldsdóttir H, Ghandi M, Mesirov JP, Tamayo P. The Molecular Signatures Database Hallmark Gene Set Collection. *Cell Syst* (2015) 1:417–25. doi: 10.1016/j.cels.2015.12.004
34. Szklarczyk D, Gable AL, Lyon D, Junge A, Wyder S, Huerta-Cepas J, et al. STRING v11: protein–protein association networks with increased coverage, supporting functional discovery in genome-wide experimental datasets. *Nucleic Acids Res* (2019) 47:D607–13. doi: 10.1093/nar/gky1131
35. Song B, Park SH, Zhao JC, Fong KW, Li S, Lee Y, et al. Targeting FOXA1-mediated repression of TGF-β signaling suppresses castration-resistant prostate cancer progression. *J Clin Invest* (2019) 129:569–82. doi: 10.1172/JCI122367
36. Gormally MV, Dexheimer TS, Marsico G, Sanders DA, Lowe C, Matak-Vinkoviä D, et al. Suppression of the FOXM1 transcriptional programme via novel small molecule inhibition. *Nat Commun* (2014) 5:1–11. doi: 10.1038/ncomms6165
37. Feng J, Jing J, Li J, Zhao H, Punj V, Zhang T, et al. BMP signaling orchestrates a transcriptional network to control the fate of mesenchymal stem cells in mice. *Dev* (2017) 144:2560–9. doi: 10.1242/dev.150136
38. Zhou BO, Yue R, Murphy MM, Peyer JG, Morrison SJ. Leptin-receptor-expressing mesenchymal stromal cells represent the main source of bone formed by adult bone marrow. *Cell Stem Cell* (2014) 15:154–68. doi: 10.1016/j.stem.2014.06.008
39. Wei N, Liu SS, Chan KKL, Ngan HYS. Tumour suppressive function and modulation of programmed cell death 4 (PDCD4) in ovarian cancer. *PLoS One* (2012) 7:e30311. doi: 10.1371/journal.pone.0030311
40. Todoerti K, Lisignoli G, Storti P, Agnelli L, Novara F, Manferdini C, et al. Distinct transcriptional profiles characterize bone microenvironment mesenchymal cells rather than osteoblasts in relationship with multiple myeloma bone disease. *Exp Hematol* (2010) 38:141–53. doi: 10.1016/j.exphem.2009.11.009
41. Gulyaeva O, Nguyen H, Sambeat A, Heydari K, Sul HS. Sox9-Meis1 Inactivation Is Required for Adipogenesis, Advancing Pref-1+ to PDGFRα+ Cells. *Cell Rep* (2018) 25:1002–17.e4. doi: 10.1016/j.celrep.2018.09.086
42. Alfares MN, Perks CM, Hamilton-Shield JP, Holly JMP. Insulin-like growth factor-II in adipocyte regulation: depot-specific actions suggest a potential role limiting excess visceral adiposity. *Am J Physiol Endocrinol Metab* (2018) 315 (6):E1098–107. doi: 10.1152/ajpendo004092017
43. Lavi N, Kessler O, Ziv K, Nir-Zvi I, Mumblat Y, Eiza N, et al. Semaphorin-3A inhibits multiple myeloma progression in a mouse model. *Carcinogenesis* (2018) 39:1283–91. doi: 10.1093/carcin/bgy106
44. Gan Q, Huang J, Zhou R, Niu J, Zhu X, Wang J, et al. PPARγ accelerates cellular senescence by inducing p16INK4α expression in human diploid fibroblasts. *J Cell Sci* (2008) 121:2235–45. doi: 10.1242/jcs.026633
45. Singhal H, Bautista DS, Tonkin KS, O'Malley FP, Tuck AB, Chambers AF, et al. Elevated Plasma Osteopontin in Metastatic Breast Cancer Associated With Increased Tumor Burden and Decreased Survival. *Clin Cancer Res* (1997) 3:605–11.
46. Agrawal U, Kumari N, Mishra AK, Vasudeva P, Kumar A, Mohanty NK, et al. Immune Signature of Urothelial Cancer Associated With Grade, Recurrence, and Invasion. *Urol Oncol* (2016) 34:418.e17–26. doi: 10.1016/J.UROLONC.2016.04.013
47. Sturtz LA, Deyarmin B, van Laar R, Yarina W, Shriver CD, Ellsworth RE. Gene expression differences in adipose tissue associated with breast tumorigenesis. *Adipocyte* (2014) 3(2):107–14. doi: 10.4161/adip.28250
48. Rayess H, Wang MB, Srivatsan ES. Cellular senescence and tumor suppressor gene p16. *Int J Cancer* (2012) 130:1715–25. doi: 10.1002/ijc.27316
49. Gao XL, Zheng M, Wang HF, Dai LL, Yu XH, Yang X, et al. NR2F1 contributes to cancer cell dormancy, invasion and metastasis of salivary adenoid cystic carcinoma by activating CXCL12/CXCR4 pathway. *BMC Cancer* (2019) 19:743. doi: 10.1186/s12885-019-5925-5
50. Robciuc MR, Skrobuk P, Anisimov A, Olkkonen VM, Alitalo K, Eckel RH, et al. Angiopoietin-Like 4 Mediates PPAR Delta Effect on Lipoprotein Lipase-Dependent Fatty Acid Uptake but Not on Beta-Oxidation in Myotubes. *PLoS One* (2012) 7:e46212. doi: 10.1371/journal.pone.0046212
51. Luan HH, Wang A, Hilliard BK, Carvalho F, Rosen CE, Ahasic AM, et al. GDF15 Is an Inflammation-Induced Central Mediator of Tissue Tolerance. *Cell* (2019) 178:1231–44.e11. doi: 10.1016/j.cell.2019.07.033
52. Levental KR, Surma MA, Skinkle AD, Lorent JH, Zhou Y, Klose C, et al. ω-3 Polyunsaturated Fatty Acids Direct Differentiation of the Membrane Phenotype in Mesenchymal Stem Cells to Potentiate Osteogenesis. *Sci Adv* (2017) 3:eaao1193. doi: 10.1126/SCIADV.AAO1193
53. Yanting C, Yang QY, Ma GL, Du M, Harrison JH, Block E. Dose- And Type-Dependent Effects of Long-Chain Fatty Acids on Adipogenesis and Lipogenesis of Bovine Adipocytes. *J Dairy Sci* (2018) 101:1601–15. doi: 10.3168/JDS.2017-13312
54. Ariazi EA, Cunliffe HE, Lewis-Wambi JS, Slifker MJ, Willis AL, Ramos P, et al. Estrogen induces apoptosis in estrogen deprivation-resistant breast cancer through stress responses as identified by global gene expression across time. *Proc Natl Acad Sci U S A* (2011) 108:18879–86. doi: 10.1073/pnas.1115188108
55. Fan P, Siwak DR, Abderrahman B, Agboke FA, Yerrum S, Jordan VC. Suppression of nuclear factor-kB by glucocorticoid receptor blocks estrogen-induced apoptosis in estrogen-deprived breast cancer cells. *Mol Cancer Ther* (2019) 18:1684–95. doi: 10.1158/1535-7163.MCT-18-1363
56. Yamaguchi N, Nakayama Y, Yamaguchi N. Down-regulation of Forkhead box protein A1 (FOXA1) leads to cancer stem cell-like properties in tamoxifen-resistant breast cancer cells through induction of interleukin-6. *J Biol Chem* (2017) 292:8136–48. doi: 10.1074/jbc.M116.763276
57. Liu Z, Liu H, He J, Lin P, Tong Q, Yang J. Myeloma cells shift osteoblastogenesis to adipogenesis by inhibiting the ubiquitin ligase MURF1 in mesenchymal stem cells. *Sci Signal* (2020) 13:eaay8203. doi: 10.1126/scisignal.aay8203
58. Farr JN, Xu M, Weivoda MM, Monroe DG, Fraser DG, Onken JL, et al. Targeting cellular senescence prevents age-related bone loss in mice. *Nat Med* (2017) 23:1072–9. doi: 10.1038/nm.4385
59. Hickson LJ, Langhi Prata LGP, Bobart SA, Evans TK, Giorgadze N, Hashmi SK, et al. Senolytics decrease senescent cells in humans: Preliminary report from a clinical trial of Dasatinib plus Quercetin in individuals with diabetic kidney disease. *EBioMedicine* (2019) 47:446–56. doi: 10.1016/j.ebiom.2019.08.069
60. Azazmeh N, Ben-Porath I. Stimulation of epidermal hyperplasia and tumorigenesis by resident p16INK4a-expressing cells. *Mol Cell Oncol* (2020) 7:1819752. doi: 10.1080/23723556.2020.1819752
61. Lawson MA, McDonald MM, Kovacic NN, Khoo WH, Terry RTL, Down J, et al. Osteoclasts Control Re-activation of Dormant Myeloma Cells by Remodeling the Endosteal Niche. *Nat Commun* (2015) 6:8983. doi: 10.1038/ncomms9983
62. Harmer D, Falank C, Reagan MR. Interleukin-6 interweaves the bone marrow microenvironment, bone loss, and multiple myeloma. *Front Endocrinol (Lausanne)* (2019) 9:788. doi: 10.3389/fendo.2018.00788
63. Azab AK, Runnels JM, Pitsillides C, Moreau A-S, Azab F, Leleu X, et al. CXCR4 inhibitor AMD3100 disrupts the interaction of multiple myeloma cells with the bone marrow microenvironment and enhances their sensitivity to therapy. *Blood* (2009) 113:4341–51. doi: 10.1182/blood-2008-10-186668
64. Liu Y, Liang HM, Lv YQ, Tang SM, Cheng P. Blockade of SDF-1/CXCR4 reduces adhesion-mediated chemoresistance of multiple myeloma cells via interacting with interleukin-6. *J Cell Physiol* (2019) 234:19702–14. doi: 10.1002/jcp.28570
65. Ghobrial IM, Liu CJ, Zavidij O, Azab AK, Baz R, Laubach JP, et al. Phase I/II trial of the CXCR4 inhibitor plerixafor in combination with bortezomib as a chemosensitization strategy in relapsed/refractory multiple myeloma. *Am J Hematol* (2019) 94:1244–53. doi: 10.1002/ajh.25627

10

A Phase 1 Study of IRX195183, a RARα-Selective CYP26 Resistant Retinoid, in Patients with Relapsed or Refractory AML

Alexander J. Ambinder[1], Kelly Norsworthy[1], Daniela Hernandez[1], Laura Palau[1], Bogdan Paun[1], Amy Duffield[2], Rosh Chandraratna[3], Martin Sanders[3], Ravi Varadhan[4], Richard J. Jones[1], B. Douglas Smith[1†] and Gabriel Ghiaur[1†]*

[1] Department of Oncology, Sidney Kimmel Comprehensive Cancer Center, Johns Hopkins University School of Medicine, Baltimore, MD, United States, [2] Department of Pathology, Johns Hopkins University School of Medicine, Baltimore, MD, United States, [3] IO Therapeutics, Santa Ana, CA, United States, [4] Division of Biostatistics and Bioinformatics, Johns Hopkins/Sidney Kimmel Comprehensive Cancer Center, Baltimore, MD, United States

***Correspondence:**
Gabriel Ghiaur
gghiaur1@jhmi.edu

†These authors share senior authorship

Subsets of non-acute promyelocytic leukemia (APL) acute myelogenous leukemia (AML) exhibit aberrant retinoid signaling and demonstrate sensitivity to retinoids *in vitro*. We present the results of a phase 1 dose-escalation study that evaluated the safety, pharmacodynamics, and efficacy of IRX195183, a novel retinoic acid receptor α agonist, in patients with relapsed or refractory myelodysplastic syndrome (MDS) or AML. In this single center, single arm study, eleven patients with relapsed or refractory MDS/AML were enrolled and treated. Oral IRX195183 was administered at two dose levels: 50 mg daily or 75 mg daily for a total of two 28-day cycles. Patients with stable disease or better were allowed to continue on the drug for four additional 28-day cycles. Common adverse events included hypertriglyceridemia, fatigue, dyspnea, and edema. Three patients at the first dose level developed asymptomatic Grade 3 hypertriglyceridemia. The maximally tolerated dose was not reached. Four of the eleven patients had (36%) stable disease or better. One had a morphological complete remission with incomplete hematologic recovery while on the study drug. Two patients had evidence of *in vivo* leukemic blast maturation, as reflected by increased CD38 expression. In a pharmacodynamics study, plasma samples from four patients treated at the lowest dose level demonstrated the capacity to differentiate leukemic cells from the NB4 cell line *in vitro*. These results suggest that IRX195183 is safe, achieves biologically meaningful plasma concentrations and may be efficacious in a subset of patients with MDS/AML.
Clinical Trial Registration: clinicaltrials.gov, identifier NCT02749708.

Keywords: acute myeloid leukemia, retinoic acid receptor agonist, differentiation therapy, microenvironment niche, phase 1 clinical trial

INTRODUCTION

Acute myeloid leukemia (AML) is a clonal process that arises out of sequential genetic and epigenetic alterations that cause an arrest of differentiation and unfettered proliferation. The retinoid signaling pathway is essential to hematopoietic differentiation and its disruption can contribute to leukemogenesis (1). This is exemplified by the t(15;17) translocation in acute promyelocytic leukemia (APL) that juxtaposes the promyelocytic leukemia protein (*PML*) gene with the retinoic acid receptor α gene. The resulting PML-RARA fusion protein acts as a dominant negative, disrupting the activities of WT RARα and RARγ, leading to a block in differentiation at the level of the promyelocyte (2). All-trans-retinoic acid (ATRA) is a natural retinoid that restores normal retinoic acid signaling and promotes the differentiation of leukemic blasts. It now forms the cornerstone of APL treatment.

Aberrant retinoic acid signaling has been demonstrated in other subsets of AML (3–5). *In vitro*, ATRA is capable of inducing differentiation and apoptosis of most non-APL AML cell lines (6). Furthermore, expression profiling predicts *in vitro* sensitivity to retinoid analogs (4). In clinical trials, however, ATRA has not shown consistent clinical benefit in non-APL AML (7–13).

These lackluster results may be a result of the unique pharmacologic properties of ATRA. ATRA induces its own catabolism by stimulating upregulation of its metabolizing enzyme, CYP26, which is most prominently expressed in the liver (14–17); this leads to a reduction in the C_{max} of ATRA with prolonged administration. CYP26 is also produced by the bone marrow stroma where it plays an essential role in endogenous retinoid homeostasis (6, 17, 18). Stromal CYP26 establishes a low retinoid environment within the stem cell niche, which is necessary for the maintenance of a pool of quiescent, long term hematopoietic stem cells (HSCs) (18). In the setting of AML, stromal upregulation of CYP26 in response to exogenous ATRA shields leukemic stem cells (LSCs) from its differentiating effects (17).

IRX195183 is a synthetic retinoid that specifically binds to the retinoic acid receptor α and is resistant to metabolism by CYP26 (17). Pharmacokinetics from the first in-human trial of IRX195183 demonstrated a steady improvement of C_{max} and AUC from D0 to D28 across a range of doses from 15mg/m^2/day to 60mg/m^2/day (described in the publicly available study protocol)[1]. This contrasts with the blunted rise in C_{max} and AUC that is observed with prolonged ATRA administration (19). suggesting that IRX195183 does not induce its own auto-catabolism. In both *in vitro* and *in vivo* mouse models, the effects of ATRA are attenuated by the presence of CYP26-producing mesenchymal stromal cells, whereas the effects of IRX195183 are unmitigated (17).

IRX195183's superior pharmacokinetic and pharmacodynamic profile make it a promising drug for the treatment of patients with myeloid malignancies. The previously conducted phase 1 study of the drug was performed in patients with hepatocellular carcinoma. Grade 3 elevations of transaminases were frequently observed in that study, but accurate attribution of this adverse effect was complicated by the high burden of liver disease in this patient population. We designed a phase I/II study of IRX195183 in the treatment of relapsed and refractory high-grade myelodysplastic syndrome (MDS) and AML. Due to the unavailability of the drug, we were unable to proceed with the phase 2 expansion cohort. Herein, we describe the design and results of the phase I portion of the study.

MATERIALS AND METHODS

The clinical trial registration number is NCT02749708. The study protocol was approved by the Johns Hopkins Institutional Review Board and was conducted in accordance with the Declaration of Helsinki.

Patient Population

Patients between the ages of 18 and 60 years of age with pathologically confirmed AML, MDS, chronic myelomonocytic leukemia (CMML), or MDS/MPN overlap syndrome were considered for enrollment. AML patients must have had either 1) relapsed or refractory disease after receiving one or more courses of induction chemotherapy, hypomethylating agent therapy, or bone marrow transplant or 2) *de novo* AML not deemed to be a candidate for conventional therapy based on age, co-morbidities, or patient preference. Patients with MDS, CMML, or MDS/MPN had to have high-risk features, defined as follows: 1) relapsed after initial response or were refractory after receiving at least four cycles of HMA therapy or 2) had *de novo* MDS but refused HMA therapy. High-risk features included at least one of the following: International Prognostic Scoring System (IPSS) of INT-2 or higher; Revised-IPSS (IPSS-R) of high or very high; secondary MDS; INT-1 IPSS or INT R-IPSS with excess blasts (≥5% blasts on bone marrow biopsy) or with transfusion dependency; or CMML or MDS/MPN with excess blasts, transfusion-dependency, abnormal karyotype, or proliferative features.

Patients were required to have an ECOG ≤ 2 or Karnofsky ≥ 60%; creatinine level of 3mg/dL or lower; total bilirubin ≤ 3mg/dL unless due to Gilbert's syndrome, hemolysis or ineffective hematopoiesis; AST (SGOT) and ALT (SGPT) ≤ 3 x the upper limit of normal (ULN); white blood cell (WBC) count ≤10,000/µl; and if the patient was a woman of childbearing age, they were required to have a negative serum or urine pregnancy test within 72 h of the start of the study drug. Patients who had received prior therapies were required to undergo a 3-week washout period and had to have recovered from all toxicities prior to the initiation of therapy. Patients requiring hydroxyurea to bring the WBC below 10,000/µl were required to have a 48 h wash out period.

Major exclusion criteria included any serious medical condition or uncontrolled concurrent illness including active infection, symptomatic congestive heart failure, unstable angina pectoris, cardiac arrhythmia, or laboratory abnormality that

[1] https://clinicaltrials.gov/ProvidedDocs/08/NCT02749708/Prot_SAP_000.pdf [Accessed February 21, 2020]

would limit compliance with the study requirements or preclude informed consent from being obtained; leukemic involvement of the central nervous system (CNS); pulmonary leukostasis; or disseminated intravascular coagulation (DIC).

Study Design and Treatment

This was a single-center, single-arm prospective phase I study. The treatment schema is summarized in **Figure 1**. The dose escalation phase used a 3 + 3 design with three dose levels (DL): DL1 was 50mg, DL2 was 75 mg, and DL3 was 100 mg. For induction therapy, IRX195183 was administered orally once daily for two 28-day cycles. Patients who had stable disease (SD) or better were eligible to continue on consolidation/maintenance, which consisted of up to four continuous 28-day cycles using the same dose they had previously received. There was no intra-patient dose escalation. IRX5183 was provided by Io Therapeutics, Inc.

Assessment of Safety and Efficacy

The primary objective was to evaluate the safety and toxicity of IRX195183 and to determine the recommended phase 2 dose. The primary endpoint was toxicity of IRX195183, determined by grading a tabulation using the National Cancer Institute Common Toxicity Criteria, Version 5.0, in order to determine dose-limiting toxicities (DLTs) and the recommended phase 2 dose. DLTs were defined as Grade 3 or higher non-hematologic toxicities, any toxicity that resulted in a delay of therapy for 2 weeks or greater, and Grade 4 treatment-associated aplasia that persists beyond 4 weeks. Exceptions included transient laboratory abnormalities that could be treated or resolved to Grade 2 or less within 1 week from holding the study drug, toxicities associated with differentiation syndrome that resolved within 2 weeks of steroid therapy to Grade 1, and asymptomatic Grade 3 hypertriglyceridemia. Grade 3 hypertriglyceridemia was initially considered a DLT, but the protocol was later amended to exclude asymptomatic Grade 3 hypertriglyceridemia. Patients with Grade 3 hypertriglyceridemia were allowed to continue on study after initiating treatment with the triglyceride lowering agent gemfibrozil.

Efficacy was a secondary endpoint of phase I and patients who received at least 1 dose were included in efficacy analyses. Bone marrow response assessments were performed at baseline and then after each cycle. Clinical responses were defined according to the Modified International Working Group-2003 criteria for AML (20) and the Modified International Working Group-2006 criteria for MDS (21).

Processing of Patient Blood Samples

Whole blood samples were centrifuged at 500 g in a clinical centrifuge, and the plasma layer was carefully removed, aliquoted, and stored at -80°C. Frozen plasma samples were thawed and clarified by centrifugation at 16,000 *g* for 2 min.

Cell Culture

The mouse mesenchymal stroma OP9 cells were cultured in in α-MEM with 2 mM L-glutamine (Life Technologies, Thermo Fisher Scientific), 100 μg/ml penicillin-streptomycin (P/S) (Gibco, Thermo Fisher Scientific), and 20% fetal calf serum (FCS) (Sigma-Aldrich). The APL cells from the NB4 cell line were cultured in RPMI 1640, L-glutamine, P/S, and with 10% and 20% FCS (R20). The cell line was purchased from ATCC and recently tested negative for Mycoplasma.

Co-Culture System

The co-culture model has previously been described (6, 22). Briefly, 24-well plates were coated with 0.1% gelatin (Sigma-Aldrich) in PBS for at least 30 min at 37°C. The gelatin was then removed and $5x10^4$ stromal cells per well were cultured overnight to obtain a confluent monolayer. At that time, media was removed, and leukemia cells were added to the culture at a density of $5x10^4$ cells/well and incubated with in various conditions for 72 h.

Flow Cytometry for Bone Marrow Aspirate Samples

Flow cytometric immunophenotyping was performed on fresh bone marrow aspirates. The material was collected in EDTA or heparin anticoagulant and processed routinely using an RBC lysis method. Cell suspensions were incubated with combinations of monoclonal antibodies (Becton Dickinson) that were used at concentrations titrated for optimal staining. Specimens were subjected to a myeloid leukemia panel that included CD7, CD10, CD11b, CD13, CD14, CD15, CD16, CD33, CD34, CD38, CD45, CD56, CD64, CD71, CD117, CD123, and HLA-DR. CD38

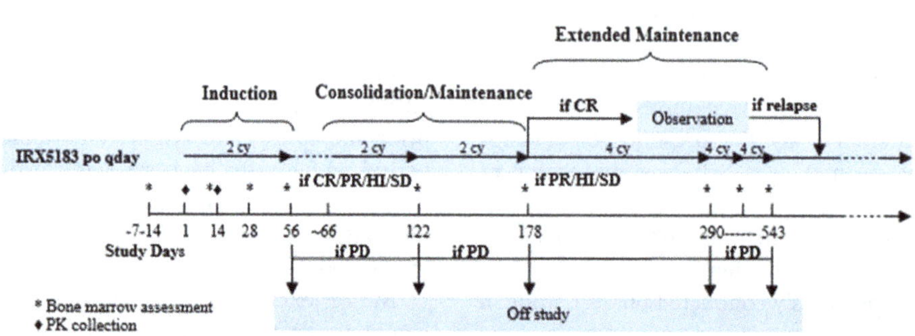

FIGURE 1 | Treatment schema of phase I clinical trial using IRX195183 in patients with high risk MDS and relapsed/refractory AML.

was conjugated to PerCP-Cy5.5. The data were analyzed on BD FACSCanto 10-color system (BD Biosciences). List mode data files were acquired and analyzed for each specimen using BD FACSDiva (BD Biosciences) and Infinicyt (Cytognos) for data acquisition and analysis, respectively.

Flow Cytometry for Cell Lines

Cell lines in the plasma differentiation assay were analyzed for expression of cell surface antigens using FACS Calibur (BD Biosciences, CA, USA). Treated cells were removed from the plate, washed with PBS and counted using Trypan Blue. For flow cytometry, cells were washed with PBS containing 0.2% BSA (Sigma-Aldrich) and stained with the appropriate antibodies for 15 min at room temperature (PE-conjugated mouse anti-human CD11b IgG1, FITC-conjugated mouse anti-human CD34 IgG1, PE-conjugated mouse anti-human CD38 IgG2α, and APC-conjugated mouse anti-human CD45 IgG2β antibodies, BD Biosciences). All antibodies were purchased from BD Biosciences. Cells were then washed with PBS and evaluated by FACS Calibur (BD Biosciences) with a minimum acquisition of 10,000 events.

In Vivo Induction of Terminal Differentiation

We performed flow cytometry to assess CD11b and CD38 expression, markers of terminal differentiation, on bone marrow biopsy specimens obtained at baseline and after each cycle of therapy for every patient enrolled in the study.

Plasma Differentiation Assay

Blood samples were collected from the first four patients enrolled in the study on day 14 of treatment, 2 h after the dose of IRX195183 was administered. NB4 cells were cultured in RPMI 1640 supplemented with L-glutamine, P/S and with 10% (R10) complete media supplemented with either 1%, 5%, or 10% patient plasma in the presence or absence of OP9 stroma cells. The degree of differentiation was then determined by measuring CD11b expression by flow cytometry and clonogenic activity in a colony forming assay. Data were normalized to NB4 cells incubated in plasma from untreated controls. For comparison, we used plasma derived from three patients with APL treated with ATRA per standard of care.

Statistical Analysis

Pre-clinical data were analyzed using unpaired, 2-tailed Student's t tests to compare differences between drug treatment groups.

RESULTS

Patient Characteristics

Eleven patients were enrolled between February 2017 and August 2018. The initial cohort of three patients received IRX195183 50 mg daily in 28-day cycles. A flow chart for the study conduct is displayed in **Figure 2**. One patient had asymptomatic Grade 3 hypertriglyceridemia triggering the enrollment of three more patients at the same dose level. The protocol was then amended to exclude asymptomatic Grade 3 hypertriglyceridemia as a DLT. Symptomatic Grade 3 hypertriglyceridemia and any Grade 4 hypertriglyceridemia remained DLTs. Using this new definition of DLT, patients were then enrolled at the next dose level.

Patient characteristics are summarized in **Table 1**. The average age was 69 years and 55% of the patients were male. Eight patients had secondary AML. The remaining three patients had primary AML, MDS with excess blasts, and CMML. All but one patient had received at least one line of prior standard-of-care therapy.

Patients were assessed regularly for safety as well as disease status. All six patients in DL1 completed at least one cycle of therapy and could be assessed for tolerability and response. After the DL1 cohort was completed and the drug was deemed to be safe at this level, three patients were enrolled in the DL2 cohort and received IRX195183 75 mg daily. One of the three went off study due to infection before DLTs could adequately be assessed, so two additional patients were enrolled before the study was terminated due to inadequate supply of the study drug. No dose escalations or reductions were made during the course of the trial for any individual patient.

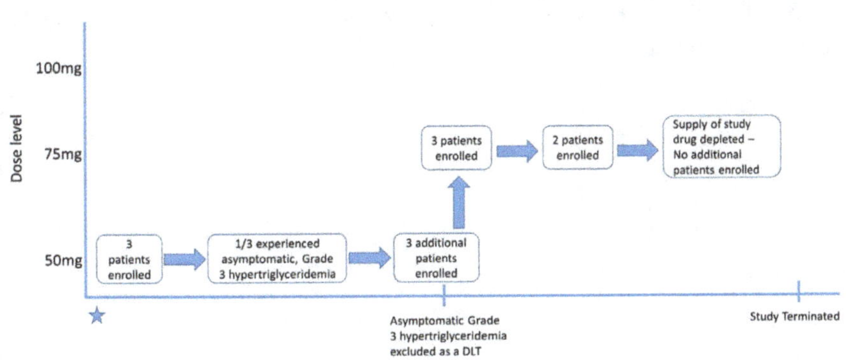

FIGURE 2 | Flow chart diagramming patient enrollment. DLT, Dose-limiting toxicity.

TABLE 1 | Baseline patient characteristics.

Patient	Dose level	Age	Gender	Diagnosis	Disease Status	No. of Prior Therapies	ECOG	Karyotype	Molecular Mutations	Days on trial	Response Duration	In Vivo Maturation	Best Response	Reason for Discontinuation
1	50 mg	70	Male	sAML	Refractory	1	1	Monosomy 7	SETBP1, ASXL1, U2AF1	48	19	No	SD	Infection
2	50 mg	58	Female	t-MN	Relapsed	2	1	11q23	FLT3, ASXL1, NUP98	56	N/A	No	PD	Progressive disease
3	50 mg	67	Female	sAML	Relapsed	4	1	5q-, trisomy 8	RUNX1, TET2, BCOR, DNMT3A, U2AF1	34	N/A	Yes	PD	Progressive disease
4	50 mg	58	Male	sAML	Relapsed	3	0	Normal	RUNX1, IDH2, DNMT3A	64	N/A	No	PD	Progressive disease
5	50 mg	75	Male	sAML	Refractory	1	1	Complex	SRSF2, TET2	69	42	Yes	CRi	Hypertriglyceridemia
6	50 mg	76	Male	CMML-2	Relapsed	2	1	Normal	ASXL1, SRSF2, TET2	63	48	No	SD	Hypertriglyceridemia
7	75 mg	64	Female	sAML	Relapsed	4	1	Normal	NPM1	63	N/A	No	PD	Progressive disease
8	75 mg	70	Male	MDS-EB1	Refractory	1	1	11q23	ETV6, ASXL1, NF1, SRSF2, KIT	112	85	No	SD	Progressive disease
9	75 mg	78	Female	sAML	Untreated	0	1	Normal	SF3B1, BCOR, BCORL1, PTPN11, RUNX1	16	N/A	No	N/A*	Infection
10	75 mg	77	Male	sAML	Relapsed	2	1	5q-	Not tested	4	N/A	No	N/A*	Infection
11	75 mg	68	Female	AML	Relapsed	2	1	5q-	p53	43	N/A	No	PD	Progressive disease

**not applicable due to inadequate duration of therapy to assess response; SD, Stable disease; PD, Progressive disease; LR, Lineage response.*

Safety and Toxicity

Table 2 summarizes the treatment-emergent adverse events at least possibly related to IRX195183. A total of six patients developed hypertriglyceridemia. Three patients had Grades 1–2 hypertriglyceridemia and three had Grades 3–4 hypertriglyceridemia. Five of the six patients were treated with lipid modifying therapies including gemfibrozil and omega-3-acid ethyl esters. Once initiated, lipid modifying therapies were continued until the study drug was discontinued. For all three patients with Grade 3 hypertriglyceridemia, the study drug was held until the hypertriglyceridemia improved. One patient was able to resume therapy after initiation of after initiating lipid modifying therapy, whereas hypertriglyceridemia led to permanent discontinuation of the study drug in the remaining two patients. All three patients who experienced grade 3 hypertriglyceridemia were treated at the first dose level, whereas none of the patients treated at the second dose level developed Grades 3–4 hypertriglyceridemia. All six patients with hypertriglyceridemia were asymptomatic and none suffered adverse consequences such as hepatosplenomegaly, acute pancreatitis, dyspnea, or neurological symptoms. There were no other DLTs and no other patients discontinued the study due to study drug-related adverse events.

Patient 2 developed Grade 3 elevations of her transaminases in the setting of hospitalization, but they returned to normal levels without discontinuation of the study drug. Two patients developed leukocytosis (>10,000/cc mm) for which hydroxyurea was initiated. Another patient, Patient 2, developed Grade 3

TABLE 2 | Treatment emergent adverse events possibly related to IRX195183.

	N = 11	
Adverse Effect:	Grade 1/2, n (%)	Grade 3/4, n (%)
Asymptomatic Hypertriglyceridemia	3 (27%)	3 (27%)
Fatigue	2 (18%)	3 (27%)
Dyspnea	3 (27%)	1 (9%)
Edema	3 (27%)	0
Hypoxia	1 (9%)	1 (9%)
Pneumonia	1 (9%)	1 (9%)
Elevated Transaminases	1 (9%)	1 (9%)
Hyponatremia	1 (9%)	1 (9%)
Anorexia	2 (18%)	0
Arthralgias	2 (18%)	0
Hypocalcemia	2 (18%)	0
Nausea/Vomiting	2 (18%)	0
Cough	1 (9%)	0
Diarrhea	1 (9%)	0
Differentiation Syndrome	1 (9%)	0
Flushing	1 (9%)	0
Headache	1 (9%)	0
Hyperglycemia	1 (9%)	0
Hypertension	1 (9%)	0
Hyperuricemia	1 (9%)	0
Hypoalbuminemia	1 (9%)	0
Hypophosphatemia	1 (9%)	0
Increased cholesterol	1 (9%)	0
Increased creatinine	1 (9%)	0
Insomnia	1 (9%)	0
Lymphedema	1 (9%)	0
Pruritus	1 (9%)	0
Rash	1 (9%)	0
Tachycardia	1 (9%)	0

hypoxia for which differentiation syndrome (DS) was considered a possible etiology. Her shortness of breath was accompanied by a small pleural effusion, but no other manifestations of DS. She was briefly treated with steroids and furosemide while the study drug was continued, and she clinically improved. Patient 6 developed grade 3 hyponatremia with a nadir sodium of 129 mmol/L. The patient's hyponatremia was preceded by several days of poor oral intake and it resolved with administration of IV fluids. Two patients experienced Grade 3 fatigue. The remainder of the Grade 3–4 AEs were hematologic and attributed to the underlying leukemia. There were no serious adverse events. Five patients died within 30 days of withdrawal from the study. Two deaths occurred as a result of infection and three were attributed to progressive leukemia.

Responses

One patient (Patient 5) achieved a morphological complete remission with incomplete hematologic recovery. He had AML secondary to MDS and had not responded to seven cycles of azacitidine 75 mg/m2, days 1-7. At baseline, he was pancytopenic, had 21% circulating blasts, and was red blood cell transfusion-dependent. Within 2 weeks of initiation of the study drug, his absolute neutrophil, and platelet counts had normalized. He also developed a leukocytosis with neutrophilic predominance, so he was treated with hydroxyurea. A bone marrow biopsy at 2 weeks demonstrated 15% blasts by immunohistochemistry and 33% by flow cytometry. At 1 month, his bone marrow biopsy demonstrated a hypercellular marrow with normal maturation and no morphological evidence of leukemia. Flow cytometric analysis detected 0.13% residual leukemic blasts, though the blasts demonstrated significantly increased expression of CD38, suggestive of maturation (**Figure 3D**). Although he developed recurrent thrombocytopenia before completion of cycle 1, he achieved transfusion independence, which he maintained for 2 months while on study. The study drug was held for Grade 3 hypertriglyceridemia on cycle 3 day 1. On cycle 3 day 9, he developed progressive disease and went off trial.

Two patients with MDS or CMML had stable disease while on IRX195183. Patient 6 had CMML with a baseline bone marrow demonstrating 2% blasts. He was treated on study for 63 days but withdrew from the study due to recurrent Grade 3 hypertriglyceridemia. His final bone marrow assessment showed CMML with no evidence of increased blasts, consistent with stable disease. Patient 8 had MDS that was unresponsive to

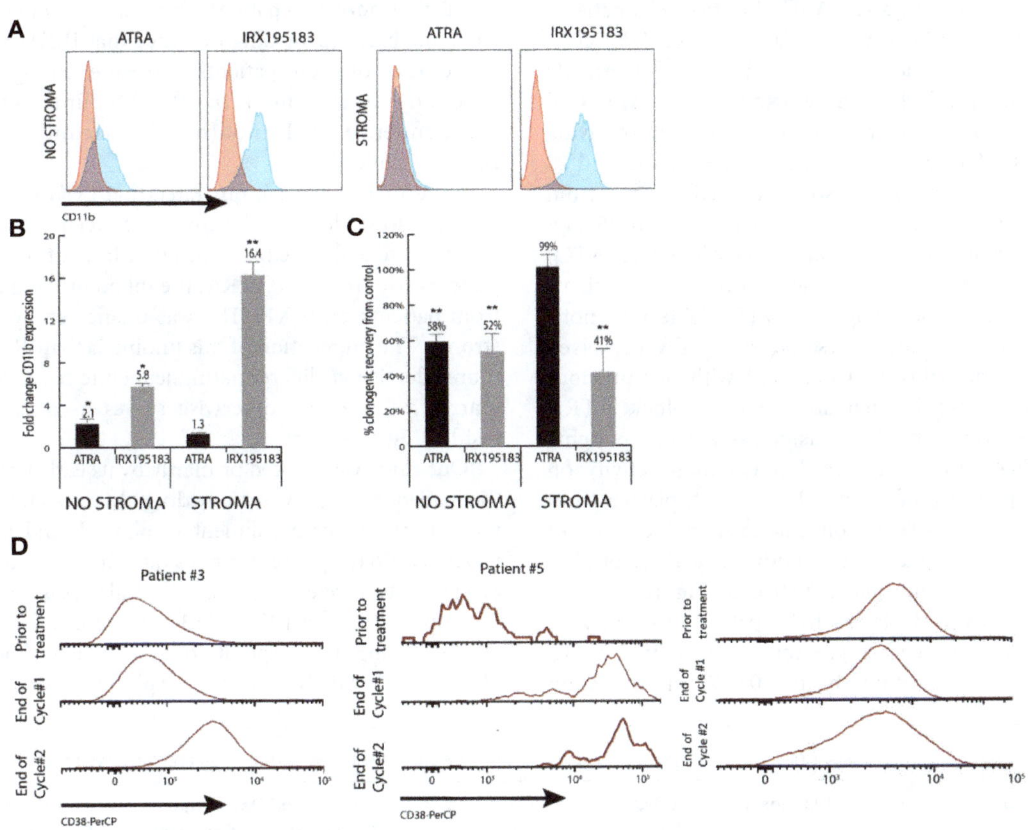

FIGURE 3 | Differentiation activity of plasma from patients treated with IRX195183. **(A)** Representative flow plots of CD11b expression of NB4 cells cultured in the presence of 10% plasma from patients treated with ATRA (1st and 3rd) or IRX195183 (2nd and 4th) in the presence or absence of bone marrow stroma. **(B, C)** Differentiation activity on plasma from patients treated with either ATRA or IRX195183 as measured by upregulation of CD11b expression **(B)** and decreased clonogenic activity **(C)** of NB4 cells. Data represents mean ± SEM, n = 4 independent patients, *$p < 0.05$, **$p < 0.01$. P was calculated using unpaired, 2-tailed Student's t test. **(D)** CD38 expression on the leukemic blasts from patient #3 and patient #5 treated with IRX195183.

six cycles of azacitidine prior to enrollment in the IRX195183 study. He was treated on study for five cycles and maintained stable disease until finally progressing to AML.

Two patients with AML had stable disease on their 1 month bone marrow specimens. Patient 1 withdrew from the study due to recurrent line-associated bacteremia. Patient 3 stopped the study drug due to hypertriglyceridemia and lack of response; however, she had evidence of significantly increased CD38 expression on the leukemic blasts from the bone marrow aspirate obtained at the end of cycle 1, suggestive of leukemic blast maturation (**Figure 3D**). Four patients discontinued the study drug due to progressive disease. Two patients were treated for less than one cycle due to infection and could not be formally evaluated for response, but they were considered non-responders for the purposes of the efficacy analysis.

Plasma Differentiation Assay

To investigate if patients receiving IRX195183 achieve biologically meaningful plasma concentrations of this drug, we designed a functional assay to determine to what extent plasma from these patients can trigger differentiation *in vitro*. Using NB4 cells as a read out, 10% plasma from patients treated with IRX195183 induced a 5.8 ± 0.2 fold upregulation of CD11b expression and 52% (± 16%) decreased clonogenic activity compared to the control (**Figures 3A–C**). Plasma from patients with APL treated with ATRA had similar effects on NB4 cells, while plasma from normal volunteers had no discernable differentiation potential. For these experiments, we used plasma from Patients 1, 2, 3, and 4 both in DL1 and receiving 50 mg daily of IRX195183 and equivalent of 25 mg/m2 and 28 mg/m2, respectively. For comparison, we used plasma from patients with low-intermediate risk APL who received 45 mg/m2 of ATRA as part of standard-of-care Arsenic Trioxide (ATO) plus ATRA. The characteristics of the ATRA-treated patients and the timing of plasma sampling is shown in **Table 3**. Of note, at the time of plasma collection, these patients had yet received treatment with arsenic trioxide. Consistent with our previous observations that mesenchymal stroma cells block ATRA induced differentiation of APL cells, plasma from patients treated with ATRA showed no pro-differentiation activity on NB4 cells in the presence of stroma. In contrast, plasma from patients treated with IRX195183 continue to show induction of CD11b expression and reduction of clonogenic activity of NB4 cells in the presence of bone marrow stroma (**Figures 3A–C**). Compared to the effects of plasma from patients treated with ATRA, IRX195183 induced a greater increase in CD11b expression (t-test $p < 0.01$, Wilcoxon $p = 0.057$) and reduction in clonogenic activity (t-test $p = 0.02$, Wilcoxon $p = 0.57$) on NB4 cells cultured on bone marrow stroma.

DISCUSSION

In this phase 1 study, IRX195183 had a manageable toxicity profile and led to one short-lived morphological CRi response. The most significant toxicity associated with the drug was hypertriglyceridemia. This adverse effect led three patients to withdraw from the study, though none of these patients suffered adverse clinical sequelae. The incidence of hypertriglyceridemia observed in this study is comparable to the 47% incidence reported in studies of single-agent ATRA for the treatment of APL and to the 64% incidence reported in studies of single agent tamibarotene in patients with relapsed/refractory AML (23, 24). Anticipation of this adverse effect and prophylactic use of lipid modifying agents may be effective in mitigating this complication in future studies. Elevated liver enzymes were rare and self-limited in this study, in contrast to the results of an unpublished phase 1 clinical trial conducted in patients with hepatocellular carcinoma. There were no other DLTs or treatment-related deaths on study. Notably, the maximally tolerated dose of the drug was not reached in this study due to limited supply.

Furthermore, two patients showed *in vivo* maturation of their leukemic blasts, providing evidence that IRX195183 is clinically active. One of these patients also experienced a CRi response with an improvement in blood counts and transfusion independence at 1 month. The second patient did not respond clinically.

Nevertheless, we demonstrated that IRX195183 administered at the lowest dose level achieves concentrations sufficient to differentiate leukemic blasts *in vitro*. In contrast to plasma from patients who received ATRA, the differentiating effect of plasma from patients on IRX195183 was unaffected by the presence of stroma. The implication of this finding is that IRX195183 may be more effective at differentiating leukemic blasts within the bone marrow, a site that otherwise serves as a sanctuary site for residual disease.

Our study was limited primarily by its early termination due to the inadequate supply of study drug. As a result, the study did not meet its target for enrollment in phase I, and it was unable to proceed onto the phase II expansion cohort. The availability of the drug for future investigative and clinical uses is uncertain, however our experience with IRX195183 may inform the design of future studies aiming to incorporate retinoid analogs into the treatment of non-APL AML. In addition, the plasma differentiation potential

TABLE 3 | Characteristics of ATRA-treated patients from whom plasma samples were obtained and the timing of plasma sampling relative to last ATRA dose.

ATRA-treated Patients	Sex	Age	Diagnosis	WBC at diagnosis	Treatment protocol	Cycle and Day at the Time of Plasma Sampling	Time of Plasma Sampling Relative to Last ATRA Dose
1	M	64	APL	0.76	ATO + ATRA	Cycle 1, Day 2	1-h post dose 3 of ATRA
2	F	69	APL	7.57	ATO + ATRA	Cycle 1, Day 2	2-h post dose 3 of ATRA
3	M	67	APL	5.89	ATO + ATRA	Cycle 2, Day 2	2-h post dose 3 of ATRA

ATO, Arsenic trioxide.

assay described here captures the significant impact that bone marrow stroma has on retinoids pharmacodynamics and may serve as a platform for interrogating the biological activity of other novel differentiating agents.

Our group has recently demonstrated the mitigating effect of bone marrow stroma on the differentiating capacity of retinoids, an effect that is mediated by CYP26 expression. IRX195183 is resistant to metabolism by CYP26 and is selective for RARα and therefore does not trigger upregulation of CYP expression in the liver and bone marrow stroma (17, 25). The result is better maintenance of the systemic C_{max} and AUC than ATRA (see protocol for NCT02749708 on Clinicaltrials.gov). These properties may translate into higher concentrations within the bone marrow microenvironment, resulting in more effective differentiation of residual leukemic blasts within this compartment (26, 27). Tamibarotene is another novel retinoid-agonist with increased specificity and potency for RARα (28). Its plasma concentrations do not decline overtime, as is seen with ATRA, and it has a lower affinity for cellular retinoic acid binding protein, which is expressed as a resistance mechanism in ATRA-resistant APL (29). Tamibarotene has shown efficacy in relapsed/refractory APL and better outcomes in the maintenance setting in comparison to ATRA (24, 30, 31). The increased selectivity demonstrated by both IRX195183 and tamibarotene may reduce off target activation of other retinoic acid receptors, reducing the burden of adverse effects associated with retinoid therapy.

Our findings suggest that IRX195183 is a safe and potentially effective agent in the treatment of retinoid-sensitive AMLs. Further studies of the efficacy of IRX195183 and other retinoic acid agonists either as single agents or in combination with other therapies in the treatment of biologically defined non-APL AML are warranted.

AUTHOR'S NOTE

RC passed away during preparation of the manuscript. Final version was approved on his behalf by MS, CEO of IO therapeutics.

ETHICS STATEMENT

The studies involving human participants were reviewed and approved by the Johns Hopkins Institutional Review Board. The patients/participants provided their written informed consent to participate in this study. Written informed consent was obtained from the individual(s) for the publication of any potentially identifiable images or data included in this article.

AUTHOR CONTRIBUTIONS

AA was involved in data collection, analysis, interpretation, and writing. KN was involved in study design, provision of study patients, data collection, analysis, interpretation, and writing. DH, LP, BP, and AD performed the correlative studies. RC and MS were involved in study design. RV was involved in data analysis and interpretation. RJ was involved in writing. BS was involved in study design, provision of study patients, data analysis, interpretation, and writing. GG was involved in study design, data analysis, interpretation, and writing. All authors contributed to the article and approved the submitted version.

REFERENCES

1. Collins SJ. Retinoic acid receptors, hematopoiesis and leukemogenesis. *Curr Opin Hematol* (2008) 15:346–51. doi: 10.1097/MOH.0b013e3283007edf
2. Wang ZY, Chen Z. Acute promyelocytic leukemia: From highly fatal to highly curable. *Blood* (2008) 111:2505–15. doi: 10.1182/blood-2007-07-102798
3. Boutzen H, Saland E, Larrue C, de Toni F, Gales L, Castelli FA, et al. Isocitrate dehydrogenase 1 mutations prime the all-trans retinoic acid myeloid differentiation pathway in acute myeloid leukemia. *J Exp Med* (2016) 213:483–97. doi: 10.1084/jem.20150736
4. McKeown MR, Corces MR, Eaton ML, Fiore C, Lee E, Lopez JT, et al. Superenhancer analysis defi nes novel epigenomic subtypes of non-APL AML, including an RARα dependency targetable by SY-1425, a potent and selective RARα agonist. *Cancer Discovery* (2017) 7:1136–53. doi: 10.1158/2159-8290.CD-17-0399
5. Mugoni V, Panella R, Cheloni G, Chen M, Pozdnyakova O, Stroopinsky D, et al. Vulnerabilities in mIDH2 AML confer sensitivity to APL-like targeted combination therapy. *Cell Res* (2019) 29:446–59. doi: 10.1038/s41422-019-0162-7
6. Su M, Alonso S, Jones JW, Yu J, Kane MA, Jones RJ, et al. All-Trans Retinoic Acid Activity in Acute Myeloid Leukemia: Role of Cytochrome P450 Enzyme Expression by the Microenvironment. *PloS One* (2015) 10:e0127790. doi: 10.1371/journal.pone.0127790
7. Venditti A, Stasi R, Del Poeta G, Buccisano F, Aronica G, Bruno A, et al. All-trans retinoic acid and low-dose cytosine arabinoside for the treatment of "poor prognosis" acute myeloid leukemia. *Leukemia* (1995) 9:1121–5. doi: 10.1200/JCO.2003.04.036
8. Estey EH, Thall PF, Pierce S, Cortes J, Beran M, Kantarjian H, et al. Randomized phase II study of fludarabine + cytosine arabinoside + idarubicin ± all-trans retinoic acid ± granulocyte colony-stimulating factor in poor prognosis newly diagnosed acute myeloid leukemia and myelodysplastic syndrome. *Blood* (1999) 93:2478–84. doi: 10.1182/blood.v93.8.2478.408k04_2478_2484
9. Schlenk RF, Fröhling S, Hartmann F, Fischer JT, Glasmacher A, del Valle F, et al. Phase III study of all-trans retinoic acid in previously untreated patients

61 years or older with acute myeloid leukemia. *Leukemia* (2004) 18:1798–803. doi: 10.1038/sj.leu.2403528

10. Milligan DW, Wheatley K, Littlewood T, Craig JIO, Burnett AKNCRI Haematological Oncology Clinical Studies Group. Fludarabine and cytosine are less effective than standard ADE chemotherapy in high-risk acute myeloid leukemia, and addition of G-CSF and ATRA are not beneficial: results of the MRC AML-HR randomized trial. *Blood* (2006) 107:4614–22. doi: 10.1182/blood-2005-10-4202
11. Burnett AK, Milligan D, Prentice AG, Goldstone AH, McMullin MF, Hills RK. Wheatley K. A comparison of low-dose cytarabine and hydroxyurea with or without all-trans retinoic acid for acute myeloid leukemia and high-risk myelodysplastic syndrome in patients not considered fit for intensive treatment. *Cancer* (2007) 109:1114–24. doi: 10.1002/cncr.22496
12. Burnett AK, Hills RK, Green C, Jenkinson S, Koo K, Patel Y, et al. The impact on outcome of the addition of all-trans retinoic acid to intensive chemotherapy in younger patients with nonacute promyelocytic acute myeloid leukemia: Overall results and results in genotypic subgroups defined by mutations in NPM1, FLT3, and CEBPA. *Blood* (2010) 115:948–56. doi: 10.1182/blood-2009-08-236588
13. Schlenk RF, Lübbert M, Benner A, Lamparter A, Krauter J, Herr W, et al. All-trans retinoic acid as adjunct to intensive treatment in younger adult patients with acute myeloid leukemia: results of the randomized AMLSG 07-04 study. *Ann Hematol* (2016) 95:1931–42. doi: 10.1007/s00277-016-2810-z
14. Muindi J, Frankel SR, Miller WH, Jakubowski A, Scheinberg DA, Young CW, et al. Continuous Treatment With All-Trans Retinoic Acid Causes a Progressive Reduction in Plasma Drug Concentrations: Implications for Relapse and Retinoid "Resistance" in Patients With Acute Promyelocytic Leukemia. Available at: https://ashpublications.org/HTTPHandlers/ArticlePdfHandler.ashx?journal=blood&volume=79&issue=2&page=299 (Accessed February 21, 2020).
15. Thatcher JE, Zelter A, Isoherranen N. The relative importance of CYP26A1 in hepatic clearance of all-trans retinoic acid. *Biochem Pharmacol* (2010) 80:903–12. doi: 10.1016/j.bcp.2010.05.023
16. Stevison F, Jing J, Tripathy S, Isoherranen N. Role of Retinoic Acid-Metabolizing Cytochrome P450s, CYP26, in Inflammation and Cancer. *Adv Pharmacol* (2015) 74:373–412. doi: 10.1016/bs.apha.2015.04.006
17. Hernandez D, Palau L, Norsworthy K, Anders NM, Alonso S, Su M, et al. Overcoming microenvironment-mediated protection from ATRA using CYP26-resistant retinoids. *Leukemia* (2020) 12:1–5. doi: 10.1038/s41375-020-0790-4
18. Ghiaur G, Yegnasubramanian S, Perkins B, Gucwa JL, Gerber JM, Jones RJ. Regulation of human hematopoietic stem cell self-renewal by the microenvironment's control of retinoic acid signaling. *Proc Natl Acad Sci U.S.A.* (2013) 110:16121–6. doi: 10.1073/pnas.1305937110
19. Jing J, Nelson C, Paik J, Shirasaka Y, Amory JK, Isoherranen N. Physiologically Based Pharmacokinetic Model of All-trans-Retinoic Acid with Application to Cancer Populations and Drug Interactions. *J Pharmacol Exp Ther* (2017) 361:246–58. doi: 10.1124/jpet.117.240523
20. Cheson BD, Bennett JM, Kopecky KJ, Büchner T, Willman CL, Estey EH, et al. Revised recommendations of the International Working Group for Diagnosis, Standardization of Response Criteria, Treatment Outcomes, and Reporting Standards for Therapeutic Trials in Acute Myeloid Leukemia. *J Clin Oncol* (2003) 21:4642–9. doi: 10.1200/JCO.2003.04.036
21. Cheson BD, Greenberg PL, Bennett JM, Lowenberg B, Wijermans PW, Nimer SD, et al. Clinical application and proposal for modification of the International Working Group (IWG) response criteria in myelodysplasia. *Blood* (2006) 108:419–25. doi: 10.1182/blood-2005-10-4149
22. Alonso S, Hernandez D, Chang Y-T, Gocke CB, McCray M, Varadhan R, et al. Hedgehog and retinoid signaling alters multiple myeloma microenvironment and generates bortezomib resistance. *J Clin Invest* (2016) 126(12):4460–8. doi: 10.1172/JCI88152
23. Kanamaru A, Takemoto Y, Tanimoto M, Murakami H, Asou N, Kobayashi T, et al. All-Trans Retinoic Acid for the Treatment of Newly Diagnosed Acute Promyelocytic Leukemia (1995). Available at: https://ashpublications.org/blood/article-pdf/85/5/1202/615263/1202.pdf (Accessed September 14, 2020).
24. Tobita T, Takeshita A, Kitamura K, Ohnishi K, Yanagi M, Hiraoka A, et al. Treatment with a new synthetic retinoid, Am80, of acute promyelocytic leukemia relapsed from complete remission induced by all-trans retinoid acid. *Blood* (1997) 90:967–73. doi: 10.1182/blood.v90.3.967.967_967_973
25. Adamson PC. All-Trans-Retinoic Acid Pharmacology and Its Impact on the Treatment of Acute Promyelocytic Leukemia (1996). Available at: http://theoncologist.alphamedpress.org/ (Accessed October 9, 2019).
26. Alonso S, Su M, Jones JW, Ganguly S, Kane MA, Jones RJ, et al. Human bone marrow niche chemoprotection mediated by cytochrome P450 enzymes. *Oncotarget* (2015) 6:14905–12. doi: 10.18632/oncotarget.3614
27. Alonso S, Jones RJ, Ghiaur G. Retinoic acid, CYP26, and drug resistance in the stem cell niche. *Exp Hematol* (2017) 54:17–25. doi: 10.1016/j.exphem.2017.07.004
28. Hashimoto Y, Kagechika H, Kawachi E, Fukasawa H, Saito G, Shudo K. Correlation of differentiation-inducing activity of retinoids on human leukemia cell lines HL-60 and NB4. *J Cancer Res Clin Oncol* (1995) 121:696–8. doi: 10.1007/BF01218530
29. Delva L, Cornic M, Balitrand N, Guidez F, Miclea JM, Delmer A, et al. Resistance to all-Trans retinoic acid (ATRA) therapy in relapsing acute promyelocytic leukemia: Study of in vitro ATRA sensitivity and cellular retinoic acid binding protein levels in leukemic cells. *Blood* (1993) 82:2175–81. doi: 10.1182/blood.v82.7.2175.bloodjournal8272175
30. Sanford D, Lo-Coco F, Sanz MA, Di Bona E, Coutre S, Altman JK, et al. Tamibarotene in patients with acute promyelocytic leukaemia relapsing after treatment with all-trans retinoic acid and arsenic trioxide. *Br J Haematol* (2015) 171:471–7. doi: 10.1111/bjh.13607
31. Takeshita A, Asou N, Atsuta Y, Sakura T, Ueda Y, Sawa M, et al. Tamibarotene maintenance improved relapse-free survival of acute promyelocytic leukemia: a final result of prospective, randomized, JALSG-APL204 study. *Leukemia* (2019) 33:358–70. doi: 10.1038/s41375-018-0233-7

11

Systematic Construction and Validation of a Metabolic Risk Model for Prognostic Prediction in Acute Myelogenous Leukemia

Yun Wang[1,2†], *Fang Hu*[1,2†], *Jin-yuan Li*[1,2†], *Run-cong Nie*[1,3†], *Si-liang Chen*[1,2], *Yan-yu Cai*[1,4], *Ling-ling Shu*[1,4], *De-jun Deng*[5], *Jing-bo Xu*[6*] *and Yang Liang*[1,2*]

[1] *Sate key Laboratory of Oncology in South China, Sun Yat-sen University Cancer Center, Collaborative Innovation Center for Cancer Medicine, Guangzhou, China,* [2] *Department of Hematologic Oncology, Sun Yat-sen University Cancer Center, Guangzhou, China,* [3] *Department of Gastric Surgery, Sun Yat-sen University Cancer Center, Guangzhou, China,* [4] *Department of VIP Region, Sun Yat-sen University Cancer Center, Guangzhou, China,* [5] *Department of Oncology and Hematology, Shenzhen Luohu District Hospital of Traditional Chinese Medicine, Shenzhen, China,* [6] *Department of Hematology, The Fifth Affiliated Hospital of Sun Yat-sen University, Zhuhai, China*

Correspondence:
Jing-bo Xu
xujingbo@mail.sysu.edu.cn
Yang Liang
liangyang@sysucc.org.cn;
liangy23@mail.sysu.edu.cn

[†] *These authors have contributed equally to this work*

Background: Acute myelogenous leukemia (AML) is a heterogeneous disease with recurrent gene mutations and variations in disease-associated gene expression, which may be useful for prognostic prediction.

Methods: RNA matrix and clinical data of AML were downloaded from GEO, TCGA, and TARGET databases. Prognostic metabolic genes were identified by LASSO analysis to establish a metabolic model. Prognostic accuracy of the model was quantified by time-dependent receiver operating characteristic curves and the area under the curve (AUC). Survival analysis was performed by log-rank tests. Enriched pathways in different metabolic risk statuses were evaluated by gene set enrichment analyses (GSEA).

Results: We identified nine genes to construct a prognostic model of shorter survival in the high-risk vs. low-risk group. The prognostic model showed good predictive efficacy, with AUCs for 5-year overall survival of 0.78 (0.73–0.83), 0.76 (0.62–0.89), and 0.66 (0.57–0.75) in the training, adult external, and pediatric external cohorts, respectively. Multivariable analysis demonstrated that the metabolic signature had independent prognostic value with hazard ratios of 2.75 (2.06–3.66), 1.89 (1.09–3.29), and 1.96 (1.00–3.84) in the training, adult external, and pediatric external cohorts, respectively. Combining metabolic signatures and classic prognostic factors improved 5-year overall survival prediction compared to the prediction by classic prognostic factors ($p < 0.05$). GSEA revealed that most pathways were metabolism-related, indicating potential mechanisms.

Conclusion: We identified dysregulated metabolic features in AML and constructed a prognostic model to predict the survival of patients with AML.

Keywords: acute myelogenous leukemia, clinical prognostic model, metabolism, nomogram, gene set enrichment analysis

INTRODUCTION

Acute myelogenous leukemia (AML) is one of the most common types of adult acute leukemia (1) and shows striking heterogeneity, with recurrent gene mutations and variations in disease-associated gene expression (2). Although intensive chemotherapy and haematopoietic stem cell transplantation are the most common treatments, AML is fatal in approximately half of younger patients and ~80% of older patients because of primary refractoriness, treatment-related death, or palindromia (3). Risk stratification of leukemia is indispensable to ensure accurate treatment. Recent studies have emphasized the vital role of cytogenetics and molecular genetic analyses in hematological malignancies as a new layer of leukemia pathogenesis. Guidelines from the European leukemia network (ELN) in 2017 indicated that molecular abnormalities in genes such as *NPM1*, *FLT3-ITD*, *CEBPA*, *RUNX1*, *TP53*, and *ASXL1* combined with karyotype abnormalities can be used as an effective and comprehensive stratification system for the diagnosis and treatment of AML (4). However, even patients in the same layer of ELN categories show different prognoses. For example, ~50% of the AML patients with t (5, 6) (q22; q22) *RUNX1-RUNX1T1* have a favorable prognosis according to ELN risk stratification but show poor prognosis after intensive chemotherapy (7). Thus, additional factors for risk stratification should be identified and combined with analyses of cytogenetic and molecular abnormalities for more accurate AML prognostic stratification.

Metabolic reprogramming has recently been recognized as a vital and distinguishing feature of tumor cells (8, 9). The pathogenesis, chemoresistance, and palindromia of leukemia are also closely related to abnormal glucose metabolism, amino acid metabolism, and lipid metabolism. It has been reported that leukemia-initiating cells preferentially perform glycolysis (5) and take up amino acids, the catabolism of which is elevated in leukemia stem cells (10). A regulator of lipid metabolism, *TPD52*, was reported to be overexpressed and related to poor prognosis in patients with AML (11). By disrupting the tricarboxylic acid cycle and eradicating leukemia stem cells, the combination of B cell lymphoma 2 inhibitor (venetoclax) and demethylated drugs (azacytidine) was found to induce more durable remission than demethylated drugs alone in older patients with AML (12–14). The first drug targeting tumor energy metabolism approved by the US Food and Drug Administration, the isocitrate dehydrogenase 2 (IDH2) enzyme inhibitor enasidenib, also showed encouraging efficacy for treating *IDH2*-mutated relapsed or refractory AML (15). Metabolic processes have been shown to play important roles in the pathogenesis and progression of leukemia. However, a metabolic signature panel has not been explored to accurately stratify patients with AML to predict prognosis and for treatment management. In this study, we constructed a metabolic prognostic model from a Gene Expression Omnibus (GEO) dataset, which was further validated in two independent adult (The Cancer Genome Atlas Acute Myeloid Leukemia, TCGA-LAML) and pediatric (Therapeutically Available Research to Generate Effective and Treatments Acute Myeloid Leukemia, TARGET-AML) databases to explore an efficient metabolic signature for the more accurate stratification management of AML.

MATERIALS AND METHODS

Datasets and Data Collection

The gene expression profiles of three AML cohorts were retrieved and downloaded from the corresponding datasets. Raw microarray data of GSE37642 (16) datasets were downloaded from the GEO database (http://www.ncbi.nlm.nih.gov/geo/) and normalized between different arrays. RNA-seq data from the TCGA-LAML dataset and TARGET-AML datasets were obtained from the UCSX Xena website (https://xenabrowser.net/datapages/). Transcripts per million normalized values were employed for further analysis. Detailed clinicopathological data including patient age, sex, leukocyte count, percentage of blast cells, French-American-British classification, genetic risk category, and survival information were download from the relevant item page on the UCSX Xena or GEO dataset website. The metabolic pathway-related gene sets of "c2.cp.kegg.v7.0.symbols" in gene set enrichment analysis (GSEA) were utilized as candidate metabolic gene lists. Genes were selected for further AML-related metabolic signature identification only when they were listed in all included cohorts.

Metabolic Signature Construction and Validation

The GSE37642 dataset was used as the training cohort to construct the metabolic risk model. Least absolute shrinkage and selection operator (LASSO) Cox regression analysis was adopted to identify the optimal weighting coefficient of the prognostic metabolic genes. The metabolic model was built according to the penalized maximum likelihood estimator with 1,000-fold cross-validation. The 1-SE criteria were employed to determine the optimal values of the penalty parameter λ. TCGA-LAML and TARGET-AML datasets served as the adult and pediatric AML validation cohorts, respectively. The metabolic risk score was generated for each patient according to the unified formula determined in the training cohort. Patients were further grouped into high- and low-risk groups according to the optimal cut-off of the metabolic risk score determined by the survminer package.

GSEA

GSEA v4.0.2 software (http://software.broadinstitute.org/gsea/login.jsp) was used to identify potential biological pathways comparing the high- and low metabolic-risk groups using the c2.cp.kegg.v7.0.symbols gene sets. A metabolic signature was generated for the GSE37642 dataset using metabolic pathway-related gene sets from c2.cp.kegg.v7.0.symbols. Only validation cohorts were included for enriched pathway analysis. A nominal $p < 0.05$ was considered statistically significant. Gene cloud biotechnology information (GCBI) and cytoscape 3.7.2 was used to explore the interactions between model-related metabolic proteins and other known related proteins.

Statistical Analysis

Time-dependent receiver operating characteristic (ROC) curves were drawn to assess the predictive performance of the metabolic signature in the three cohorts. The area under the ROC curve (AUC) was calculated using the survival ROC package. The confidence interval was measured by the bootstrap method. Overall survival (OS) was defined as the primary outcome and calculated as the date of diagnosis or study entry to death from any cause. Kaplan–Meier curves were draw using the "survival" package and compared using the log-rank test. Clinical and genetic information were explored for prognostic performance via univariable- and multivariable Cox analyses. The χ^2-test or the Fisher's exact test was performed to compare category variables. A nomogram was used to visualize and integrate the metabolic signature and classic independent risk factors, age, and genetic risk score for OS, the consistency of which was assessed by calibration. The AUC was used to evaluate and compare the prognostic value of the candidate factors. All statistical analyses were performed using R software (version 3.6.0) and SPSS version 24.0 software (SPSS, Inc., Chicago, IL, USA). A two-sided $p < 0{\cdot}05$ was considered statistically significant.

RESULTS

Patient Selection and Characteristics

Three AML cohorts including a total of 879 patients with available survival data were included in the analysis. Seven hundred and fifty-five candidate metabolic genes were retrieved from the Kyoto Encyclopedia of Genes and Genomes (KEGG) metabolic pathway-related gene sets. GSE37642 was utilized as a training cohort to estimate the prognostic metabolic model, and patients in the TCGA-LAML cohort and the TARGET-AML cohort served as external cohorts for metabolic model validation. The workflow of data collection has been shown in (**Supplemental Figure 1**). Patients from the GSE37642 and the TCGA-LAML cohorts were adults with AML with a median age of 57 (range: 18–85) years and 59 (range: 18–88) years, respectively, whereas those in the TARGET-AML datasets were pediatric patients with AML with a median age of 10 (range: 0–23) years. (**Supplemental Table 1**) shows the detailed patient characteristics of the three included cohorts.

Metabolic Risk Score Construction

The prognostic metabolic signature was trained using GSE37642 by the LASSO Cox regression. A penalized maximum likelihood estimator was performed with 1000 bootstrap replicates (**Figure 1A**). The optimal weighting coefficients were identified by the regularization parameter lambda via the 1-SE criteria (**Figures 1A,B**). Nine metabolic genes were selected for inclusion in the prognostic metabolic model. The formula for the metabolic model was as follows: metabolic risk score = 0·018 × *ALDH2* expression − 0·103 × *CYP2E1* expression + 0·078 × *DNMT3B* expression + 0·032 × *ENPP2* expression − 0·010 × *HAAO* expression − 0·039 × *ITPKA* expression − 0·007 × *PAFAH1B2* expression + 0·040 × *PHGDH* expression + 0·015 × *PSAT1* expression. The prognostic value of the selected metabolic genes was further assessed by the log-rank test after classification as high levels and low levels based on the corresponding optimal cut-off value in the training cohort (**Supplemental Figure 2**).

Evaluation of Metabolic Risk Score

The sensitivity and specificity of the metabolic risk model were assessed through time-dependent ROC analysis. The AUCs for 1-, 3-, and 5-year OS were 0.73 [95% confidence interval (CI): 0.69–0.77], 0.78 [95% CI: 0.74–0.83], and 0.78 [95% CI: 0.73–0.83] in the training cohort, respectively (**Figure 2A**). The metabolic risk score was also calculated for each patient in the other two validation cohorts by the unified formula identified in the training cohort previously mentioned herein. The AUCs for 1-, 3-, and 5-year OS were 0.68 [95% CI: 0.60–0.77], 0.71 [95% CI: 0.61–0.81], and 0.76 [95% CI: 0.62–0.89] in the adult external cohort and 0.64 [95% CI: 0.51–0.77], 0.64 [95% CI: 0.52–0.73], and 0.66 [95% CI: 0.57–0.75] in the pediatric external cohort, respectively (**Figures 2B,C**).

We further analyzed the distribution of metabolic risk scores in patients with different survival statuses using a waterfall plot. Patients with lower metabolic risk scores generally had better survival outcomes than those with high risk scores (**Figures 2D–F**). Patients were then divided into high- and low-metabolic risk groups with the optimal cut-off determined in each cohort. Patients with a low metabolic risk had a significantly longer OS survival than those with a high metabolic risk level in the training cohort, adult external cohort, and pediatric external cohort (**Figures 2G–I**). The 5-year OS rates were 14.5% [95% CI: 10.8–18.22] vs. 55.2% [95% CI: 47.6–62.8] for the high- and low-risk groups in the training cohort, 8.7% [0.0–17.5] vs. 47.4% [30.9–63.9] for the high- and low-risk groups in the adult external cohort, and 70.7% [59.3–82.1] vs. 37.7% [28.3–47.1] for the high- and low- risk groups in the pediatric cohort, respectively. Considering the potential effect of age on the metabolic gene expression, a sensitivity analysis was also performed in the younger patients (≤65 years) in both the training cohort and adult external cohort. After excluding the elder patients, those AML patients with a low metabolic risk still obtain a significantly survival advantage than those with a high metabolic risk in the population ≤65 years (**Supplemental Figure 3**).

Univariate and Multivariate Analyses

In addition to the metabolic risk score, other prognostic values included age, *RUNX1-RUX1T1* fusion and *RUNX1* mutation in the training cohort (**Figure 3A**), age and cytogenetic risk category in the adult external cohort (**Figure 3C**), *FLT3-ITD*, *WT1* mutation and cytogenetic risk category in the pediatric external cohort (**Figure 3E**). After multivariable adjustments based on the other clinical factors, the metabolic signature remained as an independent prognostic indicator with a hazard ratio of 2.75 [95% CI: 2.06–3.66] in the training cohort (**Figure 3B**), 1.89 [95% CI: 1.09–3.29] in the adult external cohort (**Figure 3D**), and 1.96 [1.00–3.84] in the pediatric external cohort (**Figure 3F**).

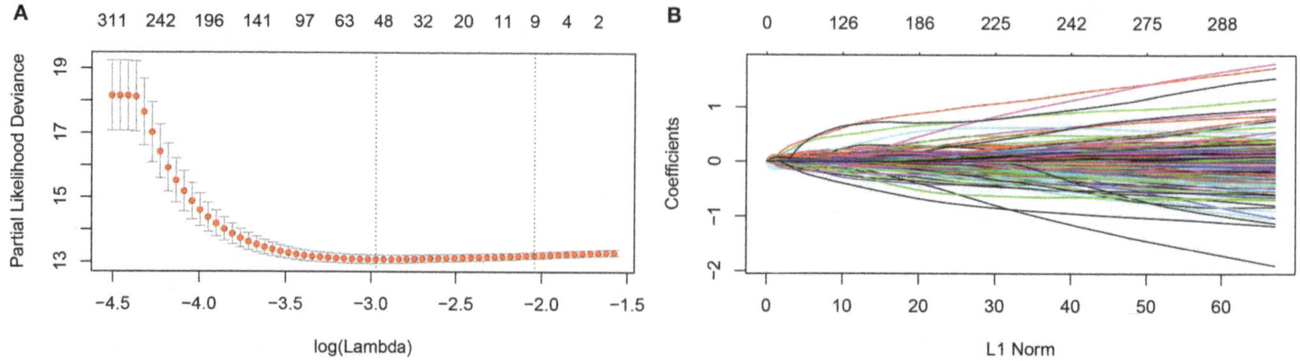

FIGURE 1 | Construction of the metabolic model. **(A)** 1,000-fold cross-validation for variable selection in the LASSO regression via 1-SE criteria. **(B)** LASSO coefficients of metabolism-related genes. Each curve represents a metabolic gene.

Clinicopathological Characteristics for Different Metabolic Risk Levels

Patients with high metabolic risk signatures were associated with an older age, lower percentage of *RUNX1_RUNX1T1*_fusion, higher percentage of *RUNX1* mutation, and higher platelet counts in the adult cohorts (including training or adult external cohort, **Figures 4A,B** and (**Supplemental Table 1**), as well as higher leukocyte counts and higher percentages of *FIL3-ITD* and blast cells in the bone marrow in the pediatric external cohort (**Figure 4C** and **Supplemental Table 1**). As expected, patients with higher metabolic risk levels had higher cytogenetic risk levels in all three cohorts (**Figure 4** and **Supplemental Table 1**). Thirty-four paired samples from TARGET dataset were further used to analyse the metabolic risk difference between the disease at diagnosis and relapse, and results showed that the patients have a higher metabolic risk at the disease relapse compared with the status at the initial diagnosis ($P = 0.022$, **Supplemental figure 4**).

GSEA

GSEA was performed in the two external cohorts to validate the metabolic-related pathway and explore other pathways enriched in different metabolic signature categories. Significantly enriched pathways were observed in the high metabolic risk group, most of which were metabolism-related pathways (**Figures 5A–D**). Among them, the biosynthesis of unsaturated fatty acids, fatty acid metabolism, and glycine, serine, and threonine metabolism were validated as enriched in the high-risk groups in both the adult and the pediatric external cohorts. Other metabolic signature-related pathways included the JAK-STAT signaling pathway, PPAR signaling pathway, mismatch repair regulation, regulation of autophagy, RNA degradation, and DNA replication (**Figures 5A–D**). Forty-eight proteins were explored from GCBI, which were interact with the 8 metabolic proteins in the model (**Figure 5E**), except for the ITPKA. In the protein-protein interaction (PPI) network, we found that the CYP2E1 and ENPP2 is interact with the proteins of phospholipase A2 family (PLA2G10, PLA2G12A, PLA2G12B, PLA2G16, PLA2G1B, PLA2G2A, PLA2G2C, PLA2G2D, PLA2G2E, PLA2G2F, PLA2G3, PLA2G4A, PLA2G4B, PLA2G4C, PLA2G4D, PLA2G4E, PLA2G4F, PLA2G5, and PLA2G6, **Figure 5E**). The interaction of nine metabolic proteins were summarized alone by STRING (**Figure 5F**).

Comparisons of Prognostic Factors and Merged Risk Scores

The prognostic sensitivity and specificity of the metabolic signature were compared to those of other potential prognostic variables. The AUC for the 5-year OS showed a significantly higher metabolic risk score (0.78 [95% CI: 0.73–0.83]) compared to that with other variables such as age 0.66 [95% CI: 0.61–0.71], *RUNX1-RUX1T1* fusion (0.47 [95% CI: 0.43–0.49]), and *RUNX1* mutation (0.58 [95% CI: 0.56–0.61]) in the training cohort (all $p < 0{\cdot}001$, **Figure 6A**). Additionally, in the adult external cohort, the metabolic risk model showed a numerically but no statistically larger AUC for the 5-year OS than the classic cytogenetic risk category (**Figure 6B**). In the pediatric external cohort, the 5-year AUC of the metabolic risk score was also equivalent to that of the cytogenetic risk category (**Figure 6C**).

Further, to generate a more accurate evaluation system, a nomogram was used to integrate the classic prognostic factors, age, and cytogenetic risk category and the present metabolic signature in the external cohorts (**Figure 7A**). The calibration plots showed that the nomogram could accurately predict the 1- and 3-year OS (**Figure 7B**). The AUC for the 5-year OS in the merged score was 0.78 [95% CI: 0.72–0.84], which was found to be significantly larger than that for the classic prognostic indicators including age (0.65 [95% CI: 0.60–0.69]) and cytogenetic risk category (0.69 [95% CI: 0.62–0.75]), indicating that adding the metabolic signature can increase the net benefit to predict OS compared to that with classic prognostic factors (**Figure 7C**).

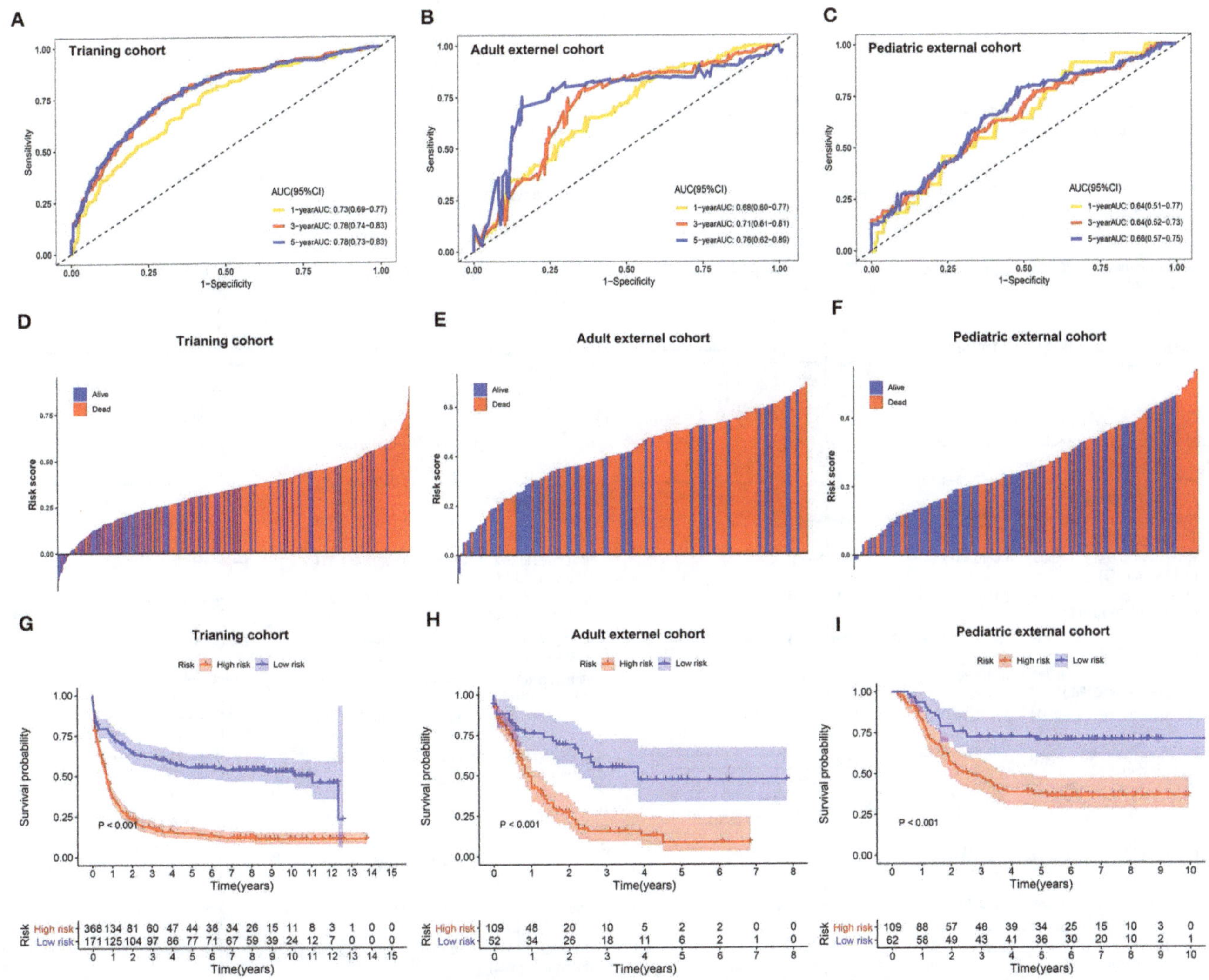

FIGURE 2 | Time-dependent receiver operating characteristic (ROC) analysis, survival outcome analysis, and Kaplan–Meier analysis of the nine-gene signature in acute myelogenous leukemia (AML). **(A–C)** Time-dependent ROC analysis for 1-, 3-, and 5-year overall survival (OS) of prognostic model in training cohort, adult external cohort, and pediatric external cohort, respectively. **(D–F)** Distribution of risk metabolic score in survival outcome analysis for training cohort, adult external cohort, and pediatric external cohort. **(G–I)** Kaplan–Meier curve of the prognostic model in the training cohort, adult external cohort, and pediatric external cohort.

DISCUSSION

Cancer cells rewire metabolic pathways to adapt to their increased nutritional demands for energy, reducing equivalents, and cellular biosynthesis (17). Leukemia cells vary the body's systemic physiology by impairing both insulin secretion and insulin sensitivity in the host to provide increased glucose to leukemia cells (18). Meanwhile, metabolism plays an important role not only in the development but also in the prognosis of leukemia (19, 20). However, prognostic models based on metabolic genes are lacking.

In the present study, a significant prognostic model based on nine metabolic genes was established in a training cohort and further verified in two independent external validation sets. The group that showed a high-risk score had poor prognosis, which was consistent across the three cohorts. The metabolic model showed a stably high prognostic value for AML, particularly for the survival of adult patients with AML. Moreover, the combination of classic prognostic factors including age and cytogenetic factors with our metabolic model improved the survival prediction compared to that with single classic risk factors, supporting the contention that the prognostic metabolic model can be utilized to supplement existing prognostic models.

In the present study, nine metabolism-related genes were identified and included in the prognostic model. The expression

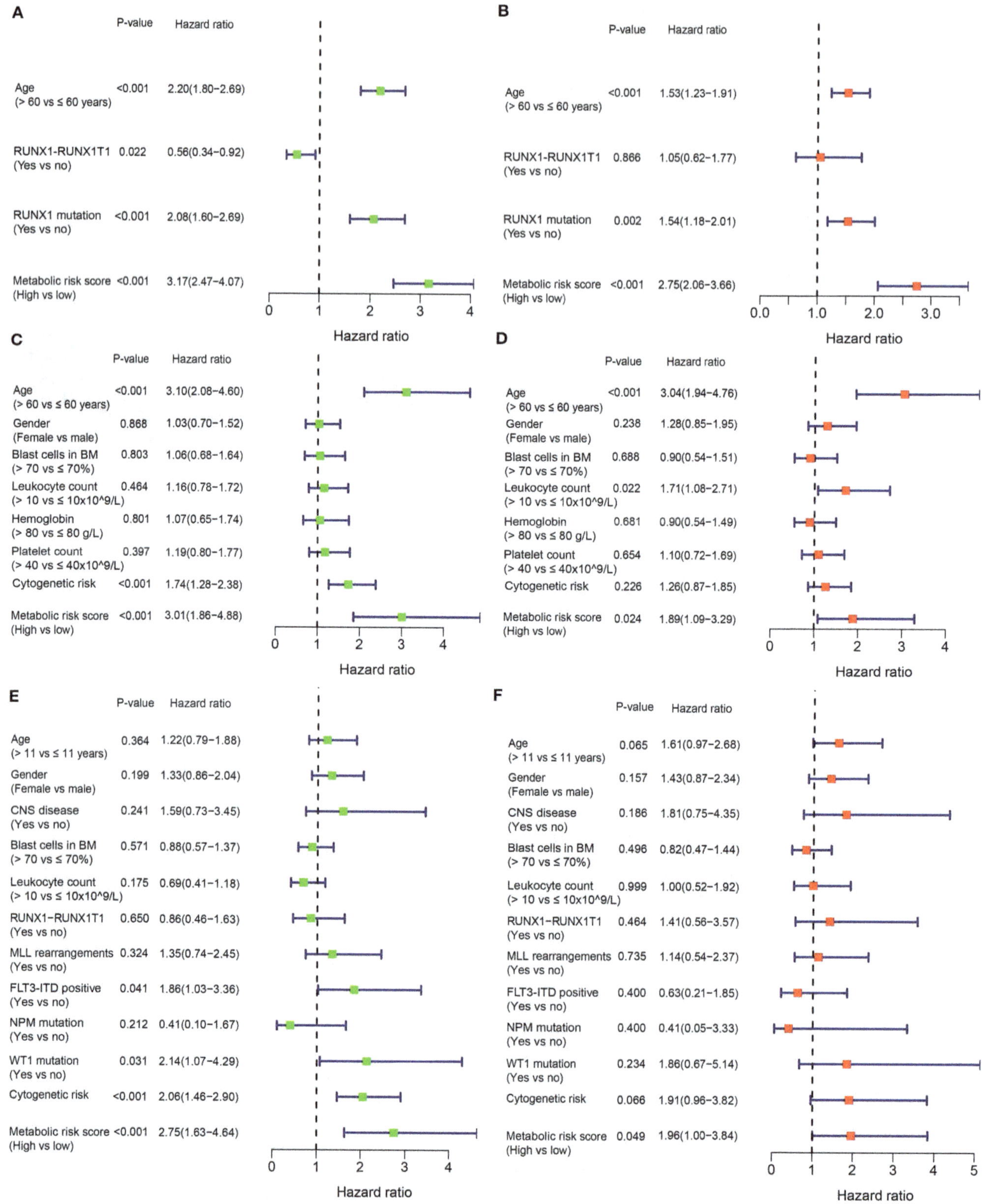

FIGURE 3 | Forest plot of the univariate (left) and multivariate (right) Cox regression analysis in the training cohort **(A,B)**, adult external cohort **(C,D)**, and pediatric external cohort **(E,F)** for acute myelogenous leukemia (AML). BM, bone marrow; CNS, central nervous system.

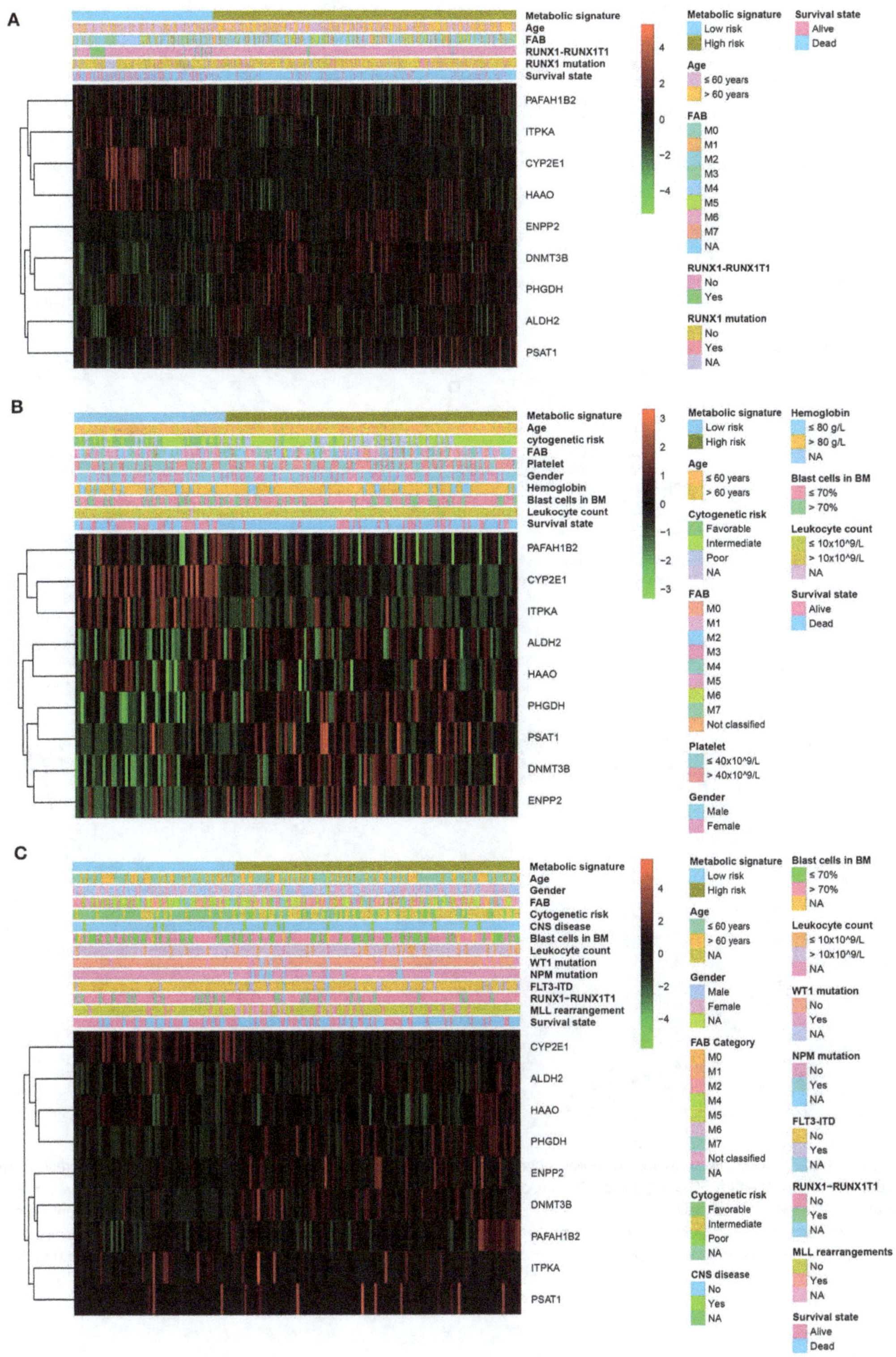

FIGURE 4 | Heatmap of the nine-gene signature and clinicopathological characteristics at different metabolic risk levels for training cohort **(A)**, adult external cohort **(B)**, and pediatric external cohort **(C)**. Each column showing gene expression or clinicopathological state represents a sample and each row represents one characteristic or gene in the model. The expression levels of the nine genes are shown in different colors. Blue and yellow indicate low- and high-risk levels, respectively. BM, bone marrow; FAB, French–American–British classification; NA, not available; CNS, central nervous system.

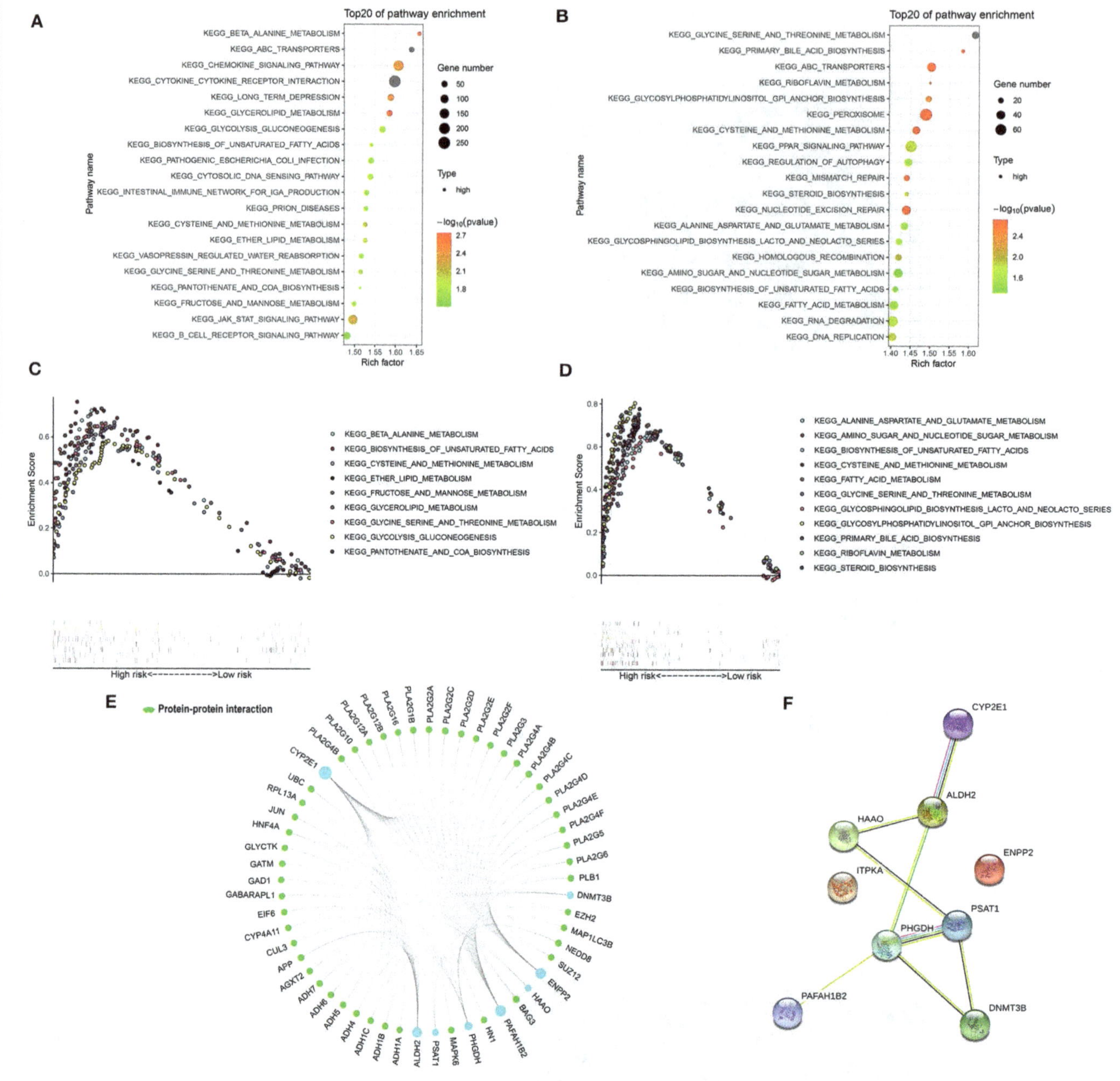

FIGURE 5 | Significantly enriched KEGG pathways in adult external cohort and pediatric external cohort based on GSEA. **(A)** Top 20 representative KEGG pathways in high-risk patients in adult external cohort ($p < 0{\cdot}05$). **(B)** Top 20 representative KEGG pathways in high-risk patients in pediatric external cohort ($p < 0{\cdot}05$). **(C)** Representative metabolic pathways in high-risk patients in adult external cohort. **(D)** Representative metabolic pathways in high-risk patients in pediatric external cohort. **(E)** The protein-protein interactions between the metabolic model related proteins and the other proteins. The model related proteins are shown in blue circles, and the size of which is determined by the number of interacting proteins. ITPKA has no known interactions with other proteins. **(F)** The interactions of 9 metabolic proteins.

of *DNMT3B*, *ALDH2*, *ENPP2*, *PHGDH*, and *PSAT1* was negatively correlated with favorable outcomes, whereas the expression of *CYP2E1*, *HAAO*, *ITPKA*, and *PAFAH1B2* was positively correlated with favorable outcomes. Most of the nine genes in our model have been reported to be involved in cancer. *DNMT3B* has been shown to play a role in genic methylation and is involved in cysteine and methionine metabolism. High expression of *DNMT3B* is independently associated with adverse outcomes in older patients with CN-AML (6, 21), which is consistent with our results. Another study verified that the ectopic expression of DNMT3B can promote the development of gastrointestinal cancers via the *de novo* methylation and transcriptional silencing of the tumor suppressor genes in mice (22). The *ITPKA* gene also participates in inositol phosphate

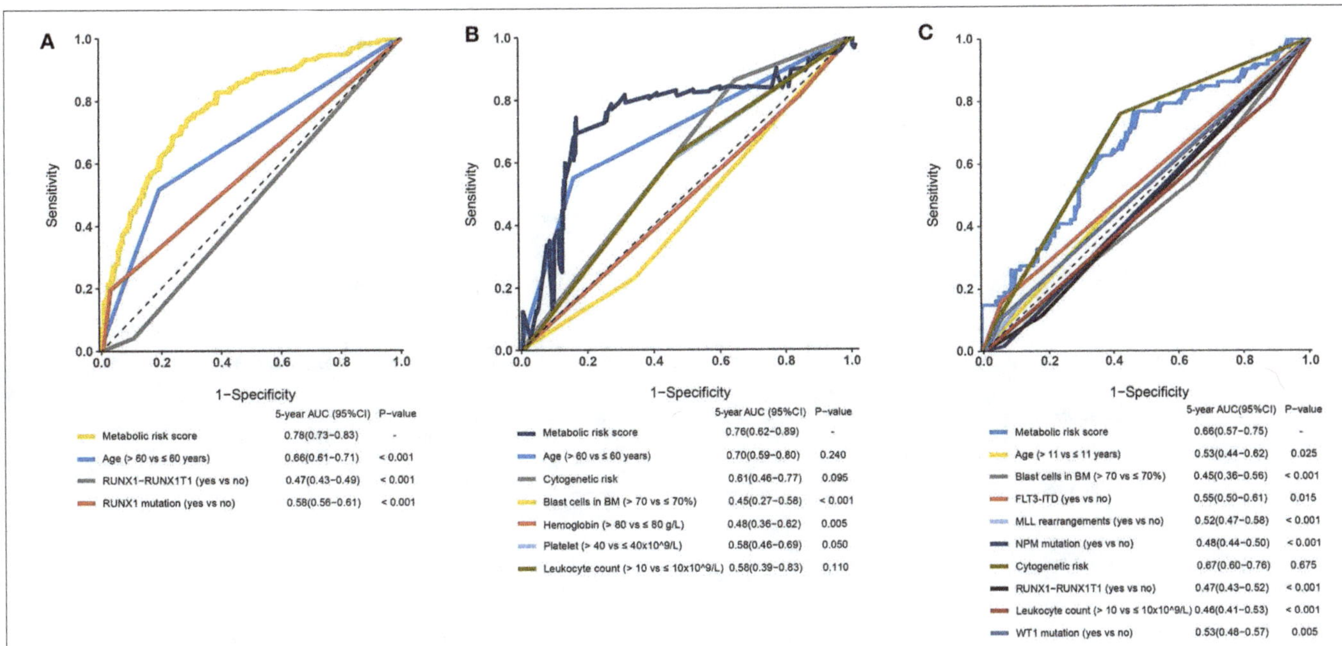

FIGURE 6 | Time-dependent receiver operating characteristic (ROC) analysis of 5-year overall survival (OS) of metabolic risk model compared to other potential prognostic factors. **(A)** Time-dependent ROC analysis for 5-year OS of metabolic risk model was compared to age, *RUNX1-RUNX1T1*, and *RUNX1* mutation in the training cohort. **(B)** Time-dependent ROC analysis for 5-year OS of metabolic risk model was compared to age, cytogenetics risk, blast cells in bone marrow, hemoglobin, platelet, and leukocyte count in the adult external cohort. **(C)** Time-dependent ROC analysis for 5-year OS of metabolic risk model compared to age, blast cells in the bone marrow, cytogenetics risk, *RUNX1-RUNX1T1* fusion, *FLT3-ITD* status, *MLL*-rearrangement, *NPM* mutation, leukocyte count, and *WT1* mutation in the pediatric external cohort. BM, bone marrow.

metabolism, and was found to be hypermethylated in patients with AML with a normal karyotype (23). *ENPP2*, which encodes the enzyme autotaxin, was found to be over-expressed in various cancers (24). A previous study reported that *FLT3-ITD* mutations in AML are closely associated with the high expression of *ENPP2* and may influence disease prognosis via the dysregulation of metabolism-related genes such as *ENPP2* (25–27). As the metabolism-associated gene with the highest weight in the model, *CYP2E* showed a positive association with the prognosis of patients with AML in our study. This enzyme plays a vital role in the production of reactive oxygen species and is involved in drug metabolism. The PPI network in our study also suggested the interaction between the phospholipase family and CYP2E1 and ENPP2. Arachidonic acid metabolism pathway and ether lipid metabolism pathway can be the potential interaction of the phospholipase family and the two metabolic genes (28, 29). Although the role of *CYP2E1* expression in the pathogenesis of AML remains unclear, polymorphisms in these gene have been shown to be associated with the risk of leukemia but not the risk of treatment-related leukemia (30–32). Decreased ALDH enzyme activity may lead to DNA damage due to the accumulation of aldehydes (33). In this study, *ALDH2* was an adverse prognostic factor in the model. A decrease in the ALDH2-GA or ALDH2-AA genotype was reported to accelerate the conversion of Fanconi anemia to MDS/AML (34). *PAFAH1B2*, which is involved in ether lipid metabolism, may also be broadly dysregulated in many types of cancer (35) and its over-expression at the transcriptional and at the protein levels in *MYC*-negative high-grade B-cell lymphomas is associated with good prognosis. Interestingly, we found different expression trends for *PAFAH1B2* between the childhood and adult leukemia metabolic profiles. This may be because of variations in the age-related regulation of the metabolism-related signature between adults and children. Other selected variables including *HAAO*, *PHGDH*, and *PSAT* were also found to predict the prognosis of AML. However, their mechanism with respect to AML remains unclear and requires further clarification.

As expected, the most significantly enriched pathways were metabolism-related in the GSEA, confirming the metabolic-related characteristics of the nine-gene signature. The high enrichment of metabolism-related and DNA repair-related pathways in the high-risk group in both independent validation cohorts indicates the potential benefit of targeting metabolism-related genes and PAPR inhibitor therapy for this population. However, the predictive value of the metabolic signature for these therapies should be further validated based on a large cohort in prospective trials.

We first focused on the role of metabolic genes in the prognosis of AML and constructed a prenotice significant model for AML stratification. However, several issues must

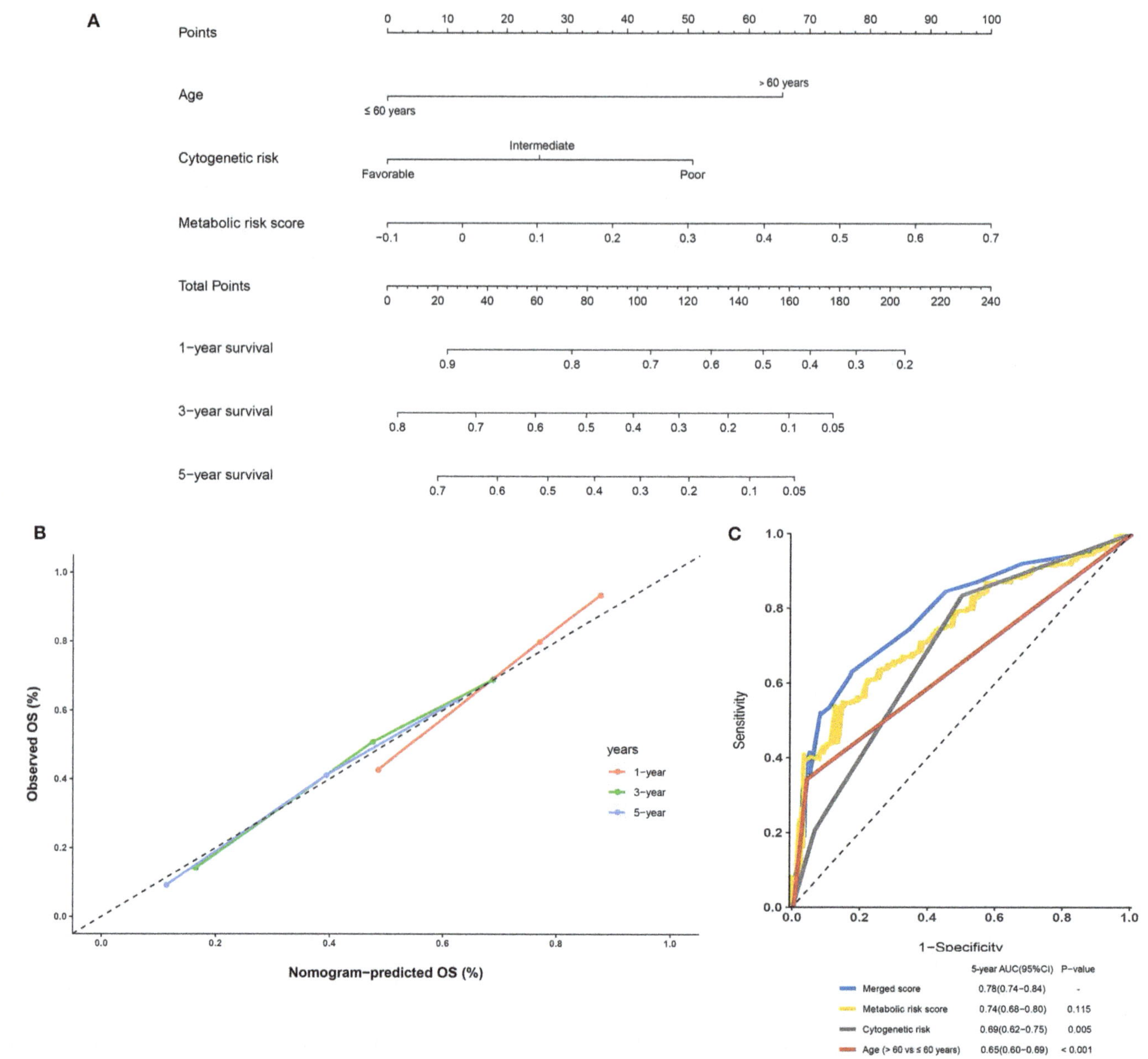

FIGURE 7 | Building and validation of the nomogram to predict the overall survival of patients with acute myelogenous leukemia (AML) combining the adult external cohort and pediatric external cohort. **(A)** Nomogram plot was built based on age, cytogenetics risk, metabolic risk score, and total points combining the adult external cohort and pediatric external cohort. **(B)** Calibration plot of the nomogram. **(C)** Time-dependent receiver operating characteristic (ROC) curves of nomograms were compared based on a 5-year OS of AML.

be resolved. First, some clinical information such as the history of metabolic disorders and therapeutic information are lacking because this information was not available in public databases. Therefore, it is difficult to evaluate the association between metabolism and therapy and to avoid the inclusion of non-leukemia-related metabolic events. Moreover, validating our model in the real world is indispensable for extrapolating the established model to other AML populations, particularly childhood AML patients. Functional experiments are also needed to determine the mechanisms underlying the effects of the prognostic metabolic genes in AML. Finally, the diagnostic value of the metabolic risk score was not evaluated in this analysis, and need to be further explored in the perspective study.

CONCLUSION

We established a prognostic metabolic model based on the metabolism-related genes in AML. The characteristic metabolic genes may reflect the disordered microenvironment of the bone marrow and may be used as potential biomarkers for AML prognosis. Validation of the model in the real world and functional experiments of the predictive metabolic genes are needed.

AUTHOR CONTRIBUTIONS

YW, JX, and YL: conceptualization. YW and FH: methodology and writing original draft. JL: validation. FH, YW, and RN: formal analysis and investigation. YL: resources, supervision, project administration, and funding acquisition. YC: data curation. YW, FH, and JL: writing, review, and editing. SC, LS, and DD: supervision.

ACKNOWLEDGMENTS

We thank platforms of TCGA, GEO, and TARGET datasets for data download and AMLCG for their work on leukemia. We also thank Herold T, Hiddemann W, and Chen J for their contributions to AML study of GSE37642.

REFERENCES

1. Ferrara F, Schiffer CA. Acute myeloid leukaemia in adults. *Lancet.* (2013) 381:484–95. doi: 10.1016/S0140-6736(12)61727-9
2. Wouters BJ, Delwel R. Epigenetics and approaches to targeted epigenetic therapy in acute myeloid leukemia. *Blood.* (2016) 127:42–52. doi: 10.1182/blood-2015-07-604512
3. Burnett A, Wetzler M, Lowenberg B. Therapeutic advances in acute myeloid leukemia. *J Clin Oncol.* (2011) 29:487–94. doi: 10.1200/Jco.2010.30.1820
4. Dohner H, Estey E, Grimwade D, Amadori S, Appelbaum FR, Buchner T, et al. Diagnosis and management of AML in adults: 2017 ELN recommendations from an international expert panel. *Blood.* (2017) 129:424–47. doi: 10.1182/blood-2016-08-733196
5. Hao XX, Gu H, Chen CQ, Huang D, Zhao YZ, Xie L, et al. Metabolic imaging reveals a unique preference of symmetric cell division and homing of leukemia-initiating cells in an endosteal niche. *Cell Metab.* (2019) 29:950–65.e6. doi: 10.1016/j.cmet.2018.11.013
6. Niederwieser C, Kohlschmidt J, Volinia S, Whitman SP, Metzeler KH, Eisfeld AK, et al. Prognostic and biologic significance of DNMT3B expression in older patients with cytogenetically normal primary acute myeloid leukemia. *Leukemia.* (2015) 29:567–75. doi: 10.1038/leu.2014.267
7. Rucker FG, Agrawal M, Corbacioglu A, Weber D, Kapp-Schwoerer S, Gaidzik VI, et al. Measurable residual disease monitoring in acute myeloid leukemia with t(8;21)(q22;q22.1): results from the AML study group. *Blood.* (2019) 134:1608–18. doi: 10.1182/blood.2019001425
8. Hanahan D, Weinberg RA. Hallmarks of cancer: the next generation. *Cell.* (2011) 144:646–74. doi: 10.1016/j.cell.2011.02.013
9. Qu W, Oya S, Lieberman BP, Ploessl K, Wang L, Wise DR, et al. Preparation and characterization of L-[5-11C]-glutamine for metabolic imaging of tumors. *J Nucl Med.* (2012) 53:98–105. doi: 10.2967/jnumed.111.093831
10. Jones CL, Stevens BM, D'Alessandro A, Reisz JA, Culp-Hill R, Nemkov T, et al. Inhibition of amino acid metabolism selectively targets human leukemia stem cells. *Cancer Cell.* (2018) 34:724–40.e4. doi: 10.1016/j.ccell.2018.10.005
11. Ha M, Han ME, Kim JY, Jeong DC, Oh SO, Kim YH. Prognostic role of TPD52 in acute myeloid leukemia: a retrospective multicohort analysis. *J Cell Biochem.* (2019) 120:3672–8. doi: 10.1002/jcb.27645
12. Huls G. Azacitidine in AML: a treatment option? *Blood.* (2015) 126:283–4. doi: 10.1182/blood-2015-06-648071
13. DiNardo CD, Pratz KW, Letai A, Jonas BA, Wei AH, Thirman M, et al. Safety and preliminary efficacy of venetoclax with decitabine or azacitidine in elderly patients with previously untreated acute myeloid leukaemia: a non-randomised, open-label, phase 1b study. *Lancet Oncol.* (2018) 19:216–28. doi: 10.1016/S1470-2045(18)30010-X
14. Pollyea DA, Stevens BM, Jones CL, Winters A, Pei SS, Minhajuddin M, et al. Venetoclax with azacitidine disrupts energy metabolism and targets leukemia stem cells in patients with acute myeloid leukemia. *Nat Med.* (2018) 24:1859–66. doi: 10.1038/s41591-018-0233-1
15. Garber K. First metabolic oncology inhibitor gets FDA green light, with record price tag. *Nat Biotechnol.* (2017) 35:895. doi: 10.1038/nbt1017-895
16. Li ZJ, Herold T, He CJ, Valk PJM, Chen P, Jurinovic V, et al. Identification of a 24-gene prognostic signature that improves the European leukemianet risk classification of acute myeloid leukemia: an international collaborative study. *J Clin Oncol.* (2013) 31:1172–81. doi: 10.1200/Jco.2012.44.3184
17. Tabe Y, Lorenzi PL, Konopleva M. Amino acid metabolism in hematologic malignancies and the era of targeted therapy. *Blood.* (2019) 134:1014–23. doi: 10.1182/blood.2019001034
18. Ye HB, Adane B, Khan N, Alexeev E, Nusbacher N, Minhajuddin M, et al. Subversion of systemic glucose metabolism as a mechanism to support the growth of leukemia cells. *Cancer Cell.* (2018) 34:659–73.e6. doi: 10.1016/j.ccell.2018.08.016
19. Herst PM, Howman RA, Neeson PJ, Berridge MV, Ritchie DS. The level of glycolytic metabolism in acute myeloid leukemia blasts at diagnosis is prognostic for clinical outcome. *J Leukoc Biol.* (2011) 89:51–5. doi: 10.1189/jlb.0710417
20. Chen WL, Wang JH, Zhao AH, Xu X, Wang YH, Chen TL, et al. A distinct glucose metabolism signature of acute myeloid leukemia with prognostic value. *Blood.* (2014) 124:1645–54. doi: 10.1182/blood-2014-02-554204
21. Mishra A, Liu SJ, Sams GH, Curphey DP, Santhanam R, Rush LJ, et al. Aberrant overexpression of IL-15 initiates large granular lymphocyte leukemia through chromosomal instability and DNA hypermethylation. *Cancer Cell.* (2012) 22:645–55. doi: 10.1016/j.ccr.2012.09.009
22. Linhart HG, Lin H, Yamada Y, Moran E, Steine EJ, Gokhale S, et al. Dnmt3b promotes tumorigenesis *in vivo* by gene-specific *de novo* methylation and transcriptional silencing. *Genes Dev.* (2007) 21:3110–22. doi: 10.1101/gad.1594007
23. Sonnet M, Claus R, Becker N, Zucknick M, Petersen J, Lipka DB, et al. Early aberrant DNA methylation events in a mouse model of acute myeloid leukemia. *Genome Med.* (2014) 6:34. doi: 10.1186/gm551
24. Argaud D, Boulanger MC, Chignon A, Mkannez G, Mathieu P. Enhancer-mediated enrichment of interacting JMJD3-DDX21 to ENPP2 locus prevents R-loop formation and promotes transcription. *Nucleic Acids Res.* (2019) 47:8424–38. doi: 10.1093/nar/gkz560

25. Schnittger S, Schoch C, Dugas M, Kern W, Staib P, Wuchter C, et al. Analysis of FLT3 length mutations in 1003 patients with acute myeloid leukemia: correlation to cytogenetics, FAB subtype, and prognosis in the AMLCG study and usefulness as a marker for the detection of minimal residual disease. *Blood.* (2002) 100:59–66. doi: 10.1182/blood.V100.1.59
26. Yanada M, Matsuo K, Suzuki T, Kiyoi H, Naoe T. Prognostic significance of FLT3 internal tandem duplication and tyrosine kinase domain mutations for acute myeloid leukemia: a meta-analysis. *Leukemia.* (2005) 19:1345–9. doi: 10.1038/sj.leu.2403838
27. Janke H, Pastore F, Schumacher D, Herold T, Hopfner KP, Schneider S, et al. Activating FLT3 mutants show distinct gain-of-function phenotypes *in vitro* and a characteristic signaling pathway profile associated with prognosis in acute myeloid leukemia. *PLoS ONE.* (2014) 9:e89560. doi: 10.1371/journal.pone.0089560
28. Spector AA, Fang X, Snyder GD, Weintraub NL. Epoxyeicosatrienoic acids (EETs): metabolism and biochemical function. *Prog Lipid Res.* (2004) 43:55–90. doi: 10.1016/s0163-7827(03)00049-3
29. Sakagami H, Aoki J, Natori Y, Nishikawa K, Kakehi Y, Natori Y, et al. Biochemical and molecular characterization of a novel choline-specific glycerophosphodiester phosphodiesterase belonging to the nucleotide pyrophosphatase/phosphodiesterase family. *J Biol Chem.* (2005) 280:23084–93. doi: 10.1074/jbc.M413438200
30. Aydin-Sayitoglu M, Hatirnaz O, Erensoy N, Ozbek U. Role of CYP2D6, CYP1A1, CYP2E1, GSTT1, and GSTM1 genes in the susceptibility to acute leukemias. *Am J Hematol.* (2006) 81:162–70. doi: 10.1002/ajh.20434
31. Bolufer P, Collado M, Barragan E, Calasanz MJ, Colomer D, Tormo M, et al. Profile of polymorphisms of drug-metabolising enzymes and the risk of therapy-related leukaemia. *Br J Haematol.* (2007) 136:590–6. doi: 10.1111/j.1365-2141.2006.06469.x
32. Vijayakrishnan J, Houlston RS. Candidate gene association studies and risk of childhood acute lymphoblastic leukemia: a systematic review and meta-analysis. *Haematologica.* (2010) 95:1405–14. doi: 10.3324/haematol.2010.022095
33. Hira A, Yabe H, Yoshida K, Okuno Y, Shiraishi Y, Chiba K, et al. Variant ALDH2 is associated with accelerated progression of bone marrow failure in Japanese Fanconi anemia patients. *Blood.* (2013) 122:3206–9. doi: 10.1182/blood-2013-06-507962
34. Yabe M, Koike T, Ohtsubo K, Imai E, Morimoto T, Takakura H, et al. Associations of complementation group, ALDH2 genotype, and clonal abnormalities with hematological outcome in Japanese patients with Fanconi anemia. *Ann Hematol.* (2019) 98:271–80. doi: 10.1007/s00277-018-3517-0
35. Kohnz RA, Mulvihill MM, Chang JW, Hsu KL, Sorrentino A, Cravatt BF, et al. Activity-based protein profiling of oncogene-driven changes in metabolism reveals broad dysregulation of PAFAH1B2 and 1B3 in cancer. *ACS Chem Biol.* (2015) 10:1624–30. doi: 10.1021/acschembio.5b00053

12

Increased Serum Level of Interleukin-10 Predicts Poor Survival and Early Recurrence in Patients with Peripheral T-Cell Lymphomas

Yan Zhang[1,2†]*, Yanlong Zheng*[1†]*, Lihong Shou*[2]*, Yuanfei Shi*[1]*, Huafei Shen*[1]*, Mingyu Zhu*[1]*, Xiujin Ye*[1]*, Jie Jin*[1] *and Wanzhuo Xie*[1*]

[1] *Department of Hematology, The First Affiliated Hospital, College of Medicine, Zhejiang University, Hangzhou, China,*
[2] *Department of Hematology, Huzhou Central Hospital, Affiliated Cent Hospital of Huzhou University, Huzhou, China*

Correspondence:
Wanzhuo Xie
xiewanzhuo@zju.edu.cn

†*These authors have contributed equally to this work*

Peripheral T cell lymphoma (PTCL) is an alloplasm group of aggressive and lymphoproliferative tumors with heterogeneous morphological changes of mature T cell immunophenotype. It has multiple subtypes and most of them have poor prognosis. Interleukin 10 (IL-10) is one kind of multi-cell-derived and multifunctional cytokine. It regulates the growth and differentiation of cells, participates in inflammation and immune response, plays an important role in tumor and infection, and is closely related to blood system diseases. Therefore, we implemented a retrospective study of 205 patients who were newly diagnosed with PTCL to explore the relationship between IL-10 and prognosis and early recurrence. We found patients with IL-10 ≥3.6 pg/ml achieved a lower CR rate and higher 1-year recurrence rate than patients with IL-10 <3.6 pg/ml (14.4 vs. 51.9%; 17.6 vs. 49.5%). On multivariate analysis, moreover, elevated IL-10 is an extremely important prognostic factor in PTCL, which can lead to worsening of overall survival (OS), low complete response (CR) rate and higher early relapse rate. Therefore, measurement of IL-10 levels in peripheral blood at the initial stage are useful for predicting the prognosis and helping us to make different treatment plans for individual patients. In the near future, IL-10 inhibitors or antagonists may become a new method of immunotargeting therapy for patients with PTCL.

Keywords: peripheral T-cell lymphoma, interleukin-10, complete response, prognosis, early recurrence

INTRODUCTION

Peripheral T cell lymphoma (PTCL) is a group of rare lymphoid malignancies with heterogeneous morphological that originating from post-thymic T cells or mature natural killer (NK) cells, accounting for about 10% of all non-Hodgkin's lymphomas (NHL) in Western countries (1). However, the morbidity of PTCL is higher in Asia, it makes up 25–30% of NHL in China (2). According to the WHO classification, PTCL can be further distinguished based on their immunophenotypical, morphological, biological, and clinical features (3). The most common subtypes include PTCL-not otherwise specified (PTCL-NOS), extra-nodal natural killer (NK)/T cell lymphoma, nasal type (ENKTL), angioimmunoblastic T-cell lymphoma (AITL), anaplastic large-cell lymphoma (ALCL), include ALCL anaplastic lymphoma kinase positive(ALCL, ALK +), and ALCL anaplastic lymphoma kinase negative

(ALCL, ALK-). Relatively uncommon subtypes include monomorphic epitheliotropic intestinal T-cell lymphoma (MEITL), T-cell Large Granular Lymphocytic Leukemia (T-LGLL), subcutaneous panniculitis like T-cell lymphoma (SPTCL), mycosisfungoides/Sezary's syndrome (MF/SS), Hepatosplenic T-cell lymphoma (HSTCL), and so on. The overall characteristics of them are aggressive clinical course and poor response to therapy. Due to its rarity and heterogeneity, prognostic studies on PTCL are relatively scarce.

The development of science and technology as a whole society has promoted the development of molecular biology and the understanding of PTCL is greatly improved, particularly in tumor micro-environment. Interleukin 10 (IL-10) is one kind of multi-cell-derived and multifunctional cytokine. It regulates the growth and differentiation of cells, participates in inflammation and immune response, plays an important role in tumor and infection, and is closely related to blood system diseases. It is mainly excreted by activated T cells, monocytes, B cells, macrophages, certain tumor cells and so on. Not only that, various studies have shown that IL-10 can promote the development of tumor cells. Studies have shown that some malignant T cells can grow and survive well, but they are mainly closely related to (M2) macrophages that are alternately activated within the microenvironment. Moreover, IL-10 will have an enhanced effect to some extent (4). In addition, the abnormality of JAK/STAT pathway will promote IL-10-mediated lymphoid hyperplasia by M2 macrophages (5). The GATA-binding protein 3 (GATA3) is a transcription factor related to the type 2 helper (Th2) cell. If GATA3 is overexpressed, it will affect the survival rate of PTCL, to be precise, it will reduce the survival rate (6). Not only that, it also induces the expression of Th2-related cytokines, such as IL-10 (7). In this way, IL-10 has more ways to help malignant lymphocytes express genetic material, achieve the purpose of reproduction, and promote immune escape of tumor. Because previous studies had shown that IL-10 is associated with abnormal proliferation of cancer cells in a variety of cancers (breast cancer, cervical cancer, thyroid cancer, etc.) (8–10). Moreover, the role of IL-10 in Hodgkin's lymphoma, diffuse large B-cell lymphoma (DLBCL) and Burkitt's lymphoma had also been extensively studied (11, 12). However, little is known about the effects of IL-10 on response and prognosis, especially the early recurrence or progression of PTCL patients. Consequently, we retrospectively analyzed 205 PTCL patients, and aimed to study the significance of IL-10 in their treatment response, survival rate, and early relapse.

The writing of our article refers to the Reporting Recommendations for Tumor Marker Prognostic Studies (REMARK): Explanation and Elaboration guidelines (13).

MATERIALS AND METHODS

Patients and Control Subjects

This is a single-center retrospective cohort analysis of 205 newly diagnosed PTCL patients at the First Affiliated Hospital of Zhejiang University School of Medicine from January 2014 to June 2019. The inclusion criteria for this retrospective study were as follows: (1) Age ≥18 years; (2) Pathological diagnosis of PTCL; (3) No long-term glucocorticoid treatment or chemotherapy before collecting clinical data; (4) Complete Clinical data. According to the Helsinki statement, all patients in our study signed an informed consent form before peripheral blood was drawn. Although the treatment regimens of PTCL patients in our study were inconsistent, most patients received combination chemotherapy, including cyclophosphamide-doxorubicin-vincristine-prednisone (CHOP) or CHOP-like regimens, and all the ENKTL patients' chemotherapy containing Pegaspargase. The final observation time was January 2020, and the median follow-up time was 14 months.

Measurement and Evaluation Indicators

We reviewed medical records, physical examinations, laboratory results, pathology reports, and radiological findings to reanalyze the clinical data of these patients. The following experimental and clinical data were collected: age at diagnosis, sex, International Prognostic Index (oncology) (IPI) score, Eastern Cooperative Oncology Group (ECOG), Ann Arbor stage, B symptoms (fever, night sweating, or weight loss), serum albumin level, bone marrow involvement, Hemophagocytic syndrome (HPS), serum interleukin-6 level (IL-6), serum interleukin-10 level (IL-10), serum interferon γ level (IFN γ), Epstein-Barr virus(EBV) infection, number of involved extra-nodal sites, serum lactate dehydrogenase (LDH), beta-2 micro-globulin(β2-MG) and serum ferritin (SF). Regular imaging examinations were performed after treatment, and disease status were recorded and analyzed. Follow-up was performed by making phone calls or reviewing medical records. Progression was defined as an increase in volume of the original focus or the development of a new focus. Early recurrence was defined as relapse or progressive disease occurrence within 1-year post-chemotherapy. OS was defined as the time from diagnosis to death for any reasons or last follow-up.

Detection of Cytokines in Peripheral Blood of Patients

The levels of cytokines in peripheral blood were detected by CBA (cytomic beam array system) flow cytometry according to the manufacturer's instructions.

Statistical Analysis

Post hoc power analyses were conducted with GPOWER (Faul, Erdfelder, Lang, & Buchner, 2007) in order to estimate the probability of occurrence of effects in the sample. The optimal cut-off values of interleukin 10, interleukin 6, and interferon gamma levels were determined by receiver operating characteristic (ROC) curve analysis. They were associated with survival status of patients. Through the normal distribution test, the continuous variables included in this study all conform to the normal distribution. Continuous variables were grouped according to the usual clinical threshold and were presented as frequencies and percentages (n, %) in company with categorical variables. All hierarchical and categorical variables were compared by Pearson's chi-square test. Among them, histological subtypes were performed bonferroni-post-hoc-correction. The survival curve was attained *via* Kaplan-Meier method and the log-rank test. Univariate and multivariate logistic regression models were used to evaluate the relevance between clinical variables and complete remission (CR) and 1-year recurrence or progression. Cox proportional hazards regression model was used to analyze univariate and multivariate of OS. All statistical analyses were calculated by statistical software package SPSS 23.0. In all comparisons, $p<0.05$ was considered to be statistically significant.

RESULTS

Patients Characteristics and Clinical Outcomes According to the Different Levels of IL-10

According to the criteria, we selected 205 patients with PTCL from January 2014 to June 2019. **Table 1** lists the clinical characteristics and laboratory data of all enrolled patients. The median age at diagnosis was 56 years (range: 18–79 years), and the ratio of male to female was 1.8:1. Eighty point five percent of these patients were in stage III-IV, and 55.1% of them had B symptoms. ENKTL accounted for 33.6% of all pathological subtypes, PTCL-NOS, AITL and ALCL accounted for 21.8, 27.5, and 12.7% respectively. In addition, there were 68 cases of bone marrow involvement, and 24 cases of HPS. More than one extranodal location was involved in 98 patients, and 120 patients were infected with EBV at the first diagnosis. The serum LDH levels were increased in 66.3% of the patients, meanwhile the levels of β2-MG were increased in 63.9%. According to the IPI risk classification, 54.1% of patients (n = 111) were at high or high-moderate risk. **Table 1** shows the clinical characteristics of patients with different IL-10 levels. It shows that patients with IL-10 levels exceeding 3.6 pg/ml have higher IPI scores and ECOG scores, and the proportion of B symptoms and HPS were significantly higher than those with IL-10 levels less than 3.6 pg/ml. Patients with IL-10 levels higher than 3.6 pg/ml had higher proportion of LDH, β2-MG, and SF. However, the different subtypes of PTCL did not show statistical significance in the stratification of IL-10 in our study, either by Pearson's chi square test (P = 0.287) or performing bonferroni-post-hoc-correction(P = 0.288).

Association of Serum Cytokines With Survival Outcome and Early Recurrence

We had analyzed six cytokines: IL-4, IL-6, IL-10, TNFα, IFNγ, and IL-17A. Only IL-6, IL-10, and IFNγ were found to have statistical significance on the survival and prognosis of PTCL patients and the median value and range of serum levels of these three cytokines were as follows: IL-10 (3.13 pg/ml, range: 0.1–8536.4 pg/ml), IL-6 (6.65 pg/ml, range: 0.1–815.2 pg/ml), and IFN-γ (1.44 pg/ml, range: 0–1330.9 pg/ml), respectively. According to the ROC curve, the cutoff values of IL-6, IL-10, and IFNγ were determined to be 2.2 pg/ml, 3.6 pg/ml and 3.0 pg/ml, respectively. The area under the curve are 0.572, 0.736, 0.634 for the IL-6, IL-10 and IFNγ (**Figure 1**). Therefore, the high group and low group were defined as being greater than or equal to the cutoff value and less than the cutoff value, respectively. Post hoc analysis demonstrated sufficient power to distinguish the significant differences (power = 0.945). Patients with IL-10 ≥3.6 pg/ml, only 14.4% of them achieved CR after treatment, but the rate of recurrence or progression within one year was nearly half, reaching 49.5%. In the group of patients with IL-10 <3.6 pg/ml, more than half of them achieved CR (51.9%) after treatment, and only 17.6% of patients relapsed or progressed within one year. Therefore, it is not difficult to speculate that patients with IL-10 ≥3.6 pg/ml may have poor therapeutic effect and are prone to early recurrence (**Table 1**). Also, the patients with IL-10 ≥3.6 pg/ml achieved lower OS and higher early recurrence or progression rate (**Figures 2A, B**, P value < 0.001). In addition, the cumulative survival rate and cumulative 1-year recurrence or progression rate between the high IL-6 and low IL-6 groups and the high IFNγ and low IFNγ groups were statistically significant (**Figures 2C–F**, all P value<0.001). To our disappointment, they were not independent factors (**Tables 3, 4**).

In univariate logistic regression analysis, lower CR rate was related to male, first diagnosis older than 60 years, stage III-IV, B symptoms, bone marrow involvement, IPI ≥3, ECOG ≥3, EBV infection, Extra-nodal ≥1, IL-10 ≥3.6 pg/ml, IL-6 ≥2.2 pg/ml, IFN γ ≥3.0 pg/ml, decreased LDH and decreased β2-MG (**Table 2**). Nevertheless, in the multivariate logistic regression analysis, only ECOG ≥3, EBV infection, IL-10 ≥3.6 pg/ml were statistically significant (**Table 2**).

In univariate logistic regression analysis, higher 1-year recurrence or progression rate was associated with stage III-IV, B symptoms, bone marrow involvement, IPI ≥3, ECOG ≥3, decreased albumin, Extra-nodal ≥1, IL-10 ≥3.6 pg/ml, IL-6 ≥2.2 pg/ml, IFN γ ≥3.0 pg/ml, decreased SF (**Table 3, Figures 2B, D, E**). However, only bone marrow involvement (OR = 3.799, 95% CI 1.630–8.854, p = 0.002), ECOG ≥3(OR = 5.873, 95% CI 2.464–13.997, p < 0.001), IL-10 ≥3.6 pg/ml(OR = 2.008, 95% CI 0.876–4.601, p = 0.009) had statistically significant in the multivariate logistic regression analysis (**Table 3**).

Univariate and Multivariate Cox Proportional Hazards Regression Analysis of OS in PTCL Patients

In our study, recurrence or progression occurred in 67 patients within one year, accounting for 32.7%. The median survival time in the groups with IL-10 ≥3.6 pg/ml and IL-10 <3.6 pg/ml were 6 months and 26 months (**Figure 2A**), respectively. Compared with patients with IL-10 <3.6 pg/ml, 1-year OS and 2-year OS were lower in patients with IL-10 ≥3.6 pg/ml (80.6 vs. 20.6%, p < 0.001; 54.6 vs. 11.3%, p < 0.001, **Figure 2A**). The univariate analysis showed that stage III-IV, B symptoms, bone marrow involvement, IPI ≥3, ECOG ≥3, decreased albumin, EBV infection, Extra-nodal ≥1, HPS, IL-10 ≥3.6 pg/ml, IL-6 ≥2.2 pg/ml, IFN γ ≥3.0 pg/ml, decreased LDH and decreased serum ferritin were prognostic indicators of OS (**Table 4, Figures 2C, E**). Then, multivariate analysis was showed that patients

TABLE 1 | Analysis of clinical and laboratory characteristics of IL-10 stratification in 205 patients with PTCL.

characteristic	total (n=205,%)	IL-10<3.6pg/ml (n=108, %)	IL-10≥3.6pg/ml (n=97, %)	p Value
Age				0.120
<60years	127(62.0)	72(66.7)	56(57.7)	
≥60years	78(38.0)	36(33.3)	41(42.3)	
Sex				0.009*
Male	132(64.4)	61(56.5)	71(73.2	
Female	73(35.6)	47(43.5)	26(26.8)	
IPI				0.000*
0-2	94(45.9)	70(64.8)	24(24.7)	
3-5	111(54.1)	38(35.2)	73(75.3)	
ECOG				0.000*
0-2	154(75.1)	94(87.0)	60(61.9)	
3-5	51(24.9)	14(13.0)	37(38.1)	
Stage				0.000*
I-II	40(19.5)	36(33.3)	4(4.1)	
III-IV	165(80.5)	72(66.7)	93(95.9)	
B symptoms				0.000*
Yes	113(55.1)	45(41.7)	68(70.1)	
No	92(44.9)	63(58.3)	29(29.9)	
Histological subtype				0.287
PTCL,NOS	57(27.8)	36(33.3)	23(23.7)	
ENKTL	69(33.6)	36(33.3)	31(32.0)	
AITL	44(21.5)	20(18.5)	24(24.7)	
ALCL,ALK+	16(7.8)	8(7.4)	8(8.3)	
ALCL,ALK-	10(4.9)	6(5.6)	4(4.1)	
Others[#]	9(4.4)	2(1.9)	7(7.2)	
Bone marrow Involvement				0.000*
Yes	68(33.2)	23(78.7)	45(46.4)	
No	137(66.8)	85(21.3)	52(53.6)	
Albumin(g/l)				0.000*
<35	58(28.3)	12(11.1)	46(47.4)	
≥35	147(71.7)	96(88.9)	51(52.6)	
HPS				0.000*
Yes	24(11.7)	3(2.8)	21(21.6)	
No	181(88.3)	105(97.2)	76(78.4)	
Elevated IL-6 level				0.000*
Yes	139(67.8)	60(55.6)	79(81.4)	
No	66(32.2)	48(44.4)	18(18.6)	
Elevated IFN γ level				0.000*
Yes	78(38.0)	23(21.3)	55(56.7)	
No	127(62.0)	85(78.7)	42(43.3)	
EBV				0.028*
Negative	85(41.5)	52(48.1)	33(34.0)	
Positive	120(58.5)	56(51.9)	64(66.0)	
Extra-nodal Involvement				0.000*
≤1	107(52.2)	71(65.7)	36(37.1)	
>1	98(47.8)	37(34.3)	61(62.9)	
Elevated LDH level				0.000*
Yes	136(66.3)	60(55.6)	76(78.4)	
No	69(33.7)	48(44.4)	21(21.6)	
Elevated β2-MG level				0.000*
Yes	131(63.9)	55(50.9)	76(78.4)	
No	74(36.1)	53(49.1)	21(21.6)	
Elevated SF level				0.004*
Yes	108(52.7)	47(43.5)	61(62.9)	
No	97(47.3)	61(56.5)	36(37.1)	
Attainment of CR				0.000*
Yes	70(34.1)	56(51.9)	14(14.4)	
No	135(65.9)	52(48.1)	83(85.6)	

(Continued)

TABLE 1 | Continued

characteristic	total (n=205,%)	IL-10<3.6pg/ml (n=108, %)	IL-10≥3.6pg/ml (n=97, %)	p Value
Recurrence/progress in one year				0.000*
Yes	67(32.7)	19(17.6)	48(49.5)	
No	138(67.3)	89(82.4)	49(50.5)	

#others: 3 cases of MEITL, 1 case of T-LGLL, 2 cases of SPTCL, 2 cases of MF/SS, 1 case of HSTCL; CR, complete response.
*Significantly different.
The classification variables are expressed by frequency and percentage. (n, %).

with poor OS had ECOG ≥3 (HR = 4.314, 95% CI 2.462–7.559, p < 0.001), Extra-nodal ≥1 (HR = 2.126, 95% CI 1.142–3.958, p = 0.017), IL-10 ≥3.6 pg/ml (HR = 6.428, 95% CI 3.369–12.266, p < 0.001), and IL-6 ≥2.2 pg/ml (HR = 2.050, 95% CI 1.122–3.745, p = 0.020).

Thus, it can be seen that among the three cytokines included in our studies, only IL-10 was significant and independent prognostic factor in both univariate and multivariate analyses of treatment response, survival, and early recurrence in PTCL patients. IL-6 had an independent effect on OS in multivariate analyses as well. The results of Cox regression analysis were present in **Table 4**.

DISCUSSION

Benefit from the oceans of studies about tumor micro-environment, tremendous progress has been made in predicting the prognosis of PTCL. Nevertheless, poor response, high mortality, and relapse remain primary challenges, so new prognostic factors need to be explored to further predict and improve the prognosis of PTCL patients. According to the established tumor models, Sato T et al. found that IL-10 has tumor-promoting and anti-tumor effects *in vivo* (14). Herein, we retrospectively analyzed six cytokines of 205 patients with PTCL and discovered that patients with IL-10 ≥3.6 pg/ml had both low CR rate, low OS rate but high 1-year recurrence or progression rate as an independent effect in multivariate analyses. Therefore, from our retrospective clinical studies, IL-10 may play a role as pro-tumor effects *in vivo*.

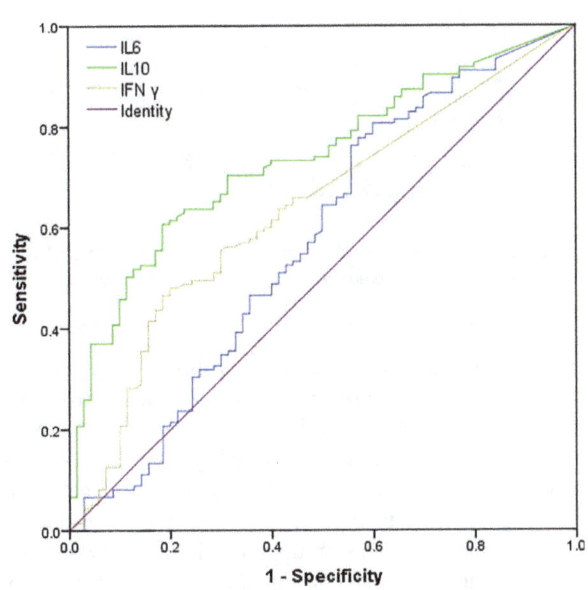

FIGURE 1 | Receiver operating characteristic (ROC) curves of serum IL-10, IL-6, and IFN γ levels of patients with PTCL. The AUC of IL-10, IL-6 and IFN γ were 0.736 (95% CI: 0.668–0.805), 0.572(95% CI: 0.485–0.659), 0.634(95% CI: 0.554–0.713)..

C. Andrew Stewart et al. observed that the majority of tumor-associated IL-10 was produced by activated Tregs. Components of the type I IFN signaling pathway, including Ifnar1, Stat1 and Stat2, were essential for the accumulation and activation of Tregs and production of IL-10 (15). In cancer-related preclinical and therapeutic models, Tregs limits the production of Th1 responses that drive CD8 + T cells and IFN γ dependent anti-tumor immunity (16, 17). Th17 cells occur in most human tumors frequently. Th17 related inflammation may lead to tumor growth or autoimmunity. The production of IL-10 limits the quantities and activity of Th17 cells in tumors, which promotes the growth of tumors (18).

The poor response of immunotherapy in most tumors were bound up with tumor-associated macrophages (TAM), Tregs and myeloid-derived suppressor cells (MDSCs). MDSCs can induce the production of Tregs and lead Tregs to tumor tissues, thus promoting the production of IL-10 (19). TAM were related to the poor clinical prognosis of various human tumors by promoting angiogenesis, local invasion and metastasis (20–23). It has been confirmed that the growth and survival of malignant T cells depend on alternately activated (M2) macrophages in the micro-environment, and the growth of alternately activated (M2) macrophages was affected by the presence of TAMs (4, 24). Sam T. Hwang found that alternately activated (M2) macrophages can affect the polarization of undifferentiated macrophages in the way specified (25). In a mouse model study, M2 macrophages can increase the secretion of IL-10 by macrophages which is necessary for the maximum growth of human cutaneous T-cell lymphoma (25). Kim SJ and Ham JS analyzed the serum cytokines and CD68- and CD163- positive macrophage in tumor tissue of 37 AITL patients after CHOP chemotherapy, and found that high IL-10 and M2 macrophage tissue infiltration all indicated low OS and poor response to treatment (26). In subsequent studies, this team further tested 34 cytokines in 121 patients with PTCL, and analyzed the correlation between overall survival rate and complete remission rate. They found that patients with AITL

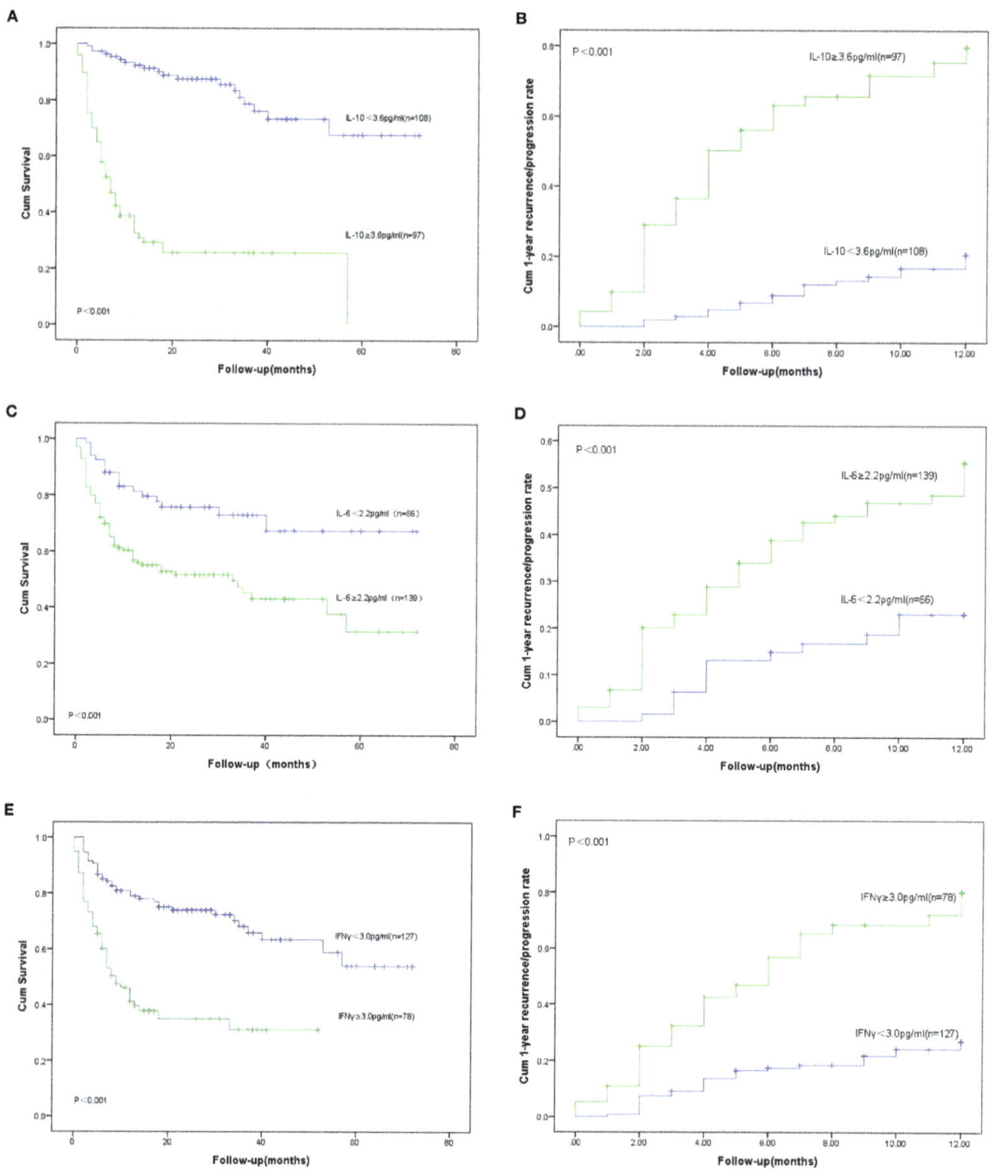

FIGURE 2 | OS: Overall survival. **(A)** OS for different serum levels of IL-10; **(B)** Recurrence/progression in one year for different serum levels of IL-10. **(C)** OS for different serum levels of IL-6; **(D)** Recurrence/progression in one year for different serum levels of IL-6; **(E)** OS for different serum levels of IFN γ; **(F)** Recurrence/progression in one year for different serum levels of IFN γ.

had higher serum cytokine levels, and IL-10 levels higher than 3.8 pg/ml were associated with adverse outcomes, which was very close to our cut-off value. In addition to IL-10, IFN γ, IL-8, IL-17, IL-23, monocyte chemoattractant protein-1 and macrophage inflammatory protein-1β, and RANTES negatively also have negative effects on clinical prognosis in patients with ALK-anaplastic large cell lymphoma (27). Li Li and Zhang Jun found that the released IL-10 made the JAK2/STAT3 pathway sensitive, leading to STAT3-induced PD-L1 expression (28). At the same time, they confirmed PD-L1 signaling network in 2 main 428 and 350 DLBCL cohorts, and showed a significant correlation among IL-10, STAT3, and PD-L1 (28). H. Dean et al. conducted genetic analysis of 20 single nucleotide polymorphisms (SNPs) in IL-10 and TNF/LTA loci in three independent case-control studies (2,635 cases and 4,234 controls), discovered IL-10 rs1800896 was related to DLBCL, as well as T-cell lymphoma (29). It was confirmed that genetic variations of immune-related genes (such as IL-10) were related to the occurrence of T-cell lymphoma in Asian populations (29). To sum up, it had been proved that IL-10 was related to the prognosis of malignant T-cell lymphoma in both gene and molecular studies and animal experimental studies. It promoted tumor cells to evade immune surveillance by regulating antigen presentation and immune cell differentiation (30). Mona R. Hassuneh et al. used LSA (a T-cell lymphoma cell line

TABLE 2 | Univariate and multivariate logistic regression models of complete response (CR) in PTCL patients.

Parameters	Univariate analysis			Multivariate analysis		
	OR	95% CI	p Value	OR	95%CI	p Value
Sex, Male	0.472	0.260-0.858	0.014*			
Age, ≥60years	2.273	1.204-4.290	0.011*			
Stage,III-IV	5.107	2.447-10.658	<0.001*			
B symptoms	2.128	1.184-3.827	0.012*			
Bone marrow Involvement	3.014	1.507-6.030	0.002*			
IPI,3-5	3.474	1.894-6.371	<0.001*			
ECOG,3-5	8.812	3.024-25.680	<0.001*	4.359	1.317-14.428	0.016*
EBV,Positive	2.667	1.473-4.827	0.001*	2.419	1.209-4.840	0.013*
Extra-nodal, >1	2.119	1.169-3.841	0.013*			
IL-10≥3.6pg/ml	6.385	3.233-12.609	<0.001*	2.973	1.344-6.578	0.015*
IL-6≥2.2pg/ml	2.271	1.236-4.175	0.008*			
IFN-γ≥3.0pg/ml	3.606	1.834-7.089	<0.001*			
Elevated LDH	2.230	1.220-4.078	0.009*			
Elevated β2-MG	2.045	1.127-3.170	0.019*			

OR, odds ratio; CI, confidence interval.
**Significantly different.*

TABLE 3 | Univariate and multivariate logistic regression models for recurrence or progression within one year in PTCL patients.

Parameters	Univariate analysis			Multivariate analysis		
	OR	95%CI	p Value	OR	95%CI	p Value
Stage,III-IV	5.559	1.888-16.364	0.002*			
B symptoms	2.106	1.145-3.873	0.017*			
Bone marrow Involvement	5.235	2.774-9.880	<0.001*	3.799	1.630-8.854	0.002*
IPI,3-5	3.008	1.605-5.636	0.001*			
ECOG,3-5	8.340	4.108-16.931	<0.001*	5.873	2.464-13.997	<0.001*
Decreased albumin	0.228	0.119-0.435	<0.001*			
Extra-nodal, >1	2.460	1.349-4.485	0.003*			
HPS	4.135	1.703-10.037	0.002*			
IL-10≥3.6pg/ml	4.589	2.431-8.663	<0.001*	2.008	0.876-4.601	0.009*
IL-6≥2.2pg/ml	2.590	1.291-5.194	0.007*			
IFN γ≥3.0pg/ml	3.536	1.920-6.512	<0.001*			
Elevated SF	1.833	1.009-3.330	0.047*			

OR, odds ratio; CI, confidence interval.
**Significantly different.*

TABLE 4 | Univariate and multivariate Cox proportional hazard regression models for overall survival (OS) in PTCL patients.

Parameters	Univariate analysis			Multivariate analysis		
	HR	95%CI	p Value	HR	95%CI	p Value
Stage,III-IV	3.079	1.486-6.382	0.002*			
B symptoms	2.483	1.547-3.985	<0.001*			
Bone marrow Involvement	2.851	1.860-4.369	<0.001*			
IPI,3-5	2.806	1.749-4.499	<0.001*			
ECOG,3-5	4.522	2.933-6.971	<0.001*	4.314	2.462-7.559	<0.001*
Decreased albumin	0.344	0.224-0.527	<0.001*			
EBV,Positive	1.671	1.060-2.637	0.027*			
Extra-nodal, >2	3.004	1.903-4.742	<0.001*	2.126	1.142-3.958	0.017*
HPS	3.678	2.176-6.218	<0.001*			
IL-10≥3.6pg/ml	8.034	4.741-13.613	<0.001*	6.428	3.369-12.266	<0.001*
IL-6≥2.2pg/ml	2.516	1.477-4.283	0.001*	2.050	1.122-3.745	0.020*
IFN-γ≥3.0pg/ml	3.249	2.095-5.037	<0.001*			
Elevated LDH	2.032	1.220-3.387	0.006*			
Elevated SF	1.605	1.041-2.476	0.032*			

HR, hazard ratio; CI, confidence interval.
**Significantly different.*

expressing IL-10) to study the role of IL-10 in tumorigenesis. Interestingly, the administration of anti-IL-10 antibodies significantly inhibited the growth of tumors in LSA (31).

Previously, stage was well recognized as having a prognostic impact in PTCL, and it had been included in previously reported indices in subsequent studies (32), indicating that it was highly significant predictor of OS. In our study, stage III–IV was associated with low response rate, early recurrence and poor OS, which was consistent with previous studies. In **Table 1**, it is easy to find that in patients with IL-10 levels higher than 3.6 pg/ml, the proportion of stage III–IV is significantly higher than that of stage I–II (95.9 vs 4.1%). It is further suggested that the increase of IL-10 levels might be related to distant metastasis and immune escape.

IL-10 has strong immunosuppression. It inhibits the proliferation of T cells (33). Thus, overexpression of IL-10 by PTCL lymphoma cells may damage the host's immune system, resulting in immunosuppression and tumor escape. At the same time, it will also provide a selective survival advantage for the PTCL cells in the host. What is more, serum IL-10 concentration is also an important prognostic factor for various tumors, such as diffuse large B-cell lymphoma (DLBCL) and adult T-cell leukemia/lymphoma (ATL) (12, 20, 34). Our study proved that IL-10 plays an important role in the treatment response, survival and early recurrence or progression of PTCL patients. In multivariate regression analysis, patients with IL-10 ≥3.6 pg/ml had a lower CR rate and a higher recurrence rate. In univariate and multivariate survival analysis, patients with IL-10 ≥3.6 pg/ml had poorer OS. To the best of our knowledge, this retrospective clinical study is the first to confirm the effect of IL-10 on the treatment response, survival, and early recurrence of Chinese PTCL patients. Insaki Atsushi et al. analyzed the serum IL-10 levels in 94 cases of ATL and found that high IL-10 levels were an important adverse prognostic factor in ATL. However, the critical value of IL-10 in our study is different from the results of Atsushi Inagaki et al. (34). They mainly target ATL patients between the ages of 38–89 and the number of cases in their study is less than 100, however our study contained the five major PTCL subtypes and the five rare subtypes of MEITL, T-LGLL, SPTCL, MF/SS, and HSTCL with age range of 18–79 years old, and we have more than twice as many cases as they have. Perhaps, the different number of cases, disease types and inclusive criteria that led to the different cutoff values. Similarly, IL-10 is still an independent prognostic factor for survival and early recurrence in patients with PTCL.

In addition, we were surprised to find that there was a gender difference between the high IL-10 group and the low IL-10 group. The proportion of female patients was significantly lower than the male patients in high IL-10 group (26.8 vs 73.2%), and the treatment response of female patients was better than that of the male (**Table 2**). It aroused our interest, and we specially reviewed some similar previous studies. Previous studies had shown the differences in immune function between age and gender. These differences were believed to be caused by hormone discrepancies, especially the loss of estradiol caused the reversal of immune response in elderly females (35). Interestingly, the inhibitory effect of female derived MDSCs on T cells proliferation were stronger than that of male. Transplantation of female derived MDSCs significantly increased the frequency and absolute number of Tregs and CD4 + IL-10 + T cells (36). However, in tumor environment, MDSCs not only have characteristics of M2 macrophages (such as the expression of arginase-1 and NOS2), but also play a role as the progenitor cells of tumor associated macrophages. Moreover, MDSCs can further regulate the cytotoxicity mediated by macrophages (37, 38).

Hemophagocytic syndrome (HPS) is an immune-mediated life-threatening disease that affects 1% of adults with hematological cancers, and its prevalence rises to 20% in patients with NHL, especially PTCL (39). Qi An et al. found that median serum concentrations of IFN γ and IL-10 were significantly higher in children with HPS compared to healthy controls (40). In our study, there were 24 patients with HPS, accounting for 11.7%, and the median serum of IL-10 and IFN γ were higher than the patients without HPS (54.02 vs. 2.70 pg/ml, $p < 0.001$; 12.42 vs. 1.02pg/ml, $p < 0.001$). Importantly, although the OS of PTCL patients with HPS decreased significantly, HPS was not an independent predictor for OS of PTCL patients after univariate and multivariate analysis in our study.

Our study still has some limitations. Firstly, the retrospective study may be biased in the selection of patients. Secondly, the dynamic changes of patients during treatment did not take into account during analysis. Thirdly, due to the limitation of the number of cases, the conclusions of this study are only verified in three common subtypes of PTCL-NOS, ENKTL, and AITL. Therefore, more in-depth studies are needed to confirm the role of IL-10 in the prognosis of patients with PTCL.

CONCLUSIONS

All in all, increased serum levels of IL-10 at diagnosis is related to the survival and early recurrence of PTCL patients. IL-10 ≥3.6 pg/ml is significantly correlated with lower CR rate, higher recurrence rate and lower OS rate. Furthermore, univariate and multivariate analysis indicated that IL-10 ≥3.6 pg/ml is an independent prognostic factor. In short, the serum level of IL-10 in the peripheral blood at the initial stage can be added to the prognostic tool to play its prognostic role in PTCL. In addition, the determination of serum cytokine levels is quick and convenient. Only a small amount of serum samples can be used to complete the detection. This is very useful to help us formulate different treatment strategies for individuals with PTCL, because it can predict the prognosis before treatment. In the near future, IL-10 inhibitors or antagonists may become a new method of Immunotargeting therapy for PTCL patients.

ETHICS STATEMENT

Written informed consent was obtained from the individual(s) for the publication of any potentially identifiable images or data included in this article.

AUTHOR CONTRIBUTIONS

WX designed the study. YZ, YLZ, LS, YS, HS, MZ, XY, and JJ collected the patients' material. YZ and YLZ analyzed data and wrote the paper. All authors contributed to the article and approved the submitted version.

ACKNOWLEDGMENTS

The authors thank the practitioners who helped to collect and sort out the patient' information and follow-up, especially Prof. Xin Huang from the Institute of Hematology, Zhejiang University, for his support in this study.

REFERENCES

1. American Society of Hematology. A clinical evaluation of the Inernational Lymphoma Study Group classification of non-Hodgkin's lymphoma. The Non-Hodgkin's Lymphoma Classification Project. *Blood* (1997) 89:3909–18. doi: 10.1182/blood.V89.11.3909
2. Shi Y. Current status and progress of lymphoma management in China. *Int J Hematol* (2018) 107(4):405–12. doi: 10.1007/s12185-018-2404-8
3. Swerdlow SH, Campo E, Harris NL. *World Health Organization classification of tumors of haematopoietic and lymphold tissues*. Lyon, France: IARC (2016).
4. Wilcox RA, Wada DA, Ziesmer SC, Elsawa SF, Comfere NF, Dietz AB, et al. Monocytes promote tumor cell survival in T-cell lymphoproliferative disorders and are impaired in their ability to differentiate into mature dendritic cells. *Blood* (2009) 114(14):2936–44. doi: 10.1182/blood-2009-05-220111
5. Staples KJ, Smallie T, Williams LM, Foey A, Burke B, Foxwell BMJ, et al. IL-10 Induces IL-10 in Primary Human Monocyte-Derived Macrophages via the Transcription Factor Stat3. *J Immunol* (2007) 178:4779–85. doi: 10.4049/jimmunol.178.8.4779
6. Iqbal J, Wright G, Wang C. Gene expression signatures delineate biological and prognostic subgroups in peripheral T-cell lymphoma. *Blood* (2014) 123:2915–23. doi: 10.1182/blood-2013-11-536359
7. Wang T, Feldman AL, Wada DA, Lu Y, Polk A, Briski R, et al. GATA-3 expression identifies a high-risk subset of PTCL, NOS with distinct molecular and clinical features. *Blood* (2014) 123:3007–15. doi: 10.1182/blood-2013-12-544809
8. Xua G, Wang F. Associations of polymorphisms in interleukins with susceptibility to breast cancer: Evidence from a meta-analysis. *Cytokine* (2020) 130:154988. doi: 10.1016/j.cyto.2020.154988
9. Lombardi Pereira AP, Paiva Trugilo K, Okuyama NCM, Mota Sena M, D'Oliveira Couto-Filho J, Watanabe MAE, et al. IL-10 c.-592C>A (rs1800872) polymorphism is associated with cervical cancer. *J Cancer Res Clin Oncol* (2020) 146(8):1971–8. doi: 10.1007/s00432-020-03256-0
10. Zhong-Wu LU, Hu J-Q, Liu W-L, Wen D, Wei W-J, Wang Y-L, et al. IL-10 restores MHC class I expression and interferes immunity in papillary thyroid cancer with Hashimoto's thyroiditis. *Endocrine Soc* (2020).
11. Sakai Y, Rezano A, Okada S, Ohtsuki T, Kawashima Y, Tsukamoto T, et al. A Novel Cytological Model of B-Cell/Macrophage Biphenotypic Cell Hodgkin Lymphoma in Ganp-Transgenic Mice. *Cancers (Basel)* (2020) 12(1):204. doi: 10.3390/cancers12010204
12. Yi JH, Yoon SE, Ryu KJ, Ko YH, Kim WS, Kim SJ. Pre-treatment serum IL-10 predicts the risk of secondary central nervous system involvement in patients with diffffuse large B-cell lymphoma. *Cytokine* (2020) 129:155048. doi: 10.1016/j.cyto.2020.155048
13. Altman DG, McShane LM, Sauerbrei W, Taube SE. Reporting Recommendations for Tumor Marker Prognostic Studies (REMARK): Explanation and Elaboration. *PloS Med* (2012) 9(5):e1001216. doi: 10.1371/journal.pmed.1001216
14. Sato T, Terai M, Tamura Y, Alexeev V, Mastrangelo MJ, Selvan SR. Interleukin 10 in the tumor microenvironment: a target for anticancer immunotherapy. *Immunol Res* (2011) 51:170–82. doi: 10.1007/s12026-011-8262-6
15. Andrew Stewart C, Muller W, Trinchieri G. Interferon-dependent IL-10 production by Tregs limits tumor Th17 inflammation. *J Clin Invest* (2013) 123(11):4859–74. doi: 10.1172/JCI65180
16. Teng MW, Ngiow SF, von Scheidt B, McLaughlin N, Sparwasser T, Smyth MJ. Conditional regulatory T-cell depletion releases adaptive immunity preventing carcinogenesis and suppressing established tumor growth. *Cancer Res* (2010) 70(20):7800–9. doi: 10.1158/0008-5472.CAN-10-1681
17. Teng MW, Ritchie DS, Neeson P, Smyth MJ. Biology and clinical observations of regulatory T cells in cancer immunology. *Curr Top Microbiol Immunol* (2011) 344:61–95. doi: 10.1007/82_2010_50
18. Wilke CM, Wang L, Wei S, Kryczek I, Zou W. Endogenous interleukin-10 constrains Th17 cells in patients with inflammatory bowel disease. *J Transl Med* (2011) 9:217. doi: 10.1186/1479-5876-9-217
19. Du J, Sun X, Song Y. The study of CD14+HLA-DR-/low myeloid-drived suppressor cell (MDSC) in peripheral blood of peripheral T-cell lymphoma patients and its biological function. *Cell Mol Biol (Noisy-le-grand)* (2017) 63 (3):62–7. doi: 10.14715/cmb/2017.63.3.12
20. Malesci A, Bianchi P, Celesti G, Basso G, Marchesi F, Grizzi F, et al. Tumor-associated macrophages and response to 5-fluorouracil adjuvant therapy in stage III colorectal cancer. *Oncoimmunology* (2017) 6(12):e1342918. doi: 10.1080/2162402X.2017.1342918
21. Qiu SQ, Waaijer SJH, Zwager MC, de Vries EGE, van der Vegt B, Schröder CP. Tumor-associated macrophages in breast cancer: Innocent bystander or important player? *Cancer Treat Rev* (2018) 70):178–89. doi: 10.1016/j.ctrv.2018.08.010
22. Futagbi G, Gyan B, Nunoo H, Tetteh JKA, Welbeck JE, Renner LA, et al. High Levels of IL-10 and CD4+CD25hi+ Treg Cells in Endemic Burkitt's Lymphoma Patients. *Biomedicines* (2015) 3:224–36. doi: 10.3390/biomedicines3030224
23. Ryder M, Ghossein RA, Ricarte-Filho JC, Knauf JA, Fagin JA. Increased density of tumor-associated macrophages is associated with decreased survival in advanced thyroid cancer. *Endocr Relat Cancer* (2008) 15(4):1069–74. doi: 10.1677/ERC-08-0036
24. Wu X, Schulte BC, Zhou Y. Depletion of M2-like tumor-associated macrophages delays cutaneous T-cell lymphoma development in vivo. *J Invest Dermatol* (2014) 134:2814–22. doi: 10.1038/jid.2014.206
25. Wu X, Hsu DK, Wang K-H, Huang Y, Mendoza L, Zhou Y, et al. IL-10 is overexpressed in human cutaneous T-cell lymphoma and is required for maximal tumor growth in a mouse model. *Leuk Lymphoma.* (2019) 60 (5):1244–52. doi: 10.1080/10428194.2018.1516037
26. Ham JS, Park HY, Ryu KJ, Ko YH, Kim WS, Kim SJ. Elevated serum interleukin-10 level and M2 macrophage infiltration are associated with poor survival in angioimmunoblastic T-cell lymphoma. *Oncotarget* (2017) 8 (44):76231–40. doi: 10.18632/oncotarget.19301
27. Yi JH, Ryu KJ, Ko YH, Kim WS, Kim SJ. Profiles of serum cytokines and their clinical implications in patients with peripheral T-cell lymphoma. *Cytokine* (2019) 113:371–9. doi: 10.1016/j.cyto.2018.10.009
28. Li L, Zhang J, Pham LV. B-cell receptor-mediated NFATc1 activation induces IL-10/STAT2/PD-L1 signaling in diffuse large B-cell lymphoma. *Blood* (2018) 132(17):1805–17. doi: 10.1182/blood-2018-03-841015
29. Dean Hosgood III H, Au W-Y, Kim HN, Liu J, Hu W, Tse J, et al. IL-10 and TNF variants and risk of non-Hodgkin lymphoma among three Asian populations. *Int J Hematol* (2013) 97:793–9. doi: 10.1007/s12185-013-1345-5
30. Mantovani A, Sozzani S, Locati M. Macrophage polarization: tumor-associated macrophages as a paradigm for polarized M2 mononuclear phagocytes. *Trends Immunol* (2002) 23:549–55. doi: 10.1016/S1471-4906 (02)02302-5

31. Hassuneh MR, Nagarkatti M, Nagarkatti PS. Role of interleukin-10 in the regulation of tumorigenicity of a T cell lymphoma. *Leuk Lymphoma* (2013) 54 (4):827–34. doi: 10.3109/10428194.2012.726721
32. Weisenburger DD, Savage KJ, Harris NL, Gascoyne RD, Jaffe ES, MacLennan KA, et al. Peripheral T-cell lymphoma, not otherwise specifified: a report of 340 cases from the International Peripheral T-cell Lymphoma Project. *Blood* (2011) 117:3402–8. doi: 10.1182/blood-2010-09-310342
33. Taga K, Mostowski H, Tosato G. Human interleukin-10 can directly inhibit T-cell growth. *Blood* (1993) 81:2964–71. doi: 10.1182/blood.V81.11.2964.bloodjournal81112964
34. Inagaki A, Ishida T, Ishii T, Komatsu H, Iida S, Ding J, et al. Clinical signifificance of serum Th1-, Th2- and regulatory T cells-associated cytokines in adult T-cell leukemia/lymphoma: High Interleukin-5 and -10 levels are signifificant unfavorable prognostic factors. *Int J Cancer* (2006) 118:3054–61. doi: 10.1002/ijc.21688
35. Kahlke V, Angele MK, Ayala A, Schwacha MG, Cioffi WG, Bland KI, et al. Immune dysfunction following traumahemorrhage: influence of gender and age. *Cytokine* (2000) 12:69–77. doi: 10.1006/cyto.1999.0511
36. Su N, Yue Y, Xiong S. Monocytic myeloid-derived suppressor cells from females, but not males, alleviate CVB3- induced myocarditis by increasing regulatory and CD4+IL-10+ T cells. *Sci Rep* (2016) 6:22658. doi: 10.1038/srep22658
37. Youn JI, Gabrilovich DI. The biology of myeloid-derived suppressor cells: the blessing and the curse of morphological and functional heterogeneity. *Eur J Immunol* (2010) 40:2969–75. doi: 10.1002/eji.201040895
38. Maeda A, Eguchi H, Nakahata K, Lo P-C, Yamanaka K, Kawamura T, et al. Monocytic MDSCs regulate macrophage-mediated xenogenic cytotoxicity. *Transpl Immunol* (2015) 33:140–5. doi: 10.1016/j.trim.2015.07.002
39. Ramos-Casals M, Brito-Zerón P, López-Guillermo A, Khamashta MA, Bosch X. Adult haemophagocytic syndrome. *Lancet* (2014) 383:1503–16. doi: 10.1016/S0140-6736(13)61048-X
40. An Q, Hu S-Y, Xuan C-M, Jin M-W, Ji Q, Wang Y. Interferon gamma and interleukin 10 polymorphisms in Chinese children with hemophagocytic lymphohistiocytosis. *Pediatr Blood Cancer* (2017) 64:9. doi: 10.1002/pbc.26505

13

Tumor Microenvironment Proteomics: Lessons from Multiple Myeloma

Rodrigo Carlini Fernando[1]*, Fabrício de Carvalho*[1]*, Adriana Franco Paes Leme*[2] *and Gisele Wally Braga Colleoni*[1*]

[1] Department of Experimental and Clinical Oncology, Discipline of Hematology and Hemotherapy, Federal University of São Paulo, UNIFESP, São Paulo, Brazil, [2] Laboratory of Mass Spectrometry, Laboratory of National Biosciences, LNBio, National Council for Research in Energy and Materials (CNPEM), Campinas, Brazil

Correspondence:
Gisele Wally Braga Colleoni
gcolleoni@unifesp.br

Although the "seed and soil" hypothesis was proposed by Stephen Paget at the end of the 19th century, where he postulated that tumor cells (seeds) need a propitious medium (soil) to be able to establish metastases, only recently the tumor microenvironment started to be more studied in the field of Oncology. Multiple myeloma (MM), a malignancy of plasma cells, can be considered one of the types of cancers where there is more evidence in the literature of the central role that the bone marrow (BM) microenvironment plays, contributing to proliferation, survival, migration, and drug resistance of tumor cells. Despite all advances in the therapeutic arsenal for MM treatment in the last years, the disease remains incurable. Thus, studies aiming a better understanding of the pathophysiology of the disease, as well as searching for new therapeutic targets are necessary and welcome. Therefore, the present study aimed to evaluate the protein expression profiling of mononuclear cells derived from BM of MM patients in comparison with these same cell types derived from healthy individuals, in order to fill this gap in MM treatment. Proteomic analysis was performed using the mass spectrometry technique and further analyses were done using bioinformatics tools, to identify dysregulated biological pathways and/or processes in the BM microenvironment of patients with MM as a result of the disease. Among the pathways identified in this study, we can highlight an upregulation of proteins related to protein biosynthesis, especially chaperone proteins, in patients with MM. Additionally, we also found an upregulation of several proteins involved in energy metabolism, which is one of the cancer hallmarks. Finally, with regard to the downregulated proteins, we can highlight mainly those involved in different pathways of the immune response, corroborating the data that has demonstrated that the immune system of MM is impaired and, therefore, the immunotherapies that have been studied recently for the treatment of the disease are extremely necessary in the search for a control and a cure for these patients who live with the disease.

Keywords: multiple myeloma, tumor microenvironment, proteome, proteomics, mass spectrometry

INTRODUCTION

Multiple myeloma (MM) is a hematologic malignancy of post-germinal center plasma cells, characterized by the infiltration of these tumor cells in the bone marrow (BM), presence of clonal immunoglobulin in the blood and/or urine of most patients, and damage to target tissues and organs, including bone lesions, hypercalcemia, kidney failure and anemia, and an increased risk of infections (1, 2). MM accounts for approximately 1% of all cancer cases and 10% of hematologic malignancies, being the second most common hematological malignancy after lymphomas (3). Over 30,000 new patients are diagnosed in the United States each year (4). The average age at diagnosis is 70 years and only 2% of patients are less than 40 years of age at diagnosis (4), which makes this disease attractive to study the interactions among tumor immunology, immunosenescence and aging, since the majority of the new cancer cases are diagnosed in people aged above 60 (4).

MM etiology is unknown, but aging and life exposure to cancer risk factors, including environment exposure to carcinogens, such as radiation, might contribute to MM development (5). Men are slightly more affected than women (4), Afro-descendants are twice as affected compared to Caucasians (4), and almost all cases of MM evolve from a premalignant condition called monoclonal gammopathy of undetermined significance (6, 7).

The treatment of MM has evolved markedly over the past few years, especially due to the introduction of high-dose of melphalan followed by autologous stem cell transplantation for eligible patients, and the introduction of immunomodulatory drugs such as thalidomide and lenalidomide, and proteasome inhibitory molecules such as bortezomib (8). More recently, several new drugs have been approved, including new immunomodulators (pomalidomide) and proteasome inhibitors (carfilzomib, ixazomib), improving the risk-benefit profile of these classes of therapies (9). Besides, monoclonal antibodies (anti-CD38 and anti-SLAMF1) was also introduced in the therapeutic MM armament, and an inhibitor of the histone deacetylase enzyme (panobinostat) (9).

These new molecules had a major impact on the survival of patients and currently younger individuals diagnosed with MM can have an average survival of ten years (10). New approaches involving immunotherapies such as CART (chimeric antigen receptor T)-cells or bi-specific antibodies (BiTEs) are underdevelopment, although they will not be available for the majority of patients worldwide (11). However, although all this progress has occurred with the expansion of the therapeutic arsenal, most patients will relapse one or more times over the course of the disease and, eventually, will become refractory to treatments available. Therefore, MM remains an incurable disease and further studies are needed to better elucidate the pathophysiology of the disease, as well to discover new potential therapeutic targets and surrogate biomarkers.

With regard to the pathophysiology of MM, BM tumor microenvironment plays a central role during disease development, and in its maintenance and progression (12). A growing body of evidence has shown that this tumor microenvironment, consisting of cellular and non-cellular elements, differs in its composition when comparing MM patients and healthy individuals (13). Regarding the cellular elements, we can highlight the mesenchymal stem cells (MSC), which have the capacity of self-renewal and differentiation in several cell types such as fibroblasts, osteoblasts, adipocytes, chondrocytes, among others (14). Through direct and indirect communication with tumor plasma cells, MSC promote their proliferation, survival, migration and drug resistance (15). Additionally, several studies, including one conducted by our group, have shown that MM MSCs differ in several aspects, including, gene expression and functional changes, in comparison to their normal counterparts derived from BM of healthy individuals (16). Other cell types are also very important to MM progression, including myeloid derived immunosuppressive cells (MDSCs), T cells, NK cells, dendritic cells, macrophages, osteoclasts and osteoblasts (13). These cells contribute to the maintenance of a tolerogenic microenvironment in BM, favoring the evasion of the immune system by tumor plasma cells. Besides, the imbalance of proliferation, differentiation and function of osteoblasts and osteoclasts are one of the most important factors for the formation of bone lesions in these patients. With regard to the non-cellular elements of the tumor microenvironment, we can mention cytokines, chemokines, growth factors and exosomes, which favor the progression of the disease, in addition to an altered composition of the extracellular matrix, which also contributes to the pathophysiology of MM (13).

Among the current therapies approved for MM, some of them also have effect on the tumor microenvironment mentioned above (17). Thus, for a better understanding of the biology of the disease and the search for new therapies, studies on the BM microenvironment of these patients are extremely relevant. In this context, proteomic studies are a very interesting approach to characterize the protein expression profiling of these cells from MM compared to BM cells from healthy individuals. In addition, evidences from the literature show that proteomic analysis gives a high confident picture of proteins differentially expressed, when compared with gene expression analysis (18).

Therefore, the present study aimed to evaluate the protein expression profiling of cells derived from BM of MM patients in comparison with these same cell types derived from healthy individuals, in order to search for potential new therapeutic targets and surrogate biomarkers, as well as to better understand the pathophysiology of the disease.

CASUISTIC AND METHODS

Ethical Aspects

This study was approved by the Institutional Review Board from Federal University of São Paulo (CAAE: 07297019.9.0000.5505). BM samples from MM patients and healthy donors were obtained after written informed consent forms by participants or legal representative, according to Helsinki Declaration and local regulations.

Subjects

Eight newly diagnosed patients with MM (and without any previous treatment for the disease) were successfully enrolled in this study and allocated in the case group. Six young healthy individuals (BM donors for allogeneic stem cell transplantation) not matched by age or gender were also enrolled in this study and allocated in the control group.

Bone Marrow Samples and Sorting of Mesenchymal Stem Cells and Mononuclear Cells

BM samples from newly diagnosed MM patients (n=8) and healthy donors (n=6) were harvested from iliac crest, through core biopsy marrow aspiration. Then, BM mononuclear cells were isolated by density gradient, using Ficoll-Paque PLUS (GE Healthcare, Little Chalfont, Bucks, GBR) and following the manufacturer's instructions. Firstly, plasma cells were sorted by Magnetic-Activated Cell Sorting (MACS) methodology, using $CD138^+$ as a positive marker (Miltenyi Biotec, Bergisch Gladbach, DEU). These cells were analyzed in another study from our group (19). Then, MSC were isolated, using $CD105^+$ as a positive marker. Due to the low number of these cells, both in patients' and controls' BM, they were expanded *in vitro* according to the protocol described in Fernando et al. (16), n=4 for each group. Finally, the flow through, i.e., the BM mononuclear cells depleted of plasma cells ($CD138^+$) and MSC ($CD105^+$) were frozen in liquid nitrogen for the following experiments. In this study, we named these cells as mononuclear cells $(MC)^{CD138\text{-}CD105\text{-}}$.

MSC Characterization

After MSC *in vitro* expansion, we characterized the MSC according to the protocol described in Fernando et al. (16). In summary, positive markers CD105, CD90 and CD73, and negative markers CD45, CD34, CD14, and HLA-DR were tested by flow cytometry. In addition, the osteoblastic differentiation capacity of these cells was also evaluated, by measuring the osteocalcin protein produced by these cells and secreted in the culture medium supernatant on days 7, 14 and 21, during the stimulus that favors the differentiation of them into osteoblasts. The Human Osteocalcin Quantikine ELISA kit (R&D Systems, Minneapolis, MN, USA) was used to perform this analysis, according to the manufacturer's instructions. All MSC from both groups used for characterization and submitted to mass spectrometry were between passages 2 to 5 of cell culture.

Protein Extraction and Quantification

We pooled the samples from each group in order to obtain the required amount of protein to perform the mass spectrometry experiment. Therefore, we obtained **1)** a pool from $MC^{CD138\text{-}CD105\text{-}}$ (n=8) and **2)** a pool from MSC (n=4), all derived from MM patients, i.e., four MM patients had both the $MC^{CD138\text{-}CD105\text{-}}$ and the MSC analyzed by mass spectrometry; and **3)** a pool from $MC^{CD138\text{-}CD105\text{-}}$ (n=6) and **4)** a pool from MSC (n=4), all from healthy donors (HD), i.e., four HD had both the $MC^{CD138\text{-}CD105\text{-}}$ and the MSC analyzed by mass spectrometry. Protein extraction and quantification were performed using the Pierce Surface Protein Isolation kit and the Pierce 660 nm Protein Assay, respectively (Thermo Scientific, Rockford, IL, USA), following the manufacturer's instructions.

Mass Spectrometry Analyses

The proteins (30μg) were reduced (5 mM dithiothreitol, 25 min at 56°C), alkylated (14 mM iodoacetamide, 30 min at room temperature in the dark), and digested with trypsin (Promega). The resulting peptides were submitted to desalting using C-18 solid phase extraction cartridges (Sep-Pak® Vac tC18 cartridge 3cc/100mg, Waters) and resuspended in dissolution buffer of iTRAQ 4-plex kit. The samples were labeled following the manufacturer's instructions: MM-$MC^{CD138\text{-}CD105\text{-}}$ was labeled with the 117 isobaric tag and the HD-$MC^{CD138\text{-}CD105\text{-}}$ with the 116. As each sample was evaluated in a technical replicate, they were also marked with the other isobaric tag, i.e., the cells from MM patients with the tag 116 and the controls with tag 117. The same rationale was used for MM-MSC and HD-MSC labeling, but, in this case, isobaric tags 114 and 115 were used.

The resulting peptide mixture (5 μg) was analyzed on an ETD enabled LTQ Velos Orbitrap mass spectrometer (Thermo Fisher Scientific) coupled with LC-MS/MS by an EASY-nLC system (Proxeon Biosystem) through a Proxeon nanoelectrospray ion source. Peptides were separated by a 2-90% acetonitrile gradient in 0.1% formic acid using an analytical column PicoFrit Column (20 cm x ID75 μm, 5 μm particle size, New objective) at a flow rate of 300 nL/min over 180 min. The nanoelectrospray voltage was set to 2.1 kV and the source temperature was 275°C. All instrument methods for the LTQ Velos Orbitrap were set up in the data dependent acquisition mode of HCD fragmentation. The resolution in the Orbitrap system was set to r= 60,000 and the 5 most intense peptide ions with charge states ≥ 2 were sequentially isolated to a target value of 50,000 and fragmented in HCD with normalized collision energy of 40% with the resolution in the Orbitrap system was set to r= 7,500 for MS/MS. The signal threshold for triggering an MS/MS event was set to 80,000 counts and activation time of 0.1 ms was used. Dynamic exclusion was enabled with exclusion size list of 400 and exclusion duration of 60 s, and repeat count of 2.

Peak lists (msf) were generated from the raw data files using Proteome Discoverer version 1.3 (Thermo Fisher Scientific) with Sequest search engine and searched against NCBI database IPI Human v3.86 (IPI Human: 91,522 sequences; 36,630,302 residues, release July 2011) with carbamidomethylation (+57.021 Da), peptide N-terminus and lysine side chains with iTRAQ as fixed modification, oxidation of methionine (+15.995 Da) and tyrosine residues with iTRAQ as variable modifications, one trypsin missed cleavage and a tolerance of 10 ppm for precursor and 0.02 Da for fragment ions.

To ensure that only one PSM per spectrum is used for protein grouping it was applied strict maximum parsimony principle to protein grouping. Protein identifications were accepted if they contained at least one identified peptide. The peptides were filtered using cutoffs to obtain a false discovery rate less than

1%. For reporter ion identification, it was chosen the most confident centroid, which is almost always the largest peak inside the integration window because of the small inclination of the Gaussian curve in the 1-sigma interval. For reporter ion quantification, the validation step ensures that only peptides that have one of the specified reporter labels as a modification are considered for protein quantification and the protein ratios are calculate by the median of the peptide ratio. The mass spectrometry raw data are available *via* ProteomeXchange with identifier PXD019126.

Bioinformatics and Statistics Analyses Workflow

In order to identify the differentially expressed proteins (DEP), we have established the following cut-off criteria: since we had to combine the samples into pools, this prevented a previous statistical analysis; therefore, the criteria used were the exclusion of the proteins that had no expression in the technical replicates and, arbitrarily, the fold-change values of 1.5 for the upregulated proteins and of 0.6 for the downregulated ones. In order to guarantee that there was no great variability among technical replicates, the coefficients of variation (CV) of the protein expression values were calculated and the CV cut-off criteria less than 15% was established to consider a DEP consistent. After identification of the DEP, we performed the bioinformatics analyses in order to extract relevant biological information from these proteins. The construction of the protein-protein interaction network and the subsequent analyzes were carried out separately for up and downregulated proteins, using the STRING tool, version 11.0 <https://string-db.org>. Then, the proteins that have no connection in the network were removed, and we performed the enrichment analyses to look for overrepresented biological function and pathways from GO (Gene Ontology) (20, 21) and KEGG (Kyoto Encyclopedia of Genes and Genomes) databases (22–25), respectively. P-value was adjusted for multiple comparisons by the FDR method (26) and values less than 0.05 was used as cut-off criteria to consider a category as significantly enriched. Finally, the function of the most relevant proteins was manually searched in the databases Gene <https://www.ncbi.nlm.nih.gov/gene>, from NCBI, and in the Gene Cards <https://www.genecards.org>, and we also made comparisons with data from previous transcriptomic and proteomic studies of our group, looking for possible overlapping of DEP. All graphs in this study, except for protein-protein interaction networks generated with the aid of STRING and Venn diagram generated with the help of <http://bioinformatics.psb.ugent.be/webtools/Venn/>, were constructed using the GraphPad Prism software version 8.0.

RESULTS

Subjects

The clinical and laboratory characteristics of MM patients enrolled in this study (n = 8) are shown in **Table 1**. All patients were classified as advanced-stage MM according to the Durie & Salmon (27) and/or International Staging System criteria (28). Most were male (75%) and the median age at diagnosis was 68.5 years.

TABLE 1 | Clinical and laboratorial characteristics of MM patients included in the study at diagnosis (N = 8).

Patients' characteristics	
Median age, years (range)	68.5 (38-80)
Sex, n (%)	
Male	06 (75)
Female	02 (25)
M-protein type, n (%)	
IgG	04 (50)
IgA	03 (37.5)
Light chain	01 (12.5)
Median tumor cells, % (range)	75 (10-90)
D&S[1] stage n (%)	
I	0 (0)
II	0 (0)
III	08 (100)
ISS[2] stage, n (%)	
1	01 (12.5)
2	01(12.5)
3	06 (75)

[1]*D&S, Durie & Salmon;* [2]*ISS, International Staging System.*

MSC Isolation, Expansion, and Characterization

In vitro expansion of MSCs was successfully performed in four MM patients and four HD. MSC from both groups were positive for the markers assessed (CD105, CD90, and CD73), and negative for the markers (CD45, CD34, CD14, and HLA-DR), and there was no difference between groups (**Supplementary Figures 1** and **2**). After *in vitro* induction for osteoblastic differentiation, it was also possible to detect osteocalcin in the medium of cell culture, and there were no difference among MM-MSC and HD-MSC in this parameter (data not shown, 16). Therefore, there were no differences between groups with regard to immunophenotype and osteoblastogenic potential after *in vitro* expansion.

Protein Isolation, Quantification, and Mass Spectrometry Analyses

As described in the methodology, in order to obtain the protein concentration required for performing mass spectrometry analyses, the samples were pooled. Between $MC^{CD138\text{-}CD105\text{-}}$, the protein concentrations from cases and controls were 67 and 99 µg, respectively, whereas between the MSC, the concentrations were 90 and 69 µg for cases and controls, respectively. 30 µg of protein from each group was used for iTRAQ kit labeling.

Bioinformatic Analyses

Our study found 75 differentially expressed proteins (DEP) between $MM\text{-}MC^{CD138\text{-}CD105\text{-}}$ and $HD\text{-}MC^{CD138\text{-}CD105\text{-}}$, being 66 upregulated and nine downregulated. Regarding MM-MSC and HD-MSC comparison, our work found 14 DEP, being 12 upregulated and two downregulated. As mentioned in the

TABLE 2 | MM-MSC and HD-MSC comparisons detected 14 differentially expressed proteins, being 12 upregulated and two downregulated.

Status	Gene Symbol	Protein Description	115/114	114/115
Upregulated	*S100A11*	Protein S100-A11	14.442	1.930
	HLA-A	HLA class I histocompatibility antigen, A alpha chain	9.565	12.014
	GAPDH	Glyceraldehyde-3-phosphate dehydrogenase	5.138	1.823
	VIM	Vimentin	2.521	2.376
	TALDO1	Transaldolase	2.280	1.908
	ANXA5	Annexin A5	2.153	2.395
	PKM	Pyruvate kinase PKM	2.105	1.972
	CANX	Calnexin	1.766	1.642
	PSMA1	Proteasome subunit alpha type-1	1.736	1.599
	ALPL	Alkaline phosphatase, tissue-nonspecific isozyme	1.731	1.817
	RAB7A	Ras-related protein Rab-7a	1.645	1.782
	CLTC	Clathrin heavy chain 1	1.522	1.543
Status	**Gene Symbol**	**Protein Description**	**115/114**	**114/115**
Downregulated	*DPYSL2*	Dihydropyrimidinase-related protein 2	0.205	0.556
	CTSZ	Cathepsin Z	0.554	0.546

methods, we chose CV values less than 15%, among technical replicates, to consider a DEP as consistent. With regard to both comparisons, 80% of the total DEP were consistent according to our cut-off. Detailed information on the up and downregulated proteins derived from both comparisons, can be seen in the supplementary material **(Supplementary Tables 1 and 2)** and in the **Table 2**.

Figures 1 and **2** show the protein-protein interaction networks for the up and downregulated proteins, respectively, between the MC of MM patients in comparison with the controls. Regarding MSC, due to the low number of DEP identified, we did not build the protein-to-protein interaction network for this comparison.

MM-MC$^{CD138-CD105-}$ *vs.* HD-MC$^{CD138-CD105-}$

We identified 68 biological processes of GO significantly unregulated between patients and controls (FDR <0.05). As the number of biological processes in the GO found was high, we chose to graphically represent only those with the highest level of significance (FDR <0.001), resulting in 24 processes **(Figure 3A).** Among the upregulated processes, we highlight three in particular - 1) Energy metabolism: which represented about

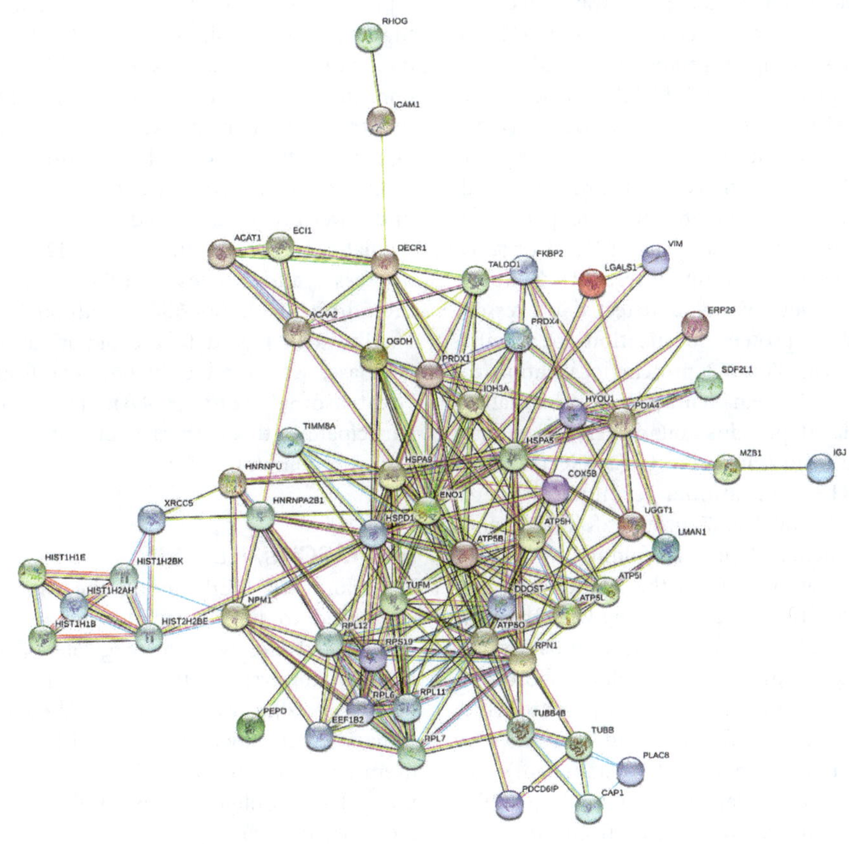

FIGURE 1 | Protein-protein interaction network in MM- MC$^{CD138-CD105-}$ *vs.* HD-MC$^{CD138-CD105-}$: upregulated proteins. Nodes represent proteins and edges represent protein-protein associations. Node color: colored nodes and white nodes represent, respectively, query proteins and first shell of interactions, and second shell of interactions. Node content: empty and filled nodes represent, respectively proteins of unknown 3D structure, and some 3D structure is known or predicted. The edges are composed of known interactions, predicted interactions, among other forms of interaction, including co-expression. (STRING https://string-db.org/).

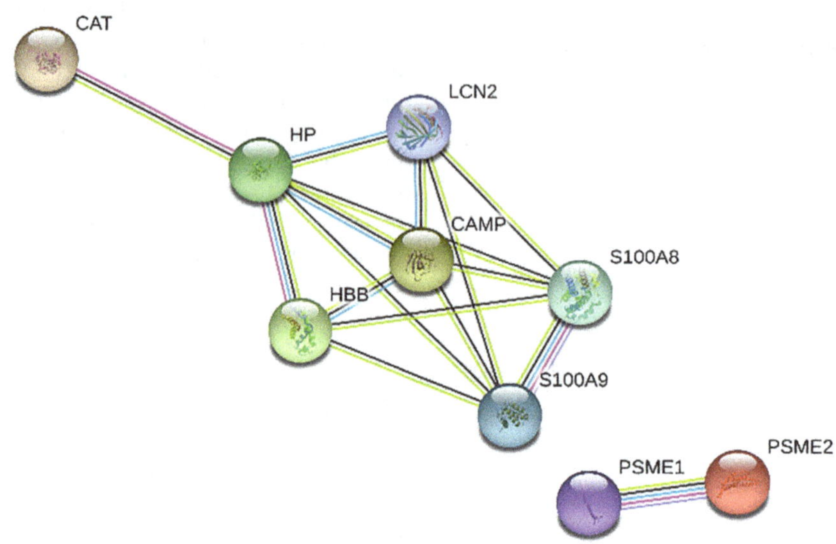

FIGURE 2 | Protein-protein interaction network in MM-MC$^{CD138-CD105-}$ *vs.* HD-MC$^{CD138-CD105-}$: downregulated proteins. Nodes represent proteins and edges represent protein-protein associations. Node color: colored nodes and white nodes represent, respectively, query proteins and first shell of interactions, and second shell of interactions. Node content: empty and filled nodes represent, respectively proteins of unknown 3D structure, and some 3D structure is known or predicted. The edges are composed of known interactions, predicted interactions, among other forms of interaction, including co-expression. (STRING https://string-db.org/).

40% of the total proteins identified, including pathways related to cellular respiration and ATP synthesis (e.g.: "GO:0042776 mitochondrial ATP synthesis coupled proton transport"; "GO: 0046034 ATP metabolic process"; " GO:0022904 respiratory electron transport chain"), oxidation reactions (e.g.: "GO:0015980 energy derivation by oxidation of organic compounds"; "GO:0055114 oxidation-reduction process"), and catabolic processes (e.g.: "GO:0009056 catabolic process"; "GO:0044248 cellular catabolic process"; "GO:1801575 organic substance catabolic process"), among others. 2) Cellular localization: representing about 13% of undetected processes, mainly pathways related to protein localization in specific regions of cells, such as "GO:0070972 protein localization to endoplasmic reticulum". 3) Protein synthesis: approximately 20% of the total upregulated proteins found were related to protein synthesis, ranging from translation (e.g.: "GO:0006412 translation", "GO:0006415 translational termination"), to protein folding, such as "GO:0006457 protein folding", and "GO:0061077 chaperone-mediated protein folding". We also identified seven biological pathways from the KEGG database significantly overrepresented **(Figure 3B),** in line with the GO biological processes, with emphasis on the following pathways: "protein processing in endoplasmic reticulum" and "ribosome" (both related to protein biosynthesis), and "oxidative phosphorylation", "fatty acid degradation", and "metabolism pathways "(all of them related to energy metabolism). In addition, we also identified an overlap of 24 upregulated DEP proteins from this study, compared to the data from our 2015 study (19), where we evaluated the protein expression of tumor plasma cells versus plasma cells from healthy donors **(Figure 5).**

Regarding downregulated proteins, we identified 27 significantly enriched biological processes. We chose to represent in **Figure 4A**, only the biological processes with the highest level of significance (FDR <0.01), resulting in 14 biological pathways. Most of the biological processes found by our study were related to the immune response, including the innate immune response, such as "GO:0070488 neutrophil aggregation", "GO:0045087 innate immune response", "GO:0030593 neutrophil chemotaxis", among others. We also find fewer processes related to cell death, such as "GO:0010941 regulation of cell death", "GO:0042981 regulation of apoptotic process", and processes related to zinc ion homeostasis, including "GO: 0006882: cellular zinc ion homeostasis". Finally, with regard to the biological pathways of the KEGG database, we found only one significantly enriched pathway "proteasome" **(Figure 4B).** Two downregulated proteins participate in this pathway: subunits 1 and 2 of the proteasome activator complex.

MM-MSC *vs.* HD-MSC

We found 14 DEP among the MSC of patients with MM compared to their normal counterpart from HD, being 12 upregulated and two downregulated **(Table 2).** Mainly due to the low number of DEP, no significantly enriched process or biological pathway was found in the GO and KEGG databases. Thus, we manually evaluated the 14 DEP through searches in the literature. In line with the results of the MC, among the upregulated proteins, some of them were involved in energy metabolism, such as glyceraldehyde-3-phosphate dehydrogenase, transaldolase 1, and pyruvate kinase M1/2, demonstrating a possible importance of the energy metabolism pathways in the pathophysiology of the disease. One upregulated protein that deserves to be highlighted is protein S100-A11. It is a member

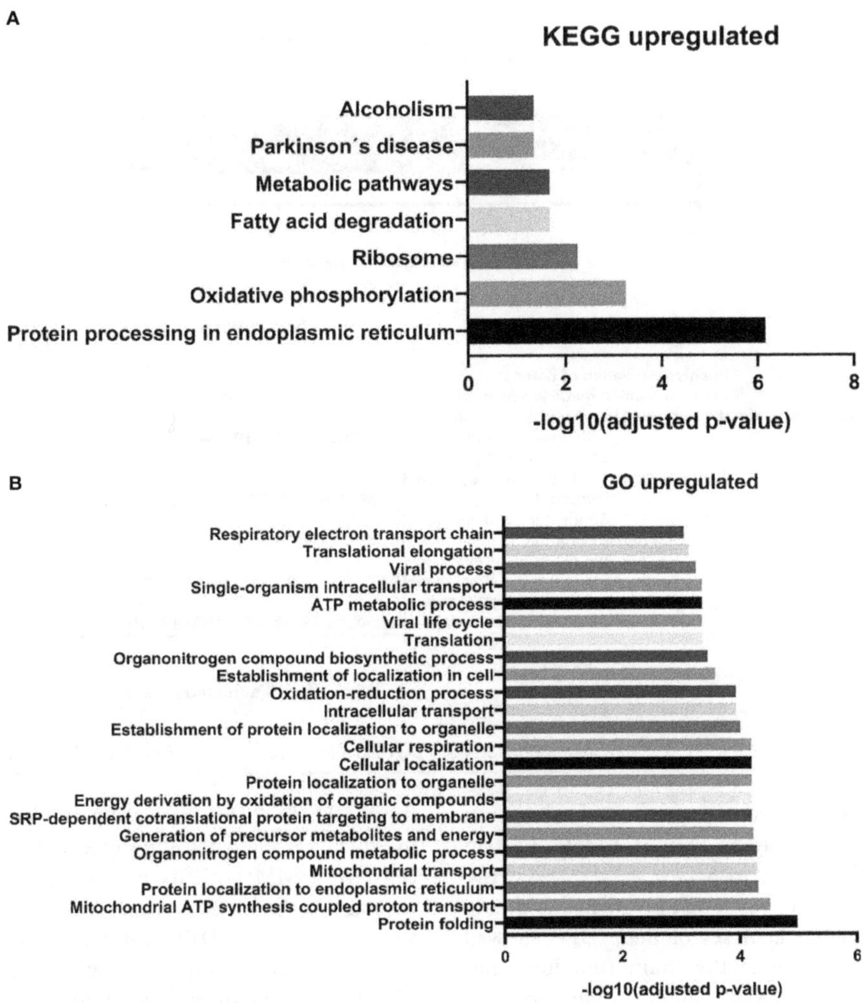

FIGURE 3 | MM-MC$^{CD138-CD105-}$ *vs.* HD-MC$^{CD138-CD105-}$ upregulated proteins. – **(A)** KEGG enriched pathways **(B)** GO enriched biological processes.

of S100 calcium-binding protein family, participating in the regulation of several cellular processes, including - but not limited to - cell cycle progression and differentiation. It has also been described in different types of cancer, playing an important role in tumorigenesis and metastasis. Another upregulated protein worth mentioning is calnexin. It is a protein that belongs to the calnexin family of molecular chaperones and plays an important role in the correct folding of proteins. Additionally, the upregulation of the proteasome subunit alpha type-1, which is a component of the proteasome complex and involved in the proteolytic degradation of intracellular proteins, has already been described in the literature in tumor plasma cells and may appear as a mechanism of resistance of these cells to effect of the proteasome inhibitor bortezomib. Finally, the RAB7A protein, member of the RAS oncogene family, was also upregulated in MM-MSC. It participates in several cellular processes, being able to perform its role as oncosuppressor or oncogenic.

DISCUSSION

The tumor microenvironment is extremely important for the development, maintenance and progression of different types of cancer, being MM one of the malignancies where its essential role has been demonstrated by several independent studies (12, 13). Despite its importance in the pathophysiology of MM, the BM tumor microenvironment of MM patients is still not so much studied. MSC are considered the most relevant player and, as a result, are the most studied cell type (29–33). However, other cell types present in BM, including lymphocytes, monocytes, dendritic cells, among others, also play an important role in the disease progression. Thus, this study aimed to analyze these cells more deeply, through a proteomic and bioinformatic analyses, in order to better understand their proteome expression profiling, aiming to identify DEP that may serve as potential biomarkers/ therapeutic targets, and/or further elucidate the pathophysiology

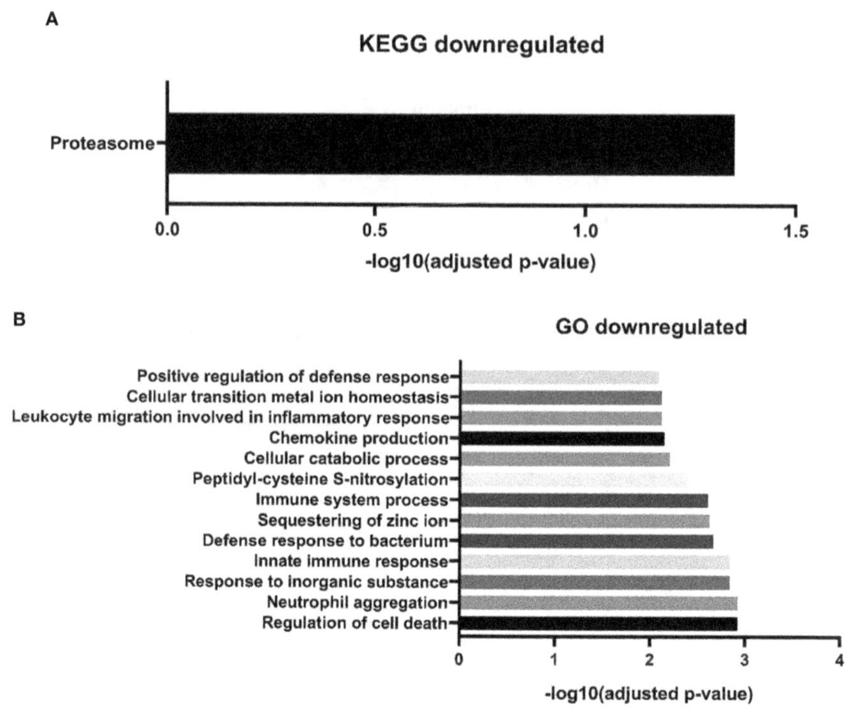

FIGURE 4 | MM-MC$^{CD138\text{-}CD105\text{-}}$ *vs.* HD-MC$^{CD138\text{-}CD105\text{-}}$ downregulated proteins. – **(A)** KEGG enriched pathways **(B)** GO enriched biological processes.

of MM. Besides, we also studied the proteome expression profiling of MM-MSC in comparison with HD-MSC. Protein expression profiling analysis of MM-MC$^{CD138\text{-}CD105\text{-}}$ *vs.* HD-MC$^{CD138\text{-}CD105}$ revealed 75 DEP, being 66 upregulated and nine downregulated. Bioinformatics analyses of these DEP showed that among upregulated proteins, the main functions and pathways were related to energy metabolism, cellular localization, and protein synthesis, whereas, among downregulated proteins, the main pathways and functions were related to the immune response, mainly to innate immunity, which raises the hypothesis of possible mechanisms of evasion of the immune response. Regarding MM-MSC vs. HD-MSC, we identified 14 DEP, being 12 upregulated and two downregulated. The search in the literature and databases showed that the most relevant proteins were among the upregulated proteins, with emphasis on the proteins S100-A11, calnexin, proteasome subunit alpha type-1, and RAB7A protein, all of them proteins described in the literature as being important in the pathophysiology of other types of cancer. Our study was the first to identify their increased expression in MM-MSC. In addition, other proteins upregulated in MM-MSC were also related to energy metabolism, as well as MM-MC$^{CD138\text{-}CD105\text{-}}$, demonstrating a potential role of this pathway in the pathophysiology of the disease.

High throughput techniques, such as mass spectrometry, microarray, RNA-seq, among others, allow the generation of an abundant amount of data, allowing to compare patient cells in pathological conditions, such as MM, in relation to cells derived from HD. In 2015, our group published a proteomics study in which we evaluated the protein expression of tumor plasma cells from MM patients in comparison to plasma cells from palatal tonsils from normal individuals (19). In this study, we identified 81 DEP among these cells (72 upregulated and nine downregulated). Among upregulated proteins, we highlighted the ones related to protein biosynthesis, while among downregulated proteins, most of them were related to the immune response. These results are in line with what we identified in this present study between MM-MC$^{CD138\text{-}CD105\text{-}}$ and HD-MC. Regarding the upregulated proteins from these two studies, we do see an overlap of 24 proteins (**Figure 5**). Among them, there are mainly proteins related to protein biosynthesis, including chaperones, for instance, the endoplasmic reticulum chaperone BiP, and hypoxia upregulated 1, ribosomal proteins, and proteins capable of post-translational modifications. On the other hand, among the downregulated proteins, no overlap was identified. Our group also published another paper in 2019, where we evaluated the MM-MSC transcriptome compared to HD-MSC (16). In this study, we identified 485 differentially expressed genes (280 up and 205 downregulated). The most significant pathways and functions were among the downregulated genes, especially genes involved in cell cycle progression, immune response, and bone metabolism. However, in this case, we did not identify any overlap with the proteins identified in this study.

In relation to upregulated DEP identified in the MM-MC$^{CD138\text{-}CD105\text{-}}$ *vs.* HD-MC$^{CD138\text{-}CD105\text{-}}$ comparison, energy metabolism was one of the enriched pathways identified

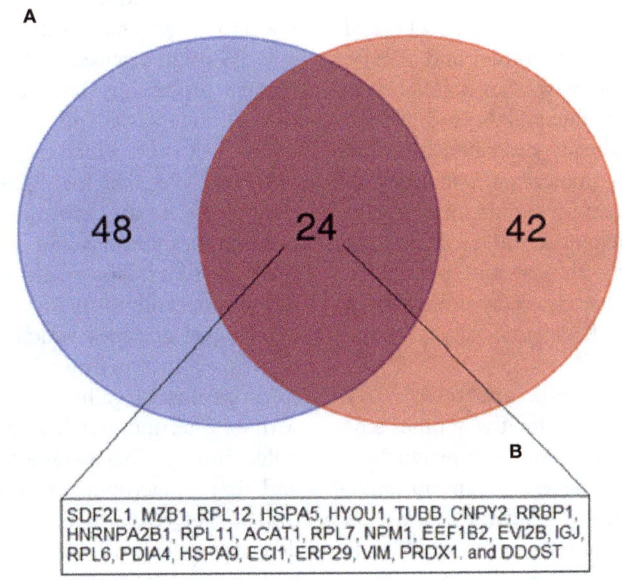

FIGURE 5 | Venn diagram showing the overlap between the upregulated DEP in the current study (MM-MC$^{CD138-CD105-}$ *vs.* HD-MC$^{CD138-CD105-}$) compared to the upregulated DEP in our previous study (MM Plasma cells *vs.* HD Plasma cells) by Fernando et al. (19). **(A)** Fernando et al. (19) study; **(B)** Current study.

through bioinformatics analysis. Ward and Thompson (34) have proposed that metabolic reprogramming, driven by activated oncogenes and inactivated tumor suppressors, is a cancer hallmark. Metabolic changes have already been described in different types of malignancies, including MM - increase in glycolysis and glutaminolysis in MM cells compared to healthy cells, among other changes (35). Some studies have demonstrated the role of these metabolic alterations in drug resistance in patients who are refractory to current available treatments (36). In another study, the authors evaluated the proteome of plasma cell from naïve MM patients, in order to identify pathways associated with good response to bortezomib-based treatment protocols. The authors reported that alternation in energy metabolism might be associated with good response to a specific bortezomib-based regime (37). Recently, Ray et al. (38) have identified Alpha-Enolase (*ENO1*), which was one of the DEP detected in our study in the mononuclear cells comparison, as a possible immunometabolic target in MM. The authors have demonstrated, through *in vitro* analyses, that BM plasmacytoid dendritic cells (pDCs) from MM patients induce *ENO1* expression in MM cells and pDCs, and they also have showed that patients with high *ENO1* expression have poor overall survival in comparison with the ones with low expression of this gene. In addition, they also reported that the inhibition of *ENO1* induces the activation of CD8$^+$ T cells and NK cells against MM cells. Another protein, IDH3A, which was connected with ENO1 in our protein-protein interaction network, might also be important for MM pathogenesis. Although its role in malignant tumors is still unclear, its overexpression was reported in hepatocellular carcinoma and in extramedullary plasmacytomas (39, 40). In addition, other two proteins, which were also connected with ENO1 in our network, might play important roles in MM: Oxoglutarate dehydrogenase (OGDH) – it is a subunit of an enzymatic complex that participates in the Krebs cycles, and it was also found that several cancer cells depend on this protein for growth and survival (41); Heterogeneous nuclear ribonucleoprotein A2/B1 (hnRNPA2B1) – it influences pre-RNA process, and mRNA metabolism and transport; Shen et al. (42) have demonstrated that a long non-coding RNA, ST3GAL6-AS1, might promote adhesion and invasion of MM cells, through binding with hnRNPA2B1, resulting in the regulation of ST3GAL6 expression (42). Therefore, studies aiming to better understand the metabolic changes, both in the tumor plasma cells as well as in the tumor microenvironment, are extremely important in the search for new therapeutic targets, especially for refractory patients.

Regarding protein biosynthesis, which was another category identified among upregulated DEP in MC, we highlight proteins related to "protein processing in endoplasmic reticulum", namely the following genes that code for these proteins *RRBP1*, *ERP29*, *PDIA4*, *LMAN1*, *DDOST*, *UGGT1*, *RPN1*, *HSPA5*, and *HYOU1*, and the ones related to "protein folding", which are *PRDX4*, *FKBP2*, *ERP29*, *PDIA4*, *LMAN1*, *HSPA5*, *UGGT1*, *HSPD1*, *HSPA9*, and *GNB2*. The HSPA5, HSPA9, and HYOU1 proteins are part of the heat shock protein 70 family, a family of chaperones involved in physiological processes, such as the assistance of general folding of unfolded and/or misfolded proteins, and which has been described as deregulated in MM patients (43, 44). Another chaperone was also identified - HSPD1 - which belongs to the HSP60 family. Recently, the HSPD1 protein has been described to regulate metabolic and protein synthesis changes in MM cells, promoting its proliferation, thus representing a potential therapeutic target (45). Moreover, we found ribosomal proteins, including RPL6, RPL7, RPL11 and RPL12, which form the 60S subunit of ribosomes, and RPS19, which form the 40S subunit. In summary, we can highlight the relevance of chaperones belonging to the HSP70 and HSP60 families, some of which have been already described by other studies as deregulated in the tumor plasma cells of patients with MM, contributing to disease progression by maintaining protein homeostasis, blocking apoptosis and helping in the stabilization of oncoproteins (44). In addition, early clinical and preclinical studies have shown that HSP inhibitors, especially inhibitors of the HSP90 family, can be promising therapeutic targets in the treatment of patients with MM (46).

In healthy individuals, plasma cells are terminally differentiated B cells which are responsible for the synthesis of immunoglobulins against pathogens. Due to the high production of proteins, these cells are naturally subject to endoplasmic reticulum (ER) stress, which activates a pathway known as UPR, helping the cell to overcome this type of stress (47). In the case of MM patients, the tumor plasma cells, in the vast majority of patients, produce a monoclonal immunoglobulin, known as paraprotein. To deal with this type of stress, that is, an extremely high production of immunoglobulin, the UPR pathway is very and constantly activated and allows the tumor cell to remain viable (47). In the case of cells in the tumor microenvironment, paraprotein is not produced. On the other hand, due to the action of tumor plasma cells on these cells, there is a production of different types of soluble elements, such as cytokines, chemokines and growth factors (13). One hypothesis is that proteins related to protein biosynthesis, as well as UPR, as is the case of chaperones, are important to keep these cells viable by producing molecules important for the maintenance and progression of MM cells. Therefore, our hypothesis is that other MM BM mononuclear cells contribute to maintenance of tumor plasma cells homeostasis, avoiding tumor cell death due to accumulation of cytoplasmic immunoglobulin overload. Other possibility is that this process is too important for MM tumor cells that, even in a more than 85% enriched pool of MCs, we can still see these proteins' expression as a sign of residual tumor plasma cells contamination.

Regarding downregulated proteins in the MC "compartment", proteasome activators complex subunits 1 and 2 proteins are components of the proteasome and play an important role in its regulation. In bortezomib-resistant patients (a class of proteasome inhibitor used in the treatment of MM), these proteins are upregulated (37). Therefore, these protein downregulation in MCs is totally in agreement with their function, not related to overexpression of proteasome pathway typically found in MM tumor cells.

Still in relation to MM-MC$^{CD138\text{-}CD105\text{-}}$, most of the downregulated proteins were related to the immune response, such as antigen processing, leukocyte recruitment, production of pro-inflammatory cytokines, and immune responses against pathogens. We can highlight the downregulation of proteins S100-A9 and S100A9, which form a complex called calprotectin and are involved in different functions, for instance, enhancing leukocyte recruitment and pro-inflammatory cytokines release. HP and CAMP have antimicrobial properties, whereas PSME1 and PSME2, discussed above, are also required for efficient antigen processing. The decrease in these proteins involved in the immune system may be related to mechanisms of tumor immune evasion, which have also been described by other groups (48, 49). We also highlight the downregulated of pathways related to innate immune response. Although the innate immune response is not as studied as adaptive response in MM patients, some studies have already demonstrated important changes in this arm of the immune response, such as changes in genes which code for innate immune response proteins, increasing the risk of developing MM (50). Additionally, Magalhães et al. (51) demonstrated that patients with long-term disease control and those with symptomatic MM differ, among other parameters, in the number of dendritic cells and tissue macrophages in BM. In addition, the number and function of NK cells is impaired in MM, and the function of dendritic cells is also altered (52). Among the new strategies to treat refractory MM cases are CART-cells and BiTEs (11). Chimeric antigen receptors (CARs) are chimeric proteins that assemble the signaling portions of the T cell receptor complex (TCR) and the variable domains of an antibody targeting an antigen of interest. A variety of targets are currently being studied in MM and include BCMA, SLAMF7, CD138, NKG2DA, kappa light chain, and CD19 ligands. Ongoing clinical trials will define its role in the coming years (11, 53). BITEs are generated to combine the specificities of two antibodies, binding simultaneously to multiple epitopes, one of which involves the activation of T cells through their CD3 molecules (54, 55). These new immunotherapies corroborate the relevance of microenvironment and strength immune system to control of refractory hematological tumors.

Finally, in relation to MM-MSC, although we have identified a low number of DEP, among the upregulated proteins, some of them are quite interesting and had not yet been described in the context of MM: Ras-related protein Rab-7a, among other functions, participate in cellular processes such as autophagy, apoptosis, signaling, and cell migration, being important for the progression and resistance to drugs in some types of cancer (56). Thus, our study suggests that further studies are needed to evaluate this molecule as a potential therapeutic target in the context of MM. In addition, we have also identified the protein S100-A11, which is a protein often upregulated in different types of human cancer, and its potential as a therapeutic target has not been evaluated yet in patients with MM. Besides, our analyses also found increased expression of the protein calnexin, a protein induced by stress in the endoplasmic reticulum. This protein has already been described in the literature as a prognostic marker and potential therapeutic target in colorectal cancer, but it has not yet been evaluated in MM (57). Finally, another protein that deserves attention is annexin V, which was upregulated in MM-MSC. Overexpression of annexin II, a protein that is related to annexin V, has already been described in plasma cells of MM patients and, in some cell lines of this disease, seems to promote proliferation, apoptosis, invasion potential and production of proangiogenic factors (58). In line with this data, Glavey et al. (59) reported that the upregulation of annexin II protein, produced by BM extracellular matrix from MM patients, is associated with a decreased overall survival.

The main limitations of this study are the low number of patients with MM enrolled. MM is a rare disease, representing only 1% of cases of cancer (3); in addition, all cases included here were seen at our public tertiary university hospital, the majority of them being severely ill patients, with advanced disease stage, often requiring immediate treatment due to medical emergencies. Since steroids or bisphosphonates could potentially alter protein expression of tumor microenvironment cells, patients who received these drugs were not eligible for the study. A possible source of bias is related to the BM biopsy site: in our study, we performed bone marrow biopsy in only one region of the iliac crest of each patient or control. However, recently, a group has demonstrated substantial intra-patient spatial heterogeneity in the bone marrow of MM patients (60). Another limitation that deserves to be highlighted is the fact that the case and control groups were not matched by sex or age, which might introduce bias in our analysis, including the relevant downregulation of immune system proteins related to physiological immunosenescence. However, several proteins identified as differentially expressed between the cells of these groups, had already been described by other groups as deregulated in MM, which increases the robustness of our data (61–63). In addition, another limitation of our study is the fact that the protein samples were analyzed in pools. This approach was necessary to obtain enough protein for the analysis proposed in this study. Although we performed experiments in technical replicates, which allowed us to verify the technical variability, we were unable to analyze possible biological variations among patients with MM. Finally, we also did not perform any functional analyses of the pathways/proteins deregulated by MM identified in our study. However, the main objective of our work was to identify molecules which can be better studied in the future as biomarkers and therapeutic targets: shifts in metabolic pathways and decrease of immune functions are among the cancer hallmarks ready to be explored in MM, which is representative of a cancer of immune system affecting elderly patients.

In summary, our study demonstrated that the BM tumor microenvironment of MM patients have a different protein expression profiling when compared to the BM micro environment of healthy individuals. Among the main altered biological pathways in MC, we can highlight the increased expression of proteins related to different functions of protein biosynthesis, especially chaperone molecules, which have been studied as potential therapeutic targets in the treatment of MM in the last years. In addition, the increased expression of proteins related to energy metabolism, which was also identified by our work, has been increasingly studied in the context of different types of cancers, including MM, being a promising therapeutic target as well. The downregulation of different proteins involved in the immune response, may contribute to escape to the maintenance and progression of the disease, in addition to drug resistance. Thus, the new immunotherapies that have been studied for the treatment of MM and other cancers, such as CART-cells and BiTEs, can be promising tools to reverse this scenario of BM immunosuppression which MM patients are subjected. Finally, with respect to MM-MSC, we have identified some potential new therapeutic targets that can be evaluated in future studies.

ETHICS STATEMENT

The studies involving human participants were reviewed and approved by Institutional Review Board from Federal University of São Paulo. Written informed consent to participate in this study was provided by the participants' legal guardian/next of kin.

AUTHOR CONTRIBUTIONS

RF: Data analysis and interpretation, and manuscript writing. FC: Study design, data collection, and review and approval of the final version of the article. AL: Data collection and analysis, and approval of the final version of the article. GC: Study design, data analysis and interpretation, and manuscript writing. All authors contributed to the article and approved the submitted version.

ACKNOWLEDGMENTS

The authors thank all the professionals who provided essential technical support during the conduction of this work.

REFERENCES

1. Kyle RA, Rajkumar SV. Multiple myeloma. *N Engl J Med* (2004) 351 (18):1860–73. doi: 10.1056/NEJMra041875
2. Palumbo A, Anderson K. Multiple myeloma. *N Engl J Med* (2011) 364 (11):1046–60. doi: 10.1056/NEJMra1011442
3. Rajkumar SV, Dimopoulos MA, Palumbo A. International myeloma working group updated criteria for the diagnosis of multiple myeloma. *Lancet Oncol* (2014) 15(12):e538–48. doi: 10.1016/S1470-2045(14)70442-5
4. Siegel RL, Miller KD, Jemal A. Cancer statistics. *CA Cancer J Clin* (2018) 68 (1):7–30. doi: 10.3322/caac.21442
5. Kumar SK, Rajkumar V, van Duin M, Sonneveld P, Mateos MV, Gay F, et al. Multiple myeloma. *Nat Rev Dis Primers* (2017) 3:17046. doi: 10.1038/nrdp.2017.46
6. Landgren O, Kyle RA, Pfeiffer RM, Katzmann JA, Caporaso NE, Hayes RB, et al. Monoclonal gammopathy of undetermined significance (MGUS) consistently precedes multiple myeloma: a prospective study. *Blood* (2009) 113(22):5412–7. doi: 10.1182/blood-2008-12-194241

7. Weiss BM, Abadie J, Verma P, Howard RS, Kuehl WM. A monoclonal gammopathy precedes multiple myeloma in most patients. *Blood* (2009) 113 (22):5418–22. doi: 10.1182/blood-2008-12-195008
8. San Miguel JF, Mateos MV, Ocio E, Garcia-Sanz R. Multiple myeloma: treatment evolution. *Hematology* (2012) 17 supl:s3–6. doi: 10.1179/102453312X13336169154971
9. Kumar SK, Anderson KC. Immune therapies in multiple myeloma. *Clin Cancer Res* (2016) 22(22):5453–60. doi: 10.1158/1078-0432.CCR-16-0868
10. Turesson I, Velez R, Kristinsson SY, Landgren O. Patterns of improved survival in patients with multiple myeloma in the twenty-first century: a population-based study. *J Clin Oncol* (2010) 28(5):830–4. doi: 10.1200/JCO.2009.25.4177
11. Hoyos V, Borrello I. The immunotherapy era of myeloma: monoclonal antibodies, vaccines, and adoptive T-cell therapies. *Blood* (2016) 128 (13):1679–87. doi: 10.1182/blood-2016-05-636357
12. Mitsiades CS, Mitsiades NS, Munshi NC, Richardson PG, Anderson KC. The role of the bone microenvironment in the pathophysiology and therapeutic management of multiple myeloma: interplay of growth factors, their receptors and stromal interactions. *Eur J Cancer* (2006) 42:1564–73. doi: 10.1016/j.ejca.2005.12.025
13. Bianchi G, Munshi NC. Pathogenesis beyond the cancer clone(s) in multiple myeloma. *Blood* (2015) 125(20):3049–58. doi: 10.1182/blood-2014-11-568881
14. Bianco P, Robey PG, Simmons PJ. Mesenchymal stem cells: revisiting history, concepts, and assays. *Cell Stem Cell* (2008) 2(4):313–9. doi: 10.1016/j.stem.2008.03.002
15. Reagan MR, Ghobrial IM. Multiple myeloma mesenchymal stem cells: characterization, origin, and tumor-promoting effects. *Clin Cancer Res* (2012) 18(2):342–9. doi: 10.1158/1078-0432.CCR-11-2212
16. Fernando RC, Mazzotti DR, Azevedo H, Sandes AF, Rizzatti EG, de Oliveira MB, et al. Transcriptome analysis of mesenchymal stem cells from multiple myeloma patients reveals downregulation of genes involved in cell cycle progression, immune response and bone metabolism. *Sci Rep* (2019) 9 (1):1056. doi: 10.1038/s41598-018-38314-8
17. Kawano Y, Moschetta M, Manier S, Glavey S, Gorgun GT, Roccaro AM, et al. Targeting the bone marrow microenvironment in multiple myeloma. *Immunol Rev* (2015) 263(1):160–72. doi: 10.1111/imr.12233
18. Cox J, Mann M. Is proteomics the new genomics? *Cell* (2007) 130(3):395–8. doi: 10.1016/j.cell.2007.07.032
19. Fernando RC, de Carvalho F, Mazzotti DR, Evangelista AF, Braga WMT, de Lourdes Chauffaille M, et al. Multiple myeloma cell lines and primary tumors proteoma: protein biosynthesis and immune system as potential therapeutic targets. *Genes Cancer* (2015) 6(11-12):462–71. doi: 10.18632/genesandcancer.88
20. Ashburner M, Ball CA, Blake JA, Botstein D, Butler H, Cherry JM, et al. Gene ontology: tool for the unification of biology. The Gene Ontology Consortium. *Nat Genet* (2000) 25(1):25–9. doi: 10.1038/75556
21. Gene Ontology Consortium: going forward. *Nucleic Acids Res* (2015) 43 (Database issue):D1049–56. doi: 10.1093/nar/gku1179
22. Kanehisa M, Goto S. KEGG: kyoto encyclopedia of genes and genomes. *Nucleic Acids Res* (2000) 28(1):27–30. doi: 10.1093/nar/28.1.27
23. Kanehisa M, Goto S, Sato Y, Kawashima M, Furumichi M, Tanabe M. Data, information, knowledge and principle: back to metabolism in KEGG. *Nucleic Acids Res* (2014) 42(Database issue):D199–205. doi: 10.1093/nar/gkt1076
24. Kanehisa M, Sato Y, Kawashima M, Furumichi M, Tanabe M. KEGG as a reference resource for gene and protein annotation. *Nucleic Acids Res* (2016) 44(D1):D457–62. doi: 10.1093/nar/gkv1070
25. Kanehisa M, Furumichi M, Tanabe M, Sato Y, Morishima K. KEGG: new perspectives on genomes, pathways, diseases and drugs. *Nucleic Acids Res* (2017) 45(D1):D353–d61. doi: 10.1093/nar/gkw1092
26. Benjamini Y, Hochberg Y. Controlling the false discovery rate: a practical and powerful approach to multiple testing. *J R Stat Soc Ser B (Methodol)* (1995) 57 (1):289–300. doi: 10.1111/j.2517-6161.1995.tb02031.x
27. Durie BG, Salmon SE. A clinical staging system for multiple myeloma. Correlation of measured myeloma cell mass with presenting clinical features, response to treatment, and survival. *Cancer* (1975) 36:842–54. doi: 10.1002/1097-0142(197509)36:3<842::AID-CNCR2820360303>3.0.CO;2-U
28. Greipp PR, San Miguel J, Durie BG, Crowley JJ, Barlogie B, Bladé J, et al. International staging system for multiple myeloma. *J Clin Oncol* (2005) 23 (15):3412–20. doi: 10.1200/JCO.2005.04.242
29. Arnulf B, Lecourt S, Soulier J, Ternaux B, Lacassagne MN, Crinquette A, et al. Phenotypic and functional characterization of bone marrow mesenchymal stem cells derived from patients with multiple myeloma. *Leukemia* (2007) 21 (1):158–63. doi: 10.1038/sj.leu.2404466
30. Corre J, Mahtouk K, Atta M, Gadelorge M, Huynh A, Fleury-Cappellesso S, et al. Bone marrow mesenchymal stem cells are abnormal in multiple myeloma. *Leukemia* (2007) 21(5):1079–88. doi: 10.1038/sj.leu.2404621
31. Garayoa M, Garcia JL, Santamaria C, Garcia-Gomez A, Blanco JF, Pandiella A, et al. Mesenchymal stem cells from multiple myeloma patients display distinct genomic profile as compared with those from normal donors. *Leukemia* (2009) 23(8):1515–27. doi: 10.1038/leu.2009.65
32. André T, Meuleman N, Stamatopoulos B, De Bryun C, Pieters K, Bron D, et al. Evidences of early senescence in multiple myeloma bone marrow mesenchymal stromal cells. *PloS One* (2013) 8(3):e59756. doi: 10.1371/journal.pone.0059756
33. Garcia-Gomez A, De Las Rivas J, Ocio M, Díaz-Rodríguez E, Montero JC, Martin M, et al. Transcriptomic profile induced in bone marrow mesenchymal stromal cells after interaction with multiple myeloma cells: implications in myeloma progression and myeloma bone disease. *Oncotarget* (2014) 5(18):8284–305. doi: 10.18632/oncotarget.2058
34. Ward PS, Thompson CB. Metabolic reprogramming: a cancer hallmark even Warburg did not anticipate. *Cancer Cell* (2012) 21(3):297–308. doi: 10.1016/j.ccr.2012.02.014
35. Ei Arfani C, De Veirman K, De Bruyne E, Menu E. Metabolic features of multiple myeloma. *Int J Mol Sci* (2018) 19(4):E1200. doi: 10.3390/ijms19041200
36. Maiso P, Huynh D, Moschetta M, Sacco A, Aljawai Y, Mishima Y, et al. Metabolic signature identifies novel targets for drug resistance in Multiple Myeloma. *Cancer Res* (2015) 75(10):2071–82. doi: 10.1158/0008-5472.CAN-14-3400
37. Dytfeld D, Rosebeck S, Kandarpa M, Mayampurath A, Mellacheruvu D, Alonge MM, et al. Proteomic profilling of naïve multiple myeloma patient plasma cells identifies pathways associated with favourable response to bortezomib-based treatment regimens. *Br J Haematol* (2015) 170(1):66–79. doi: 10.1111/bjh.13394
38. Ray A, Song Y, Du T, Chauhan D, Anderson KC. Preclinical validation of Alpha-Enolase (ENO1) as a novel immunometabolic target in multiple myeloma. *Oncogene* (2020) 39:2786–96. doi: 10.1038/s41388-020-1172-0
39. Liu X, Qiao Y, Ting X, Si W. Isocitrate dehydrogenase 3A, a rate-limiting enzyme of the TCA cycle, promotes hepatocellular carcinoma migration and invasion through regulation of MTA1, a core component of the NuRD complex. *Am J Cancer Res* (2020) 10(10):3212–29.
40. Hedvat CV, Comenzo RL, Teruya-Feldstein J, Olshen AB, Ely SA, Osman K, et al. Insights into extramedullary tumour cell growth revealed by expression profiling of human plasmacytomas and multiple myeloma. *Br J Haematol* (2003) 122(5):728–44. doi: 10.1046/j.1365-2141.2003.04481.x
41. Allen EL, Ulanet DB, Pirman D, Mahoney CE, Coco J, Si Y, et al. Differential aspartate usage identifies a subset of cancer cells particularly dependent on OGDH. *Cell Rep* (2016) 17:876–90. doi: 10.1016/j.celrep.2016.09.052
42. Shen Y, Feng Y, Li F, Jia Y, Peng Y, Zhao W, et al. lncRNA ST3GAL6-AS1 promotes invasion by inhibiting hnRNPA2B1-mediated ST3GAL6 expression in multiple myeloma. *Int J Oncol* (2021) 58(4):1. doi: 10.3892/ijo.2021.5185
43. Chatterjee M, Andrulis M, Stuhmer T, Muller E, Hofmann C, Steinbrunn T, et al. The PI3K/Akt signaling pathway regulates the expression of Hsp70, which critically contributes to Hsp90-chaperone function and tumor cell survival in multiple myeloma. *Haematologica* (2012) 98(7):1132–41. doi: 10.3324/haematol.2012.066175
44. Zhang L, Fok JHL, Davies FE. Heat shock proteins in multiple myeloma. *Oncotarget* (2014) 5(5):1132–48. doi: 10.18632/oncotarget.1584
45. Wu X, Guo J, Chen Y, Liu X, Yang G, Wu Y, et al. The 60-kDa heat shock protein regulates energy rearrangement and protein synthesis to promote proliferation of multiple myeloma cells. *Br J Haematol* (2020) 190(5):741–52. doi: 10.1111/bjh.16569
46. Grosicki S, Bednarczyk M, Janikowska G. Heat shock proteins as a new, promising target of multiple myeloma therapy. *Expert Rev Hematol* (2020) 13 (2):117–26. doi: 10.1080/17474086.2020.1711730

47. Nikesitch N, Lee JM, Ling S, Roberts TL. Endoplasmic reticulum stress in the development of multiple myeloma and drug resistance. *Clin Transl Immunol* (2018) 7(1):e1007. doi: 10.1002/cti2.1007
48. Romano A, Conticello C, Cavalli M, Vetro C, La Fauci A, Parrinello NL, et al. Immunological dysregulation in mutliple myeloma microenvironment. *Biomed Res Int* (2014) 2014:198539. doi: 10.1155/2014/198539
49. Kawano Y, Roccaro AM, Ghobrial IM, Azzu J. Multiple myeloma and the immune microenvironment. *Curr Cancer Drug Targets* (2017) 17(9):806–18. doi: 10.2174/1568009617666170214102301
50. Purdue MP, Lan Q, Menashe I, Zheng T, Zhang Y, Yeager M, et al. Variation in innate immunity genes and risk of multiple myeloma. *Hematol Oncol* (2011) 29(1):42–6. doi: 10.1002/hon.954
51. Pessoa de Magalhães RJ, Vidriales MB, Fernandez-Gimenez C, García-Sanz R, Mateos MV, Gutierrez NC, et al. Analysis of the immune system of multiple myeloma patients achieving long-term disease control by multidimensional flow cytometry. *Haematologica* (2013) 98(1):79–86. doi: 10.3324/haematol.2012.067272
52. Tamura H. Immunopathogenesis and immunotherapy of multiple myeloma. *Int J Hematol* (2018) 107:278–85. doi: 10.1007/s12185-018-2405-7
53. Timmers M, Roex G, Wang Y, Campillo-Davo D, Van Tendeloo VFI, Chu Y, et al. Chimeric antigen receptor-modified T cell therapy in multiple myeloma: beyond B cell maturation antigen. *Front Immunol* (2019) 10:1613. doi: 10.3389/fimmu.2019.01613
54. Neri P, Bahlis NJ, Lonial S. New strategies in multiple myeloma: Immunotherapy as a novel approach to treat patients with multuple myeloma. *Clin Cancer Res* (2016) 22(24):5959–65. doi: 10.1158/1078-0432.CCR-16-0184
55. Shah N, Chari A, Scott E, Mezzi K, Usmani SZ. B-cell maturation antigen (BCMA) in multiple myeloma: rationale for targeting and current therapeutic approaches. *Leukemia* (2020) 34(4):985–1005. doi: 10.1038/s41375-020-0734-z
56. Guerra F, Bucci C. Role of the RAB7 protein in tumor progression and cisplatin chemoresistance. *Cancers (Basel)* (2019) 11(8):1096. doi: 10.3390/cancers11081096
57. Ryan D, Carberry S, Murphy AC, Lindner AU, Fay J, Hector S, et al. Calnexin, an ER-induced protein, is a prognostic marker and potential therapeutic target in colorectal cancer. *J Transl Med* (2016) 14:196. doi: 10.1186/s12967-016-0948-z
58. Bao H, Jiang M, Zhu M, Sheng F, Ruan J, Ruan C. Overexpression of annexin II affects the proliferation, apoptosis, invasion and production of proangiogenic factors in multiple myeloma. *Int J Hematol* (2009) 90 (2):177–85. doi: 10.1007/s12185-009-0356-8
59. Glavey SV, Naba A, Manier S, Clauser K, Tahri S, Park J, et al. Proteomic characterization of human multiple myeloma bone marrow extracellular matrix. *Leukemia* (2017) 31(11):2426–34. doi: 10.1038/leu.2017.102
60. Rasche L, Chavan SS, Stephens OW, Patel PH, Tytarenko R, Ashby C, et al. Spatial genomic heterogeneity in multiple myeloma revealed by multi-region sequencing. *Nat Commun* (2017) 8(1):268. doi: 10.1038/s41467-017-00296-y
61. Felix RS, Colleoni GW, Caballero OL, Yamamoto M, Almeida M, Andrade VC, et al. SAGE analysis highlights the importance of p53csv, ddx5, mapkapk2 and ranbp2 to multiple myeloma tumorigenesis. *Cancer Lett* (2009) 278(1):41–8. doi: 10.1016/j.canlet.2008.12.022
62. Demasi AP, Martinez EF, Napimoga MH, Freitas LL, Vassallo J, Duarte AS, et al. Expression of peroxiredoxins I and IV in multiple myeloma: association with immunoglobulin accumulation. *Virchows Arch* (2013) 463(1):47–55. doi: 10.1007/s00428-013-1433-1
63. Azab AK, Hu J, Quang P, Azab F, Pitsillides C, Awwad R, et al. H Hypoxia promotes dissemination of multiple myeloma through acquisition of epithelial to mesenchymal transition-like features. *Blood* (2012) 119(24):5782–94. doi: 10.1182/blood-2011-09-380410

14

Long-Term Remission Achieved by Ponatinib and Donor Lymphocytes Infusion in a Ph+ Acute Lymphoblastic Leukemia Patient in Molecular Relapse After Allogenic Stem Cell Transplant and Dasatinib

Cirino Botta [1,2], Nadia Caruso [2], Sabrina Bossio [2], Francesca Storino [2], Giuseppe Console [3], Massimo Martino [3], Francesco Mendicino [1], Eugenio Lucia [1], Rosellina Morelli [4], Pierpaolo Correale [5], Fortunato Morabito [2,6], Massimo Gentile [1,2] and Ernesto Vigna [1,2]*

[1] Hematology Unit, Hematology and Oncology Department, "Annunziata" Hospital of Cosenza, Cosenza, Italy, [2] Biotechnology Research Unit, Hematology and Oncology Department, "Annunziata" Hospital of Cosenza, Cosenza, Italy, [3] Stem Cell Transplant Program, Clinical Section, Department of Hemato-Oncology and Radiotherapy, "Grande Ospedale Metropolitano Bianchi-Melacrino-Morelli", Reggio Calabria, Italy, [4] Medicine Department, "Annunziata" Hospital of Cosenza, Cosenza, Italy, [5] Medical Oncology Unit, Department of Hemato-Oncology and Radiotherapy, "Grande Ospedale Metropolitano Bianchi-Melacrino-Morelli", Reggio Calabria, Italy, [6] Hematology Department and Bone Marrow Transplant Unit, Cancer Care Center, Augusta Victoria Hospital, East Jerusalem, Israel

***Correspondence:**
Cirino Botta
cirino.botta@gmail.com

Currently, the prognosis of Ph+ acute lymphoblastic leukemia (Ph+ ALL) patients relapsing after an allogenic hematopoietic stem cell transplantation (allo-SCT) remains poor, with few therapeutic options available. Here we present the case of a 32 years old patient with dasatinib-resistant post-transplant molecular relapse of ALL, who received, as second-line therapy, the combination of ponatinib and donor lymphocyte infusion (DLI). The therapy was safe and the patient achieved a sustained minimal residual disease negative disease, still ongoing after 22 months, which was accompanied by several changes in the immune populations distribution within the bone marrow (i.e., the increase in the CD8/CD4 lymphocytes ratio). Our report provides evidence of the efficacy of the third generation TKI inhibitor ponatinib in combination with DLI as second line therapy for Ph+ ALL relapsing after an allo-SCT.

Keywords: T lymphocytes, donor lymphocyte infusion (DLI), ponatinib, bone marrow microenviroment, acute lymhoblastic leukemia

BACKGROUND

B cell Acute lymphoblastic leukemia (B-ALL) is a hematologic malignancy arising from B-cell progenitors that accounts for 20% of adult leukemias (1). Among ALL adult patients, approximately 25% presents an acquired chromosomal abnormality, the Philadelphia chromosome (Ph), resulting from a balanced translocation between chromosome 9 and 22 (2, 3), which leads to the formation of the hybrid BCR-ABL transcript. The occurrence of Ph chromosome increases with age and is associated with a worse prognosis (4). From a clinical point of view, Ph+ ALL usually presents with a higher white blood cell count (as compare to Ph- ALL) and with a 5% risk of central nervous system involvement at diagnosis (3). The 5 year survival rate range from about 40% for people aged 25–64 years to <15% for patients over 65 years (1). Tyrosine kinase inhibitors (TKIs) directed to BCR-ABL fusion protein (imatinib, dasatinib, ponatinib) represent the backbone of current therapy, achieving, when used alone or in combinatory schedules including chemotherapy, a hematological remission rate of about 90%. Allogenic hematopoietic stem cell transplantation (allo-SCT) still remains the only potentially curative treatment for patients in first remission; it should be noted, however, that it relies on patient "fitness" as well as on the availability of suitable donors, and is associated with a significant risk of morbidity and mortality (1). Despite the advances made since TKIs introduction, disease relapse remains the main cause of treatment failure. Indeed, relapsed or refractory ALL patients have dismal outcome with a median overall survival (OS) shorter than 1 year and a 3 year OS of <25% (5). To date, various therapeutic strategies are available for these patients including immunotherapy [donor lymphocyte infusions (DLI), blinatumomab, inotuzumab ozogamicin, or chimeric antigen receptor T cells (CAR-T)] as well as conventional cytarabine-based chemotherapy (CHT) regimens, a second allo-SCT, participation in a clinical trial or supportive care (5). DLI could induce remission in some patients by restoring the graft-vs.-tumor response; the anti-CD22 antibody-drug-conjugated (ADC) inotuzumab and the bispecific T cell engager (BiTE) blinatumomab demonstrated improved outcome as compared to standard salvage chemotherapy; the CD19-directed CAR-T tisagenlecleucel achieved 83% remission rate in pluri-treated young and adult patients with precursor B-ALL (5). Any of the previously described new drugs brings a series of new adverse events spanning from graft-vs.-host disease (GVHD) (with DLI) to cytokine release syndrome (CRS) and neurotoxicity (with blinatumomab and CAR-T) that could be life-threatening and should be carefully took into account during the decision-making phase.

In this case report, we describe a young woman presenting with molecular relapsed Ph+ B-cell ALL initially treated with CHT+TKI induction regimen followed by a matched related donor allo-SCT and maintenance treatment with TKI until relapse occurred. The patient achieved then a long term complete molecular and cytogenetic remission following Ponatinib+DLI with minimal toxicity.

TABLE 1 | Patient's main characteristics at baseline and along the treatment.

Case presentation	
Classification	B-precursor ALL Ph+
WBC (μl)/Hb (g/dl)/platelets (μl)	40,000/8.7/87,000
Blasts	80%
Blasts phenotypes	CD19+, CD20–, CD10bright, CD45dim, CD34+, CD58+, CD5–, CD38low
BCR-ABL isoform	P210
Induction regimen	Vincristine + Dasatinib
CD34+ cell dose during transplant	4.6×10^6/kg
GVHD prophylaxis	Cyclosporin, MTX
Time from transplantation to relapse (months)	16
Treatment after relapse	DLI + ponatinib
Current status	Alive in molecular remission
Time from diagnosis (months)	45

CASE PRESENTATION

A 32 year-old woman without significant comorbidities (with the exception of favism) presented to the emergency room with asthenia in March 2016 (all information reported in **Table 1**). Routine blood count showed lymphocytosis (white blood cell count: 40,000/mmc; platelets: 87,000/mmc; hemoglobin: 8.7 g/dl) with 80% lymphoid blasts in a peripheral blood smear. The subsequent bone marrow (BM) aspiration confirmed the diagnosis, showing the presence of aberrant cells with a B precursor immunophenotype (CD19+CD20–CD10brightCD45dimCD34+CD58+CD5–CD38low) (**Figure 1A**) and expression of the BCR-ABL1 p210 fusion gene. Flow cytometric analysis of cerebrospinal fluid revealed no central nervous system involvement. On May 5, 2016, the patient started an induction treatment with Vincristine 2 mg weekly (4 administrations), methylprednisolone (60 mg/m^2/day for 28 days) and dasatinib 140 mg daily (early switch from imatinib due to intolerance after the first 7 days of treatment), associated with the intrathecal administration of cytarabine and methylprednisolone as a prophylaxis, which resulted in a rapid hematological complete response and BM negative minimal residual disease (MRD) ($10^{-4.2}$ in PCR, $10^{-4.5}$ in FCM) after 5 months (**Figure 1B**). On October 2016, the patient underwent an allo-SCT (4.6×10^6 CD34+ cells /Kg) from a HLA-matched relative (brother), after a myeloablative conditioning regimen that included busulfan and cyclophosphamide (BuCy2) plus antithymoglobulin (ATG). As graft-vs.-host disease (GVHD) prophylaxis the patient received cyclosporine and methotrexate. Grade 2 fever and grade 1 mucositis and diarrhea were the main acute toxicities observed during hospitalization. On February 2017, for the reappearance of BCR-ABL1 transcript (BCR-ABL/ABL ratio in peripheral blood: 0.079%), the patient stopped (progressively) cyclosporine treatment and re-started dasatinib. On day 200 after transplant the detected chimerism was 100%. MRD negativity was then maintained until February 2018, when the patient experienced a molecular relapse while staying in morphological CR (BCR-ABL/ABL ratio in peripheral blood: 0.025%). Of note, the patient was negative for the T315I mutation (conventional Sanger sequencing). The therapeutic decision, at this point, was to change the TKI, by switching to ponatinib (45 mg once a day), and to begin DLI (5 consecutive infusions until September 2018). The patient quickly achieved a complete molecular response (CMR) (MR4.5) but experienced signs of GVHD with the development of progressively expanding dyskeratosis and dry eye (confirmed with Schirmer test) for

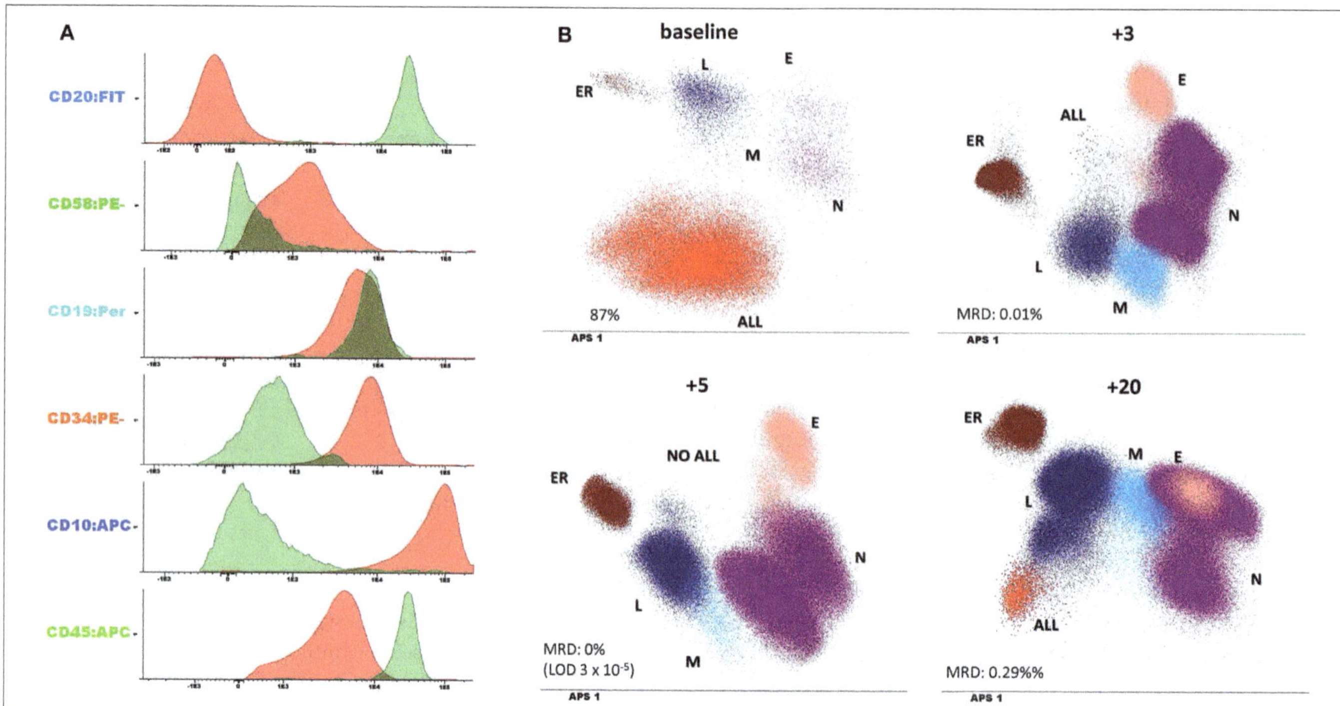

FIGURE 1 | **(A)** Leukemic phenotype at baseline. The histograms report both the leukemic clone (in red) and the normal B cell compartment (in green) to underscore the expression of aberrant markers. **(B)** minimal residual disease (MRD) evaluation performed at 4 different timepoints (the number on the top of each panel represents the number of months from diagnosis) and compared with baseline phenotype. Dotplots are represented with a dimensionality reduction approach (principal component analysis or automatic population separator (APS) in infinicyt software, Cytognos) which allow the identification of the different immune population within the bone marrow (L, lymphocytes; ER, erythroblasts; N, granulocytes; M, monocytes; E, eosinophils; ALL, leukemic clone).

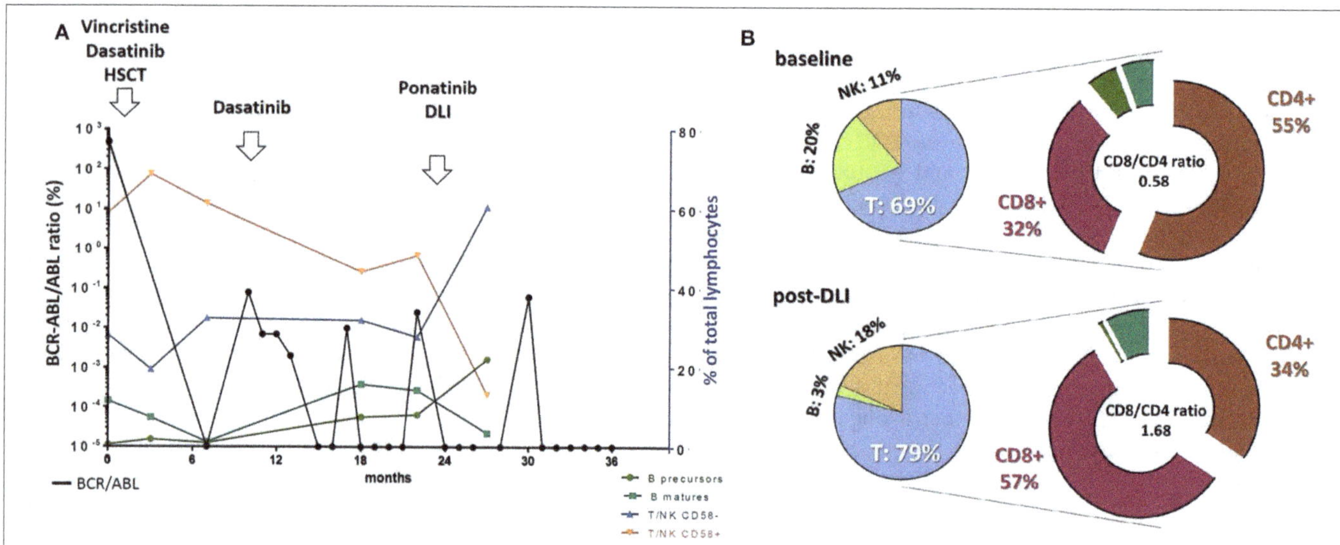

FIGURE 2 | **(A)** Trends in BCR-ABL transcript levels in peripheral blood coupled with different normal immune populations distribution within the bone marrow along disease evolution and in response to different treatments. BCR-ABL/ABL ratio values are reported on the left vertical axis while cell population abundance refers to the right axis. **(B)** T, NK, and B cell representation within the whole lymphocyte group at baseline and after ponatinib + donor lymphocytes infusion (DLI). Notably, within the T cell compartment we observed an inversion in the CD8/CD4 ratio, favoring the CD8 compartment after DLI treatment.

which begun a treatment with steroids and cyclosporin. Central nervous system evaluation through MNR and cerebrospinal fluid analysis reveal no signs of leukemic involvement. Interestingly, this clinical picture was accompanied by a substantial increase in normal B cell progenitors, an inversion between CD58+ and CD58− T/NK lymphocytes distribution (**Figure 2A**) and

TABLE 2 | Comparison of published case reports on the combination of DLI+TKI in T-ALL.

	Yoshimitsu et al. (15)	Tiribelli et al. (16)	Tachibana et al. (17)	Maharaj et al. (5)
WBC (μl)/Hb (g/dl)/platelets (μl) at diagnosis	11,700/10.2/28,000	NA	40,800/NA/NA	67,000/12.3/49,000
BM Blasts	98.6%	NA	97%	NA
Blasts phenotypes	CD10$^+$, CD13$^+$, CD19$^+$, CD34$^+$,CD33$^+$	NA	CD10$^+$, CD13$^+$, CD19$^+$, CD34$^+$, HLA-DR$^+$	NA
BCR-ABL isoform	p190	p190	NA	p190
SNC involvement	NA	Meningeal and ocular	NA	NA
1th Induction regimen	ALL202 (prednisolone, CPA, daunorubicin, VCR) + imatinib + intrathecal CHT (methotrexate, ARA-C and DEX)	VCR, daunorubicin, l-asparaginase and prednisone + intrathecal CHT (methotrexate, ARA-C and DEX)	Prednisolone, DXR, vindesine and CPA + imatinib	UKALL14 (PEG-asparaginase, daunorubicin, VCR, CPA, ARA-C, mercapopurine, DEX + + intrathecal CHT (methotrexate)
1th consolidation regimen	HD MTX and HD ARA-C	HAM protocol (HD ARA-C and mitoxantrone) + CNS radiotherapy	MTX, ARA-C, and methylprednisolone	CPA + total body irradiation
Response to 1th treatment	CCR	CCR	CMR	CMR
CD34+ cell dose during transplant	5.0 × 10^6/kg	3.0 × 10^6/kg	NA	NA
Time from allo-SCT to first relapse (months)	4.5	5.5	3.0	6
Treatment after relapse	Imatinib ± DLI	Imatinib BFM protocol (VCR, ifosfamide, MTX, ARA-C, and teniposide) DLI + VCR + prednisone Nilotinib ± DLI	imatinib, CPA, DXR, VCR and prednisolone Imatinib ± DLI imatinib, CPA, DXR, VCR, and prednisolone Dasatinib	Dasatinib ± DLI Dasatinib + IL-2
Best response to TKI + DLI	CMR	CMR	CCR maintenance	CCR
Signs of GVHD	ANA+	grade I skin and liver GVHD	None	NA
Last reported status	CMR at 24 months after Imatinib + DLI start	CMR at 10 months after Nilotinib + DLI start	Relapse at 8 months after Imatinib + DLI start	Relapse at 6 months after Dasatinib + DLI start

HD, high doses; MTX, methotrexate; ARA-C, cytarabine; VCR, vincristine; CPA, cyclophosophamide; DEX, dexamethasone; DXR, doxorubicin; DLI, donor lymphocytes infusion; CCR, complete cytogenetic remission, CMR, complete molecular remission; allo-SCT, allogenic stem cell transplant; NA, not available.

by an inversion of the CD8/CD4 ratio (**Figure 2B**) within the BM. At the last evaluation, done on December 2019, the patient is continuing therapy with ponatinib 45 mg once a day with reasonable tolerance and still maintains a MR4.5 (response maintained for 22+ months).

DISCUSSION

The management of allo-SCT relapsed Ph+ ALL patients represents a great challenge due to few active therapeutic regimens that rarely are successful, rendering the prognosis very poor (6). Indeed, contrary to what happens in chronic myelogenous leukemia (CML), TKIs are less effective in B-ALL scenario due to the rapid onset of drug resistance (7). Additionally, molecular detection of relapse (such as in the case of MRD reappearance) could help to identify patients who could potentially benefit from an early salvage therapy. This point is currently under active investigation, with increasing data suggesting that after an allo-SCT, the loss of MRD negativity, as measured by reappearance of BCR-ABL transcript within the bone marrow, precedes hematologic relapse, therefore justifying an early initiation of the treatment (8, 9). In this regard, in both Ph− and Ph+ ALL and detectable MRD, therapy with blinatumomab (alone or in combination with TKI, respectively) has shown encouraging results, and larger clinical trials are ongoing (10, 11). However, as previously discussed, Ph+ ALL patients relapsing after an allo-SCT, currently undergo a second line therapy which could include (1) an alternative TKI (alone or in combination with chemotherapy or steroids); (2) blinatumumab; or (3) the anti-CD22 (if present on leukemic clone) inotuzumab ozogamicin, being the latter two indicated for TKIs intolerant or refractory patients only. Tisagenlecleucel represents a further therapeutic option for Ph+ ALL patients up to 25 years after at least 2 relapses or failure of 2 TKIs. Additionally, a second allogenic allo-SCT or DLI could be considered for relapsed patients, even if data are currently unclear. Here we reported a case of a post-transplant molecular relapsed ALL patient treated with the combo ponatinib-DLI, who achieved a sustained long-term response with MRD negativity (+22 months). TKI inhibitors are known to be unable to eradicate leukemic clones, mainly due to the fact that stem leukemic clones are often Ph- or BCR-ABL independent, thus being not targetable with current drugs (12). On the other hands, the infusion of DLI from an allogeneic donor could induce deep remissions but at the cost of significant toxicity (such as GVHD) (13, 14). On these bases, the combination of a TKI inhibitor (to deeply reduce tumor burden) with DLI (to try to eradicate residual clonal cells) could represent a reasonable option to produce long lasting remissions. Previous case reports explored the feasibility of the combination of both 1st and 2nd generation TKI with DLI (5, 15–17), with alternate results (**Table 2**). Specifically, imatinib + DLI used at first relapse after allo-SCT (but not at late relapse) was followed by CMR achievement lasting over 24 months with negligible signs of GVHD (15). Furthermore, in imatinib resistant patients, the combination of 2nd generation TKI Dasatinib or Nilotinib + DLI achieved MRD negativity and CMR, respectively. Interestingly, Nilotinib + DLI used at 4th relapse, surprisingly induced a CMR lasting over 10 months, with a manageable grade 1 cutaneous and hepatic GVHD (16). Along this line, in our scenario (Dasatinib-resistant patient), the combination of the 3rd generation TKI inhibitor ponatinib with DLI represented an attractive therapeutic opportunity.

Accordingly, we quickly achieved a molecular response with no signs of acute GVHD other than a manageable cutaneous dyskeratosis, and the patients received 5 consecutive DLI injections, continuing to maintain a complete molecular response. Interestingly, the treatment combination produced several immune changes within the BM, that are in line with the reported immunomodulatory activity of this class of drugs (18, 19). We indeed observed a "normalization" in bone marrow composition (including a repopulation in precursor and naïve b and T cells) coupled with an unbalance in the CD8/CD4 ratio in favor of the cytotoxic CD8 T cell population, known to be essential for anticancer response (20). As a result, the patient achieved a quick and sustained complete molecular response with the development along the time, of manageable dyskeratosis and is still in complete molecular remission. Summarizing, we believe ponatinib in combination with DLI a very active regimen in ALL patients after the failure of a first line TKI and allo-SCT. Clinical trials are eagerly awaited to confirm its therapeutic potential in this setting.

ETHICS STATEMENT

Written informed consent was obtained from the individual for the publication of any potentially identifiable images or data included in this article.

AUTHOR CONTRIBUTIONS

CB composed the manuscript and performed literature review. NC, SB, and FS did the acquisition and analysis of laboratory data for the work. CB and EV critically revised and interpreted the data. EV, GC, MM, FMe, EL, RM, FMo, MG, and CB took care of the patient from the clinical point of view. CB and EV wrote the manuscript while MG and PC fully revised and improved it. All authors contributed to the article and approved the submitted version.

REFERENCES

1. Stevenson M, Pandor A, Hamilton J, Stevens J, Rowntree C, Martyn-St James M, et al. Ponatinib for treating acute lymphoblastic leukaemia: an evidence review group perspective of a NICE single technology appraisal. *Pharmacoeconomics*. (2018) 36:759–68. doi: 10.1007/s40273-018-0624-7
2. Fielding AK, Richards SM, Chopra R, Lazarus HM, Litzow MR, Buck G, et al. Outcome of 609 adults after relapse of acute lymphoblastic leukemia (ALL); an MRC UKALL12/ECOG 2993 study. *Blood*. (2007) 109:944–50. doi: 10.1182/blood-2006-05-018192
3. Petrungaro A, Gentile M, Mazzone C, Greco R, Uccello G, Recchia AG, et al. Ponatinib-induced graft-versus-host disease/graft-versus-leukemia effect in a patient with philadelphia-positive acute lymphoblastic leukemia without the T315I mutation relapsing after allogeneic transplant. *Chemotherapy*. (2017) 62:353–6. doi: 10.1159/000477714
4. Fielding AK. The treatment of adults with acute lymphoblastic leukemia. *Hematol Am Soc Hematol Educ Prog*. (2008) 2008:381–9. doi: 10.1182/asheducation-2008.1.381
5. Maharaj D, Vianna P, DeCarvalho G, Pourkalbassi D, Hickey C, Gouvea J. Molecular remission using low-dose immunotherapy for relapsed refractory Philadelphia chromosome-positive precursor B-cell acute lymphoblastic leukemia post-allogeneic stem cell transplant. *Fut Sci OA*. (2019) 5:FSO380. doi: 10.2144/fsoa-2019-0009
6. Spyridonidis A, Labopin M, Schmid C, Volin L, Yakoub-Agha I, Stadler M, et al. Outcomes and prognostic factors of adults with acute lymphoblastic leukemia who relapse after allogeneic hematopoietic cell transplantation. An analysis on behalf of the acute leukemia working party of EBMT. *Leukemia*. (2012) 26:1211–7. doi: 10.1038/leu.2011.351
7. Leoni V, Biondi A. Tyrosine kinase inhibitors in BCR-ABL positive acute lymphoblastic leukemia. *Haematologica*. (2015) 100:295–9. doi: 10.3324/haematol.2015.124016
8. Lee S, Kim DW, Cho B, Kim YJ, Kim YL, Hwang JY, et al. Risk factors for adults with philadelphia-chromosome-positive acute lymphoblastic leukaemia in remission treated with allogeneic bone marrow transplantation: the potential of real-time quantitative reverse-transcription polymerase chain reaction. *Br J Haematol*. (2003) 120:145–53. doi: 10.1046/j.1365-2141.2003.03988.x
9. Pemmaraju N, Kantarjian H, Jorgensen JL, Jabbour E, Jain N, Thomas D, et al. Significance of recurrence of minimal residual disease detected by multi-parameter flow cytometry in patients with acute lymphoblastic leukemia in morphological remission. *Am J Hematol*. (2017) 92:279–85. doi: 10.1002/ajh.24629
10. Kantarjian HM, Stein AS, Bargou RC, Grande Garcia C, Larson RA, Stelljes M, et al. Blinatumomab treatment of older adults with relapsed/refractory B-precursor acute lymphoblastic leukemia: results from 2 phase 2 studies. *Cancer*. (2016) 122:2178–85. doi: 10.1002/cncr.30031
11. King AC, Pappacena JJ, Tallman MS, Park JH, Geyer MB. Blinatumomab administered concurrently with oral tyrosine kinase inhibitor therapy is a well-tolerated consolidation strategy and eradicates measurable residual disease in adults with Philadelphia chromosome positive acute lymphoblastic leukemia. *Leuk Res*. (2019) 79:27–33. doi: 10.1016/j.leukres.2019.02.009
12. Walter MJ. Antecedent CHIP in CML?. *Blood*. (2017) 129:3–4. doi: 10.1182/blood-2016-11-746842

13. Loren AW, Porter DL. Donor leukocyte infusions for the treatment of relapsed acute leukemia after allogeneic stem cell transplantation. *Bone Marrow Transplant.* (2008) 41:483–93. doi: 10.1038/sj.bmt.1705898
14. Lu YF, Gavrilescu LC, Betancur M, Lazarides K, Klingemann H, Van Etten RA. Distinct graft-versus-leukemic stem cell effects of early or delayed donor leukocyte infusions in a mouse chronic myeloid leukemia model. *Blood.* (2012) 119:273–84. doi: 10.1182/blood-2011-01-331009
15. Yoshimitsu M, Fujiwara H, Ozaki A, Hamada H, Matsushita K, Arima N, et al. Case of a patient with Philadelphia-chromosome-positive acute lymphoblastic leukemia relapsed after myeloablative allogeneic hematopoietic stem cell transplantation treated successfully with imatinib and sequential donor lymphocyte infusions. *Int J Hematol.* (2008) 88:331–5. doi: 10.1007/s12185-008-0150-z
16. Tiribelli M, Sperotto A, Candoni A, Simeone E, Buttignol S, Fanin R. Nilotinib and donor lymphocyte infusion in the treatment of Philadelphia-positive acute lymphoblastic leukemia (Ph+ ALL) relapsing after allogeneic stem cell transplantation and resistant to imatinib. *Leuk Res.* (2009) 33:174–7. doi: 10.1016/j.leukres.2008.03.031
17. Tachibana T, Numata A, Tanaka M, Motohashi K, Fujisawa S, Fujita H, et al. Successful treatment with dasatinib and allogeneic peripheral blood stem cell transplant for imatinib-resistant Philadelphia chromosome-positive acute lymphoblastic leukemia relapsing after bone marrow transplant and donor lymphocyte infusion. *Leuk Lymph.* (2011) 52:1376–9. doi: 10.3109/10428194.2011.566395
18. Hughes A, Yong ASM. Immune effector recovery in chronic myeloid leukemia and treatment-free remission. *Front Immunol.* (2017) 8:469. doi: 10.3389/fimmu.2017.00469
19. Loscocco F, Visani G, Galimberti S, Curti A, Isidori A. BCR-ABL independent mechanisms of resistance in chronic myeloid leukemia. *Front Oncol.* (2019) 9:939. doi: 10.3389/fonc.2019.00939
20. Botta C, Misso G, Martino EC, Pirtoli L, Cusi MG, Tassone P, et al. The route to solve the interplay between inflammation, angiogenesis and anti-cancer immune response. *Cell Death Dis.* (2016) 7:e2299. doi: 10.1038/cddis.2016.211

15

FtH-Mediated ROS Dysregulation Promotes CXCL12/CXCR4 Axis Activation and EMT-Like Trans-Differentiation in Erythroleukemia K562 Cells

Roberta Chirillo [1†], Ilenia Aversa [1†], Anna Di Vito [1], Alessandro Salatino [1], Anna Martina Battaglia [1], Alessandro Sacco [1], Maddalena Adriana Di Sanzo [1], Maria Concetta Faniello [1,2], Barbara Quaresima [1], Camillo Palmieri [1], Flavia Biamonte [1,2] and Francesco Costanzo [2,3]*

[1] Department of Experimental and Clinical Medicine, "Magna Græcia" University of Catanzaro, Catanzaro, Italy, [2] Department of Experimental and Clinical Medicine, Research Center of Biochemistry and Advanced Molecular Biology, "Magna Græcia" University of Catanzaro, Catanzaro, Italy, [3] Interdepartmental Center of Services (CIS), "Magna Græcia" University of Catanzaro, Catanzaro, Italy

***Correspondence:**
Flavia Biamonte
flavia.biamonte.fb@gmail.com

† These authors have contributed equally to this work

The cell-microenvironment communication is essential for homing of hematopoietic stem cells in stromal niches. Recent evidences support the involvement of epithelial-to-mesenchymal (EMT) process in hematopoietic stem cell homeostasis as well as in leukemia cells invasiveness and migration capability. Here, we demonstrate that the alteration of iron homeostasis and the consequent increase of redox metabolism, mediated by the stable knock down of ferritin heavy chain (FtH), enhances the expression of CXCR4 in K562 erythroleukemia cells, thus promoting CXCL12-mediated motility. Indeed, addition of the CXCR4 receptor antagonist AMD3100 reverts this effect. Upon FtH knock down K562 cells also acquire an "EMT-like" phenotype, characterized by the increase of *Snail*, *Slug* and Vimentin with the parallel loss of E-cadherin. By using fibronectin as substrate, the cell adhesion assay further shows a reduction of cell adhesion capability in FtH-silenced K562 cells. Accordingly, confocal microscopy shows that adherent K562 control cells display a variety of protrusions while FtH-silenced K562 cells remain roundish. These phenomena are largely due to the reactive oxygen species (ROS)-mediated up-regulation of HIF-1α/CXCR4 axis which, in turn, promotes the activation of NF-κB and the enhancement of EMT features. These data are confirmed by treatments with either N-acetylcysteine (NAC) or AMD3100 or NF-κB inhibitor IκB-alpha which revert the FtH-silenced K562 invasive phenotype. Overall, our findings demonstrate the existence of a direct relationship among iron metabolism, redox homeostasis and EMT in the hematological malignancies. The effects of FtH dysregulation on CXCR4/CXCL12-mediated K562 cell motility extend the meaning of iron homeostasis in the leukemia cell microenvironment.

Keywords: ferritin heavy chain, ROS, CXCR4, EMT, NF-κB, leukemia, tumor microenvironment, hematological malignancies

INTRODUCTION

The tumor microenvironment (TME) is a major player in cancer progression and several signals, such as oxygen supply, cytokines, and chemokines drive the communication between TME and tumor cells (1–3). The CXCL12/CXCR4 axis promotes tumor cell growth and propagation of distant metastases through the activation of epithelial-to-mesenchymal transition (EMT) (4). During EMT, cancer cells acquire features of mesenchymal-like cells including enhanced migratory and invasive abilities, changes in cellular adhesion and remodeling of the extracellular matrix (5, 6). Cancer cells expressing CXCR4 tend to home to secondary organs where its ligand CXCL12 is actively secreted, mainly by mesenchymal stromal cells (7).

Tumors rapidly exhaust the local oxygen supply creating a hypoxic environment which, in turn, promotes the overproduction of reactive oxygen species (ROS) (8). ROS can induce EMT, but the specificity of their action in the regulation of given EMT markers is dependent on the cellular context and the type of tissue (9–12). Numerous studies have explored the role of ROS in inducing both cell migration and EMT in solid cancer (13, 14). In this regard, we and others have previously reported that the knock down of ferritin heavy chain (FtH), the catalytic subunit of the human ferritin, promotes cell motility through either the activation of CXCR4 signaling or the induction of EMT in a variety of solid cancer *in vitro* models including breast and lung cancer cell lines (15–17).

The trafficking of tumor cells represents a key process that contributes to progression also of hematological malignancies such as myeloid and lymphoid leukemias or multiple myeloma (18, 19). A common feature of these tumors is the homing and infiltration of hematological cancer cells into the bone marrow (BM) which supports initiation, maintenance and proliferation of the malignant cells (7). Both homing and migration of leukemic stem cells are regulated by niche cells living in the BM through the activation of the CXCL12/CXCR4 axis signaling (20–22). Indeed, blocking CXCL12 binding to CXCR4 with the specific CXCR4 inhibitor AMD3100 disrupts hematological neoplastic cells interaction with the BM microenvironment (21).

In chronic myelogenous leukemia (CML) cells, CXCR4 activates PI3K/AKT signaling pathway and promotes the translocation of NF-κB complexes into nucleus thereby decreasing the expression of pro-apoptotic proteins (23, 24). Moreover, CXCL12 activates pro-survival signal pathways including those mediated by MAPK, S-6-kinase, STAT3 and STAT5, and *in vitro* treatment with CXCR4 antagonists inhibits cell growth and induces cell death (25, 26). The molecular mechanisms regulating the expression of CXCR4 in hematological malignancies have therefore been largely investigated. Numerous evidences show that hypoxia in BM leads to increased HIF-1α transcriptional activity on CXCR4 expression resulting in enhanced migration and homing of circulating malignant cells to new BM niches (27–29).

During the last decade, EMT has gained increasing attention also in hematological malignancies. Few reports indicate that EMT-transcription factors (TFs), including Twist-1 and Slug, are implicated in hematopoietic stem cell self-renewal by interacting with stemness signaling key factors c-Myc and c-Kit (30, 31) while Slug up-regulation promotes leukemogenesis and confers resistance to apoptosis in leukemia cells (32). In addition, imatinib-resistant CML cells exhibit a so-called "EMT-like" phenotype along with increased invasion and migration properties both *in vitro* and *in vivo* (33). Overall these data suggest that EMT might play significant role in inducing tumor dissemination and thus chemoresistance also in hematological malignancies; however, this topic still has remarkable gaps to overwhelm.

In this study, we address for the first time the role of FtH-induced ROS increase in bestowing mesenchymal properties to hematological cells. To achieve this goal, we defined the effects of FtH knock down in the induction of EMT markers, activation of CXCR4/CXCL12 signaling pathway and migration of K562 erythroleukemia cells, and further attempted to understand the molecular mechanisms involved.

MATERIALS AND METHODS

Cell Culture and Treatment

K562, a human erythroleukemia cell line (ATCC number CCL-243), was cultured as described in Di Sanzo et al. (34). The human stromal cells HS5, were cultured in DMEM medium supplemented with 10% fetal bovine serum and antibiotics at 37°C in an atmosphere of humidified air containing 5% CO_2. Lentiviral preparations and transductions were performed as previously described using a shRNA as control ($K562^{shRNA}$) or a shRNA that targets the 196–210 region of the *FtH* mRNA ($K562^{shFtH}$) (35). All the experiments were performed using a puromycin-selected pool of clones (1 μg/mL) (Sigma Aldrich, St. Louis, MI, USA). K562 cells were transfected using the Nucleofector system from Amaxa (Lonza, Basel, Switzerland) according to the manufacturer's optimized protocol. To evaluate the role of NF-κB in inducing EMT-like features, we over-expressed the NF-κB inhibitor IκB-α using a homemade pRc/CMV-HA-IκB-α plasmid and its empty control kindly provided by Prof. Ileana Quinto (Magna Graecia University of Catanzaro, Italy) as previously described by Aversa et al. (36). CXCL12 was added to K562 cell culture medium at a final concentration of 100 ng/ml. N-acetylcysteine (NAC) was added to the K562 cell culture medium at a final concentration of 5 mM for 2 h. Plerixafor (AMD3100) was added to the K562 cell culture medium at a final concentration of 10 μM for 1 h.

Protein Extractions

Protein extractions were performed on $K562^{shRNA}$, $K562^{shFtH}$, $K562^{shFtH/pRc/CMV}$, $K562^{shFtH/pRc/CMV-3HA-I\kappa B}$ and NAC treated cells. Briefly, for total protein extractions, K562 cells were lysed in ice-cold radioimmunoprecipitation assay (RIPA) buffer containing protease inhibitors as described by Zolea et al. (37). For the quantification of nuclear p65 amounts, protein extraction from nucleus was performed as previously described by Aversa et al. (36).

Western Blotting Analysis

A total of 40 μg protein extract was boiled for 10 min in SDS sample buffer, separated by 12% SDS-PAGE and transferred to a nitrocellulose membrane by electroblotting as reported in Di Sanzo et al. (38). The nitrocellulose membranes were incubated overnight at 4°C with the following antibodies: (a) anti-CXCR4 (1:500; Abcam), (b) anti-HIF-1α (H-206) (1:200; Santa Cruz Biotechnology), (c) anti-p65 (C-20) (sc-372, 1:1,000; Santa Cruz Biotechnology), (d) anti-HDAC (1:5,000; Sigma-Aldrich), (e) anti-HA probe (F-7) (1:1,000; Santa Cruz Biotechnology), (f) anti-Vimentin, (g) anti-E-cadherin, (h) anti-Snail, (i) anti-Slug (1:1,000; Cell Signaling Technology, Danvers, MA, USA), (l) anti-FtH (1:200; Santa Cruz Biotechnology), (m) anti-γ-Tubulin (C-20) (1:2,000; Santa Cruz Biotechnology), (n) anti-Nucleolin (D4C7O) (1:1,000; Cell Signaling Technology) over-night at 4°C, followed by incubation with goat anti-rabbit and mouse anti-goat secondary antibodies (1:5,000; Santa Cruz Biotechnology). Membranes were incubated with horseradish peroxidase (HRP)-conjugated secondary antibodies and immunoreactive bands were visualized with the ECL Western blotting detection system (BioRad, Hercules, CA, USA).

Quantification of CXCR4 Surface Expression

K562 cells (2×10^5) were harvested and rinsed once. Then, the cells were incubated with anti-CXCR4 antibody (1:400; Abcam) for 1 h at 4°C. After primary antibody incubation, the cells were rinsed with 1X PBS and incubated for 30 min with Alexa Fluor 633 donkey anti-goat antibody (H+L) (1:400) resuspended in 5 mg/ml BSA and 0.76 mg/ml EDTA. The cells were rinsed with 1X PBS, resuspended in 300 μl 1X PBS and evaluated by a FACS BD LSRFortessa^{TM} X-20 cytofluorometer (BD Biosciences, San Jose, CA, USA).

Immunofluorescence

K562 cells were cultured on cover slip coated with fibronectin for 24 h. Samples preparation was performed as reported in Biamonte et al. (39). Thereafter, these cover slips were incubated for 1 h with primary antibodies anti-Vimentin (clone V9, ready to use, Dako) and 1 h with secondary antibody FITC-conjugated anti-mouse diluted in blocking buffer. For E-cadherin staining, the cover slips were incubated overnight at 4°C with primary antibody (clone 24E10, 1:200, Cell Signaling) in a humidified room, and for 1 h with Alexa Fluor 488-conjugated anti-rabbit, both diluted in blocking buffer. To stain actin filaments, cells were incubated for 30 min in this buffer containing Alexa Fluor 488 phalloidin at 1:40 dilution (Thermo Fisher Scientific, Waltham, Massachusetts, USA). After 3 washes with PBS, nuclear DAPI (1:500, Invitrogen, Carlsbad, CA) was added for 20 min. The samples were mounted on microscope slides using a mounting solution ProLong Gold antifade reagent (Thermo Fisher Scientific). Images were collected using a Leica DM-IRB/TC-SP2 confocal microscopy system (63× objective).

Cell Adhesion Assay

K562^{shRNA}, K562^{shFtH} and K562^{shFtH} NAC-treated cells were subjected to adhesion assays using Fibronectin as an adhesion substrate. Briefly, 6-well flat-bottom plates were incubated overnight at 37°C with 5 μg/cm^2 of Fibronectin in PBS. After gentle washing with PBS and incubation with 1% BSA for 1 h at room temperature, cells (3×10^4 cells/well) were added and allowed to adhere for 24 h at 37°C. Non-adherent cells were then removed by washing each well with PBS and adherent cells were counted using the cell count function in Image J 1.42 software, on ten fields per well. Each field consisted of a photo obtained at 200× magnification.

Migration Assay

K562^{shRNA}, K562^{shFtH} and K562^{shFtH} NAC-treated cells were used to the migration assay using as chemoattractant CXCL12 chemokine as already described by Aversa et al. (15). After 18 h of incubation, the upper chambers were removed, and the cells in the lower chambers were counted using an optical microscope. Migration assay using the conditioned media derived from stromal cells HS5 (HS5-CM) was assessed in 24-well plate and polycarbonate filters with an 8.0 μm pore size. First, the supernatant media of HS5 cells was collected after 12 h and passed through a 0.45 μm filter. Briefly, 2×10^5 K562 cells were harvested, suspended in 200 μl serum-free RPMI with 1% BSA and placed in the upper chamber. The lower chambers contained 500 μl of HS5-CM. The plates were incubated at 37°C in 5 % CO2 for 8 h. The upper chambers were removed, and the cells in the lower chambers were counted using an optical microscope. The cell migration is expressed as the percentage of increase compared with the corresponding control.

ROS Detection

ROS were determined by incubating 2×10^5 K562^{shRNA}, K562^{shFtH} and K562^{shFtH} cells NAC-treated with 1μM redox-sensitive probe 2′-7′-DCF (CM-H2CFDA; MolecularProbes, Eugene, OR, USA) for 30 min at 37°C. Afterward, pellet was washed twice with 1X PBS, then the pellet was resuspended in 1X PBS and analyzed using a FACS BD LSRFortessa^{TM} X-20 cytofluorometer (BD Biosciences).

RNA Isolation and qPCR Analysis

Total RNA isolation was performed as previously reported in Sottile et al. (40). Gene expression analysis was assessed by real-time PCR using the cDNA obtained from K562^{shRNA}, K562^{shFtH}, K562$^{shFtH/pRc/CMV}$, K562$^{shFtH/pRc/CMV-3HA-I\kappa B}$ cells and K562^{shFtH} cells treated with NAC.

Real time PCR was performed ad reported in Biamonte et al. (41). Briefly, 50 ng of cDNA was amplified in 20 μl of reaction mix containing Power SYBR Green PCR Master mix (Thermo Fisher Scientific) and the expression of *CXCR4, FtH, E-cadherin, HIF-1α, Snail, Slug* and *Vimentin* were analyzed. The human *GAPDH* cDNA fragment was amplified as the internal control. Data analysis was performed using the $2^{-\Delta\Delta Ct}$.

Statistical Analysis

All experiments were conducted at least three times, and the results are reported as mean values ± standard deviations

(SD). Data analysis was performed by Student's-t-test assuming equal variances. p-values $\leq$ 0.05 were considered statistically significant.

RESULTS

FtH Knock Down Promotes CXCL12/CXCR4 Axis Activation and Motility in K562 Cells

Earlier studies by others and us indicate that FtH interacts with internalized olo-CXCR4 receptor thereby suppressing the downstream signaling pathway in a variety of epithelial tumor cells (15, 16). As experimental model we used a pool of erythroleukemia K562 cell clones stably silenced for *FtH* ($K562^{shFtH}$). FtH mRNA and protein expression levels in $K562^{shFtH}$ and in $K562^{shRNA}$ control cells are reported in **Figure S1A**. To assess the role of FtH on CXCR4 signaling in hematological tumors, we first measured CXCR4 levels in $K562^{shFtH}$ and in $K562^{shRNA}$ and we found that *FtH* knock down significantly enhanced CXCR4 expression at both mRNA and protein levels (**Figure 1A**). Flow cytometry analysis revealed an increase of about 25% in CXCR4 cell surface expression in $K562^{shFtH}$ cells compared to $K562^{shRNA}$ control cells (**Figure 1B**). Next, to determine whether the CXCR4 increase modulates the cell migration ability, we cultured both $K562^{shRNA}$ and $K562^{shFtH}$ cells either in RPMI medium supplemented with 100 ng/ml CXCL12 or in a HS5 mesenchymal stromal cells-conditioned medium for 8 h. As controls, we prepared parallel cultures of K562 cells with RPMI complete medium alone (data not shown). Cell migration assays demonstrate that $K562^{shFtH}$ cells exhibit a higher migration ability of about 5-fold compared to K562 control cells upon exposure to both CXCL12 or HS5-conditioned medium. Accordingly, treatment with the specific CXCR4 inhibitor AMD3100 (10 μM for 8 h) significantly decreased the migration of $K562^{shFtH}$ in both modified culture media (**Figures 1C,D**).

FtH Silencing Induces Mesenchymal-Like Features in K562 Cells

We then explored the effect of *FtH* knock down on the classic EMT markers E-cadherin and Vimentin, as well as on the two EMT-transcription factors (EMT-Tfs) Snail and Slug. Real-time PCR and WB analyses clearly indicate a consistent increase in the steady-state amounts of both EMT-Tfs in $K562^{shFtH}$ cells compared to $K562^{shRNA}$ cells (**Figures 2A,B**).

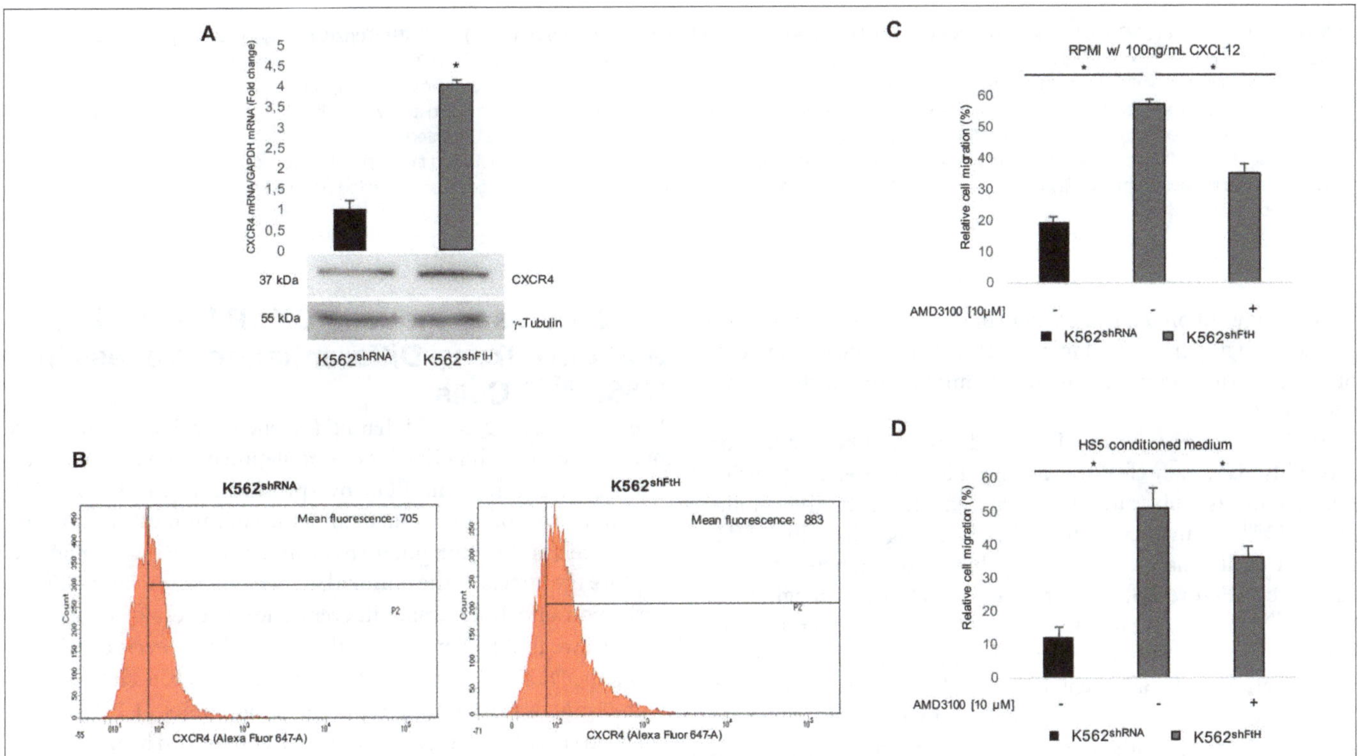

FIGURE 1 | CXCR4/CXCL12 axis is activated in $K562^{shFtH}$ cells. **(A)** qPCR and western blot analysis of CXCR4 in $K562^{shRNA}$ and $K562^{shFtH}$ cells. Final results represent mean ± SD of three independent experiments, $^{*}p < 0.05$. γ-Tubulin was used as loading control in WB experiments **(B)** Flow cytometry analysis of CXCR4 in $K562^{shRNA}$ and $K562^{shFtH}$ cells. Data are representative of three independent experiments **(C)** CXCL12 dependent-cell migration was examined in 24-well plates. Cells were placed in the upper chamber (8 μm) in nude RPMI. After 8 h, cells migrated toward medium containing CXCL12 (100 ng/ml) were counted using an optical microscope. Data are reported percentage of migrated cells. Final results represent mean ± SD of three independent experiments, $^{*}p < 0.05$. **(D)** Migration analysis of $K562^{shRNA}$ and $K562^{shFtH}$ cells performed in 24-well plates. Cells were allowed to migrate for 8 h into the lower chamber containing conditioned medium of HS5 cells. Migrated cells were counted, and the percentage of migrated cells was calculated. Final results represent mean ± SD of three independent experiments, $^{*}p < 0.05$.

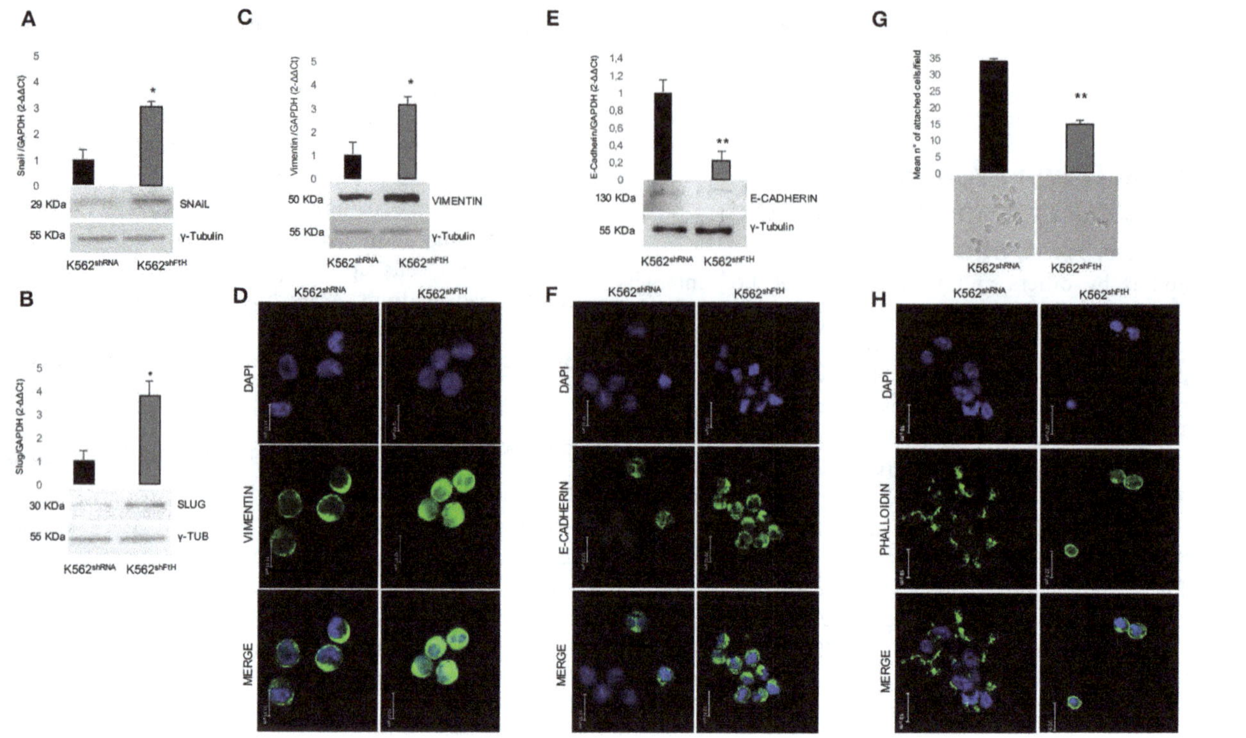

FIGURE 2 | Analysis of EMT markers in K562 cells upon FtH silencing. qPCR and Western Blot analysis of **(A)** Snail, **(B)** Slug, **(C)** Vimentin and **(E)** E-Cadherin in K562^{shRNA} and K562^{shFtH} cells. Final results are reported as mean ± SD of three independent experiments, $^{*}p < 0.05$. γ-Tubulin was used as loading control in WB experiments. Immunofluorescence staining for **(D)** Vimentin and **(F)** E-Cadherin in K562^{shRNA} and K562^{shFtH} cells. Images were collected using a Leica TCS SP2 confocal microscopy system (63X). Data are representative of three independent experiments **(E)**. **(G)** Cell adhesion assay in K562^{shRNA} and K562^{shFtH} cells performed in a 6-well plate coated with 5 μg/mL fibronectin. Results are reported as the mean number of adherent cells counted per field upon 24 h through the optical microscope, $^{**}p < 0.01$ (upper panel). A representative image of adherent K562^{shRNA} and K562^{shFtH} cells obtained from optical microscope (lower panel). **(H)** Representative images of immunofluorescence staining for Phalloidin in K562^{shRNA} and K562^{shFtH} cells. Images were collected using a Leica TCS SP2 confocal microscopy system (63X).

Accordingly, upon *FtH* silencing, the expression of Vimentin appears roughly triplicated in parallel with a significant decrease of E-cadherin amounts either at mRNA or protein level (**Figures 2C–F**).

Besides increased motility, reduced cell-cell adhesion capability is a key feature of the EMT process. By using fibronectin as substrate, we analyzed the adhesion ability of K562^{shFtH} and control cells, founding that the FtH-silenced cells halved their capability to adhere to the substrate (**Figure 2G**, upper panel). Optical imaging of K562^{shRNA} cells reveals that they behave as adherent cells stucking to fibronectin through cell protrusion, while the fraction of adherent K562^{shFtH} remains roundish (**Figure 2G**, lower panel). Confocal microscopy shows F-actin aggregates, cell-surface protrusions and/or extensions with a complex network of actin filaments (pseudopodia, lamellipodia) and actin bundles (filopodia) in K562^{shRNA} cells. In K562^{shFtH} cells, instead, F-actin is organized in a three-dimensional network beneath the plasma membrane, which likely accounts for the rounded shape of these cells (**Figure 2H**).

ROS Increase Induces CXCR4 Signaling and EMT *Trans*-Differentiation Process in K562^{shFtH} Cells

We have already reported that *FtH*-silencing induces, in a variety of cell types including K562, a dysregulation of redox homeostasis ending in a consistent ROS overproduction (15, 36, 42, 43). Given the role of ROS in mediating the communication between tumor cell and tumor microenvironment (TME), we sought to explore the effects of the antioxidant agent NAC on both CXCR4 activation and EMT trans-differentiation process of K562^{shFtH}. To this, we first re-determined the intracellular levels of ROS by using the DCF-DA assay. As shown in **Figure 3A**, a 4 h treatment with 5 mM NAC strongly reduced the amounts of ROS in the silenced cells. The decrease of ROS is accompanied by the reversal of the majority of the phenomena induced by FtH-silencing; indeed, the intracellular protein amount of CXCR4 is consistently reduced (**Figure 3B**) as well as its messenger RNA (**Figure 3C**) while its cell surface expression is only slightly affected (data not shown). Accordingly, EMT markers expression is down-regulated, with the exception of *E-cadherin* (**Figure 3D**), and the

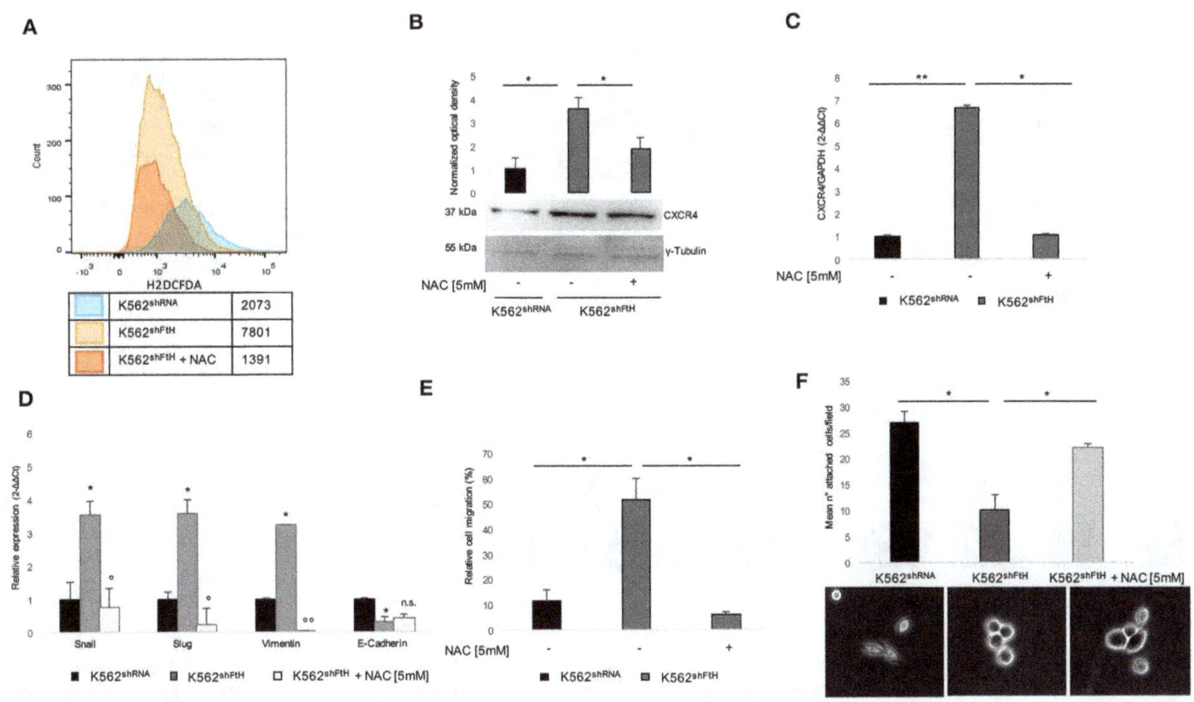

FIGURE 3 | Effects of NAC treatment on EMT transdifferentiation in K562^{shFtH} cells. **(A)** Flow cytometry analysis of ROS in K562^{shRNA} and K562^{shFtH} cells treated and not treated with 5 mM NAC for 2 h. Cells were labeled with H2DCFDA and the assay was performed in triplicate. **(B)** Western blot analysis (lower panel) and optical densitometry (upper panel) of CXCR4 in K562^{shRNA} and K562^{shFtH} cells treated and not treated with 5 mM NAC. Final results are reported as mean ± SD of three independent experiments, $^{*}p < 0.05$. γ-Tubulin was used as loading control. **(C)** qPCR analysis of *CXCR4* in K562^{shRNA} and K562^{shFtH} cells treated and not treated with 5 mM NAC. Final results represent mean ± SD of three independent experiments, $^{*}p < 0.05$; $^{**}p < 0.01$. **(D)** qPCR analysis of *Snail*, *Slug*, *Vimentin*, and *E-Cadherin* mRNA expression in K562^{shRNA}, K562^{shFtH} and K562^{shFtH} cells treated with NAC. Final results represent mean ± SD of three independent experiments, $^{*}p < 0.05$ compared to K562^{shRNA} cells. $^{\circ}p < 0.05$, $^{\circ\circ}p < 0.01$ compared to K562^{shFtH} cells. n.s., not significant. **(E)** Migration analysis in K562^{shRNA} and K562^{shFtH} cells treated and not treated with NAC was examined in 24-well plates. After 8 h, cells migrated toward CXCL12 (100 ng/ml) were counted using an optical microscope. Data are reported as the percentage of migrated cells. Final results represent mean ± SD of three independent experiments, $^{*}p < 0.05$. **(F)** Cell adhesion assay in K562^{shRNA}, K562^{shFtH} and K562^{shFtH} cells treated with NAC were cultured in a 6-well plate coated with 5 μg/mL fibronectin. After 24 h adherent cells were counted using an optical microscope; data are reported as mean of the number of adherent cells per field (upper panel), $^{*}p < 0.05$. A representative image of adherent K562^{shRNA}, K562^{shFtH} and K562^{shFtH} cells treated with NAC obtained from optical microscope (lower panel).

migratory ability is also consistently impaired (**Figure 3E**). The percentage of K562^{shFtH} cells adherent to fibronectin substrate is increased (**Figure 3F**, upper panel), together with the lack of roundish morphology and with a partial recovery of cell protrusions (**Figure 3F**, lower panel).

ROS Orchestrate EMT *Trans*-Differentiation Process by Acting on HIF-1α/CXCR4/NF-κB Axis in K562^{shFtH} Cells

Next, we analyzed HIF-1α expression levels in the *FtH* silenced cells, given its function as transcriptional factor of CXCR4. As shown in **Figures 4A,B**, *FtH* silencing induced HIF-1α up-regulation at both mRNA and protein levels and this effect was significantly attenuated by treatment with 5 mM NAC for 2 h. It has been recently found that CXCR4 modulates PI3K/Akt/NF-κB signaling pathway and that both NF-κB and CXCR4 belong to a regulatory network driving the migration of cancer stem cells (24). Moreover, NF-κB is currently considered a master regulator of cancer cells aggressive phenotype through the direct transcriptional activation of EMT genes in solid tumors (10, 44, 45), and we recently demonstrated its ROS-mediated activation in K562^{shFtH} cells (36).

Therefore, we assessed the effects of the CXCR4 inhibitor AMD3100 on the phenotype acquired by K562 cells upon *FtH* silencing. As shown in **Figures 4C,D**, p65 nuclear accumulation in K562^{shFtH} cells was significantly reduced upon AMD3100 treatment and this was accompanied by a consistent decrease of all the EMT markers except for *E-Cadherin* that appeared unaffected. This effect was dependent on NF-κB transcriptional activity since blocking NF-κB with the specific inhibitor Ik-Bα suppressed *Snail, Slug* and *Vimentin* upregulation in K562^{shFtH} cells (**Figure 4E**). The expression of Ik-Bα in K562^{shFtH} cells is reported in **Figure S1B**.

These results strongly suggest that FtH is involved in bestowing K562 cells with more migratory and more mesenchymal-like features through the hypoxia-induced activation of CXCR4 and p65 transcriptional activation of selected EMT markers (**Figure 4F**).

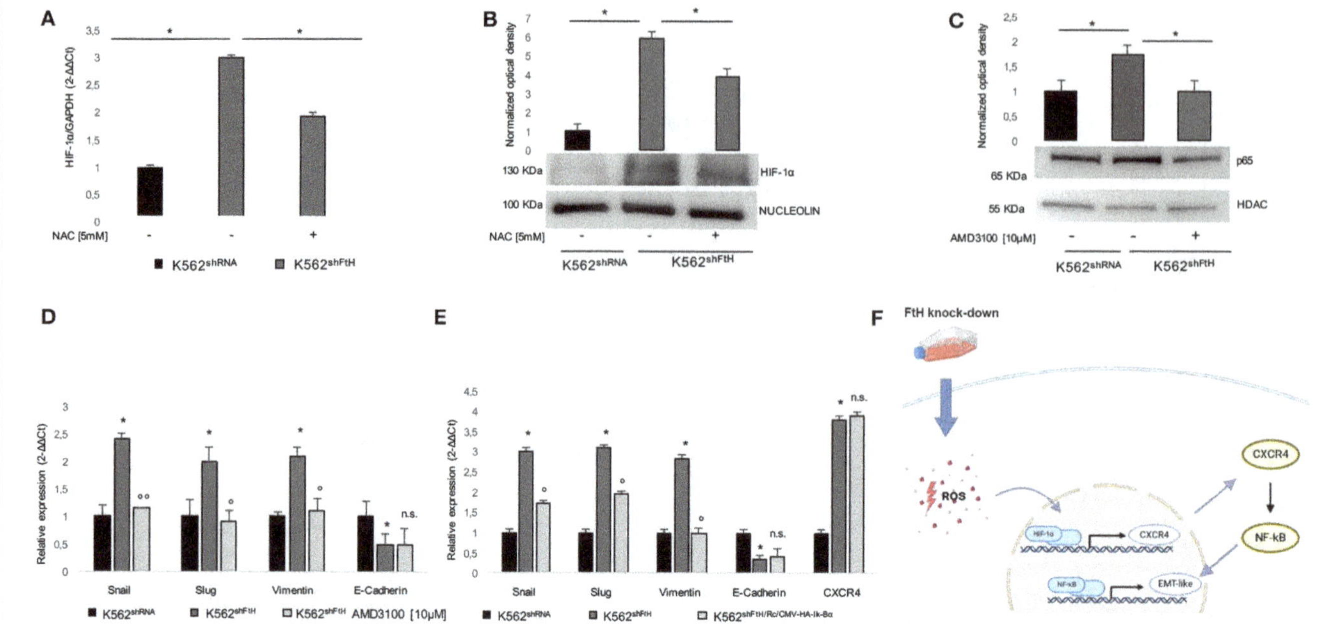

FIGURE 4 | ROS/ HIF-1α/ CXCR4/ NF-kB axis activates EMT in K562^{shFtH} cells. **(A)** qPCR analysis of *HIF-1α* in K562^{shRNA} and K562^{shFtH} cells treated and not treated with NAC. Final results represent mean ± SD of three independent experiments, $^{*}p < 0.05$. **(B)** Western Blot analysis of HIF-1α (lower panel) and optical densitometry (upper panel) in K562^{shRNA} and K562^{shFtH} cells treated and not treated with NAC. Final results are reported as mean ± SD of three independent experiments, $^{*}p < 0.05$. γ-Tubulin was used as loading control. **(C)** Western Blot analysis of p65 (lower panel) and optical densitometry (upper panel) in K562^{shRNA} and K562^{shFtH} cells treated and not treated with AMD3100. Final results are reported as mean ± SD of three independent experiments, $^{*}p < 0.05$. HDAC was used as loading control of nuclear protein fraction. **(D)** qPCR analysis of *Snail*, *Slug*, *Vimentin*, and *E-Cadherin* mRNA expression in K562^{shRNA} and K562^{shFtH} cells treated and not treated with AMD3100. Final results represent mean ± SD of three independent experiments, $^{*}p < 0.05$, compared to K562^{shRNA} cells. $^{\circ}p < 0.05$, $^{\circ\circ}p < 0.01$, compared to KK562^{shFtH} cells. n.s., not significant. **(E)** qPCR analysis of *Snail*, *Slug*, *Vimentin*, *E-Cadherin*, and *CXCR4* mRNA expression in K562^{shRNA}, K562^{shFtH} and K562$^{shFtH/Rc/CMV-HA-Ik-B\alpha}$ cells. Final results represent mean ± SD of three independent experiments, $^{*}p < 0.05$, compared to K562^{shRNA} cells. $^{\circ}p < 0.05$, compared to K562^{shFtH} cells. n.s., not significant. **(F)** Cartoon of ROS/ HIF-1α/ CXCR4/ NF-kB axis activating EMT in K562^{shFtH} cells.

DISCUSSION

Tumor cell migration is a critical process that contributes to the development and progression of both solid and hematological malignancies (46, 47). In solid tumors, the EMT process enhances the metastatic potential converting polarized epithelial cells into non-polarized mesenchymal cells thus promoting cell mobility, invasion and resistance to apoptotic stimuli (48–50). In hematological malignancies, the blasts move from BM into peripheral blood and colonize distant sites such as liver and spleen, a process reminiscent of EMT in metastatic solid tumors (51–53). Moreover, it has been recently demonstrated that EMT transcription factors are critical in promoting leukemia and lymphoma progression (6, 18).

Many of the molecules driving homing and retention of leukemic cells in tissues have been identified (54, 55); among them, the CXCL12/CXCR4 axis has been shown to be essential for hematopoietic stem cell (HSC) migration and homing and also for cancer cell migration and metastasis (3, 20, 56). In particular, CXCR4 expression is necessary to keep the leukemic cells in the CXCL12-enriched BM microenvironment, and the efficient blockade of CXCR4 mobilizes the cells from the BM into the circulation (3, 19, 22).

In solid cancers, a tumor microenvironment that is rich in reactive oxygen species (ROS) promotes the binding of the hypoxia inducible factor subunit HIF-1α to its response element (HRE) in the promoter region of CXCR4, thus critically influencing CXCR4-mediated expression and functions, and ultimately encouraging cancer metastasis (27, 28). Hypoxia represents a key driver of metabolic reprograming also in the leukemic BM niche where it is often associated with increased production of ROS (27, 57). This feature has been observed in numerous leukemic cell lines and also in cells from patients with CML and AML (58–60). Growing evidences suggest the role of ROS-mediated metabolic alterations in triggering hematopoietic cancer cell mobilization (54, 61).

In the last years, we and others have demonstrated that the knock down of ferritin heavy chain (FtH) induces EMT in epithelial derived cell lines, mainly though not exclusively by increasing ROS production (15, 17). The role of ferritin in hematological malignancies has been explored as well (42, 62, 63). In chronic myelogenous leukemia K562 cells *FtH*-silencing, by altering the redox metabolism, triggers p65 nuclear activation and resistance to doxorubicin (36).

In this study, we demonstrate that *FtH* knock-down promotes a quasi-mesenchymal phenotype and enhances mobility in K562 cells through the activation of a molecular axis arising from

ROS mediated-induction of HIF-1α/CXCR4 and ending in p65-mediated transcriptional activation of the mesenchymal markers *Snail*, *Slug* and *Vimentin*.

In detail, K562 cells react to *FtH* knock down-induced oxidative stress by enhancing the expression of the regulatory HIF-1α subunit that, in turn, acts as a transcription factor for *CXCR4*. According to these results, ROS attenuation with NAC specifically reduced CXCR4 mRNA and protein levels induced by hypoxia. In $K562^{shFtH}$ cells, CXCR4 up-regulation promotes the nuclear translocation of p65 subunit belonging to the transcriptional complex NF-κB. There is increasing evidence suggesting a reciprocal interplay between CXCR4 and NF-κB signaling in fine tuning cancer cellular signaling pathways (23, 24). Although the vast majority of data report that NF-κB contributes to the increase in CXCR4 expression (64), few recent reports suggest the possible existence of a regulatory feedback loop (24). Our results highlight that, besides being redox sensitive, the activation of NF-κB in $K562^{shFtH}$ cells is also dependent on CXCR4 increase, being reversible upon AMD3100 inhibitor treatment.

A positive correlation between NF-κB activation and EMT has been described in several human solid tumors including breast cancer (44), prostate cancer (65), renal carcinoma (66) and head and neck squamous cell carcinomas (67). A number of studies have also recently demonstrated that NF-κB regulates the transcription of EMT-inducing factors *Slug*, *Twist* and *Sip1* (68). Our results provide further evidence regarding NF-κB's involvement in EMT regulation also in the hematological malignancies since, in $K562^{shFtH}$ cells, p65 nuclear translocation is accompanied by the over expression of the two key EMT-TF *Snail* and *Slug* and of the major mesenchymal marker *Vimentin* in association with the break-down of the epithelial marker *E-cadherin*. These molecular rearrangements are mirrored by cytoskeletal remodeling along with increased cell motility and reduced cell adhesion capability to fibronectin substrate. The assessment of the EMT transdifferentiation highlights that either NAC or AMD3100 or IκB alpha treatment is able to attenuate the increase of *Snail*, *Slug* and *Vimentin* as well as the migratory and the adhesion abilities of K562 lacking of FtH expression. On the contrary, none of the above mentioned treatments restore *E-cadherin* levels in $K562^{shFtH}$ cells suggesting the non-involvement of ROS/CXCR4/NF-κB molecular axis in the regulation of this marker but rather the existence of other underlying molecular regulatory mechanisms such as the previously reported epigenetic imprinting (69).

To the best of our knowledge this is one of the few reports highlighting the role of ROS in the acquisition of characteristics ascribable to EMT phenotype in cells of hematological origins. Moreover, we describe a link between iron metabolism and CXCR4 in the hematological malignancies which may suggest a potential mechanism through which leukemic cells acquire a metastatic phenotype and a tendency to move to a distal organ. Finally, we believe that iron metabolism might be considered as part of the dynamic crosstalk between hematopoietic cancer cells and their microenvironment and that a perturbation of this crosstalk affects the metastatic potential in the hematological malignancies. Clearly, the cellular context of iron/redox metabolism in the modulation of this phenotype is important; hence, cell- or leukemia-subtype specific dependence of this new molecular axis would be the focus of future studies.

AUTHOR CONTRIBUTIONS

RC, IA, FB, and FC conceived and designed the study. RC, IA, AD, ASal, AB, ASac, MD, and FB performed the experiments. RC, IA, MF, BQ, CP, FB, and FC analyzed the data. RC, IA, FB, and FC wrote the first draft of the manuscript. All authors contributed to manuscritp revision, read and approved the submitted version.

ACKNOWLEDGMENTS

We thank Caterina Alessi for the administrative support. We thank the Interdipartimental Centre of Services (CIS) for the flow cytometry facilities.

REFERENCES

1. Bissell MJ, Radisky DC, Rizki A, Weaver VM, Petersen OW. The organizing principle: microenvironmental influences in the normal and malignant breast. *Differentiation.* (2002) 70:537–46. doi: 10.1046/j.1432-0436.2002.700907.x
2. Bardaweel SK, Gul M, Alzweiri M, Ishaqat A, Alsalamat HA, Bashatwah RM. Reactive oxygen species: the dual role in physiological and pathological conditions of the human body. *Eurasian J Med.* (2018) 50:193–201. doi: 10.5152/eurasianjmed.2018.17397
3. Weisberg E, Azab AK, Manley PW, Kung AL, Christie AL, Bronson R, et al. Inhibition of CXCR4 in CML cells disrupts their interaction with the bone marrow microenvironment and sensitizes them to nilotinib. *Leukemia.* (2012) 26:985–90. doi: 10.1038/leu.2011.360
4. Hu TH, Yao Y, Yu S, Han LL, Wang WJ, Guo H, et al. SDF-1/CXCR4 promotes epithelial-mesenchymal transition and progression of colorectal cancer by activation of the Wnt/??-catenin signaling pathway. *Cancer Lett.* (2014) 354:417–26. doi: 10.1016/j.canlet.2014.08.012
5. Yang J, Mani SA, Weinberg RA. Exploring a new twist on tumor metastasis. *Cancer Res.* (2006) 66:4549–52. doi: 10.1158/0008-5472.CAN-05-3850
6. Kahlert UD, Joseph JV, Kruyt FAE. EMT- and MET-related processes in nonepithelial tumors: importance for disease progression, prognosis, and therapeutic opportunities. *Mol Oncol.* (2017) 11:860–77. doi: 10.1002/1878-0261.12085
7. Singh P, Pelus LM. CXCR4 expression in the bone marrow microenvironment is required for hematopoietic stem and progenitor cell maintenance and

early hematopoietic regeneration after myeloablation. *Stem Cells.* (2020) 1–15. doi: 10.1002/stem.3174. [Epub ahead of print].

8. Yu LM, Zhang WH, Han XX, Li YY, Lu Y, Pan J, et al. Hypoxia-Induced ROS contribute to myoblast pyroptosis during obstructive sleep apnea via the NF-κ B/HIF-1 signaling pathway. *Oxid Med Cell Longev.* (2019) 2019:4596368. doi: 10.1155/2019/4596368
9. Wang Z, Li Y, Sarkar F. Signaling mechanism(S) of reactive oxygen species in epithelial-mesenchymal transition reminiscent of cancer stem cells in tumor progression. *Curr Stem Cell Res Ther.* (2010) 5:74–80. doi: 10.2174/157488810790442813
10. Cichon MA, Radisky DC. ROS-induced epithelial-mesenchymal transition in mammary epithelial cells is mediated by NF-κB-dependent activation of Snail. *Oncotarget.* (2014) 5:2827–38. doi: 10.18632/oncotarget.1940
11. Li W, Cao L, Han L, Xu Q, Ma Q. Superoxide dismutase promotes the epithelial-mesenchymal transition of pancreatic cancer cells via activation of the H_2O_2ERK/NF-κB axis. *Int J Oncol.* (2015) 46:2613–20. doi: 10.3892/ijo.2015.2938
12. Sioutas A, Vainikka LK, Kentson M, Dam-Larsen S, Wennerström U, Jacobson P, et al. Oxidant-induced autophagy and ferritin degradation contribute to epithelial–mesenchymal transition through lysosomal iron. *J Inflamm Res.* (2017) 10:29–39. doi: 10.2147/JIR.S128292
13. Cannito S, Novo E, di Bonzo LV, Busletta C, Colombatto S, Parola M. Epithelial-mesenchymal transition: from molecular mechanisms, redox regulation to implications in human health and disease. *Antioxid Redox Signal.* (2010) 12:1383–430. doi: 10.1089/ars.2009.2737
14. Storz P. Reactive oxygen species in tumor progression. *Front Biosci.* (2005) 10:1881–96. doi: 10.2741/1667
15. Aversa I, Zolea F, Ieranò C, Bulotta S, Trotta AM, Faniello MC, et al. Epithelial-to-mesenchymal transition in FHC-silenced cells: The role of CXCR4/CXCL12 axis. *J Exp Clin Cancer Res.* (2017) 36:1–15. doi: 10.1186/s13046-017-0571-8
16. Li R, Luo C, Mines M, Zhang J, Fan GH. Chemokine CXCL12 induces binding of ferritin heavy chain to the chemokine receptor CXCR4, alters CXCR4 signaling, and induces phosphorylation and nuclear translocation of ferritin heavy chain. *J Biol Chem.* (2006) 281:37616–27. doi: 10.1074/jbc.M607266200
17. Zhang KH, Tian HY, Gao X, Lei WW, Hu Y, Wang DM, et al. Ferritin heavy chain-mediated iron homeostasis and subsequent increased reactive oxygen species production are essential for epithelial-mesenchymal transition. *Cancer Res.* (2009) 69:5340–48. doi: 10.1158/0008-5472.CAN-09-0112
18. Chen SC, Liao TT, Yang MH. Emerging roles of epithelial-mesenchymal transition in hematological malignancies. *J Biomed Sci.* (2018) 25:37. doi: 10.1186/s12929-018-0440-6
19. Roccaro AM, Mishima Y, Sacco A, Moschetta M, Tai YT, Shi J, et al. CXCR4 regulates extra-medullary myeloma through epithelial-mesenchymal-transition-like transcriptional activation. *Cell Rep.* (2015) 12:622–35. doi: 10.1016/j.celrep.2015.06.059
20. Dewan MZ, Ahmed S, Iwasaki Y, Ohba K, Toi M, Yamamoto N. Stromal cell-derived factor-1 and CXCR4 receptor interaction in tumor growth and metastasis of breast cancer. *Biomed Pharmacother.* (2006) 60:273–6. doi: 10.1016/j.biopha.2006.06.004
21. D'Alterio C, Barbieri A, Portella L, Palma G, Polimeno M, Riccio A, et al. Inhibition of stromal CXCR4 impairs development of lung metastases. *Cancer Immunol Immunother.* (2012) 61:1713–20. doi: 10.1007/s00262-012-1223-7
22. Peled A, Klein S, Beider K, Burger JA, Abraham M. Role of CXCL12 and CXCR4 in the pathogenesis of hematological malignancies. *Cytokine.* (2018) 109:11–6. doi: 10.1016/j.cyto.2018.02.020
23. Jiang C, Ma S, Hu R, Wang X, Li M, Tian F, et al. Effect of CXCR4 on apoptosis in osteosarcoma cells via the PI3K/Akt/NF-κβ signaling pathway. *Cell Physiol Biochem.* (2018) 46:2250–60. doi: 10.1159/000489593
24. Es-haghi M, Soltanian S, Dehghani H. Perspective: cooperation of nanog, NF-κB, and CXCR4 in a regulatory network for directed migration of cancer stem cells. *Tumor Biol.* (2016) 37:1559–65. doi: 10.1007/s13277-015-4690-6
25. Liu X, Xiao Q, Bai X, Yu Z, Sun M, Zhao H, et al. Activation of STAT3 is involved in malignancy mediated by CXCL12-CXCR4 signaling in human breast cancer. *Oncol Rep.* (2014) 32:2760–8. doi: 10.3892/or.2014.3536
26. Delgado-Martín C, Escribano C, Pablos JL, Riol-Blanco L, Rodríguez-Fernández JL. CXCL12 uses CXCR4 and a signaling core formed by bifunctional Akt, Erk1/2 and mTORC1 to control simultaneously chemotaxis and survival in mature dendritic cells. *J Biol Chem.* (2011) 286:37222–36. doi: 10.1074/jbc.M111.294116
27. Gu Q, He Y, Ji J, Yao Y, Shen W, Luo J, et al. Hypoxia-inducible factor 1α (HIF-1α) and reactive oxygen species (ROS) mediates radiation-induced invasiveness through the SDF-1α/CXCR4 pathway in non-small cell lung carcinoma cells. *Oncotarget.* (2015) 6:10893–907. doi: 10.18632/oncotarget.3535
28. Barriga EH, Maxwell PH, Reyes AE, Mayor R. The hypoxia factor Hif-1α controls neural crest chemotaxis and epithelial to mesenchymal transition. *J Cell Biol.* (2013) 201:759–76. doi: 10.1083/jcb.201212100
29. Chetram MA, Hinton CV. ROS-mediated regulation of CXCR4 in cancer. *Front Biol.* (2013) 8273Ű-8. doi: 10.1007/s11515-012-1204-4
30. Dong CY, Liu XY, Wang N, Wang LN, Yang BX, Ren Q, et al. Twist-1, A novel regulator of hematopoietic stem cell self-renewal and myeloid lineage development. *Stem Cells.* (2014) 32:3173–82. doi: 10.1002/stem.1803
31. Zhang Z, Zhu P, Zhou Y, Sheng Y, Hong Y, Xiang D, et al. A novel slug-containing negative-feedback loop regulates SCF/c-Kit-mediated hematopoietic stem cell self-renewal. *Leukemia.* (2017) 31:403–13. doi: 10.1038/leu.2016.201
32. Wei CR, Liu J, Yu XJ. Targeting SLUG sensitizes leukemia cells to ADR-induced apoptosis. *Int J Clin Exp Med.* (2015) 8:22139–48.
33. Puissant A, Dufies M, Fenouille N, Ben Sahra I, Jacquel A, Robert G, et al. Imatinib triggers mesenchymal-like conversion of CML cells associated with increased aggressiveness. *J Mol Cell Biol.* (2012) 4:207–20. doi: 10.1093/jmcb/mjs010
34. Di Sanzo M, Aversa I, Santamaria G, Gagliardi M, Panebianco M, Biamonte F, et al. FTH1P3, a novel H-ferritin pseudogene transcriptionally active, is ubiquitously expressed and regulated during cell differentiation. *PLoS ONE.* (2016) 11:e0151359. doi: 10.1371/journal.pone.0151359
35. Zolea F, Battaglia AM, Chiarella E, Malanga D, De Marco C, Bond HM, et al. Ferritin heavy subunit silencing blocks the erythroid commitment of K562 cells via miR-150 up-regulation and GATA-1 repression. *Int J Mol Sci.* (2017) 18:2167. doi: 10.3390/ijms18102167
36. Aversa I, Chirillo R, Chiarella E, Zolea F, Di Sanzo M, Biamonte F, et al. Chemoresistance in H-ferritin silenced cells: The role of NF-κB. *Int J Mol Sci.* (2018) 19:2969. doi: 10.3390/ijms19102969
37. Zolea F, Biamonte F, Battaglia AM, Faniello MC, Cuda G, Costanzo F. Caffeine positively modulates ferritin heavy chain expression in H460 cells: effects on cell proliferation. *PLoS ONE.* (2016) 11:e0163078. doi: 10.1371/journal.pone.0163078
38. Di Sanzo M, Gaspari M, Misaggi R, Romeo F, Falbo L, De Marco C, et al. H ferritin gene silencing in a human metastatic melanoma cell line: a proteomic analysis. *J Proteome Res.* (2011) 10:5444–53. doi: 10.1021/pr200705z
39. Biamonte F, Santamaria G, Sacco A, Perrone FM, Di Cello A, Battaglia AM, et al. MicroRNA let-7g acts as tumor suppressor and predictive biomarker for chemoresistance in human epithelial ovarian cancer. *Sci Rep.* (2019) 9:1–12. doi: 10.1038/s41598-019-42221-x
40. Sottile R, Federico G, Garofalo C, Tallerico R, Faniello MC, Quaresima B, et al. Iron and ferritin modulate MHC class I expression and NK cell recognition. (2019) 10:1–12. doi: 10.3389/fimmu.2019.00224
41. Biamonte F, Battaglia AM, Zolea F, Oliveira DM, Aversa I, Santamaria G, et al. Ferritin heavy subunit enhances apoptosis of non-small cell lung cancer cells through modulation of miR-125b/p53 axis. *Cell Death Dis.* (2018) 9:1174. doi: 10.1038/s41419-018-1216-3
42. Zolea F, Biamonte F, Candeloro P, Di Sanzo M, Cozzi A, Di Vito A, et al. H ferritin silencing induces protein misfolding in K562 cells: A Raman analysis. *Free Radic Biol Med.* (2015) 89:614–23. doi: 10.1016/j.freeradbiomed.2015.07.161
43. Di Sanzo M, Chirillo R, Aversa I, Biamonte F, Santamaria G, Giovannone ED, et al. shRNA targeting of ferritin heavy chain activates H19/miR-675 axis in K562 cells. *Gene.* (2018) 657:92–9. doi: 10.1016/j.gene.2018.03.027
44. Huber MA, Azoitei N, Baumann B, Grünert S, Sommer A, Pehamberger H, et al. NF-κB is essential for epithelial-mesenchymal transition and metastasis in a model of breast cancer progression. *J Clin Invest.* (2004) 114:569–81. doi: 10.1172/JCI200421358
45. Nomura A, Majumder K, Giri B, Dauer P, Dudeja V, Roy S, et al. Inhibition of NF-kappa B pathway leads to deregulation of epithelial – mesenchymal

transition and neural invasion in pancreatic cancer. *Lab Invest.* (2016) 96:1268–78. doi: 10.1038/labinvest.2016.109
46. Redondo-muñoz J, García-pardo A, Teixidó J. Molecular players in hematologic tumor cell trafficking. *Front Immunol.* (2019) 10:156. doi: 10.3389/fimmu.2019.00156
47. Kuznetsov M, Kolobov A. Mathematical biology investigation of solid tumor progression with account of proliferation / migration dichotomy via Darwinian mathematical model. *J Math Biol.* (2019) 80:601–26. doi: 10.1007/s00285-019-01434-4
48. Chen CC, You JY, Gau JP, Huang CE, Chen YY, Tsai YH, et al. Favorable clinical outcome and unique characteristics in association with Twist1 overexpression in de novo acute myeloid leukemia. *Blood Cancer J.* (2015) 5:e339. doi: 10.1038/bcj.2015.67
49. Jordan NV, Johnson GL, Abell AN. Tracking the intermediate stages of epithelial-mesenchymal transition in epithelial stem cells and cancer. *Cell Cycle.* (2011) 10:2865–73. doi: 10.4161/cc.10.17.17188
50. Kalluri R, Weinberg RA. The basics of epithelial-mesenchymal transition. *J Clin Invest.* (2009) 119:1420–28. doi: 10.1172/JCI39104
51. Percival M, Lai C, Estey E, Hourigan CS, Hutchinson F, Section M, et al. Bone marrow evaluation for diagnosis and monitoring of acute myeloid leukemia. *HHS Public Access Blood Rev.* (2018) 31:185–92. doi: 10.1016/j.blre.2017.01.003
52. Al-katari MS. Acute lymphoblastic leukemia presenting with liver infiltration and severe lactic acidosis. *Am J Case Rep.* (2018) 19:453–7. doi: 10.12659/AJCR.907383
53. Fracchiolla NS, Fattizzo B, Cortelezzi A. Review article mesenchymal stem cells in myeloid malignancies : a focus on immune escaping and therapeutic implications. *Stem Cells Int.* (2017) 2017::6720594. doi: 10.1155/2017/6720594
54. Schroeder MA, Dipersio JF. Mobilization of hematopoietic stem and leukemia cells. *J Leukoc Biol.* (2012) 91:47–57. doi: 10.1189/jlb.0210085
55. Burger JA. Mechanisms of leukemia cell trafficking, homing, and tissue retention in chronic lymphocytic leukemia. *Chronic Lymph Leuk.* (2011) 5:91–9.
56. Tavor S, Petit I, Porozov S, Avigdor A, Dar A, Leider-Trejo L, et al. CXCR4 regulates migration and development of human acute myelogenous leukemia stem cells in transplanted NOD/SCID mice. *Cancer Res.* (2004) 64:2817–24. doi: 10.1158/0008-5472.CAN-03-3693
57. Testa U, Labbaye C, Castelli G, Pelosi E. Oxidative stress and hypoxia in normal and leukemic stem cells. *Exp Hematol.* (2016) 44:540–60. doi: 10.1016/j.exphem.2016.04.012
58. Validity RM. The influence of hypoxia on CML trafficking through modulation of CXCR4 and E-cadherin expression. *Leukemia.* (2013) 27:961–4. doi: 10.1038/leu.2012.353
59. Prieto-bermejo R, Romo-gonzález M, Pérez-fernández A, Ijurko C. Reactive oxygen species in haematopoiesis : leukaemic cells take a walk on the wild side. *J Exp Clin Cancer Res.* (2018) 37:125. doi: 10.1186/s13046-018-0797-0
60. Muz B, Puente P De, Azab F, Luderer M, Azab AK. The role of hypoxia and exploitation of the hypoxic environment in hematologic malignancies. *Mol Cancer Res.* (2014) 12:1347–55. doi: 10.1158/1541-7786.MCR-14-0028
61. Self-renewal SC, Gur-cohen S, Golan K, Kaufmann KB, Itkin T. Reactive oxygen species regulate hematopoietic stem cell self-renewal, migration and development,as well as their bone marrow microenvironment. *Antioxid Redox Signal.* (2014) 21:1605–19. doi: 10.1089/ars.2014.5941
62. Biamonte F, Zolea F, Bisognin A, Di Sanzo M, Saccoman C, Scumaci D, et al. H-ferritin-regulated microRNAs modulate gene expression in K562 cells. *PLoS ONE.* (2015) 10:e0122105. doi: 10.1371/journal.pone.0122105
63. Bertoli S, Paubelle E, Bérard E, Saland E, Thomas X et al. Ferritin heavy/light chain (FTH1/FTL) expression, serum ferritin levels, and their functional as well as prognostic roles in acute myeloid leukemia. *Eur J Haematol.* (2019) 102:131–42. doi: 10.1111/ejh.13183
64. Penzo M, Habiel DM, Ramadass M, Kew RR, Marcu KB. Cell migration to CXCL12 requires simultaneous IKK α and IKK β -dependent NF- κ B signaling?. *Biochim Biophys Acta.* (2014) 1843:1796–804. doi: 10.1016/j.bbamcr.2014.04.011
65. Zhang Q, Helfand BT, Jang TL, Zhu LJ, Chen L, Yang XJ, et al. Nuclear factor-κB-mediated transforming growth factor-beta-induced expression of vimentin is an independent predictor of biochemical recurrence after radical prostatectomy nuclear factor- κ b-mediated transforming growth factor- β - induced expression of vimentin is an independent predictor of biochemical recurrence after radical prostatectomy. *Clin Cancer Res.* (2009) 15:3557–67. doi: 10.1158/1078-0432.CCR-08-1656
66. Pantuck AJ, An J, Liu H, Rettig MB. NF- κ B – dependent plasticity of the epithelial to mesenchymal transition induced by von hippel-lindau inactivation in renal cell carcinomas. *Cancer Res.* (2010) 70:752–62. doi: 10.1158/0008-5472.CAN-09-2211
67. Chung CH, Parker JS, Ely K, Carter J, Yi Y, Murphy BA, et al. Gene expression profiles identify epithelial-to-mesenchymal transition and activation of nuclear factor- K B signaling as characteristics of a high-risk head and neck squamous cell carcinoma. *Cancer Res.* (2006) 66:8210–9. doi: 10.1158/0008-5472.CAN-06-1213
68. Pires BRB, Mencalha AL, Ferreira GM, Souza WF De. NF-kappaB is involved in the regulation of EMT genes in breast cancer cells. *PLoS ONE.* (2017) 12:e0169622. doi: 10.1371/journal.pone.0169622
69. Zha L, Cao Q, Cui X, Li F, Liang H. Epigenetic regulation of E-cadherin expression by the histone demethylase UTX in colon cancer cells. *Med Oncol.* (2016) 33:21. doi: 10.1007/s12032-016-0734-z

16

Identification and Validation of a Prognostic Gene Signature for Diffuse Large B-Cell Lymphoma Based on Tumor Microenvironment-Related Genes

Tao Pan[1,2†], *Yizi He*[1†], *Huan Chen*[1], *Junfei Pei*[3], *Yajun Li*[1], *Ruolan Zeng*[1], *Jiliang Xia*[4], *Yilang Zuo*[1], *Liping Qin*[1], *Siwei Chen*[5], *Ling Xiao*[5*] and *Hui Zhou*[1*]

[1] Department of Lymphoma & Hematology, Hunan Cancer Hospital, The Affiliated Cancer Hospital of Xiangya School of Medicine, Central South University, Changsha, China, [2] The Third Xiangya Hospital, Central South University, Changsha, China, [3] Department of Gastrointestinal Surgery, First Hospital of Jilin University, Changchun, Jilin, China, [4] Hunan Province Key Laboratory of Tumor Cellular & Molecular Pathology, Cancer Research Institute, Hengyang School of Medicine, University of South China, Hengyang, China, [5] Department of Histology and Embryology of School of Basic Medical Science, Central South University, Changsha, China

***Correspondence:**
Ling Xiao
xiaolingcsu@csu.edu.cn
Hui Zhou
zhouhui9403@126.com

†These authors have contributed equally to this work

Diffuse large B-cell lymphoma (DLBCL) is an extremely heterogeneous tumor entity, which makes prognostic prediction challenging. The tumor microenvironment (TME) has a crucial role in fostering and restraining tumor development. Consequently, we performed a systematic investigation of the TME and genetic factors associated with DLBCL to identify prognostic biomarkers for DLBCL. Data for a total of 1,084 DLBCL patients from the Gene Expression Omnibus database were included in this study, and patients were divided into a training group, an internal validation group, and two external validation groups. We calculated the abundance of immune–stromal components of DLBCL and found that they were related to tumor prognosis and progression. Then, differentially expressed genes were obtained based on immune and stromal scores, and prognostic TME-related genes were further identified using a protein–protein interaction network and univariate Cox regression analysis. These genes were analyzed by the least absolute shrinkage and selection operator Cox regression model to establish a seven-gene signature, comprising *TIMP2*, *QKI*, *LCP2*, *LAMP2*, *ITGAM*, *CSF3R*, and *AAK1*. The signature was shown to have critical prognostic value in the training and validation sets and was also confirmed to be an independent prognostic factor. Subgroup analysis also indicated the robust prognostic ability of the signature. A nomogram integrating the seven-gene signature and components of the International Prognostic Index was shown to have value for prognostic prediction. Gene set enrichment analysis between risk groups demonstrated that immune-related pathways were enriched in the low-risk group. In conclusion, a novel and reliable TME relevant gene signature was proposed and shown to be capable of predicting the survival of DLBCL patients at high risk of poor survival.

Keywords: diffuse large B-cell lymphoma, tumor microenvironment, Gene Expression Omnibus database, signature, prognostic

INTRODUCTION

Diffuse large B-cell lymphoma (DLBCL) is a heterogeneous tumor entity with a striking degree of genetic and clinical heterogeneity. Although more than half of DLBCL patients may achieve long-term remission, the disease remains a major clinical challenge, with approximately 30% of patients not being cured (1, 2). The heterogeneity of the tumor, in particular, poses a major barrier to understanding the genetic basis of the disease and its response to therapy (3). Therefore, there is an urgent need to identify new individual prognostic and risk-stratified biomarkers.

In recent years, the role of the tumor microenvironment (TME) in tumorigenesis has gradually been discovered (4). Studies have revealed that tumor cells are targets of the immune system in the early stages of tumor development; however, over time, these cells begin to resist the innate immune response and then gradually weaken and adapt to it (5–7). Thus, a better understanding of the interactions between the TME and the immune response may provide new approaches to improve the efficiency of current immunotherapies, especially immune checkpoint inhibitor and chimeric antigen receptor (CAR) T cell therapies (8). Several studies have considered the latent role of the TME in the occurrence and development of DLBCL, but their results were controversial (9).

In the era of rituximab and immunotherapy, the ability of the International Prognostic Index (IPI) to predict the prognosis of individual DLBCL patients has decreased (10). A better understanding of the interactions between the TME and IPI scores may provide new approaches to improve response rates to current treatment strategies. Thus, incorporating a prognostic factor from the TME into the existing IPI system would help greatly in the development of prognostic stratification of DLBCL. Here, we propose a compound prognostic nomogram combining a TME-related prognostic model with clinical features. This approach provides a basis for better understanding the molecular mechanisms underlying the prognoses of DLBCL patients.

MATERIALS AND METHODS

Data Sources

Gene expression profiling and clinical data of patients with DLBCL were obtained from the Gene Expression Omnibus (GEO) database (https://www.ncbi.nlm.nih.gov/geo/). Data series were downloaded in a normalized expression matrix file format and were used directly for the analyses. Patients in the GSE31312 dataset were randomly divided into a training group (N = 282) and an internal validation group (N = 188) in a 6:4 ratio. In addition, two DLBCL microarray datasets were used for validation, including 414 DLBCL patients from the GSE10846 dataset and 200 DLBCL patients from the GSE11318 dataset.

Generation and Analysis of ImmuneScore, StromalScore, and ESTIMATEScore

The ESTIMATE (Estimation of STromal and Immune cells in MAlignant Tumors using Expression data) package in R version 3.6.3 was used to evaluate the abundance of immune and stromal components of the TME from expression data (11). We obtained three scores, ImmuneScore, StromalScore, and ESTIMATEScore, which respectively represent the immune abundance, the stromal abundance, and the sum of both in the TME; for instance, a higher ImmuneScore means a higher abundance of immune components in the TME.

Identification of Differentially Expressed Genes

To obtain DEGs between high- and low-scoring samples, microarray data from GEO were analyzed using NCBI GEO2R (https://www.ncbi.nlm.nih.gov/geo/geo2r/). 470 patients with GSE31312 were divided by the median of ImmuneScore (StromalScore), and the high and low ImmuneScore (StromalScore) groups were obtained, respectively. Based on comparisons of the high- and low-scoring groups, Adj. $P < 0.05$ and fold change >1.05 were set as the thresholds for DEG identification to obtain differential immune and stromal genes. We then took the intersection of immune differential genes and stromal differential genes. The DEGs were visualized using heatmaps (https://software.broadinstitute.org/morpheus/) and Venn plots (http://bioinformatics.psb.ugent.be/webtools/Venn/).

Functional Enrichment Analyses

DAVID (https://david.ncifcrf.gov/summary.jsp), an online tool for gene functional enrichment, was used for gene ontology (GO) analysis (with respect to cellular component, molecular function, and biological process) and Kyoto Encyclopedia of Genes and Genomes (KEGG) pathway analysis of the 183 DEGs shared between the ImmuneScore groups and the StromalScore groups. The results were displayed using the ggplot2 R package. $P < 0.05$ was considered statistically significant.

Gene set enrichment analysis (GSEA) was performed using the gsea-4.0.3 software downloaded from https://www.gsea-msigdb.org/gsea/index.jsp to explore whether immune pathways were significantly different between the high-risk and low-risk groups.

Protein–Protein Interaction Network Construction and Univariate Cox Regression Analysis

The PPI network was obtained from the STRING database (https://string-db.org/) and reconstructed with version 3.7.2 of Cytoscape. Univariate Cox analysis of overall survival (OS) was used to determine the relationships between expression of 183 DEGs and prognosis. In order to obtain the most critical and meaningful genes to construct the model, we used a method from Bi et al. (12) to further screen the genes. In the PPI network, we kept the core gene located in the center by eliminating genes with fewer peripheral nodes. In univariate Cox regression, the smaller the p-value, the more significant the prognosis. Therefore, the sharing factors between the degree of the nodes ≥3 in PPI and the $p < 0.0001$ of univariate Cox regression analysis were carried out.

Generation of the Risk Prediction Model

The training dataset GSE31312 was used to establish the TME risk model. The R package "glmnet" was used for least absolute shrinkage and selection operator (LASSO) Cox regression analysis. A risk formula for predicting prognosis was established by LASSO Cox regression analysis. Then, we calculated the individualized risk score of each patient by dividing all patients into high-risk and low-risk groups using the median risk score as the cut-off value. Kaplan–Meier survival analysis and log-rank test were used to evaluate the difference in OS between the high- and low-risk groups. Time-dependent receiver operating characteristic (ROC) curves were plotted to evaluate prognostic value (13). The analysis was performed using SangerBox (http://sangerbox.com/Tool).

Univariate and Multivariate Cox Regression for IPI Components and the Seven-Gene Signature

To assess whether the risk prediction model could be used as an independent prognostic indicator for DLBCL patients, univariate and multivariate Cox regression analyses were performed with SPSS 26.

Construction and Validation of the Nomogram

A nomogram integrating IPI components and the seven-gene model was established based on the GSE31312 cohort to assess the probability of 1-, 3-, and 5-year individualized OS *via* the rms R package (https://cran.r-project.org/web/packages/rms/). In addition, the discriminatory ability of the nomogram was graphically evaluated using a calibration map.

CIBERSORT and Tumor-Infiltrating Immune Cell Profile

We used the CIBERSORT computational method to estimate the abundance distribution of TICs in GSE31312. The abundance of 22 immune cells was detected by t-test to observe the differences among risk groups. All analyses were performed with R (version 3.6.3, https://www.r-project.org/).

RESULTS

Identification of Scores Associated With Survival and Clinical Features

The clinical information of DLBCL patients from the GSE31312, GSE10846, and GSE11318 datasets is summarized in **Table 1**. To determine the correlations of ImmuneScore, StromalScore, and ESTIMATEScore with clinical features of DLBCL, clinical data from the GSE31312 dataset were analyzed. As shown in **Figure 1A**, the high-scoring group had longer OS than the low-scoring group for ImmuneScore, StromalScore, and ESTIMATEScore. Significant differences in ImmuneScore, StromalScore, and ESTIMATEScore were found at different stages of DLBCL by Kruskal–Wallis rank sum test (**Figure 1B**). On average, stage IV ranked the lowest among all stages with respect to ImmuneScore, StromalScore, and ESTIMATEScore (**Figure 1B**). Moreover, the scores showed a negative correlation with IPI scores by Kruskal–Wallis rank sum test (**Figure 1C**). Taken together, these results show that the immune and stromal components of the TME are related to prognosis and progression of DLBCL.

TABLE 1 | The clinical characteristics of the DLBCL patients from GEO.

Characteristics	GSE31312 (N = 470)	GSE10846 (N = 414)	GSE11318 (N = 200)
Age			
<=60	200 (42.55)	188 (45.41)	69 (34.5)
>60	270 (57.45)	226 (54.59)	94 (47)
NA			37 (18.5)
Gender			
Male	271 (57.66)	224 (54.11)	110 (55)
Female	199 (42.34)	172 (41.55)	90 (45)
NA		18 (4.34)	
Subtype			
GCB	227 (48.30)	183 (44.20)	70 (35)
ABC	199 (42.34)	167 (40.34)	73 (36.5)
NA	44 (9.36)	64 (15.46)	57 (28.5)
Stage			
I–II	220 (46.81)	189 (45.65)	75 (37.5)
IIII–IV	229 (48.72)	217 (52.42)	87 (43.5)
NA	21 (4.47)	8 (1.93)	38 (19)
ECOG			
<2	374 (79.57)	296 (71.50)	122 (61)
≥2	96 (20.43)	93 (22.46)	39 (19.5)
NA		25 (6.04)	39 (19.5)
LDH			
Normal	148 (31.50)	173 (41.78)	69 (34.5)
Elevated	278 (59.14)	178 (43.00)	78 (39)
NA	44 (9.36)	63 (15.22)	53 (26.5)
Extranodal sites			
<2	194 (41.28)	238 (57.49)	NA
≥2	276 (58.72)	145 (35.02)	
NA		31 (7.49)	
IPI score			
<2	169 (35.96)	NA	NA
≥2	255 (54.25)		
NA	46 (9.79)		

DEGs AND ENRICHMENT ANALYSIS

To gain insight into the role of the TME in DLBCL, we divided patients into high-scoring and low-scoring groups according to the median ImmuneScore (StromalScore). The number of patients in the high ImmuneScore group who also had a high StromalScore group was 147, and the number of patients in the low ImmuneScore group who also had a low StromalScore group was also 147. Therefore, 294 patients had consistent ImmuneScore and StromalScore subgroups, representing 62.5% of all patients (**Supplementary Table S1**). We next investigated the changes in immune (or stromal) score-related DEGs between high-scoring and low-scoring samples. A total of 865 ImmuneScore-related DEGs were identified among which 836 genes were upregulated and 29 genes were downregulated (**Figure 2A**). Similarly, there were 597 StromalScore-related DEGs, including 569 upregulated and 28 downregulated genes (**Figure 2A**). A Venn diagram was used to depict the co-up/

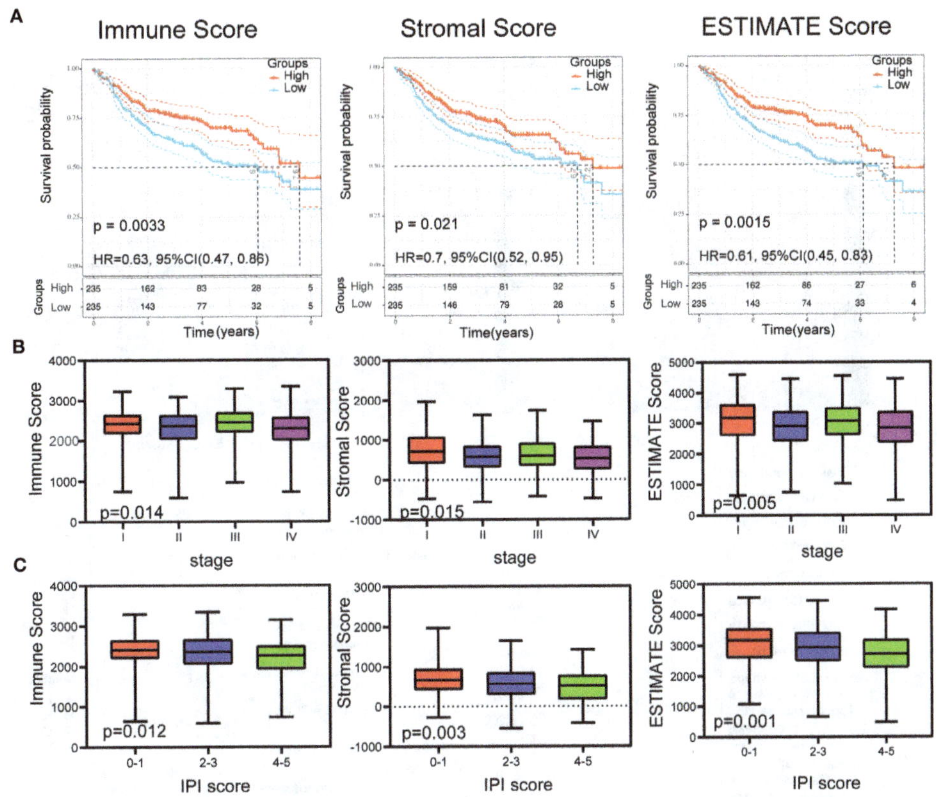

FIGURE 1 | Relationship of scores with the survival and important clinical factor of patients with DLBCL. **(A)** Kaplan–Meier analysis for DLBCL patients grouped by ImmuneScores, StromalScores and ESTIMATEScore, and the differences between the two curves were determined by the logrank test. **(B)** The distribution of ImmuneScores, StromalScores and ESTIMATEScore in stages using Kruskal–Wallis rank sum test. **(C)** The distribution of ImmuneScores, StromalScores and ESTIMATEScore in IPI scores using Kruskal–Wallis rank sum test.

downregulated genes associated with the different score groups (N = 183, **Figure 2B**, **Supplementary Table S2**). Enrichment analyses showed that these DEGs were related to immune-related GO terms, including immune response and informatory response (**Figure 2C**, **Supplementary Table S3**). KEGG pathway analyses also indicated that the genes were mainly involved in cytokine-cytokine receptor interaction pathways (**Figure 2D**, **Supplementary Table S3**).

Sharing of PPI Network and Univariate Cox Regression

A total of 183 DEGs were used to construct the PPI network, which is shown in **Figure 3A**. Univariate Cox regression was performed on 183 genes, and the genes with p <0.0001 were selected (**Figure 3B**). Then, intersection analysis was performed between the degree of the nodes ≥3 in the PPI and p <0.0001, resulting in 18 overlapping genes (**Figure 3C**).

Construction of a Risk Prediction Model Based on the TME

According to the characteristics of variable selection and regularization, LASSO Cox regression was used to determine the optimal weight coefficient for the prognostic TME-related genes. Using one standard error of the best penalty parameter λ value and 1,000-fold cross-validation (**Figure 4A**), we obtained a seven-gene prognostic signature from the 18 genes identified above (**Figure 4B**). The left line indicated the optimal values by λ.min criteria (**Figure 4B**). Then, coefficient values were extracted, and the coefficients of the seven genes were multiplied by their mRNA expression levels to calculate individual risk scores using the following formula: Risk score = the mRNA expression level of *CSF3R** (−0.06993781) + the mRNA expression level of *QKI** (−0.76400334) + the mRNA expression level of *LAMP2** (−2.14079252) + the mRNA expression level of *TIMP2** (−0.98332426) + the mRNA expression level of *LCP2** (−1.23980147) + the mRNA expression level of *AAK1** (−0.46856491) + the mRNA expression level of *ITGAM** (−0.20720812). Patients from the training group were divided into high-risk and low-risk groups based on the median risk score. The distributions of risk scores, survival status, and expression levels in the training set are presented in **Figure 4C**. Time-dependent ROC curve analysis showed that during 1-, 3-, and 5-year follow-up, the area under the curve (AUC) values were 0.71, 0.68, and 0.67 (**Figure 4D**). Survival analysis showed that patients in the high-risk group had significantly shorter median OS

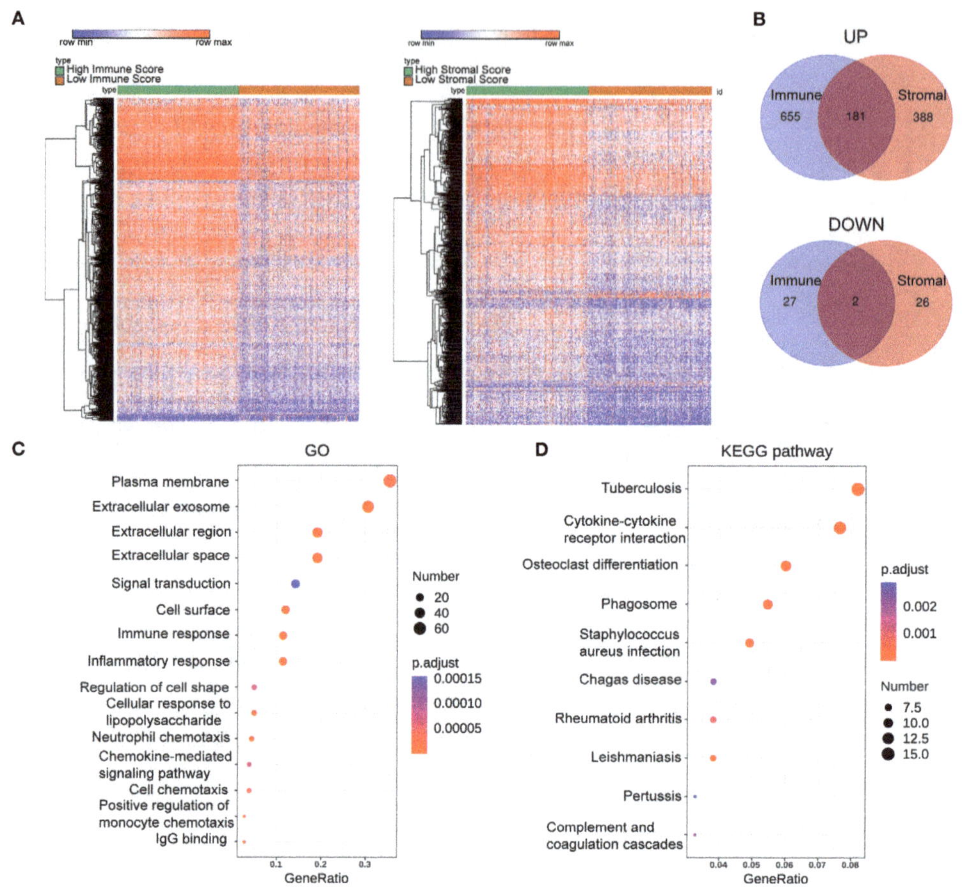

FIGURE 2 | Heatmaps, Venn plots, and enrichment analysis. **(A)** The DEGs heatmaps are obtained by comparing the high score group and the low group in Immunescores and Stromalscores. **(B)** Venn diagram shows that there are 181 co-up-regulated gene and 2 co-down-regulated genes. **(C, D):** GO **(C)** and KEGG **(D)** analysis for 183 TME-related DEGs. number: Number of genes enriched. GO, Gene Ontology; KEGG, Kyoto Encyclopedia of Genes and Genomes.

compared with the low-risk group (hazard ratio (HR) = 4.63; 95% confidence interval (CI) = 2.85–7.54; $p < 0.0001$; **Figure 4E**).

Internal Validation of our Signature in GSE31312 Cohort

To verify the robustness of the seven-gene prognostic signature, we used the signature to calculate individual risk scores and divided patients from the GSE31312 cohort into high-risk and low-risk groups using the same cutoff value determined in the training set. The distributions of risk scores, survival status, and expression levels were consistent with those obtained in the training set (**Supplementary Figure S1A**). The verification results demonstrated that the AUC values were 0.71, 0.68, and 0.61 during 1-, 3-, and 5-year follow-up, respectively (**Supplementary Figure S1B**). The prognosis of the low-risk group was significantly better than that of the high-risk group (HR = 4.1; 95% CI = 2.3–7.33; $p = 0.001$; **Supplementary Figure S1C**). Finally, we also applied the seven-gene signature to all GSE31312 samples and found that the relationships between the distributions of risk scores, survival status, and expression levels were again consistent with those obtained in the training set (**Supplementary Figure S2A**). Time-dependent ROC curve analysis showed that in predicting 1-, 3-, and 5-year OS, the AUC values were 0.71, 0.68, and 0.65, respectively, indicating an acceptable degree of distinction (**Supplementary Figure S2B**). Similarly, the prognosis of the low-risk group was significantly better than that of the high-risk group (HR = 4.45; 95% CI = 3.07–6.47; $p < 0.0001$; **Supplementary Figure S2C**). Thus, the model effectively provided prognostic classifications within the GSE31312 dataset.

External Validation of our Signature in GSE10846 and GSE11318 Cohorts

The seven-gene prognostic signature was validated in the GSE10846 and GSE11318 datasets. The results are presented in **Figure 5** as Kaplan–Meier curves. Consistent with the above findings, there were significant differences in survival outcomes among different risk groups in both GSE10846 (HR = 1.96; 95% CI = 1.42–2.7; $p < 0.0001$; **Supplementary Figure S1D**) and GSE11318 (HR = 1.66; 95% CI = 1.14–2.42; $p = 0.008$; **Supplementary Figure S1E**). Thus, the signature was predictive in both internal and external datasets.

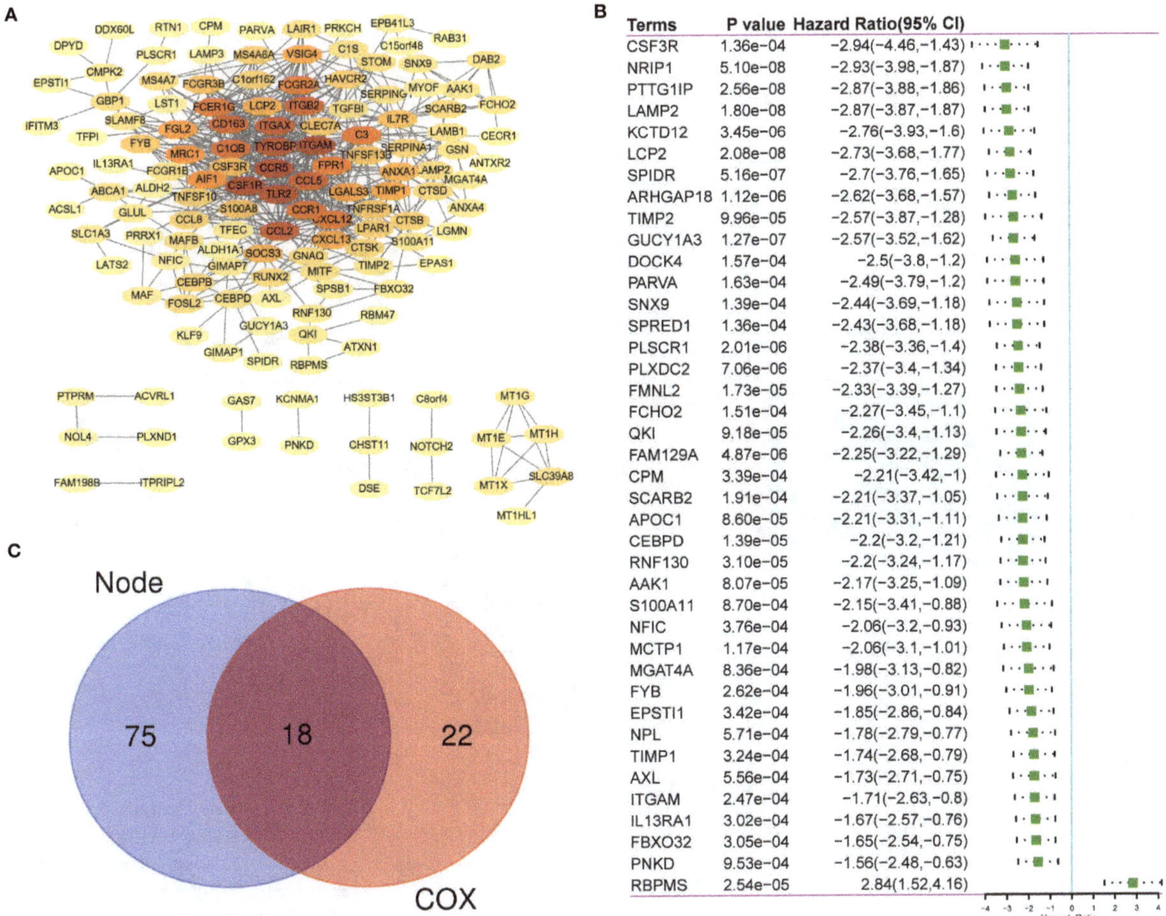

FIGURE 3 | The sharing of PPI Network and Univariate COX Regression. **(A)** 183 TME-related DEGs were used to construct PPI network. **(B)** 183 DEGs was analyzed by univariate cox analysis, selecting the top significant factors with $p < 0.0001$. **(C)** 18 factors of overlap are obtained by venn map. PPI, Protein–protein interaction network.

Validation of the Seven-Gene Signature Using Clinical Parameters and Patient Outcomes

To further understand the relationship between the seven-gene signature and other clinical data, including pathologic subtype, clinical stage, and IPI score, we performed survival analysis using clinical parameters. The results demonstrated that low-risk patients had significantly favorable OS compared to high-risk patients with the activated B-cell-like (ABC) subtype of DLBCL ($p = 0.0014$; HR = 2.04; 95% CI = 1.31–3.19; **Figure 5A**). Similar results were obtained in germinal center B-cell-like (GCB) patients ($p < 0.0001$; HR = 2.85; 95% CI = 1.7–4.48; **Figure 5B**). An analogous result was also obtained in patients at different stages; the low-risk group had a favorable prognosis compared with the high-risk group (**Figures 5C, D**). Moreover, patients in the low-risk group had significantly favorable OS compared with high-risk patients in both the IPI<2 group and the IPI≥2 group (**Figures 5E, F**). These results demonstrate the independent predictive ability of our signature in clinical applications.

Univariate and Multivariate Cox Regression for IPI Components and the Risk Prediction Model

To evaluate whether the risk prediction model could be used as an independent prognostic index for DLBCL patients, analyses were performed to identify the factors affecting the prognosis of DLBCL patients. These analyses were performed only on the datasets that included clinical IPI components data (GSE31312 and GSE10846), and the results showed that the seven-gene signature was an independent prognostic factor in these datasets (**Table 2**).

Construction and Validation of the Nomogram

A nomogram was established to forecast 1-, 3-, and 5-year survival based on IPI components and the seven-gene model (**Figure 6A**). The nomogram demonstrated that high total points predicted worse survival. The calibration chart showed an acceptable agreement between the predicted survival rate and

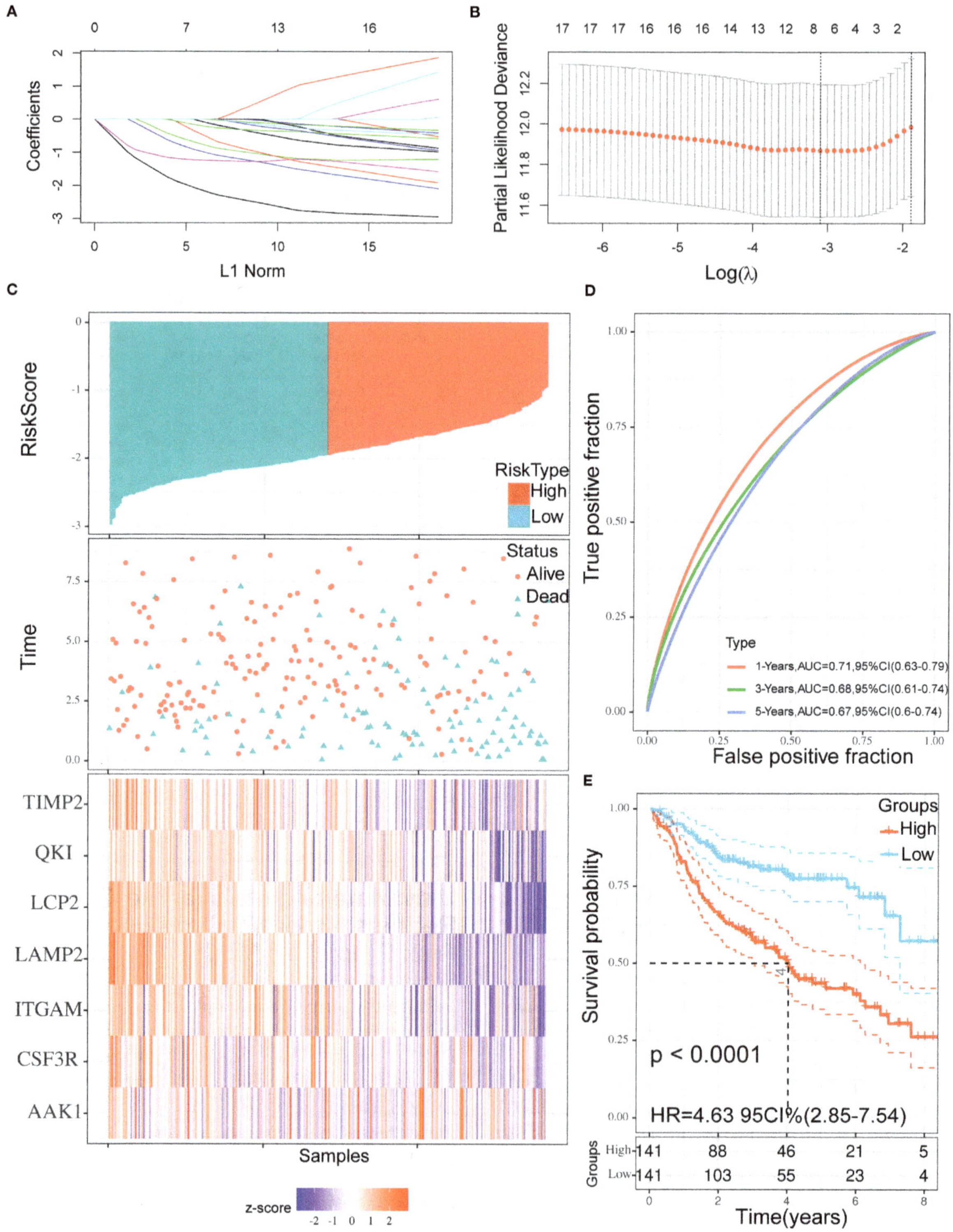

FIGURE 4 | Construction of the prognostic signature. **(A, B)** Using 18 genes to perform a LASSO COX regression **(A)** and obtaining the seven-gene prognostic signature **(B)**. **(C)** The distribution of risk scores, the survival status of patients, and expression levels in training set were presented. **(D)** The time-dependent ROC curve and AUC of the signature. **(E)** Kaplan–Meier plots of overall survival between high- *vs* low-risk groups in training set by the logrank test. LASSO, Least absolute shrinkage and selection operator; ROC, Receiver operating characteristic curve; AUC, Area under curve.

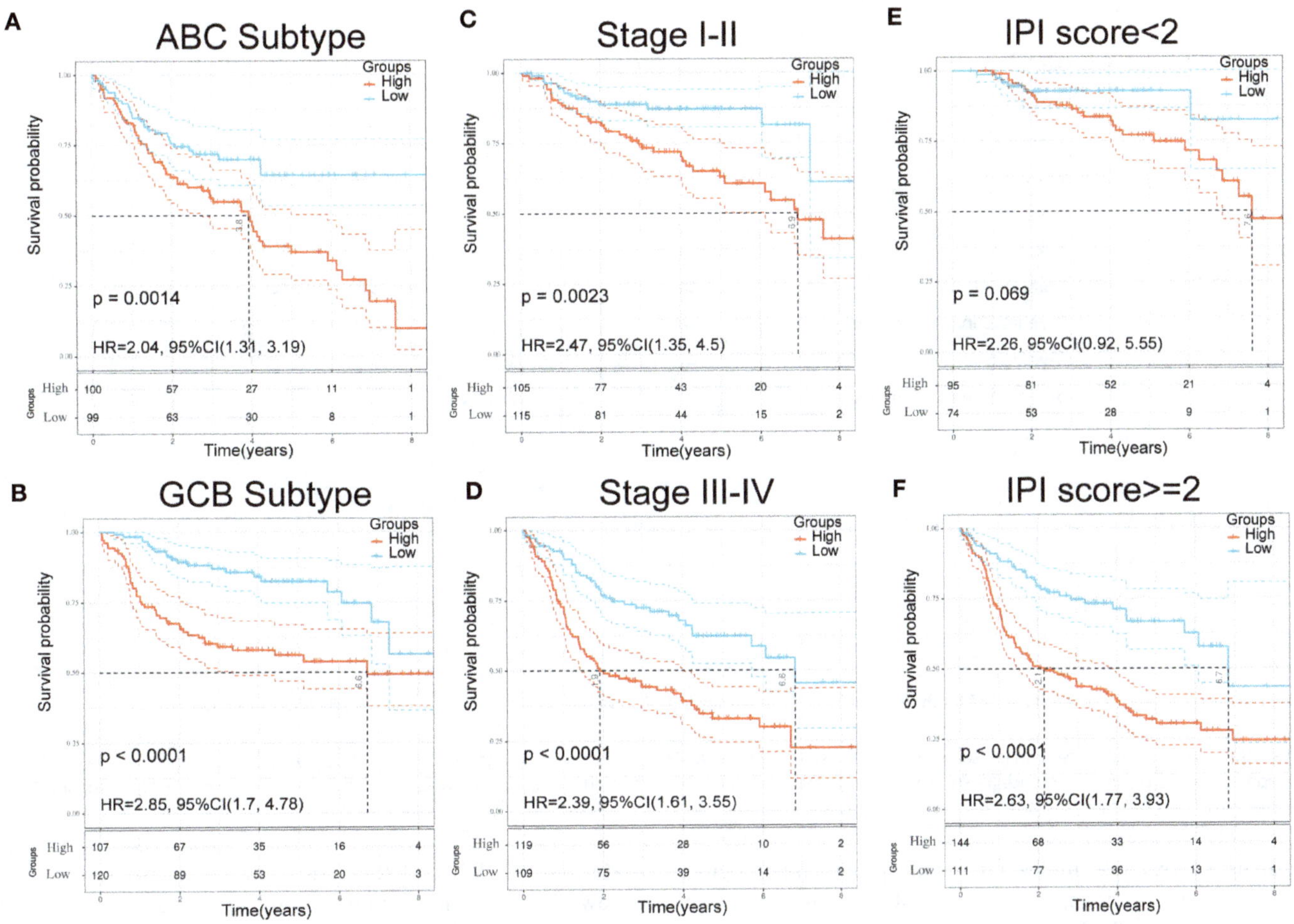

FIGURE 5 | Validation of seven-gene signature in significant clinical subgroups. **(A, B)** Kaplan–Meier plots of overall survival between high and low risk groups in ABC subtype **(A)** and GCB subtype **(B)** by the logrank test. **(C, D):** Kaplan–Meier plots of overall survival between high- and low-risk groups in stages I–II **(C)** and III–IV **(D)** by the logrank test. **(E, F)** Kaplan–Meier plots of overall survival between high- and low-risk groups in IPI<2 **(E)** and IPI≥2 **(F)** by the logrank test.

TABLE 2 | Univariable and multivariable Cox regression analysis in DLBCL.

Variable	Univariate analysis			Multivariate analysis		
	HR	95% CI	P value	HR	95% CI	P value
GSE31312						
Our signature	2.603	1.878–3.608	0.000	2.954	2.058–4.24	0.000
Age (>60 vs. <=60 years)	1.849	1.336–2.56	0.000	1.871	1.319–2.655	0.000
ECOG (>=2 vs. <2)	2.036	1.46–2.84	0.000	1.617	1.107–2.363	0.013
Stage (III/IV vs. I/II)	2.337	1.687–3.237	0.000	2.08	1.406–3.077	0.000
LDH (Elevated vs. Normal)	2.129	1.452–3.121	0.000	1.496	1.003–2.231	0.048
Extranodal sites (>=2 vs. <2)	2.202	1.596–3.037	0.000	1.519	1.053–2.192	0.025
GSE10846						
Our signature	1.957	1.42–2.698	0.000	2.275	1.559–3.32	0.000
Age (>60 vs. <=60 years)	2.209	1.59–3.069	0.000	2.292	1.587–3.309	0.000
ECOG (>=2 vs. <2)	2.835	2.049–3.921	0.000	2.082	1.413–3.067	0.000
Stage (III/IV vs. I/II)	1.834	1.326–2.537	0.000	1.481	1.022–2.147	0.038
LDH (Elevated vs. Normal)	2.67	1.87–3.812	0.000	1.836	1.244–2.711	0.002
Extranodal sites (>=2 vs. <2)	1.927	1.144–3.246	0.014	1.095	0.575–2.085	0.782

CI, confidence interval; HR, hazard ratio.

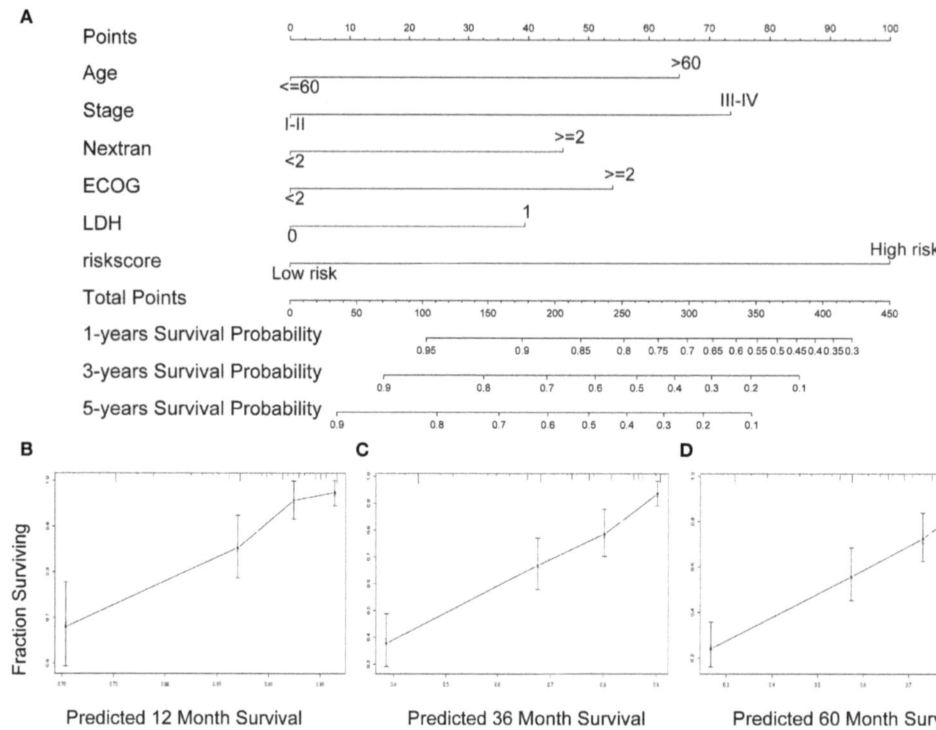

FIGURE 6 | A nomogram Based on the seven-gene prognostic signature. **(A)** Construction of a nomogram to forecast 12-, 36-, and 60-month survival by the IPI components & the seven-gene model. **(B–D)** The calibration chart shows that the predicted survival rate is consistent with the actual survival rate for 12 months **(B)**, 36 months **(C)**, and 60 months **(D)**. IPI, International Prognostic Index.

the actual survival rate, indicating that our proposed nomogram has stability in predicting DLBCL patient prognosis in clinical practice (**Figures 6B–D**).

Immune-Infiltrating Cells and GSEA in Different Groups

In order to further verify the relationship between TME and DLBCL, we used CIBERSORT to analyze the proportions of 22 immune-infiltrating cells in GSE31312 samples between different risk groups. **Figure 7A** shows the compositions of immune cells in 470 patients, and **Figure 7B** shows the differences in the proportion of each immune cell type between the high-risk and low-risk groups. The results showed that 12 types of immune-infiltrating cells were correlated with the risk group. Specifically, the proportions of naïve B cells, memory B cells, regulatory T cells, resting natural killer (NK) cells, and monocytes were significantly higher in the high-risk group compared with the low-risk group, whereas the proportions of CD8+ T cells, activated CD4+ memory T cells, gamma delta T cells, activated NK cells, M1 macrophages, M2 macrophages, and neutrophils were significantly lower (**Figure 7B**). These results further confirmed that the prognostic signature was related to the immune activity of the TME. GSEA was used to probe the potential mechanism for the two risk groups to identify the enriched KEGG pathway. Two immune-related pathways were enriched in the low-risk group: intestinal immune network for IgA production and primary immunodeficiency diseases (**Figures 7C, D**), and the rest of the enrichment results are shown in the **Supplementary Figure S1**. The immune pathway of the intestinal immune network for IgA production is associated with central deficits in the pathogenesis of the disease (14). Primary immunodeficiency is a pathway associated with primary immunodeficiency (15). These results suggest that the prognosis of DLBCL may be closely related to immune regulation in the TME.

DISCUSSION

DLBCL is characterized by a heterogeneous tumor entity with variable therapeutic outcomes. Risk stratification and prognosis of DLBCL patients remain challenges for clinicians and researchers (1, 16). In the rituximab era, IPI, R-IPI, and NCCN-IPI risk scores are calculated using easily obtained clinical features that are part of standard diagnostic procedures. However, all three scoring systems fail to identify a very high-risk group with long-term OS clearly below 50% (10). Moreover, the progression of a tumor is affected not only by its intrinsic characteristics but also by the extrinsic TME. Immune system accumulation and immune cell infiltration could have a profound impact on carcinogenesis and prognosis (17). There is also increasing evidence that the microenvironment has an important role in predicting tumor progression and prognosis (17, 18). Consequently, screening for a gene prognostic signature

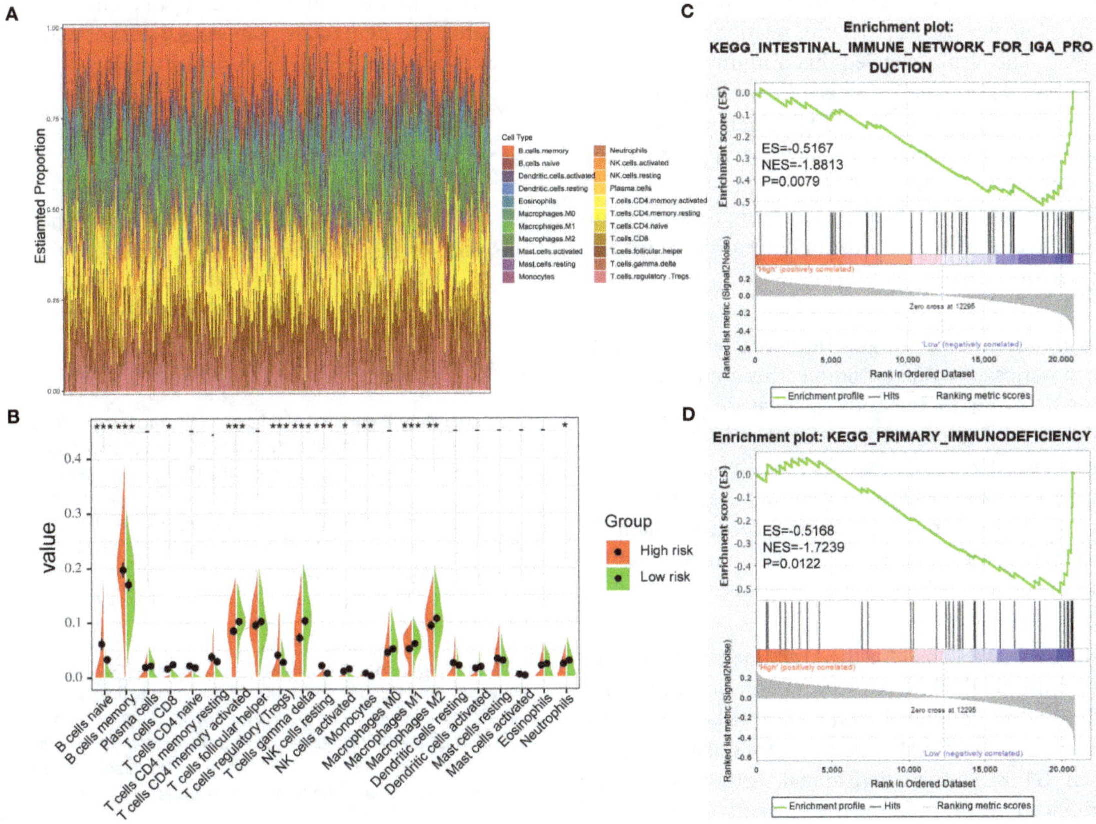

FIGURE 7 | Immune-Infiltrating Cells and GSEA in Difference of Groups. **(A)** The landscape of immune cell infiltration of DLBCL patients in GSE31312. **(B)** the difference of 22 immune-infiltrating cells in GSE31312 samples among risk groups. **(C, D)** GSEA was performed between high-risk and low-risk groups based on the seven-gene signature. (*p < 0.05; **p < 0.01; ***p < 0.001).

that adequately reflects the TME would be of great significance for individualized prevention and treatment of DLBCL patients (16, 19). In this study, we established seven prognostic gene markers which robustly and reliably predicted an individualized immune prognostic model for DLBCL patients on the basis of immune genes. The seven-gene prognostic signature was combined with IPI components to build a composite prognostic nomogram, which was capable of accurate prediction and showed positive net benefit in DLBCL.

The seven genes in our signature were *TIMP2*, *QKI*, *LCP2*, *LAMP2*, *ITGAM*, *CSF3R*, and *AAK1*. Although these genes are differentially expressed in immune cells or stromal cells, the expression of these genes in normal germinal center B cells and in a subset of DLBCL is uncertain, and our sequencing data comes from tumor tissues, so we cannot distinguish whether the expression level is caused by stromal or tumor components. High expression of *TIMP2* has been reported to inhibit matrix metalloproteinases to produce anti-tumor activity (20). *TIMP2* was also demonstrated to interact with multiple integrin pathways and is involved in angiogenesis in gastric cancer (21). *LCP2* encodes a protein of 533 amino acids that participates in T cell activation and increases the activity of the *IL-2* gene promoter through its transient overexpression (22). High expression of *LCP2* is associated with better outcomes in DLBCL patients (17, 18). *CSF3R* is closely related to prognosis of patients with chronic neutrophilic leukemia or atypical chronic myeloid leukemia and thus represents a potentially useful criterion for disease diagnosis (23). *QKI* gene encodes an RNA-binding protein that regulates the functions of diverse mRNAs, which play critical parts in tumorigenesis through inactivation of tumor suppressor genes in multiple tumors (24, 25). *LAMP2* is essential for maintaining the structural integrity of the lysosomal compartment and relocalizes to the cell surface of some highly metastatic tumor cells. *LAMP2* has been functionally validated as an essential mediator of drug resistance and tumor recurrence in hematological diseases (26–28). *ITGAM* and *AAK1* have not been previously reported to be related to cancer, and our study is the first to suggest that they could be used as new prognostic markers of DLBCL. Furthermore, the GSEA results showed that enrichment of the seven-gene signature was significantly correlated with immune-related signaling pathways, indicating that this model has potential clinical applications in predicting survival outcomes of patients.

Zamani-Ahmadmahmudi et al. constructed an independent seven-gene prognostic signature that could distinguish low-risk patients with DLBCL from high-risk ones (29). In our study, we not only constructed a risk prediction model for the prognosis of DLBCL patients, but we also explore the relationship between TME and DLBCL. The results showed that immune and stromal components in the TME were negatively correlated with the prognosis of DLBCL patients. Our TME-related seven-gene prognostic signature was shown to have strong predictive power and to represent an independent prognostic factor. In the era of immune targeting, distinguishing high-risk patients from the perspective of TME can inform clinical decisions and lead to better outcomes.

Although our TME-based prognostic model was shown to predict tumor prognosis in a large sample, this study had some limitations. First, owing to the retrospective design and the unavailability of control group samples in the GEO databases, the results were biased to some extent. Thus, a well-designed, prospective, international, multicenter clinical trial is needed to verify our findings in the future. In addition, further functional research is warranted to explore the molecular functions of the identified immune genes during DLBCL progression.

In conclusion, we established for the first time a TME-related prognostic signature in DLBCL patients, which is a promising prognostic model when combined with clinical IPI components. The results presented here not only help to clarify immune responses in the DLBCL microenvironment but also indicate new clinical applications for immune therapy and individualized therapy in patients with DLBCL.

AUTHOR CONTRIBUTIONS

HZ and LX conceived and designed the study and reviewed the manuscript. TP and YH collected, arranged, and analyzed the data and wrote the manuscript. HC, YL, RZ, and JX revised the statistical methodology. JP, SC, YZ, and LQ designed and prepared the figures and tables. All authors contributed to the article and approved the submitted version.

ACKNOWLEDGMENTS

We would like to thank Yongzi Xie from The Third Xiangya Hospital for his valuable lessons in writing.

SUPPLEMENTARY MATERIAL

Supplementary Figure 1 | Validation of the prognostic signature. **(A)** The distribution of risk scores, the survival status of patients, and expression levels in internal validation set were presented. **(B)** The time-dependent ROC curve and AUC in internal validation set. **(C)** Kaplan-Meier plots of overall survival between high- *vs* low-risk internal validation groups by the logrank test. **(D)** Kaplan–Meier plots of overall survival between high- and low-risk groups in GSE10846 by the logrank test. **(E)** Kaplan–Meier plots of overall survival between high- and low-risk groups in GSE11318 by the logrank test. ROC, receiver operating characteristic curve; AUC, area under curve.

Supplementary Figure 2 | Validation of the prognostic signature in all GSE31312 tumor samples. **(A)** The distribution of risk scores, the survival status of patients, and expression levels were presented. **(B)** The time-dependent ROC curve and AUC in all GSE31312 patients. **(C)** Kaplan–Meier plots of overall survival between high- and low-risk groups in GSE31312 by the logrank test. ROC, receiver operating characteristic curve; AUC, area under curve.

Supplementary Table 1 | ImmuneScores, StromalScores, and ESTIMATEScore.

Supplementary Table 2 | The list of 183 DEGs.

Supplementary Table 3 | The results of the gene enrichment analysis.

Supplementary Picture 1 | GSEA enrichment results.

REFERENCES

1. Miao Y, Medeiros LJ, Li Y, Li J, Young KH. Genetic alterations and their clinical implications in DLBCL. *Nat Rev Clin Oncol* (2019) 16(10):634–52. doi: 10.1038/s41571-019-0225-1
2. Mulder TA, Wahlin BE, Österborg A, Palma M. Targeting the immune microenvironment in lymphomas of B-cell origin: from biology to clinical application. *Cancers* (2019) 11(7):915–46. doi: 10.3390/cancers11070915
3. Höpken UE, Rehm A. Targeting the tumor microenvironment of leukemia and lymphoma. *Trends Cancer* (2019) 5(6):351–64. doi: 10.1016/j.trecan.2019.05.001
4. Leone RD, Powell JD. Metabolism of immune cells in cancer. *Nat Rev Cancer* (2020) 20(9):516–31. doi: 10.1038/s41568-020-0273-y
5. Angell H, Galon J. From the immune contexture to the Immunoscore: the role of prognostic and predictive immune markers in cancer. *Curr Opin Immunol* (2013) 25(2):261–7. doi: 10.1016/j.coi.2013.03.004
6. Dong H, Strome SE, Salomao DR, Tamura H, Hirano F, Flies DB, et al. Tumor-associated B7-H1 promotes T-cell apoptosis: a potential mechanism of immune evasion. *Nat Med* (2002) 8(8):793–800. doi: 10.1038/nm730
7. Wang T, Niu G, Kortylewski M, Burdelya L, Shain K, Zhang S, et al. Regulation of the innate and adaptive immune responses by Stat-3 signaling in tumor cells. *Nat Med* (2004) 10(1):48–54. doi: 10.1038/nm976
8. Binnewies M, Roberts EW, Kersten K, Chan V, Fearon DF, Merad M, et al. Understanding the tumor immune microenvironment (TIME) for effective therapy. *Nat Med* (2018) 24(5):541–50. doi: 10.1038/s41591-018-0014-x
9. Tamma R, Ranieri G, Ingravallo G, Annese T, Oranger A, Gaudio F, et al. Inflammatory cells in diffuse large B cell lymphoma. *J Clin Med* (2020) 9 (8):2418–35. doi: 10.3390/jcm9082418
10. Ruppert AS, Dixon JG, Salles G, Wall A, Cunningham D, Poeschel V, et al. International prognostic indices in diffuse large B-cell lymphoma: a comparison of IPI, R-IPI, and NCCN-IPI. *Blood* (2020) 135(23):2041–8. doi: 10.1182/blood.2019002729
11. Yoshihara K, Shahmoradgoli M, Martínez E, Vegesna R, Kim H, Torres-Garcia W, et al. Inferring tumour purity and stromal and immune cell admixture from expression data. *Nat Commun* (2013) 4:2612. doi: 10.1038/ncomms3612

12. Bi K-W, Wei X-G, Qin X-X, Li B. BTK has potential to be a prognostic factor for lung adenocarcinoma and an indicator for tumor microenvironment remodeling: a study based on TCGA data mining. *Front Oncol* (2020) 10:424:424. doi: 10.3389/fonc.2020.00424
13. Heagerty PJ, Lumley T, Pepe MS. Time-dependent ROC curves for censored survival data and a diagnostic marker. *Biometrics* (2000) 56(2):337–44. doi: 10.1111/j.0006-341x.2000.00337.x
14. Kiryluk K, Li Y, Scolari F, Sanna-Cherchi S, Choi M, Verbitsky M, et al. Discovery of new risk loci for IgA nephropathy implicates genes involved in immunity against intestinal pathogens. *Nat Genet* (2014) 46(11):1187–96. doi: 10.1038/ng.3118
15. Amaya-Uribe L, Rojas M, Azizi G, Anaya J-M, Gershwin ME. Primary immunodeficiency and autoimmunity: a comprehensive review. *J Autoimmun* (2019) 99:52–72. doi: 10.1016/j.jaut.2019.01.011
16. Schmitz R, Wright GW, Huang DW, Johnson CA, Phelan JD, Wang JQ, et al. Genetics and pathogenesis of diffuse large B-cell lymphoma. *N Engl J Med* (2018) 378(15):1396–407. doi: 10.1056/NEJMoa1801445
17. Ohtani H, Jin Z, Takegawa S, Nakayama T, Yoshie O. Abundant expression of CXCL9 (MIG) by stromal cells that include dendritic cells and accumulation of CXCR3+ T cells in lymphocyte-rich gastric carcinoma. *J Pathol* (2009) 217 (1):21–31. doi: 10.1002/path.2448
18. Thompson ED, Zahurak M, Murphy A, Cornish T, Cuka N, Abdelfatah E, et al. Patterns of PD-L1 expression and CD8 T cell infiltration in gastric adenocarcinomas and associated immune stroma. *Gut* (2017) 66(5):794–801. doi: 10.1136/gutjnl-2015-310839
19. Reddy A, Zhang J, Davis NS, Moffitt AB, Love CL, Waldrop A, et al. Genetic and functional drivers of diffuse large B cell lymphoma. *Cell* (2017) 171 (2):481–494.e15. doi: 10.1016/j.cell.2017.09.027
20. Peeney D, Fan Y, Nguyen T, Meerzaman D, Stetler-Stevenson WG. Matrisome-associated gene expression patterns correlating with TIMP2 in cancer. *Sci Rep* (2019) 9(1):20142. doi: 10.1038/s41598-019-56632-3
21. Wang W, Zhang Y, Liu M, Wang Y, Yang T, Li D, et al. TIMP2 is a poor prognostic factor and predicts metastatic biological behavior in gastric cancer. *Sci Rep* (2018) 8(1):9629. doi: 10.1038/s41598-018-27897-x
22. Sunden SL, Carr LL, Clements JL, Motto DG, Koretzky GA. Polymorphism in and localization of the gene LCP2 (SLP-76) to chromosome 5q33.1-qter. *Genomics* (1996) 35(1):269–70. doi: 10.1006/geno.1996.0354
23. Maxson JE, Gotlib J, Pollyea DA, Fleischman AG, Agarwal A, Eide CA, et al. Oncogenic CSF3R mutations in chronic neutrophilic leukemia and atypical CML. *N Engl J Med* (2013) 368(19):1781–90. doi: 10.1056/NEJMoa1214514
24. Mo HY, Jo YS, Yoo NJ, Kim MS, Song SY, Lee SH. Frameshift mutation of candidate tumor suppressor genes QK1 and TMEFF2 in gastric and colorectal cancers. *Cancer Biomark* (2019) 24(1):1–6. doi: 10.3233/CBM-160559
25. Schaid DJ, McDonnell SK, FitzGerald LM, DeRycke L, Fogarty Z, Giles GG, et al. Two-stage Study of familial prostate cancer by whole-exome sequencing and custom capture identifies 10 novel genes associated with the risk of prostate cancer. *Eur Urol* (2020) S0302-2838(20)30614-X. doi: 10.1016/j.eururo.2020.07.038
26. Damaghi M, Tafreshi NK, Lloyd MC, Sprung R, Estrella V, Wojtkowiak JW, et al. Chronic acidosis in the tumour microenvironment selects for overexpression of LAMP2 in the plasma membrane. *Nat Commun* (2015) 6:8752. doi: 10.1038/ncomms9752
27. Huang P-S, Lin Y-H, Chi H-C, Tseng Y-H, Chen CY, Lin T-K, et al. Dysregulated FAM215A stimulates LAMP2 expression to confer drug-resistant and malignant in human liver cancer. *Cells* (2020) 9(4):961–83. doi: 10.3390/cells9040961
28. Robert G, Auberger P. Azacitidine resistance caused by LAMP2 deficiency: a therapeutic window for the use of autophagy inhibitors in MDS/AML patients? *Autophagy* (2019) 15(5):927–9. doi: 10.1080/15548627.2019.1586259
29. Zamani-Ahmadmahmudi M, Nassiri SM. Development of a reproducible prognostic gene signature to predict the clinical outcome in patients with diffuse large B-cell lymphoma. *Sci Rep* (2019) 9(1):12198. doi: 10.1038/s41598-019-48721-0

17

Neoantigens in Hematologic Malignancies

Melinda A. Biernacki[1,2]* and *Marie Bleakley*[1,3]

[1] Clinical Research Division, Fred Hutchinson Cancer Research Center, Seattle, WA, United States, [2] Department of Medicine, University of Washington, Seattle, WA, United States, [3] Department of Pediatrics, University of Washington, Seattle, WA, United States

***Correspondence:**
Melinda A. Biernacki
mbiernac@fredhutch.org

T cell cancer neoantigens are created from peptides derived from cancer-specific aberrant proteins, such as mutated and fusion proteins, presented in complex with human leukocyte antigens on the cancer cell surface. Because expression of the aberrant target protein is exclusive to malignant cells, immunotherapy directed against neoantigens should avoid "on-target, off-tumor" toxicity. The efficacy of neoantigen vaccines in melanoma and glioblastoma and of adoptive transfer of neoantigen-specific T cells in epithelial tumors indicates that neoantigens are valid therapeutic targets. Improvements in sequencing technology and innovations in antigen discovery approaches have facilitated the identification of neoantigens. In comparison to many solid tumors, hematologic malignancies have few mutations and thus fewer potential neoantigens. Despite this, neoantigens have been identified in a wide variety of hematologic malignancies. These include mutated nucleophosmin1 and PML-RARA in acute myeloid leukemia, ETV6-RUNX1 fusions and other mutated proteins in acute lymphoblastic leukemia, BCR-ABL1 fusions in chronic myeloid leukemia, driver mutations in myeloproliferative neoplasms, immunoglobulins in lymphomas, and proteins derived from patient-specific mutations in chronic lymphoid leukemias. We will review advances in the field of neoantigen discovery, describe the spectrum of identified neoantigens in hematologic malignancies, and discuss the potential of these neoantigens for clinical translation.

Keywords: neoantigen, hematologic malignancies, human leukocyte antigen, T cell receptor, immunotherapy, mutations, fusion proteins

INTRODUCTION

Neoantigens are composed of peptides derived from full-length aberrant cancer-specific proteins through a multi-step intracellular process that has been extensively reviewed (1–3) and presented in complex with human leukocyte antigen (HLA) molecules. This peptide-HLA complex is recognized by T cell receptors (TCRs). Non-viral neoantigens can be potentially be generated from any protein-coding mutations, fusion proteins, and cancer-specific splice isoforms (**Figure 1**), although not every aberrant protein will yield neoantigens. In the treatment of solid tumors, clinical successes have been seen with adoptive transfer of neoantigen-specific tumor-infiltrating lymphocytes (TIL) (4–7) and neoantigen vaccines (8–10), highlighting the importance of this class of antigens in effective anti-tumor immunity. T cell responses against neoantigens also appear to contribute to the efficacy of immune checkpoint blockade therapy (11, 12) and allogeneic hematopoietic cell transplantation (HCT) (13). Therapies targeting a neoantigen derived from an oncogenic driver

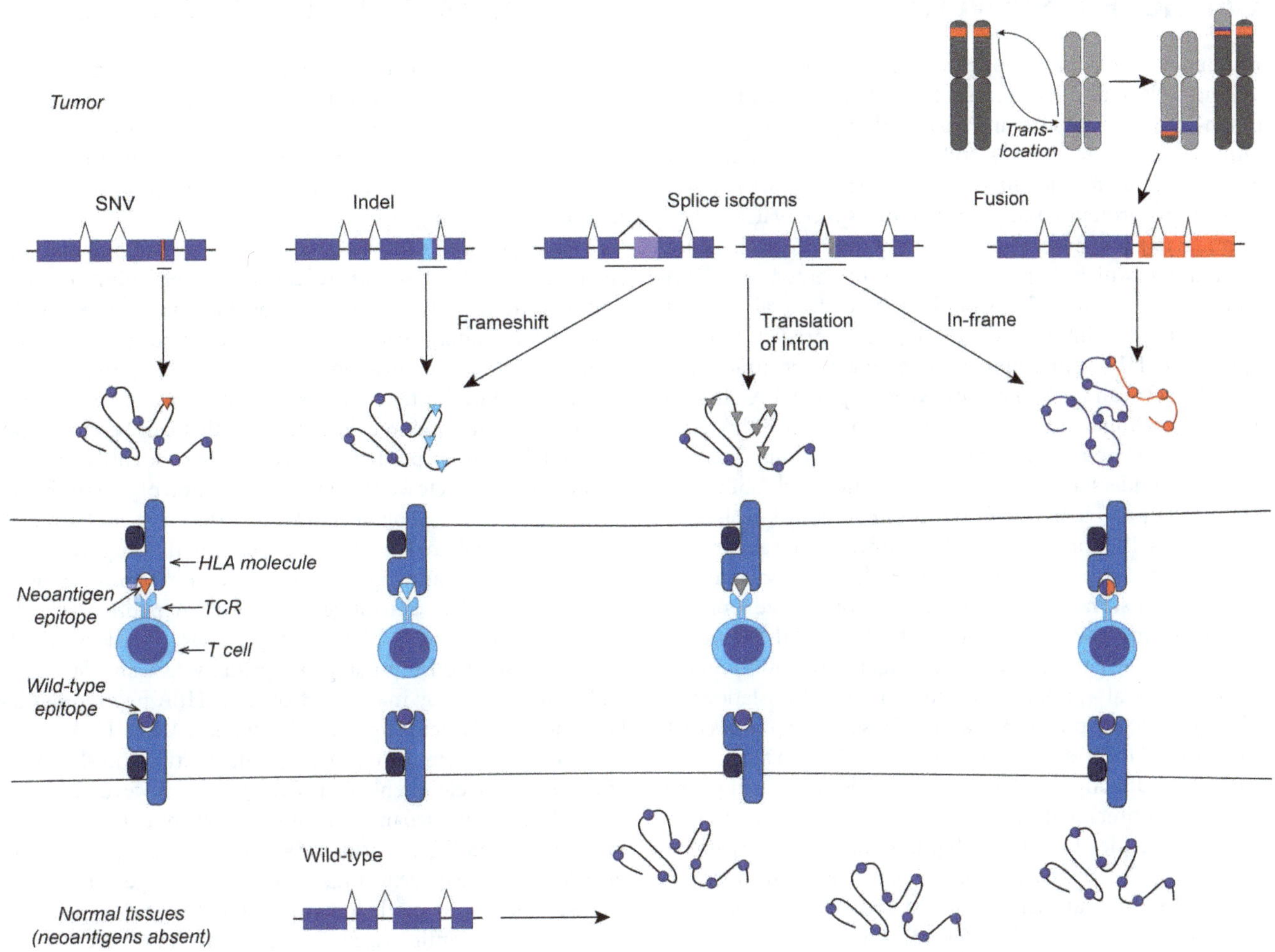

FIGURE 1 | Schematic representation of different classes of non-viral neoantigens. From left to right: Protein-coding single nucleotide variants (SNV) lead to neoantigens that differ from the wild-type antigen by a single amino acid that alters HLA and/or TCR binding. Frameshift insertion-deletion (indels) mutations result in a novel amino acid sequence downstream of the indel. Cancer-specific splice isoforms can lead to frameshifts, if the splice is out of frame, or, like genomic fusions, juxtapose two usually separate amino acid sequences, or produce entirely novel amino acid sequence from introns or other portions of the genome that are not normally translated.

in the founding clone could be curative, and tumor escape through loss of the target protein is unlikely when the neoantigen is from a protein critical for maintaining the malignant phenotype. As neoantigens are presented solely on malignant cells and not on healthy equivalents, the risk of "on-target, off-tumor" toxicity is minimized.

There are three major limitations to therapeutically targeting neoantigens in hematologic malignancies. First, most hematologic malignancies have relatively few protein-coding mutations and/or gene fusions, and thus fewer potential neoantigens than solid tumors, which may carry hundreds or even thousands of mutations in an individual patient (14). Second, therapies directed against any one neoantigen will apply only to the subset of patients who have both the mutation or fusion and restricting HLA allele, making neoantigens a less broadly applicable target than antigens from overexpressed wild-type proteins. However, in contrast to most solid tumors, many hematologic malignancies have recurrent mutations and/or fusions that are common within subgroups of patients and represent shared neoantigens. Finally, though targeting driver-derived neoantigens may prevent escape through loss of the target protein, other mechanism of escape from neoantigen-directed immunotherapy are possible, including downregulation or loss of HLA expression (15–24) or altered proteasomal processing of the epitope (25) by the malignant cell. However, the potential limitations of neoantigens as therapeutic targets are outweighed by their benefits: the high specificity for tumor and absent expression on normal cells; the ability to target intracellular as well as cell surface proteins; and, in some cases, the indispensable role of the aberrant protein in the malignant phenotype (26). Targeting a single high-quality neoantigen can be sufficient for disease control or even cure (4, 6, 7).

NEOANTIGEN DISCOVERY

Innovations in high-throughput genomic and transcriptomic sequencing techniques have greatly facilitated the identification of protein-coding mutations and fusions that produce potential neoantigens. However, there is still no reliable comprehensive *in silico* method for identifying immunogenic neoantigen epitopes from protein-coding mutations, splice variants, or other amino acid sequence-altering abnormalities. One challenge is determining which peptides will be presented on HLA molecules (27). *In silico* HLA-binding prediction algorithms [including but not limited to (28–36)] can predict binding of peptides to HLA molecules with reasonable accuracy and thereby identify candidate neoantigen epitopes. HLA-binding prediction algorithms are quite robust for prevalent HLA class I molecules, and active research by multiple groups has led to a greater understanding of and an improved ability to reliably predict peptide binding to uncommon class I molecules and most class II molecules (37–44). However, HLA-binding predictions do not specify whether the peptides are processed and presented on cell surfaces, although separate predictive tools for antigen processing have been developed (45–53). HLA-binding prediction from the parent amino acid sequence will additionally miss non-canonical epitopes (54), such as post-translationally modified or spliced peptides (55), and will also miss epitopes that are not predicted to bind HLA but actually do (56). An alternative approach is to directly determine the peptidome of malignant cells by immunoprecipitating HLA complexes and then to elute and identify peptides by tandem liquid chromatography–mass spectrometry (57–59). This unbiased approach can identify peptides as they are naturally presented on cells of interest but has significant technical hurdles (60–63). Modifications, such as the use of monoallelic cells (43, 60) should help to overcome some of these technical issues. Since predictive algorithms rely on datasets of peptides that are naturally processed and HLA-binding, improvements to direct identification of HLA ligands will in turn increase the reliability of predictive tools (64).

Determining which epitopes are immunogenic is also a challenge. Presentation of a peptide epitope on an HLA molecule is necessary but not sufficient for T cell recognition. Currently there are no reliable *in silico* tools to assess the immunogenicity of a neoantigen peptide, although this is an active area of research (65–70). There are three starting pools of cells in which one can assess the immunogenicity of a putative neoantigen: patient TIL or marrow-infiltrating lymphocytes (MIL), patient peripheral blood T cells, and healthy donor peripheral blood T cells after primary *in vitro* stimulation. The T cell repertoire of patients may be enriched for neoantigen-specific T cells (71, 72) due to antigen-induced expansion, but immunosuppressive tumor environments can render such T cells dysfunctional (73) or even absent (74). Finally, while neoantigen-specific T cells may exist in the repertoires of patients, unbiased methods to determine the cognate antigens of TCRs from their sequence are still in their infancy (23, 75). Stimulating healthy donor T cells with neoantigen-bearing antigen-presenting cells *in vitro* can be used to isolate reactive T cells without confounding T cell dysfunction (76, 77).

SHARED VS. PERSONAL NEOANTIGENS

Shared or public neoantigens derive from aberrant proteins that are present in all or a sizeable subset of patients with a given disease. In contrast, private or personal neoantigens are those that result from mutations, fusions, or other abnormal amino acid sequences that occur rarely in a disease or are idiosyncratic to an individual's malignancy.

Whole genome and whole exome sequencing of hematologic malignancies (78–85) has revealed the spectrum of fusions and mutations (also referred to as the mutanome) of these diseases, including events that range from rare to highly recurrent. Many of these genetic abnormalities may give rise to neoantigens. Mutanomes provide a rich source of cancer-specific aberrant amino acid sequences that can be interrogated with HLA-binding prediction algorithms to identify candidate neoantigens (70). However, with the exception of one study in the myeloproliferative neoplasms (MPNs) (85), the mutanomes of hematologic malignancies have not yet been thoroughly explored as sources of neoantigens. Another source of both public and personal candidate neoantigens is the HLA peptidome, which is the comprehensive library of peptides eluted from HLA molecules isolated from malignant primary cells and/or cell lines and characterized by mass spectrometry. HLA peptidomes have been defined in acute myeloid leukemia (AML) (57), chronic lymphocytic leukemia (CLL) (59, 86), multiple myeloma (87), and chronic myeloid leukemia (CML) (58). However, mutation-derived candidate neoantigen epitopes have only been identified in more focused HLA peptidome studies [for example, in a subset of AML (74, 88)], reflecting both the heterogeneity of these diseases and the currently limited sensitivity of this approach.

Personal neoantigens can arise from truly patient-specific gene mutations and fusions. In addition, some recurrently affected single genes and gene fusions are highly heterogenous across individuals and would be expected to yield semi-personal rather than shared neoantigens. For example, fusions involving the mixed lineage leukemia (MLL)/ histone-lysine N-methyltransferase 2A (KMT2A) gene in acute lymphoblastic leukemia (ALL) and AML produce diverse amino acid sequences among patients because the fusions may occur at multiple breakpoints in the MLL/KMT2A genes and with multiple (>100) partner genes (89, 90). Recurrently mutated gene in hematologic malignancies that are likely to produce semi-personal rather than shared neoantigens include Wilms tumor 1 (WT1) in AML (91–94) and T cell ALL (95), Notch1 and FBXW7 in T cell ALL (96–98), and TP53 in multiple malignancies (99–101). In these examples, mutations occur at a variety of sites in the gene and involve multiple different nucleotide substitutions, insertions, and/or deletions, such that few, if any, of the resulting amino acid sequences and resulting potential neoantigens would be shared among patients even with the same disease.

At the other end of the spectrum are highly recurrent fusions and mutations, exemplified by the RUNX1-RUNX1T1 fusion (89) and exon 12 mutations in nucleophosmin1 (NPM1) (102, 103) in AML. Virtually all patients with such fusions or mutations will have identical aberrant amino acid sequences. Neoantigens created from these abnormalities are shared among patients who have the mutations or fusions and are potential therapeutic targets for these individuals as a group.

Whether optimal therapies should target shared neoantigens, personal neoantigens, or both is currently unknown. Some key features of neoantigen quality have been postulated [reviewed in (104)], including: clonality, dissimilarity to self-antigens, similarity to microbial antigens (105), high protein expression, binding to HLA, and low likelihood that genetic abnormality yielding the neoantigen will be lost (for example, driver mutations or genes involved in cell survival where loss would harm cancer fitness) through deletion or transcriptional repression. Neoantigens with high-quality features are likely to be suitable therapeutic targets whether they are personal or shared. One note of caution with personal neoantigens is that unless autologous tumor is available, there may be no way to validate that a given putative neoantigen is in fact presented on primary tumor, and thus no way to confidently predict therapeutic efficacy.

The feasibility of targeting personal neoantigens is currently under investigation. As the accessibility of whole genome and whole exome sequencing increases, defining an individual patient's mutanome is becoming increasingly practical, although the ability to reliably predict personal neoantigens remains imperfect (27). Personalized neoantigen vaccines based on patient mutanomes have shown efficacy in solid tumors (8–10), and as of December 2019, 14 clinical trials of personalized neoantigen vaccines were recruiting in the United States, although only one of these studies includes patients with a hematologic malignancy (NCT03631043, multiple myeloma). In addition, increasingly sophisticated T cell engineering technologies have made the production of personalized neoantigen-specific engineered T cell therapies more practical; currently three trials of such therapies for patients with advanced solid tumors (NCT03412877, NCT04102436, NCT03970382) are enrolling.

Although both personal and shared neoantigens have therapeutic promise, in this review we will focus primarily on shared neoantigens (summarized in **Table 1**), which make up the bulk of the data to date.

NEOANTIGENS IN SPECIFIC HEMATOLOGIC MALIGNANCIES

Acute Myeloid Leukemia

AML is the most common acute leukemia in adults, and mutations in nucleophosmin1 (NPM1) occur in 30–35% of adult patients (102, 103). The majority of NPM1 mutations are insertions of four nucleotides in exon 12, resulting in a frameshift that produces a novel C-terminal 11 amino acid sequence (123). NPM1 mutations are stable across the disease course and considered to be driver events, thus an optimal immunotherapy target. Eighty-five percent of patients with NPM1-mutated ($NPM1^{mut}$) AML share the type A/D mutations that produce an identical abnormal amino acid sequence. Epitopes from the mutated region were independently identified as HLA ligands by two groups that used mass spectrometry to determine the amino acid sequences of peptides eluted off HLA molecules from primary leukemic blasts (74, 88) or AML cell lines (88).

Van der Lee et al. subsequently identified $CD8^+$ T cell clones from healthy donors that were specific for the $NPM1^{mut}$ HLA-A*02:01-restricted epitopes CLAVEEVSL and C*LAVEEVSL (74). These clones specifically recognized HLA-A*02:01$^+$ peptide-pulsed targets and $NPM1^{mut}$ AML blasts. One C*LAVEEVSL-specific TCR was sequenced and transferred into $CD8^+$ T cells using a viral vector. T cells with transferred $NPM1^{mut}$ TCRs could lyse $NPM1^{mut}$ but not NPM1 wild-type AML *in vitro* and partially controlled leukemia *in vivo* in an $NPM1^{mut}$ OCI-AML3 cell-line-derived xenograft murine model. These results convincingly demonstrate that CLAVEEVSL and C*LAVEEVSL are naturally presented on HLA-A*02:01 on leukemic blasts, are immunogenic, and are thus *bona fide* AML neoantigens. Curiously, although the peptide was immunogenic, the authors were unable to identify naturally occurring epitope-specific T cell responses in HLA-A*02:01$^+$ patients with $NPM1^{mut}$ AML. While a subsequent publication (123) suggested that $NPM1^{mut}$ -specific responses could be elicited *ex vivo* in patients, these studies were less stringently controlled.

Earlier studies identified candidate $NPM1^{mut}$-derived epitopes predicted to bind HLA-A*02:01 (106–108), against which the authors elicited $CD8^+$ T cells responses in patients and healthy donors after *ex vivo* stimulation. $CD8^+$ T cells specific for two epitopes (AIQDLCLAV and AIQDLCVAV) identified in these publications lysed an $NPM1^{mut}$ AML sample (106), suggesting that these epitopes were naturally processed and presented. However, these peptides were not identified among HLA-A*02:01 ligands in either of two subsequent studies that directly examined peptide epitopes eluted from HLA-A*02:01 on $NPM1^{mut}$ primary blasts (74, 88) or cell lines (88), and identification of AIQDLCL/VAV-specific $CD8^+$ T cells has not been reproduced by other groups.

In around 13% of AML cases (124, 125), a fusion of the retinoic acid receptor (RARA) gene on chromosome 17 and the promyelocytic leukemia (PML) gene on chromosome 15 occurs as a result of the chromosomal translocation, t(15; 17)(q24.1;q21.1), the classic translocation that produces the distinct entity of acute promyelocytic leukemia (APL). The resulting PML-RARA fusion protein not only serves as a driver of the leukemic phenotype but also represents a potential shared neoantigen at the fusion junction. Gambacorti-Passerini et al. investigated the immunogenicity of the PML-RARA fusion region by stimulating peripheral blood mononuclear cells (PBMC) from healthy volunteer donors with a 25mer peptide spanning the fusion (110, 126). $CD4^+$ T cell clones from one donor proliferated specifically in response to exogenous PML-RARA peptide presented on HLA-DR*11 in autologous target cells. One T cell clone could lyse peptide-pulsed autologous target cells and recognize autologous target cells transduced to express the PML-RARA fusion protein. However, in a subsequent study, no PML-RARA-specific $CD4^+$ T cell responses could be elicited from any of four HLA-DR*11$^+$ individuals in remission after treatment for APL (111). Since neither study evaluated whether PML-RARA-specific T cells could recognize primary APL cells, the PML-RARA/HLA-DR*11 epitope would still currently be

TABLE 1 | Shared or potentially shared neoantigens relevant in hematologic malignancies (fs, frameshift).

Disease	Parent protein	Epitope	HLA restriction	Level of evidence for neoantigen status	Reference(s)
AML	NPM1 fs (type A/D)	C*LAVEESL	A*02:01	Definite	(74, 88)
		CLAVEEVSL			
		AIQDLCLAV		Possible	(106–109)
	NPM1 fs (type C)	AIQDLCVAV		Possible	
	PML-RARA	NSNHVASGAGEAAIETQSSSSEEIV	DR*11	Possible	(110, 111)
ALL	ETV6-RUNX1	RIAECILGM	A*02:01	Conflicting	(112–114)
MPN	CALR fs	KMRMRRMRR	A*03:01	Possible	(85, 109, 115)
		RMRRTRRKM	B*07:02	Possible	
		Multiple	B*08:01	Candidate	(85)
		RMMRTKMRM	C*03:03	Possible	(109)
	JAK2 V617F	VLNYGVCFC	A*02:01	Possible	(116)
	MPL	Multiple	A*03:01	Candidate	(85, 116)
CML	BCR-ABL1	KQSSKALQR	A*03:01	Possible	(117)
	BCR-ABL1 E255K	KVYEGVWKK	A*03:01	Possible	(118)
B cell lymphomas	D393-CD20	(P)LFRRMSSLEVIA	DRB1*04	Possible	(119)
Multiple tumors	KRAS G12D	GADGVGKSA(L)	C*08:02	Definite	(6)
		VVVGADGVGK	A*11:01	Possible	(120)
	KRAS G12V	(V)VVGAVGVGK		Possible	
	BRAF V600E	GDFGLATEKSRWSGS	DQA1*03/ DQB1*03	Possible	(71)
	TP53 R175H	HMTEVVRHC	A*02:01	Possible	(121, 122)
		YKQSQHMTEVVRHCPHHERCSDSDG	Class II	Possible	(121)
	TP53 R248Q	YMCNSSCMGGMNQRPILTIITLEDS	Class I & II	Possible	
	TP53 R248W	SSCMGGMNWR	A*68:01	Possible	
		SSCMGGMNWRPILTII	DPB1*02:01	Possible	
	TP53 R282W	FEVRVCACPGRDWRTEEENLRKKGE	Classs II	Possible	

For levels of evidence:

"Definite" indicates that the epitope is immunogenic and that epitope-specific T cells clearly and consistently recognize primary malignant cells in a mutation/fusion- and HLA-specific manner.

"Possible" indicates epitopes that have demonstrated immunogenicity but either lack direct evidence of specific recognition of primary malignant cells (i.e., cell lines only) or data is inconsistent.

"Candidate" indicates that the peptide epitope has been demonstrated to bind the restricting HLA in vitro.

"Controversial" indicates conflicting data between groups.

considered a possible, rather than definite, AML neoantigen pending confirmation that the epitope is naturally presented on APL cells.

Acute Lymphoblastic Leukemia

ALL is the most common childhood cancer. Like other hematologic and pediatric malignancies, there are few non-synonymous mutations (14, 127) and thus few potential neoantigens. However, in recent studies, Zamora et al. found surprisingly abundant neoantigen-specific CD8$^+$ T cell responses in MIL from pediatric patients with ALL (112). To identify putative patient-specific neoantigens, cancer-specific mutations were identified from genomic sequencing of diagnostic biopsies and matched germline tissues from six patients. HLA typing was extrapolated from sample mRNA sequencing data, and the amino acid sequences of protein-coding mutations were interrogated using HLA-binding prediction algorithms. Mutation- or fusion-derived 15mer synthetic peptides were used to evaluate patient T cell specificity *ex vivo*. Functional CD8$^+$ T cell responses against at least one neoantigen were detected in all patients and encompassed 31 of 36 putative neoantigens mostly originating from patient-specific single gene mutations.

The Zamora study also identified T cells responsive to several epitopes from the recurrent ETV6-RUNX1 fusion in five patients. The ETV6-RUNX1 fusion results from the t(12; 21)(p13.2;q22.1) chromosomal translocation and is the most common genetic event in childhood B-lineage ALL, occurring in 15–20% of patients (128–131). ETV6-RUNX1 epitopes eliciting T cell responses in this study were predicted to bind to HLA-A*02:01, HLA-A*11:01, and HLA-B*15:01, and ETV6-RUNX1-specific T cells were identified by positive staining with HLA-A*02:01 or HLA-A*11:01 peptide/HLA tetramers. In earlier studies, the same HLA-A*02:01 epitope (RIAECILGM) was identified as binding stably to HLA-A2 in *in vitro* competitive-binding assays by a group that also isolated CD8$^+$ T cell lines specific for the epitope (113). The two RIAECILGM-specific lines that were isolated from healthy donors lysed fusion-expressing cell lines, and one T cell line from a patient with ETV6-RUNX1$^+$ ALL lysed autologous leukemic blasts at low levels. However, a subsequent study disputed whether the ETV6-RUNX1 epitope is in fact naturally processed and presented, as it showed that the native RIAECILGM peptide had virtually no binding to HLA-A*02:01 *in vitro*, was not processed by cells transduced to express the ETV6-RUNX1 epitope, and was not cleaved at the relevant position by human proteasomes *in vitro* (114). Given the conflicting data, it remains unclear whether the RIAECILGM epitope is truly an ALL neoantigen.

Myeloproliferative Neoplasms

Philadelphia (Ph) chromosome-negative myeloproliferative neoplasms (MPNs) comprise a group of disorders, including essential thrombocytosis (ET), polycythemia vera (PV), and primary myelofibrosis (PMF). MPNs arise from an abnormal hematopoietic progenitor cell, in most cases consequent to the acquisition of one of three driver mutations in JAK2 (Janus kinase 2), CALR (calreticulin), or MPL (c-mpl proto-oncogene; thrombopoietin receptor), along with a variety of passenger mutations (132) that can all produce neoantigens. Recently, Schischlik et al. comprehensively evaluated potential neoantigens in 113 patients with MPNs (85). Using whole-transcriptome sequencing to define the MPN mutanome, they identified 13 fusions, 221 non-synonymous single nucleotide variants, 31 insertion or deletion mutations, and 20 frameshift-producing splicing abnormalities. HLA-binding predictions for the 12 most prevalent HLA-A, -B, and -C alleles in their patient cohort yielded 541 patient-specific peptides predicted to bind to at least one of the HLA alleles. Subsequent *in vitro* HLA binding studies of 35 peptides derived from aberrantly spliced proteins associated with SF3B1 mutations and from mutated CALR (CALR^{mut}) and MPL validated binding of 23 peptides to HLA-A*03:01, -A*11:01, -B*07:02, and -B*08:01.

Although Schischlik et al. did not evaluate processing or immunogenicity of their putative neoantigens, others have identified T cell responses to CALR^{mut} and JAK2 V617F. Cimen Bozkus et al. used *in vitro* stimulation to elicit T cell responses to CALR^{mut} peptides that were primarily CD4$^+$ T cells in patients with MPNs and both CD4$^+$ and CD8$^+$ in healthy donors. Inhibition of the PD-1 and CTLA-4 immune checkpoint molecules *in vitro*, and PD-1 *in vivo* (in a patient treated with pembrolizumab), enhanced T cell responses. An immunogenic HLA-C*03:03-restricted 10mer epitope was identified, and T cells specific for this epitope produced cytokine in response to antigen-presenting cells pulsed with a 15mer peptide, indicating that the epitope was processed from the longer peptide (109). While this finding is encouraging, data conclusively demonstrating that the CALR^{mut} epitope is processed from the full-length protein and presented on HLA-C*03:03 on primary MPN cells is currently lacking. Another group described cytokine production, primarily by CD4$^+$ T cells, in response to *ex vivo* stimulation of peripheral blood mononuclear cells from patients with MPNs with long (31mer) CALR^{mut} peptides (133). CD8$^+$ T cells specific for CALR^{mut} peptides presented on HLA-A*03:01 and -B*07:02 were identified by another group, but the low avidity of the T cells prevented them from assessing whether the epitopes were naturally processed and presented on CALR^{mut} cells (115). Additionally, a 9mer peptide spanning the JAK2 V617F mutation (VLNYGVCFC) was identified as a ligand of HLA-A*02:01 by HLA-binding prediction; epitope-specific CD8$^+$ T cells lysed target cells either pulsed with the mutant peptide or naturally expressing JAK2 V617F, but also recognized targets pulsed with wild-type JAK2 peptide with lower efficiency (116). While this is a promising possible neoantigen with broad applicability for patients with MPNs, especially PV, further study is needed to definitively show that VLNYGVCFC is presented on primary malignant cells.

Philadelphia Chromosome-Positive Malignancies

The BCR-ABL1 fusion derives from translocation t(9; 22)(q34;q11), also called the Ph chromosome, which is highly recurrent in chronic myeloid leukemia (CML) and Ph-positive ALL (Ph$^+$-ALL). Most patients have one of two fusions resulting from different breakpoints, namely ^{P210}BCR-ABL1 and ^{P190}BCR-ABL1. ^{P210}BCR-ABL1 is found in both CML and Ph$^+$-ALL, while ^{P190}BCR-ABL1 is primarily associated with Ph$^+$-ALL (134). As an oncogenic driver, the BCR-ABL1 fusion is essential to the malignant phenotype and an ideal therapeutic target. Small molecule tyrosine kinase inhibitors (TKIs) are now key components of therapy for Ph$^+$ malignancies, but resistance does occur. Because the fusion is highly recurrent and disease-specific, it is a potential source for shared neoantigens. BCR-ABL1 was first described as a neoantigen in 1992 (135), and additional BCR-ABL1 epitopes were subsequently investigated by multiple groups [reviewed in (136)]. However, evidence for the natural CML presentation of BCR-ABL1 fusion peptides is conflicting: one group eluted an immunogenic fusion peptide from HLA-A*03:01 in primary CML (117), but a recent comprehensive evaluation of the HLA-ligandome in CML found no BCR-ABL1 epitopes presented on class I or class II molecules (58). Because the biology and specific fusions differ in the two diseases, the CML and Ph$^+$-ALL peptidomes may differ. Interestingly, adoptive transfer of *ex vivo*-expanded ^{P190}BCR-ABL1-specific CD8$^+$ T cells showed encouraging anti-leukemic activity in three patients with Ph$^+$-ALL (137). Specific BCR-ABL1 mutations that confer TKI resistance might also serve as neoantigens; one group identified donor-derived CD8$^+$ T cell responses to an HLA-A*03:01-restricted epitope from BCR-ABL1 E255K in a patient with the mutation who had achieved remission after HCT (118). While the BCR-ABL1 E255K-specific T cell clones could recognize minigene-transduced target cells, recognition of primary CML was not tested and thus it remains unclear whether the epitope represents a *bona fide* CML neoantigen.

Lymphomas and Chronic Lymphocytic Leukemia

In B cell malignancies, such as lymphomas and myelomas, neoplastic B cell-produced clonal immunoglobulin (Ig) was first described as a tumor-specific antigen in 1972 (138). Ig idiotypes have been extensively investigated as neoantigens with varying degrees of success, including in clinical trials (139). More recently, Khodadoust et al. recovered peptides representing somatic mutations in Ig heavy and light chain genes from the peptidomes of both class I and class II molecules in 17 primary mantle cell lymphomas (MCL) and two MCL cell lines, and detected circulating functional CD4$^+$ T cells specific for one Ig neoantigen that could kill autologous lymphoma (140). Subsequent studies by this group identified primarily class II-restricted Ig-derived neoantigens in other B cell malignancies, including follicular lymphoma, diffuse large B cell lymphoma, and chronic lymphocytic leukemia (CLL) (141). A cytoplasmic variant of CD20 (D393-CD20), produced by alternative splicing of the CD20 transcript, is detectable in malignant primary B cells and B cell lines, but not normal resting B cells (142). CD4$^+$ T cell responses to an epitope of D393-CD20 could be elicited from both healthy donors and patients with B cell lymphomas after *in vitro* peptide stimulation and blocked with anti-HLA-DR monoclonal antibody, but the exact HLA restriction could not be determined (119). *MYD88* is recurrently mutated in a variety of B cell malignancies and has been proposed as a potential neoantigen (143). Separately, in a small cohort of CLL patients evaluated after HCT, CD8$^+$ responses to neoantigens created from patient-specific non-Ig somatic mutations were identified; one well-studied patient-derived T cell clone could lyse autologous primary CLL cells, indicating that the epitope the clone recognized was a true personal neoantigen (13).

Neoantigens With General Applicability in Hematologic Malignancies

While some genetic abnormalities are specific to or even defining of particular cancer types, others, especially mutations in oncogenes or tumor suppressor genes, can be found in numerous cancers with a wide variety of cellular origins, including hematopoietic tissues. For example, somatic mutations affecting members of the Ras-MAPK pathway are among the most common in human cancers and are found across diverse cancer types (144–147). Similarly, TP53 is the most commonly mutated gene in human cancer, with TP53 mutations estimated to occur in ~25% of all cancers (99). Neoantigens derived from these mutations may thus be shared not just among patients with a single disease but across patients with many different cancers, including hematologic cancers (**Table 2**).

Mutations in KRAS or NRAS are found in ~5–26% of hematologic malignancies (146, 148) (**Table 2**). The most recurrent oncogenic mutations that occur in the RAS genes (NRAS, KRAS, HRAS) across cancers occur at codons 12, 13, and 61. As such, neoantigens derived from these recurrent mutations in RAS genes are attractive therapeutic targets with applicability in multiple diseases, including blood cancers. Moreover, the amino acid sequences of RAS family members are highly similar, such that identical epitopes may be derived from different proteins. Although there are no publications specifically investigating RAS-derived neoantigens in hematologic malignancies, findings from studies in solid tumors have potential applicability. For example, Tran et al. studied tumor-infiltrating lymphocytes (TIL) from a patient with metastatic KRAS G12D-mutated colorectal cancer and identified CD8$^+$ T cell clones specific for a KRAS G12D epitope presented on HLA-C*08:02 (6). KRAS G12D specific T cells expanded in the patient's peripheral blood after re-infusion of TIL, were persistently detectable ~9 months after TIL infusion, and mediated at least a transient regression of metastatic lung lesions. Subsequently, Cafri et al. performed *in vitro* stimulation of memory T cells isolated from two patients with KRAS-mutated solid tumors (one with endometrial cancer, one with rectal cancer) and identified CD8$^+$ T cells specific for an HLA-A*11:01-restricted epitope from KRAS G12V and CD4$^+$ T cells specific for an HLA-DRB1*08:01 restricted epitope from KRAS G12D (156). Earlier studies also identified murine TCRs with specificity for HLA-A*11:01-restricted epitopes from KRAS G12D and G12V in HLA-A*11:01$^+$ transgenic mice immunized with KRAS peptides (120). Retroviral transfer of the KRAS-specific TCRs into human T cells conferred KRAS neoantigen-specific anti-tumor activity *in vitro* and *in vivo*. These findings have been translated into clinical trials of transgenic TCR T cell immunotherapy for HLA-A*11:01$^+$ patients with certain KRAS G12D- or G12V-mutated solid tumors (NCT03190941 and NCT03745326). Although this clinical trial is directed toward patients with solid tumors, such therapies also have applicability to those with hematologic malignancies; for example, alterations at codon G12 of NRAS occur in a subset of patients with AML and produce identical amino acid sequences to the equivalent KRAS mutations, and so should yield the same epitope that could be targeted with KRAS G12D or G12V-directed T cells.

Mutations in BRAF, another component of the Ras-MAPK pathway, are present in about 8% of all human cancers (150). While the majority of BRAF-mutated malignancies are solid tumors, BRAF mutations do occur in a subset of hematologic malignancies. The BRAF V600E mutation is highly prevalent in hairy cell leukemia (151–153) and systemic histiocytoses (Erdheim-Chester disease and Langerhans cell histiocytosis) (154) and have also been identified in CLL (148) (**Table 2**). BRAF-derived neoantigens, particularly those originating from the V600E mutation, thus have applicability in a subset of hematologic malignancies. By examining peripheral blood lymphocytes from a patient with BRAF V600E$^+$ melanoma who had a clinical response after TIL therapy, Veatch et al. identified a CD4$^+$ T cell clone specific for an HLA-DQB1*03-restricted epitope of BRAF V600E (71). Lentiviral transfer of the BRAF V600E-specific TCR to donor CD4$^+$ conferred recognition of BRAF V600E-expressing target cells. An earlier study also detected CD4$^+$ T cell responses to HLA class II-restricted epitopes from BRAF V600E in patients with BRAF V600E melanoma, although not in the context of clinical response after immunotherapy (157).

TP53 mutations occur in malignancies of all origins (99), including all types of hematologic malignancies (100, 101, 158) (**Table 2**). While TP53 mutations can be quite heterogeneous,

TABLE 2 | Recurrently mutated genes in cancers, including hematologic malignancies, for which possible or definite public neoantigens have been identified.

Gene/gene family	Overall prevalence of any mutation in the gene/gene family in human cancers	Prevalence of any mutation in the gene/gene family in hematologic malignancies	Mutation hotspots (all cancers including hematologic)	Mutations yielding possible/definite neoantigens*	References
KRAS/ NRAS/HRAS	~25% (all RAS genes)	~26% multiple myeloma ~16% AML ~14% ALL ~10% CLL ~5% MDS (~30% CMML)	G12, G13, Q61	G12D, G12V	(146, 148, 149).
BRAF	~8%	~100% hairy cell leukemia ~40–60% systemic histiocytoses ~5% CLL	V600	V600E	(148, 150–154)
TP53	~25%	14% AL 12% AML 7–10% CLL 6% MDS 6–24% B cell lymphoma 7–40% non-B cell lymphoma 6% myeloma and other plasma cell dyscrasias	R175, R245, R248, R273, R282	R175H, R248Q, R248W, R282W	(99–101, 155)

*See **Table 1** for specific details about neoantigens.*

there are mutation hotspots at R175, R245, R248, R273, and R282 that are shared across multiple kinds of cancers, including hematologic cancers (99, 101). Neoantigens created from TP53 mutations thus have broad potential applicability in blood cancers as well as solid tumors. Malekzadeh et al. isolated T cells specific for HLA class I- and class II-restricted epitopes from five different recurrent TP53 mutations from TIL generated from patients with a variety of epithelial tumors (colorectal, ovarian, and pancreatic) (121). Both this publication and a subsequent report from the same group (122) identified an HLA-A*02:01-restricted epitope from TP53 R175H that appears to be naturally presented on a number of tumor cell lines. $CD4^+$ and $CD8^+$ responses to epitopes from patient-specific TP53 mutations have also been identified (122, 159, 160). Because the codon distribution of TP53 mutations is not specific to the tissue origin of a cancer, therapy targeting the TP53 R175H epitope, for example, should be equally applicable in a TP53 $R175H^+$ hematologic cancer as in a TP53 $R175H^+$ solid tumor, assuming the epitope is processed and presented appropriately. Similarly, specific mutations that are identical in many different malignancies, like the ones described in this section, are sources for neoantigens that are shared across cancers.

THERAPEUTIC APPLICATIONS OF NEOANTIGENS

While neoantigens are attractive targets for therapy because of their high specificity for malignant cells, there are challenges in translating neoantigen-directed immunotherapies to the clinic and the best approach to neoantigen-directed therapy is currently unknown. One strategy is to adoptively transfer neoantigen-specific T cells. T cells can be isolated from patient peripheral blood, TIL, or MIL (in hematologic malignancies), then expanded *ex vivo* non-specifically or against a defined antigen and re-infused (4, 6, 7, 161). Alternatively, T cells can be engineered to express a transgenic neoantigen-specific TCR (TCR-T), allowing infusion of a rapidly generated product with defined specificity and composition. Preclinical studies have shown that transfer of neoantigen-specific TCR-Ts is feasible (71, 74, 122), and two clinical trials of autologous TCR-T targeting HLA-A*11:01-restricted epitopes derived from point mutations in KRAS are enrolling (NCT03190941 and NCT03745326). Although TCR-T targeting epitopes from wild-type WT1 have shown safety (162–164) and efficacy (165), no clinical trials of neoantigen-specific TCR-T immunotherapy for hematologic malignancies have opened to date. TCR constructs can be modified to include other features to improve TCR-T safety and function: a CD8 co-stimulatory receptor enables $CD4^+$ T cells to function with a class I-restricted TCR and provide targeted help to neoantigen-specific $CD8^+$ T cells (166–168), a safety switch (167, 169) enables rapid removal of transgenic TCR-T cells in the event of toxicity, and other elements have been advanced [reviewed in (170)]. Lastly, vaccines do not require adoptive cell transfer, have shown clinical efficacy in solid tumors (8–10), and are particularly attractive for targeting highly immunogenic but less prevalent neoantigens.

Many factors influence which immunotherapy strategy is optimal for a given antigen. For neoantigens, the relatively low prevalence of each neoantigen among individuals with a given hematologic malignancy is a significant consideration, as immunotherapy for one neoantigen will apply only to a subset of patients. For example, the $NPM1^{mut}$ epitope described above (74) is only presented by the ~15% of AML patients with NPM1^{mut} (30–35%) and HLA-A*02:01 (~50% in the U.S.A.) and this represents one of the most broadly applicable recurrent neoantigens in hematologic malignancies. Producing neoantigen-directed TCR-T therapies using currently standard viral transfer methods is probably not cost-effective for less common neoantigens given their narrow applicability, but vaccines could be. Moreover, the growing use of non-viral techniques for TCR gene transfer, such as transposon-based technologies (159, 171, 172), nanoparticles (173), and RNA electroporation (174) should facilitate the development of TCR-T immunotherapy for all neoantigens, as illustrated by a recently opened clinical trial of gene-edited TCR-T immunotherapy for personal neoantigens (NCT03970382). The use of "universal donor cells" that have been engineered to be HLA-negative and express natural killer (NK) cell inhibitory molecules (175), in combination with silencing or editing the endogenous TCR (163), could also facilitate neoantigen-directed TCR-T immunotherapy.

Another consideration is the natural immunologic landscape of a particular malignancy. *Ex vivo* expansion and vaccination rely largely on the presence of existing anti-tumor responses that can be boosted *in vivo* or *ex vivo* and would be challenging in an immunosuppressive environment. Because hematologic malignancies have multiple mechanisms for blocking effective naturally occurring anti-leukemic immune responses (11, 176–183), TCR-T immunotherapy may be preferable for these diseases. For example, transgenic TCRs can used to modify selected virus-specific memory T cells for therapeutic transfer (165). Immune checkpoint blockade has been used alone in MPNs (109); combining them with neoantigen-specific immunotherapies could potentiate their effect in these and other hematological malignancies.

DISCUSSION

Much progress has been made in the field of neoantigens generally and in hematologic malignancies specifically. A number of promising *bona fide* and potential shared neoantigens have been identified for hematologic malignancies, most of which are derived from well-established mutations and fusions. However, growing access to comprehensive sequencing technologies has greatly enhanced the ability to define disease- and patient-specific mutanomes, which are valuable sources of potential neoantigens. Combined with improvements in T cell antigen discovery approaches, sequencing advances will facilitate the discovery of additional shared and personal neoantigens derived from known as well as new genetic abnormalities, expanding the repertoire of potential targets and moving the field forward. While there are a number of challenges in translating neoantigen-directed immunotherapies to the clinic, the rapid evolution of neoantigen discovery methods and the immunotherapy field is making barriers to clinical translation surmountable. Experience gained from T cell immunotherapy and vaccine studies in solid tumors and from cell therapy engineering for non-neoantigen targets will provide a critical foundation for building potent neoantigen-directed immunotherapies that are viable treatment strategies for hematologic malignancies.

AUTHOR CONTRIBUTIONS

MAB and MB reviewed the literature and wrote and edited the manuscript.

FUNDING

This work was supported by Hyundai Hope on Wheels (TE 6705) and by a Stand Up To Cancer Innovative Research Grant, Grant Number SU2C-AACR-IRG 14-17. Stand Up To Cancer is a division of the Entertainment Industry Foundation. Research grants are administered by the American Association for Cancer Research, the scientific partner of SU2C. MAB received additional support from a National Cancer Institute Paul Calabresi Career Development Award for Clinical Oncology (5 K12 CA076930-18) and from Alex's Lemonade Stand-Foundation for Childhood Cancer.

ACKNOWLEDGMENTS

We thank Drs. Deborah Banker and Michelle Brault for the editorial assistance.

REFERENCES

1. Cresswell P. Antigen processing and presentation. *Immunol Rev.* (2005) 207:5–7. doi: 10.1111/j.0105-2896.2005.00320.x
2. Vyas JM, Van der Veen AG, Ploegh HL. The known unknowns of antigen processing and presentation. *Nat Rev Immunol.* (2008) 8:607–18. doi: 10.1038/nri2368
3. Blum JS, Wearsch PA, Cresswell P. Pathways of antigen processing. *Annu Rev Immunol.* (2013) 31:443–73. doi: 10.1146/annurev-immunol-032712-095910
4. Tran E, Turcotte S, Gros A, Robbins PF, Lu YC, Dudley ME, et al. Cancer immunotherapy based on mutation-specific CD4+ T cells in a patient with epithelial cancer. *Science.* (2014) 344:641–5. doi: 10.1126/science.1251102
5. Robbins PF, Lu YC, El-Gamil M, Li YF, Gross C, Gartner J, et al. Mining exomic sequencing data to identify mutated antigens recognized by adoptively transferred tumor-reactive T cells. *Nat Med.* (2013) 19:747–52. doi: 10.1038/nm.3161
6. Tran E, Robbins PF, Lu YC, Prickett TD, Gartner JJ, Jia L, et al. T-Cell Transfer Therapy Targeting Mutant KRAS in Cancer. *N Engl J Med.* (2016) 375:2255–62. doi: 10.1056/NEJMoa1609279
7. Zacharakis N, Chinnasamy H, Black M, Xu H, Lu YC, Zheng Z, et al. Immune recognition of somatic mutations leading to complete durable regression in metastatic breast cancer. *Nat Med.* (2018) 24:724–30. doi: 10.1038/s41591-018-0040-8
8. Ott PA, Hu Z, Keskin DB, Shukla SA, Sun J, Bozym DJ, et al. An immunogenic personal neoantigen vaccine for patients with melanoma. *Nature.* (2017) 547:217–21. doi: 10.1038/nature22991
9. Sahin U, Derhovanessian E, Miller M, Kloke BP, Simon P, Lower M, et al. Personalized RNA mutanome vaccines mobilize poly-specific

therapeutic immunity against cancer. *Nature.* (2017) 547:222–6. doi: 10.1038/nature23003
10. Keskin DB, Anandappa AJ, Sun J, Tirosh I, Mathewson ND, Li S, et al. Neoantigen vaccine generates intratumoral T cell responses in phase Ib glioblastoma trial. *Nature.* (2019) 565:234–9. doi: 10.1038/s41586-018-0792-9
11. Yarchoan M, Johnson BA III, Lutz ER, Laheru DA, Jaffee EM. Targeting neoantigens to augment antitumour immunity. *Nat Rev Cancer.* (2017) 17:209–22. doi: 10.1038/nrc.2016.154
12. Yang W, Lee KW, Srivastava RM, Kuo F, Krishna C, Chowell D, et al. Immunogenic neoantigens derived from gene fusions stimulate T cell responses. *Nat Med.* (2019) 25:767–75. doi: 10.1038/s41591-019-0434-2
13. Rajasagi M, Shukla SA, Fritsch EF, Keskin DB, DeLuca D, Carmona E, et al. Systematic identification of personal tumor-specific neoantigens in chronic lymphocytic leukemia. *Blood.* (2014) 124:453–62. doi: 10.1182/blood-2014-04-567933
14. Lawrence MS, Stojanov P, Polak P, Kryukov GV, Cibulskis K, Sivachenko A, et al. Mutational heterogeneity in cancer and the search for new cancer-associated genes. *Nature.* (2013) 499:214–8. doi: 10.1038/nature12213
15. Koopman LA, Corver WE, van der Slik AR, Giphart MJ, Fleuren GJ. Multiple genetic alterations cause frequent and heterogeneous human histocompatibility leukocyte antigen class I loss in cervical cancer. *J Exp Med.* (2000) 191:961–76. doi: 10.1084/jem.191.6.961
16. Campoli M, Chang CC, Ferrone S. HLA class I antigen loss, tumor immune escape and immune selection. *Vaccine.* (2002) 20 (Suppl. 4):A40–5. doi: 10.1016/S0264-410X(02)00386-9
17. Garrido F, Ruiz-Cabello F, Aptsiauri N. Rejection versus escape: the tumor MHC dilemma. *Cancer Immunol Immunother.* (2017) 66:259–71. doi: 10.1007/s00262-016-1947-x
18. Shukla SA, Rooney MS, Rajasagi M, Tiao G, Dixon PM, Lawrence MS, et al. Comprehensive analysis of cancer-associated somatic mutations in class I HLA genes. *Nat Biotechnol.* (2015) 33:1152–8. doi: 10.1038/nbt.3344
19. Benitez R, Godelaine D, Lopez-Nevot MA, Brasseur F, Jimenez P, Marchand M, et al. Mutations of the β2-microglobulin gene result in a lack of HLA class I molecules on melanoma cells of two patients immunized with MAGE peptides. *Tissue Antigens.* (1998) 52:520–9. doi: 10.1111/j.1399-0039.1998.tb03082.x
20. Sade-Feldman M, Jiao YJ, Chen JH, Rooney MS, Barzily-Rokni M, Eliane JP, et al. Resistance to checkpoint blockade therapy through inactivation of antigen presentation. *Nat Commun.* (2017) 8:1136. doi: 10.1038/s41467-017-01062-w
21. Gettinger S, Choi J, Hastings K, Truini A, Datar I, Sowell R, et al. Impaired HLA class I antigen processing and presentation as a mechanism of acquired resistance to immune checkpoint inhibitors in lung cancer. *Cancer Discov.* (2017) 7:1420–35. doi: 10.1158/2159-8290.CD-17-0593
22. McGranahan N, Rosenthal R, Hiley CT, Rowan AJ, Watkins TBK, Wilson GA, et al. Allele-specific HLA loss and immune escape in lung cancer evolution. *Cell.* (2017) 171:1259–71.e11. doi: 10.1016/j.cell.2017.10.001
23. Paulson KG, Voillet V, McAfee MS, Hunter DS, Wagener FD, Perdicchio M, et al. Acquired cancer resistance to combination immunotherapy from transcriptional loss of class I HLA. *Nat Commun.* (2018) 9:3868. doi: 10.1038/s41467-018-06300-3
24. Christopher MJ, Petti AA, Rettig MP, Miller CA, Chendamarai E, Duncavage EJ, et al. Immune escape of relapsed AML cells after allogeneic transplantation. *N Engl J Med.* (2018) 379:2330–41. doi: 10.1056/NEJMoa1808777
25. Ebstein F, Keller M, Paschen A, Walden P, Seeger M, Burger E, et al. Exposure to Melan-A/MART-126–35 tumor epitope specific CD8(+)T cells reveals immune escape by affecting the ubiquitin-proteasome system (UPS). *Sci Rep.* (2016) 6:25208. doi: 10.1038/srep25208
26. Yamamoto TN, Kishton RJ, Restifo NP. Developing neoantigen-targeted T cell-based treatments for solid tumors. *Nat Med.* (2019) 25:1488–99. doi: 10.1038/s41591-019-0596-y
27. The problem with neoantigen prediction. *Nat Biotechnol.* (2017) 35:97. doi: 10.1038/nbt.3800
28. Bocchia M, Wentworth PA, Southwood S, Sidney J, McGraw K, Scheinberg DA, et al. Specific binding of leukemia oncogene fusion protein peptides to HLA class I molecules. *Blood.* (1995) 85:2680–4. doi: 10.1182/blood.V85.10.2680.bloodjournal85102680
29. Sturniolo T, Bono E, Ding J, Raddrizzani L, Tuereci O, Sahin U, et al. Generation of tissue-specific and promiscuous HLA ligand databases using DNA microarrays and virtual HLA class II matrices. *Nat Biotechnol.* (1999) 17:555–61. doi: 10.1038/9858
30. Singh H, Raghava GP. ProPred: prediction of HLA-DR binding sites. *Bioinformatics.* (2001) 17:1236–7. doi: 10.1093/bioinformatics/17.12.1236
31. Peters B, Sette A. Generating quantitative models describing the sequence specificity of biological processes with the stabilized matrix method. *BMC Bioinformatics.* (2005) 6:132. doi: 10.1186/1471-2105-6-132
32. Guan P, Hattotuwagama CK, Doytchinova IA, Flower DR. MHCPred 2.0: an updated quantitative T-cell epitope prediction server. *Appl Bioinformatics.* (2006) 5:55–61. doi: 10.2165/00822942-200605010-00008
33. Sidney J, Assarsson E, Moore C, Ngo S, Pinilla C, Sette A, et al. Quantitative peptide binding motifs for 19 human and mouse MHC class I molecules derived using positional scanning combinatorial peptide libraries. *Immunome Res.* (2008) 4:2. doi: 10.1186/1745-7580-4-2
34. Wang P, Sidney J, Dow C, Mothe B, Sette A, Peters B. A systematic assessment of MHC class II peptide binding predictions and evaluation of a consensus approach. *PLoS Comput Biol.* (2008) 4:e1000048. doi: 10.1371/journal.pcbi.1000048
35. Hoof I, Peters B, Sidney J, Pedersen LE, Sette A, Lund O, et al. NetMHCpan, a method for MHC class I binding prediction beyond humans. *Immunogenetics.* (2009) 61:1–13. doi: 10.1007/s00251-008-0341-z
36. Kim Y, Ponomarenko J, Zhu Z, Tamang D, Wang P, Greenbaum J, et al. Immune epitope database analysis resource. *Nucleic Acids Res.* (2012) 40:W525–30. doi: 10.1093/nar/gks438
37. Jurtz V, Paul S, Andreatta M, Marcatili P, Peters B, Nielsen M. NetMHCpan-4.0: Improved peptide-MHC class I interaction predictions integrating eluted ligand and peptide binding affinity data. *J Immunol.* (2017) 199:3360–8. doi: 10.4049/jimmunol.1700893
38. Jensen KK, Andreatta M, Marcatili P, Buus S, Greenbaum JA, Yan Z, et al. Improved methods for predicting peptide binding affinity to MHC class II molecules. *Immunology.* (2018) 154:394–406. doi: 10.1111/imm.12889
39. Barra C, Alvarez B, Paul S, Sette A, Peters B, Andreatta M, et al. Footprints of antigen processing boost MHC class II natural ligand predictions. *Genome Med.* (2018) 10:84. doi: 10.1186/s13073-018-0594-6
40. Bulik-Sullivan B, Busby J, Palmer CD, Davis MJ, Murphy T, Clark A, et al. Deep learning using tumor HLA peptide mass spectrometry datasets improves neoantigen identification. *Nat Biotechnol.* (2018) 37, 55–63. doi: 10.1038/nbt.4313
41. Chen B, Khodadoust MS, Olsson N, Wagar LE, Fast E, Liu CL, et al. Predicting HLA class II antigen presentation through integrated deep learning. *Nat Biotechnol.* (2019) 37, 1332–43. doi: 10.1038/s41587-019-0280-2
42. Racle J, Michaux J, Rockinger GA, Arnaud M, Bobisse S, Chong C, et al. Robust prediction of HLA class II epitopes by deep motif deconvolution of immunopeptidomes. *Nat Biotechnol.* (2019) 37, 1283–6. doi: 10.1038/s41587-019-0289-6
43. Abelin JG, Harjanto D, Malloy M, Suri P, Colson T, Goulding SP, et al. Defining HLA-II ligand processing and binding rules with mass spectrometry enhances cancer epitope prediction. *Immunity.* (2019) 51:766–79.e17. doi: 10.1016/j.immuni.2019.08.012
44. Garde C, Ramarathinam SH, Jappe EC, Nielsen M, Kringelum JV, Trolle T, et al. Improved peptide-MHC class II interaction prediction through integration of eluted ligand and peptide affinity data. *Immunogenetics.* (2019) 71:445–54. doi: 10.1007/s00251-019-01122-z
45. Besser H, Louzoun Y. Cross-modality deep learning-based prediction of TAP binding and naturally processed peptide. *Immunogenetics.* (2018) 70:419–28. doi: 10.1007/s00251-018-1054-6
46. Tenzer S, Peters B, Bulik S, Schoor O, Lemmel C, Schatz MM, et al. Modeling the MHC class I pathway by combining predictions of proteasomal cleavage, TAP transport and MHC class I binding. *Cell Mol Life Sci.* (2005) 62:1025–37. doi: 10.1007/s00018-005-4528-2
47. Calis JJ, Reinink P, Keller C, Kloetzel PM, Kesmir C. Role of peptide processing predictions in T cell epitope identification: contribution

of different prediction programs. *Immunogenetics.* (2015) 67:85–93. doi: 10.1007/s00251-014-0815-0
48. Diez-Rivero CM, Lafuente EM, Reche PA. Computational analysis and modeling of cleavage by the immunoproteasome and the constitutive proteasome. *BMC Bioinformatics.* (2010) 11:479. doi: 10.1186/1471-2105-11-479
49. Paul S, Karosiene E, Dhanda SK, Jurtz V, Edwards L, Nielsen M, et al. Determination of a predictive cleavage motif for eluted major histocompatibility complex class II ligands. *Front Immunol.* (2018) 9:1795. doi: 10.3389/fimmu.2018.01795
50. Zhang GL, Petrovsky N, Kwoh CK, August JT, Brusic V. PRED(TAP): a system for prediction of peptide binding to the human transporter associated with antigen processing. *Immunome Res.* (2006) 2:3. doi: 10.1186/1745-7580-2-3
51. Boehm KM, Bhinder B, Raja VJ, Dephoure N, Elemento O. Predicting peptide presentation by major histocompatibility complex class I: an improved machine learning approach to the immunopeptidome. *BMC Bioinformatics.* (2019) 20:7. doi: 10.1186/s12859-018-2561-z
52. Larsen MV, Lundegaard C, Lamberth K, Buus S, Lund O, Nielsen M. Large-scale validation of methods for cytotoxic T-lymphocyte epitope prediction. *BMC Bioinformatics.* (2007) 8:424. doi: 10.1186/1471-2105-8-424
53. Nielsen M, Lundegaard C, Lund O, Kesmir C. The role of the proteasome in generating cytotoxic T-cell epitopes: insights obtained from improved predictions of proteasomal cleavage. *Immunogenetics.* (2005) 57:33–41. doi: 10.1007/s00251-005-0781-7
54. Liepe J, Ovaa H, Mishto M. Why do proteases mess up with antigen presentation by re-shuffling antigen sequences? *Curr Opin Immunol.* (2018) 52:81–6. doi: 10.1016/j.coi.2018.04.016
55. Liepe J, Marino F, Sidney J, Jeko A, Bunting DE, Sette A, et al. A large fraction of HLA class I ligands are proteasome-generated spliced peptides. *Science.* (2016) 354:354–8. doi: 10.1126/science.aaf4384
56. Fritsch EF, Rajasagi M, Ott PA, Brusic V, Hacohen N, Wu CJ. HLA-binding properties of tumor neoepitopes in humans. *Cancer Immunol Res.* (2014) 2:522–9. doi: 10.1158/2326-6066.CIR-13-0227
57. Berlin C, Kowalewski DJ, Schuster H, Mirza N, Walz S, Handel M, et al. Mapping the HLA ligandome landscape of acute myeloid leukemia: a targeted approach toward peptide-based immunotherapy. *Leukemia.* (2015) 29:647–59. doi: 10.1038/leu.2014.233
58. Bilich T, Nelde A, Bichmann L, Roerden M, Salih HR, Kowalewski DJ, et al. The HLA ligandome landscape of chronic myeloid leukemia delineates novel T-cell epitopes for immunotherapy. *Blood.* (2019) 133:550–65. doi: 10.1182/blood-2018-07-866830
59. Nelde A, Kowalewski DJ, Backert L, Schuster H, Werner JO, Klein R, et al. HLA ligandome analysis of primary chronic lymphocytic leukemia (CLL) cells under lenalidomide treatment confirms the suitability of lenalidomide for combination with T-cell-based immunotherapy. *Oncoimmunology.* (2018) 7:e1316438. doi: 10.1080/2162402X.2017.1316438
60. Abelin JG, Keskin DB, Sarkizova S, Hartigan CR, Zhang W, Sidney J, et al. Mass Spectrometry profiling of HLA-associated peptidomes in mono-allelic cells enables more accurate epitope prediction. *Immunity.* (2017) 46:315–26. doi: 10.1016/j.immuni.2017.02.007
61. Hawkins OE, Vangundy RS, Eckerd AM, Bardet W, Buchli R, Weidanz JA, et al. Identification of breast cancer peptide epitopes presented by HLA-A*0201. *J Proteome Res.* (2008) 7:1445–57. doi: 10.1021/pr700761w
62. Trolle T, McMurtrey CP, Sidney J, Bardet W, Osborn SC, Kaever T, et al. The length distribution of class I-restricted T cell epitopes is determined by both peptide supply and MHC allele-specific binding preference. *J Immunol.* (2016) 196:1480–7. doi: 10.4049/jimmunol.1501721
63. Bassani-Sternberg M, Pletscher-Frankild S, Jensen LJ, Mann M. Mass spectrometry of human leukocyte antigen class I peptidomes reveals strong effects of protein abundance and turnover on antigen presentation. *Mol Cell Proteomics.* (2015) 14:658–73. doi: 10.1074/mcp.M114.042812
64. Gfeller D, Bassani-Sternberg M. Predicting antigen presentation-what could we learn from a million peptides? *Front Immunol.* (2018) 9:1716. doi: 10.3389/fimmu.2018.01716
65. Luksza M, Riaz N, Makarov V, Balachandran VP, Hellmann MD, Solovyov A, et al. A neoantigen fitness model predicts tumour response to checkpoint blockade immunotherapy. *Nature.* (2017) 551:517–20. doi: 10.1038/nature24473
66. Smith CC, Chai S, Washington AR, Lee SJ, Landoni E, Field K, et al. Machine-learning prediction of tumor antigen immunogenicity in the selection of therapeutic epitopes. *Cancer Immunol Res.* (2019) 7:1591–604. doi: 10.1158/2326-6066.CIR-19-0155
67. Riley TP, Keller GLJ, Smith AR, Davancaze LM, Arbuiso AG, Devlin JR, et al. Structure based prediction of neoantigen immunogenicity. *Front Immunol.* (2019) 10:2047. doi: 10.3389/fimmu.2019.02047
68. Richman LP, Vonderheide RH, Rech AJ. Neoantigen dissimilarity to the self-proteome predicts immunogenicity and response to immune checkpoint blockade. *Cell Syst.* (2019) 9:375–82.e4. doi: 10.1016/j.cels.2019.08.009
69. Kosaloglu-Yalcin Z, Lanka M, Frentzen A, Logandha Ramamoorthy Premlal A, Sidney J, Vaughan K, et al. Predicting T cell recognition of MHC class I restricted neoepitopes. *Oncoimmunology.* (2018) 7:e1492508. doi: 10.1080/2162402X.2018.1492508
70. Yadav M, Jhunjhunwala S, Phung QT, Lupardus P, Tanguay J, Bumbaca S, et al. Predicting immunogenic tumour mutations by combining mass spectrometry and exome sequencing. *Nature.* (2014) 515:572–6. doi: 10.1038/nature14001
71. Veatch JR, Lee SM, Fitzgibbon M, Chow IT, Jesernig B, Schmitt T, et al. Tumor-infiltrating BRAFV600E-specific CD4+ T cells correlated with complete clinical response in melanoma. *J Clin Invest.* (2018) 128:1563–8. doi: 10.1172/JCI98689
72. Gros A, Parkhurst MR, Tran E, Pasetto A, Robbins PF, Ilyas S, et al. Prospective identification of neoantigen-specific lymphocytes in the peripheral blood of melanoma patients. *Nat Med.* (2016) 22:433–8. doi: 10.1038/nm.4051
73. Sakuishi K, Apetoh L, Sullivan JM, Blazar BR, Kuchroo VK, Anderson AC. Targeting Tim-3 and PD-1 pathways to reverse T cell exhaustion and restore anti-tumor immunity. *J Exp Med.* (2010) 207:2187–94. doi: 10.1084/jem.20100643
74. van der Lee DI, Reijmers RM, Honders MW, Hagedoorn RS, de Jong RC, Kester MG, et al. Mutated nucleophosmin 1 as immunotherapy target in acute myeloid leukemia. *J Clin Invest.* (2019) 129:774–85. doi: 10.1172/JCI97482
75. Kula T, Dezfulian MH, Wang CI, Abdelfattah NS, Hartman ZC, Wucherpfennig KW, et al. T-Scan: a genome-wide method for the systematic discovery of T cell epitopes. *Cell.* (2019) 178:1016–28.e13. doi: 10.1016/j.cell.2019.07.009
76. Bleakley M, Otterud BE, Richardt JL, Mollerup AD, Hudecek M, Nishida T, et al. Leukemia-associated minor histocompatibility antigen discovery using T-cell clones isolated by *in vitro* stimulation of naive CD8+ T cells. *Blood.* (2010) 115:4923–33. doi: 10.1182/blood-2009-12-260539
77. Stronen E, Toebes M, Kelderman S, van Buuren MM, Yang W, van Rooij N, et al. Targeting of cancer neoantigens with donor-derived T cell receptor repertoires. *Science.* (2016) 352:1337–41. doi: 10.1126/science.aaf2288
78. Ding LW, Sun QY, Tan KT, Chien W, Mayakonda A, Yeoh AEJ, et al. Mutational landscape of pediatric acute lymphoblastic leukemia. *Cancer Res.* (2017) 77:390–400. doi: 10.1158/0008-5472.CAN-16-1303
79. Iacobucci I, Mullighan CG. Genetic basis of acute lymphoblastic leukemia. *J Clin Oncol.* (2017) 35:975–83. doi: 10.1200/JCO.2016.70.7836
80. Bolouri H, Farrar JE, Triche T Jr, Ries RE, Lim EL, Alonzo TA, et al. The molecular landscape of pediatric acute myeloid leukemia reveals recurrent structural alterations and age-specific mutational interactions. *Nat Med.* (2018) 24:103–12. doi: 10.1038/nm.4439
81. Cancer Genome Atlas Research N. Genomic and epigenomic landscapes of adult de novo acute myeloid leukemia. *N Engl J Med.* (2013) 368:2059–74. doi: 10.1056/NEJMoa1301689
82. Landau DA, Tausch E, Taylor-Weiner AN, Stewart C, Reiter JG, Bahlo J, et al. Mutations driving CLL and their evolution in progression and relapse. *Nature.* (2015) 526:525–30. doi: 10.1038/nature15395
83. Puente XS, Bea S, Valdes-Mas R, Villamor N, Gutierrez-Abril J, Martin-Subero JI, et al. Non-coding recurrent mutations in chronic lymphocytic leukaemia. *Nature.* (2015) 526:519–24. doi: 10.1038/nature14666
84. Bose P, Nazha A, Komrokji RS, Patel KP, Pierce SA, Al-Ali N, et al. Mutational landscape of myelodysplastic/myeloproliferative neoplasm-unclassifiable. *Blood.* (2018) 132:2100–3. doi: 10.1182/blood-2018-05-848473

85. Schischlik F, Jager R, Rosebrock F, Hug E, Schuster M, Holly R, et al. Mutational landscape of the transcriptome offers putative targets for immunotherapy of myeloproliferative neoplasms. *Blood.* (2019) 134:199–210. doi: 10.1182/blood.2019000519
86. Kowalewski DJ, Schuster H, Backert L, Berlin C, Kahn S, Kanz L, et al. HLA ligandome analysis identifies the underlying specificities of spontaneous antileukemia immune responses in chronic lymphocytic leukemia (CLL). *Proc Natl Acad Sci USA.* (2015) 112:E166–75. doi: 10.1073/pnas.1416389112
87. Walz S, Stickel JS, Kowalewski DJ, Schuster H, Weisel K, Backert L, et al. The antigenic landscape of multiple myeloma: mass spectrometry (re)defines targets for T-cell-based immunotherapy. *Blood.* (2015) 126:1203–13. doi: 10.1182/blood-2015-04-640532
88. Narayan R, Olsson N, Wagar LE, Medeiros BC, Meyer E, Czerwinski D, et al. Acute myeloid leukemia immunopeptidome reveals HLA presentation of mutated nucleophosmin. *PLoS ONE.* (2019) 14:e0219547. doi: 10.1371/journal.pone.0219547
89. van Dongen JJ, Macintyre EA, Gabert JA, Delabesse E, Rossi V, Saglio G, et al. Standardized RT-PCR analysis of fusion gene transcripts from chromosome aberrations in acute leukemia for detection of minimal residual disease. Report of the BIOMED-1 Concerted Action: investigation of minimal residual disease in acute leukemia. *Leukemia.* (1999) 13:1901–28. doi: 10.1038/sj.leu.2401592
90. Meyer C, Burmeister T, Groger D, Tsaur G, Fechina L, Renneville A, et al. The MLL recombinome of acute leukemias in 2017. *Leukemia.* (2018) 32:273–84. doi: 10.1038/leu.2017.213
91. King-Underwood L, Renshaw J, Pritchard-Jones K. Mutations in the Wilms' tumor gene WT1 in leukemias. *Blood.* (1996) 87:2171–9. doi: 10.1182/blood.V87.6.2171.bloodjournal8762171
92. Pronier E, Bowman RL, Ahn J, Glass J, Kandoth C, Merlinsky TR, et al. Genetic and epigenetic evolution as a contributor to WT1-mutant leukemogenesis. *Blood.* (2018) 132:1265–78. doi: 10.1182/blood-2018-03-837468
93. Niktoreh N, Walter C, Zimmermann M, von Neuhoff C, von Neuhoff N, Rasche M, et al. Mutated WT1, FLT3-ITD, and NUP98-NSD1 fusion in various combinations define a poor prognostic group in pediatric acute myeloid leukemia. *J Oncol.* (2019) 2019:1609128. doi: 10.1155/2019/1609128
94. Potter N, Miraki-Moud F, Ermini L, Titley I, Vijayaraghavan G, Papaemmanuil E, et al. Single cell analysis of clonal architecture in acute myeloid leukaemia. *Leukemia.* (2019) 33:1113–23. doi: 10.1038/s41375-018-0319-2
95. Tosello V, Mansour MR, Barnes K, Paganin M, Sulis ML, Jenkinson S, et al. WT1 mutations in T-ALL. *Blood.* (2009) 114:1038–45. doi: 10.1182/blood-2008-12-192039
96. Weng AP, Ferrando AA, Lee W, Morris JPt, Silverman LB, Sanchez-Irizarry C, et al. Activating mutations of NOTCH1 in human T cell acute lymphoblastic leukemia. *Science.* (2004) 306:269–71. doi: 10.1126/science.1102160
97. Grabher C, von Boehmer H, Look AT. Notch 1 activation in the molecular pathogenesis of T-cell acute lymphoblastic leukaemia. *Nat Rev Cancer.* (2006) 6:347–59. doi: 10.1038/nrc1880
98. Girardi T, Vicente C, Cools J, De Keersmaecker K. The genetics and molecular biology of T-ALL. *Blood.* (2017) 129:1113–23. doi: 10.1182/blood-2016-10-706465
99. Bykov VJN, Eriksson SE, Bianchi J, Wiman KG. Targeting mutant p53 for efficient cancer therapy. *Nat Rev Cancer.* (2018) 18:89–102. doi: 10.1038/nrc.2017.109
100. Stengel A, Kern W, Haferlach T, Meggendorfer M, Fasan A, Haferlach C. The impact of TP53 mutations and TP53 deletions on survival varies between AML, ALL, MDS and CLL: an analysis of 3307 cases. *Leukemia.* (2017) 31:705–11. doi: 10.1038/leu.2016.263
101. Xu-Monette ZY, Medeiros LJ, Li Y, Orlowski RZ, Andreeff M, Bueso-Ramos CE, et al. Dysfunction of the TP53 tumor suppressor gene in lymphoid malignancies. *Blood.* (2012) 119:3668–83. doi: 10.1182/blood-2011-11-366062
102. Falini B, Martelli MP, Bolli N, Sportoletti P, Liso A, Tiacci E, et al. Acute myeloid leukemia with mutated nucleophosmin (NPM1): is it a distinct entity? *Blood.* (2011) 117:1109–20. doi: 10.1182/blood-2010-08-299990
103. Falini B, Mecucci C, Tiacci E, Alcalay M, Rosati R, Pasqualucci L, et al. Cytoplasmic nucleophosmin in acute myelogenous leukemia with a normal karyotype. *N Engl J Med.* (2005) 352:254–66. doi: 10.1056/NEJMoa041974
104. McGranahan N, Swanton C. Neoantigen quality, not quantity. *Sci Transl Med.* (2019) 11:eaax7918. doi: 10.1126/scitranslmed.aax7918
105. Balachandran VP, Luksza M, Zhao JN, Makarov V, Moral JA, Remark R, et al. Identification of unique neoantigen qualities in long-term survivors of pancreatic cancer. *Nature.* (2017) 551:512–6. doi: 10.1038/nature24462
106. Greiner J, Schneider V, Schmitt M, Gotz M, Dohner K, Wiesneth M, et al. Immune responses against the mutated region of cytoplasmatic NPM1 might contribute to the favorable clinical outcome of AML patients with NPM1 mutations (NPM1mut). *Blood.* (2013) 122:1087–8. doi: 10.1182/blood-2013-04-496844
107. Hofmann S, Gotz M, Schneider V, Guillaume P, Bunjes D, Dohner H, et al. Donor lymphocyte infusion induces polyspecific $CD8^+$ T-cell responses with concurrent molecular remission in acute myeloid leukemia with NPM1 mutation. *J Clin Oncol.* (2013) 31:e44–7. doi: 10.1200/JCO.2011.41.1116
108. Schneider V, Zhang L, Bullinger L, Rojewski M, Hofmann S, Wiesneth M, et al. Leukemic stem cells of acute myeloid leukemia patients carrying NPM1 mutation are candidates for targeted immunotherapy. *Leukemia.* (2014) 28:1759–62. doi: 10.1038/leu.2014.116
109. Cimen Bozkus C, Roudko V, Finnigan JP, Mascarenhas J, Hoffman R, Iancu-Rubin C, et al. Immune checkpoint blockade enhances shared neoantigen-induced T-cell immunity directed against mutated calreticulin in myeloproliferative neoplasms. *Cancer Discov.* (2019) 9:1192–207. doi: 10.1158/2159-8290.CD-18-1356
110. Gambacorti-Passerini C, Grignani F, Arienti F, Pandolfi PP, Pelicci PG, Parmiani G. Human CD4 lymphocytes specifically recognize a peptide representing the fusion region of the hybrid protein pml/RAR alpha present in acute promyelocytic leukemia cells. *Blood.* (1993) 81:1369–75. doi: 10.1182/blood.V81.5.1369.1369
111. Dermime S, Bertazzoli C, Marchesi E, Ravagnani F, Blaser K, Corneo GM, et al. Lack of T-cell-mediated recognition of the fusion region of the pml/RAR-alpha hybrid protein by lymphocytes of acute promyelocytic leukemia patients. *Clin Cancer Res.* (1996) 2:593–600.
112. Zamora AE, Crawford JC, Allen EK, Guo XJ, Bakke J, Carter RA, et al. Pediatric patients with acute lymphoblastic leukemia generate abundant and functional neoantigen-specific $CD8^+$ T cell responses. *Sci Transl Med.* (2019) 11:eaat8549. doi: 10.1126/scitranslmed.aat8549
113. Yotnda P, Garcia F, Peuchmaur M, Grandchamp B, Duval M, Lemonnier F, et al. Cytotoxic T cell response against the chimeric ETV6-AML1 protein in childhood acute lymphoblastic leukemia. *J Clin Invest.* (1998) 102:455–62. doi: 10.1172/JCI3126
114. Popovic J, Li LP, Kloetzel PM, Leisegang M, Uckert W, Blankenstein T. The only proposed T-cell epitope derived from the TEL-AML1 translocation is not naturally processed. *Blood.* (2011) 118:946–54. doi: 10.1182/blood-2010-12-325035
115. Tubb VM, Schrikkema DS, Croft NP, Purcell AW, Linnemann C, Freriks MR, et al. Isolation of T cell receptors targeting recurrent neoantigens in hematological malignancies. *J Immunother Cancer.* (2018) 6:70. doi: 10.1186/s40425-018-0386-y
116. Holmstrom MO, Hjortso MD, Ahmad SM, Met O, Martinenaite E, Riley C, et al. The JAK2V617F mutation is a target for specific T cells in the JAK2V617F-positive myeloproliferative neoplasms. *Leukemia.* (2017) 31:495–8. doi: 10.1038/leu.2016.290
117. Clark RE, Dodi IA, Hill SC, Lill JR, Aubert G, Macintyre AR, et al. Direct evidence that leukemic cells present HLA-associated immunogenic peptides derived from the BCR-ABL b3a2 fusion protein. *Blood.* (2001) 98:2887–93. doi: 10.1182/blood.V98.10.2887
118. Cai A, Keskin DB, DeLuca DS, Alonso A, Zhang W, Zhang GL, et al. Mutated BCR-ABL generates immunogenic T-cell epitopes in CML patients. *Clin Cancer Res.* (2012) 18:5761–72. doi: 10.1158/1078-0432.CCR-12-1182
119. Vauchy C, Gamonet C, Ferrand C, Daguindau E, Galaine J, Beziaud L, et al. CD20 alternative splicing isoform generates immunogenic CD4 helper T epitopes. *Int J Cancer.* (2015) 137:116–26. doi: 10.1002/ijc.29366
120. Wang QJ, Yu Z, Griffith K, Hanada K, Restifo NP, Yang JC. Identification of T-cell receptors targeting KRAS-mutated human tumors. *Cancer Immunol Res.* (2016) 4:204–14. doi: 10.1158/2326-6066.CIR-15-0188

121. Malekzadeh P, Pasetto A, Robbins PF, Parkhurst MR, Paria BC, Jia L, et al. Neoantigen screening identifies broad TP53 mutant immunogenicity in patients with epithelial cancers. *J Clin Invest.* (2019) 129:1109–14. doi: 10.1172/JCI123791
122. Lo W, Parkhurst M, Robbins PF, Tran E, Lu YC, Jia L, et al. Immunologic recognition of a shared p53 mutated neoantigen in a patient with metastatic colorectal cancer. *Cancer Immunol Res.* (2019) 7:534–43. doi: 10.1158/2326-6066.CIR-18-0686
123. Forghieri F, Riva G, Lagreca I, Barozzi P, Vallerini D, Morselli M, et al. Characterization and dynamics of specific T cells against nucleophosmin-1 (NPM1)-mutated peptides in patients with NPM1-mutated acute myeloid leukemia. *Oncotarget.* (2019) 10:869–82. doi: 10.18632/oncotarget.26617
124. Grimwade D, Hills RK, Moorman AV, Walker H, Chatters S, Goldstone AH, et al. Refinement of cytogenetic classification in acute myeloid leukemia: determination of prognostic significance of rare recurring chromosomal abnormalities among 5876 younger adult patients treated in the United Kingdom Medical Research Council trials. *Blood.* (2010) 116:354–65. doi: 10.1182/blood-2009-11-254441
125. Grimwade D, Ivey A, Huntly BJ. Molecular landscape of acute myeloid leukemia in younger adults and its clinical relevance. *Blood.* (2016) 127:29–41. doi: 10.1182/blood-2015-07-604496
126. Papaemmanuil E, Gerstung M, Malcovati L, Tauro S, Gundem G, Van Loo P, et al. Clinical and biological implications of driver mutations in myelodysplastic syndromes. *Blood.* (2013) 122:3616–27; quiz 99. doi: 10.1182/blood-2013-08-518886
127. Chalmers ZR, Connelly CF, Fabrizio D, Gay L, Ali SM, Ennis R, et al. Analysis of 100,000 human cancer genomes reveals the landscape of tumor mutational burden. *Genome Med.* (2017) 9:34. doi: 10.1186/s13073-017-0424-2
128. Shurtleff SA, Buijs A, Behm FG, Rubnitz JE, Raimondi SC, Hancock ML, et al. TEL/AML1 fusion resulting from a cryptic t(12;21) is the most common genetic lesion in pediatric ALL and defines a subgroup of patients with an excellent prognosis. *Leukemia.* (1995) 9:1985–9.
129. Romana SP, Mauchauffe M, Le Coniat M, Chumakov I, Le Paslier D, Berger R, et al. The t(12;21) of acute lymphoblastic leukemia results in a tel-AML1 gene fusion. *Blood.* (1995) 85:3662–70. doi: 10.1182/blood.V85.12.3662.bloodjournal85123662
130. Romana SP, Poirel H, Leconiat M, Flexor MA, Mauchauffe M, Jonveaux P, et al. High frequency of t(12;21) in childhood B-lineage acute lymphoblastic leukemia. *Blood.* (1995) 86:4263–9. doi: 10.1182/blood.V86.11.4263.bloodjournal86114263
131. Rubnitz JE, Downing JR, Pui CH, Shurtleff SA, Raimondi SC, Evans WE, et al. TEL gene rearrangement in acute lymphoblastic leukemia: a new genetic marker with prognostic significance. *J Clin Oncol.* (1997) 15:1150–7. doi: 10.1200/JCO.1997.15.3.1150
132. Vainchenker W, Kralovics R. Genetic basis and molecular pathophysiology of classical myeloproliferative neoplasms. *Blood.* (2017) 129:667–79. doi: 10.1182/blood-2016-10-695940
133. Holmstrom MO, Riley CH, Svane IM, Hasselbalch HC, Andersen MH. The CALR exon 9 mutations are shared neoantigens in patients with CALR mutant chronic myeloproliferative neoplasms. *Leukemia.* (2016) 30:2413–6. doi: 10.1038/leu.2016.233
134. Voncken JW, Kaartinen V, Pattengale PK, Germeraad WT, Groffen J, Heisterkamp N. BCR/ABL P210 and P190 cause distinct leukemia in transgenic mice. *Blood.* (1995) 86:4603–11. doi: 10.1182/blood.V86.12.4603.bloodjournal86124603
135. Chen W, Peace DJ, Rovira DK, You SG, Cheever MA. T-cell immunity to the joining region of p210BCR-ABL protein. *Proc Natl Acad Sci USA.* (1992) 89:1468–72. doi: 10.1073/pnas.89.4.1468
136. Riley CL, Mathieu MG, Clark RE, McArdle SE, Rees RC. Tumour antigen-targeted immunotherapy for chronic myeloid leukaemia: is it still viable? *Cancer Immunol Immunother.* (2009) 58:1489–99. doi: 10.1007/s00262-009-0675-x
137. Comoli P, Basso S, Riva G, Barozzi P, Guido I, Gurrado A, et al. BCR-ABL-specific T-cell therapy in Ph+ ALL patients on tyrosine-kinase inhibitors. *Blood.* (2017) 129:582–6. doi: 10.1182/blood-2016-07-731091
138. Lynch RG, Graff RJ, Sirisinha S, Simms ES, Eisen HN. Myeloma proteins as tumor-specific transplantation antigens. *Proc Natl Acad Sci USA.* (1972) 69:1540–4. doi: 10.1073/pnas.69.6.1540
139. Bendandi M. Idiotype vaccines for lymphoma: proof-of-principles and clinical trial failures. *Nat Rev Cancer.* (2009) 9:675–81. doi: 10.1038/nrc2717
140. Khodadoust MS, Olsson N, Wagar LE, Haabeth OA, Chen B, Swaminathan K, et al. Antigen presentation profiling reveals recognition of lymphoma immunoglobulin neoantigens. *Nature.* (2017) 543:723–7. doi: 10.1038/nature21433
141. Khodadoust MS, Olsson N, Chen B, Sworder B, Shree T, Liu CL, et al. B-cell lymphomas present immunoglobulin neoantigens. *Blood.* (2019) 133:878–81. doi: 10.1182/blood-2018-06-845156
142. Henry C, Deschamps M, Rohrlich PS, Pallandre JR, Remy-Martin JP, Callanan M, et al. Identification of an alternative CD20 transcript variant in B-cell malignancies coding for a novel protein associated to rituximab resistance. *Blood.* (2010) 115:2420–9. doi: 10.1182/blood-2009-06-229112
143. Nelde A, Walz JS, Kowalewski DJ, Schuster H, Wolz OO, Peper JK, et al. HLA class I-restricted MYD88 L265P-derived peptides as specific targets for lymphoma immunotherapy. *Oncoimmunology.* (2017) 6:e1219825. doi: 10.1080/2162402X.2016.1219825
144. Malumbres M, Barbacid M. RAS oncogenes: the first 30 years. *Nat Rev Cancer.* (2003) 3:459–65. doi: 10.1038/nrc1097
145. Schubbert S, Shannon K, Bollag G. Hyperactive Ras in developmental disorders and cancer. *Nat Rev Cancer.* (2007) 7:295–308. doi: 10.1038/nrc2109
146. Ward AF, Braun BS, Shannon KM. Targeting oncogenic Ras signaling in hematologic malignancies. *Blood.* (2012) 120:3397–406. doi: 10.1182/blood-2012-05-378596
147. Prior IA, Lewis PD, Mattos C. A comprehensive survey of Ras mutations in cancer. *Cancer Res.* (2012) 72:2457–67. doi: 10.1158/0008-5472.CAN-11-2612
148. Vendramini E, Bomben R, Pozzo F, Benedetti D, Bittolo T, Rossi FM, et al. KRAS, NRAS, and BRAF mutations are highly enriched in trisomy 12 chronic lymphocytic leukemia and are associated with shorter treatment-free survival. *Leukemia.* (2019) 33:2111–5. doi: 10.1038/s41375-019-0444-6
149. Hobbs GA, Der CJ, Rossman KL. RAS isoforms and mutations in cancer at a glance. *J Cell Sci.* (2016) 129:1287–92. doi: 10.1242/jcs.182873
150. Holderfield M, Deuker MM, McCormick F, McMahon M. Targeting RAF kinases for cancer therapy: BRAF-mutated melanoma and beyond. *Nat Rev Cancer.* (2014) 14:455–67. doi: 10.1038/nrc3760
151. Tiacci E, Trifonov V, Schiavoni G, Holmes A, Kern W, Martelli MP, et al. BRAF mutations in hairy-cell leukemia. *N Engl J Med.* (2011) 364:2305–15. doi: 10.1056/NEJMoa1014209
152. Arcaini L, Zibellini S, Boveri E, Riboni R, Rattotti S, Varettoni M, et al. The BRAF V600E mutation in hairy cell leukemia and other mature B-cell neoplasms. *Blood.* (2012) 119:188–91. doi: 10.1182/blood-2011-08-368209
153. Chung SS, Kim E, Park JH, Chung YR, Lito P, Teruya-Feldstein J, et al. Hematopoietic stem cell origin of BRAFV600E mutations in hairy cell leukemia. *Sci Transl Med.* (2014) 6:238ra71. doi: 10.1126/scitranslmed.3008004
154. Berres ML, Lim KP, Peters T, Price J, Takizawa H, Salmon H, et al. BRAF-V600E expression in precursor versus differentiated dendritic cells defines clinically distinct LCH risk groups. *J Exp Med.* (2014) 211:669–83. doi: 10.1084/jem.20130977
155. Bouaoun L, Sonkin D, Ardin M, Hollstein M, Byrnes G, Zavadil J, et al. TP53 Variations in human cancers: new lessons from the IARC TP53 database and genomics data. *Hum Mutat.* (2016) 37:865–76. doi: 10.1002/humu.23035
156. Cafri G, Yossef R, Pasetto A, Deniger DC, Lu YC, Parkhurst M, et al. Memory T cells targeting oncogenic mutations detected in peripheral blood of epithelial cancer patients. *Nat Commun.* (2019) 10:449. doi: 10.1038/s41467-019-08304-z
157. Sharkey MS, Lizee G, Gonzales MI, Patel S, Topalian SL. $CD4^+$ T-cell recognition of mutated B-RAF in melanoma patients harboring the V599E mutation. *Cancer Res.* (2004) 64:1595–9. doi: 10.1158/0008-5472.CAN-03-3231
158. Kandoth C, McLellan MD, Vandin F, Ye K, Niu B, Lu C, et al. Mutational landscape and significance across 12 major cancer types. *Nature.* (2013) 502:333–9. doi: 10.1038/nature12634

159. Deniger DC, Pasetto A, Tran E, Parkhurst MR, Cohen CJ, Robbins PF, et al. Stable, nonviral expression of mutated tumor neoantigen-specific t-cell receptors using the sleeping beauty transposon/transposase system. *Mol Ther.* (2016) 24:1078–89. doi: 10.1038/mt.2016.51
160. Yossef R, Tran E, Deniger DC, Gros A, Pasetto A, Parkhurst MR, et al. Enhanced detection of neoantigen-reactive T cells targeting unique and shared oncogenes for personalized cancer immunotherapy. *JCI Insight.* (2018) 3:e122467. doi: 10.1172/jci.insight.122467
161. Noonan KA, Huff CA, Davis J, Lemas MV, Fiorino S, Bitzan J, et al. Adoptive transfer of activated marrow-infiltrating lymphocytes induces measurable antitumor immunity in the bone marrow in multiple myeloma. *Sci Transl Med.* (2015) 7:288ra78. doi: 10.1126/scitranslmed.aaa7014
162. Chapuis AG, Ragnarsson GB, Nguyen HN, Chaney CN, Pufnock JS, Schmitt TM, et al. Transferred WT1-reactive CD8+ T cells can mediate antileukemic activity and persist in post-transplant patients. *Sci Transl Med.* (2013) 5:174ra27. doi: 10.1126/scitranslmed.3004916
163. Ochi T, Fujiwara H, Okamoto S, An J, Nagai K, Shirakata T, et al. Novel adoptive T-cell immunotherapy using a WT1-specific TCR vector encoding silencers for endogenous TCRs shows marked antileukemia reactivity and safety. *Blood.* (2011) 118:1495–503. doi: 10.1182/blood-2011-02-337089
164. Ohminami H, Yasukawa M, Fujita S. HLA class I-restricted lysis of leukemia cells by a $CD8^+$ cytotoxic T-lymphocyte clone specific for WT1 peptide. *Blood.* (2000) 95:286–93. doi: 10.1182/blood.V95.1.286
165. Chapuis AG, Egan DN, Bar M, Schmitt TM, McAfee MS, Paulson KG, et al. T cell receptor gene therapy targeting WT1 prevents acute myeloid leukemia relapse post-transplant. *Nat Med.* (2019) 25:1064–72. doi: 10.1038/s41591-019-0472-9
166. Hung K, Hayashi R, Lafond-Walker A, Lowenstein C, Pardoll D, Levitsky H. The central role of $CD4^+$ T cells in the antitumor immune response. *J Exp Med.* (1998) 188:2357–68. doi: 10.1084/jem.188.12.2357
167. Dossa RG, Cunningham T, Sommermeyer D, Medina-Rodriguez I, Biernacki MA, Foster K, et al. Development of T-cell immunotherapy for hematopoietic stem cell transplantation recipients at risk of leukemia relapse. *Blood.* (2018) 131:108–20. doi: 10.1182/blood-2017-07-791608
168. Sommermeyer D, Hudecek M, Kosasih PL, Gogishvili T, Maloney DG, Turtle CJ, et al. Chimeric antigen receptor-modified T cells derived from defined CD8+ and CD4+ subsets confer superior antitumor reactivity *in vivo.* *Leukemia.* (2016) 30:492–500. doi: 10.1038/leu.2015.247
169. Di Stasi A, Tey SK, Dotti G, Fujita Y, Kennedy-Nasser A, Martinez C, et al. Inducible apoptosis as a safety switch for adoptive cell therapy. *N Engl J Med.* (2011) 365:1673–83. doi: 10.1056/NEJMoa1106152
170. Biernacki MA, Brault M, Bleakley M. T-cell receptor-based immunotherapy for hematologic malignancies. *Cancer J.* (2019) 25:179–90. doi: 10.1097/PPO.0000000000000378
171. Kebriaei P, Singh H, Huls MH, Figliola MJ, Bassett R, Olivares S, et al. Phase I trials using Sleeping Beauty to generate CD19-specific CAR T cells. *J Clin Invest.* (2016) 126:3363–76. doi: 10.1172/JCI86721
172. Bishop DC, Xu N, Tse B, O'Brien TA, Gottlieb DJ, Dolnikov A, et al. PiggyBac-engineered T cells expressing CD19-specific CARs that Lack IgG1 Fc spacers have potent activity against B-ALL xenografts. *Mol Ther.* (2018) 26:1883–95. doi: 10.1016/j.ymthe.2018.05.007
173. Wang J, Ma Z, Carr SA, Mertins P, Zhang H, Zhang Z, et al. Proteome profiling outperforms transcriptome profiling for coexpression based gene function prediction. *Mol Cell Proteomics.* (2017) 16:121–34. doi: 10.1074/mcp.M116.060301
174. Campillo-Davo D, Fujiki F, Van den Bergh JMJ, De Reu H, Smits E, Goossens H, et al. Efficient and non-genotoxic RNA-based engineering of human T cells using tumor-specific T cell receptors with minimal TCR mispairing. *Front Immunol.* (2018) 9:2503. doi: 10.3389/fimmu.2018.02503
175. Torikai H, Reik A, Soldner F, Warren EH, Yuen C, Zhou Y, et al. Toward eliminating HLA class I expression to generate universal cells from allogeneic donors. *Blood.* (2013) 122:1341–9. doi: 10.1182/blood-2013-03-478255
176. Lemos H, Huang L, Prendergast GC, Mellor AL. Immune control by amino acid catabolism during tumorigenesis and therapy. *Nat Rev Cancer.* (2019) 19:162–75. doi: 10.1038/s41568-019-0106-z
177. van der Burg SH, Arens R, Ossendorp F, van Hall T, Melief CJ. Vaccines for established cancer: overcoming the challenges posed by immune evasion. *Nat Rev Cancer.* (2016) 16:219–33. doi: 10.1038/nrc.2016.16
178. Fukuno K, Hara T, Tsurumi H, Shibata Y, Mabuchi R, Nakamura N, et al. Expression of indoleamine 2,3-dioxygenase in leukemic cells indicates an unfavorable prognosis in acute myeloid leukemia patients with intermediate-risk cytogenetics. *Leuk Lymphoma.* (2015) 56:1398–405. doi: 10.3109/10428194.2014.953150
179. Mussai F, De Santo C, Abu-Dayyeh I, Booth S, Quek L, McEwen-Smith RM, et al. Acute myeloid leukemia creates an arginase-dependent immunosuppressive microenvironment. *Blood.* (2013) 122:749–58. doi: 10.1182/blood-2013-01-480129
180. Zhang L, Gajewski TF, Kline J. PD-1/PD-L1 interactions inhibit antitumor immune responses in a murine acute myeloid leukemia model. *Blood.* (2009) 114:1545–52. doi: 10.1182/blood-2009-03-206672
181. Buggins AG, Milojkovic D, Arno MJ, Lea NC, Mufti GJ, Thomas NS, et al. Microenvironment produced by acute myeloid leukemia cells prevents T cell activation and proliferation by inhibition of NF-kappaB, c-Myc, and pRb pathways. *J Immunol.* (2001) 167:6021–30. doi: 10.4049/jimmunol.167.10.6021
182. Bruck O, Blom S, Dufva O, Turkki R, Chheda H, Ribeiro A, et al. Immune cell contexture in the bone marrow tumor microenvironment impacts therapy response in CML. *Leukemia.* (2018) 32:1643–56. doi: 10.1038/s41375-018-0175-0
183. Burger JA, Gribben JG. The microenvironment in chronic lymphocytic leukemia (CLL) and other B cell malignancies: insight into disease biology and new targeted therapies. *Semin Cancer Biol.* (2014) 24:71–81. doi: 10.1016/j.semcancer.2013.08.011

18

Clinical Value of ctDNA in Hematological Malignancies (Lymphomas, Multiple Myeloma, Myelodysplastic Syndrome and Leukemia)

Xiangyu Tan[1], *Han Yan*[1], *Lei Chen*[1], *Yuyang Zhang*[1] *and Chunyan Sun*[1,2*]

[1] *Department of Hematology, Union Hospital, Tongji Medical College, Huazhong University of Science and Technology, Wuhan, China,* [2] *Collaborative Innovation Center of Hematology, Huazhong University of Science and Technology, Wuhan, China*

Correspondence:
Chunyan Sun
suncy0618@163.com

Background: Circulating tumor DNA (ctDNA) has offered a minimally invasive approach for the detection and measurement of cancer. However, its diagnostic and prognostic value in hematological malignancies remains unclear.

Materials and methods: Pubmed, Embase, and Cochrane Library were searched for relating literature. Diagnostic accuracy variables and disease progression prediction data were pooled by the Meta-Disc version 1.4 software. Review Manager version 5.4 software was applied for prognostic data analysis.

Results: A total of 11 studies met our inclusion criteria. In terms of diagnosis, the pooled sensitivity and specificity were 0.51 (95% confidence intervals (CI) 0.38–0.64) and 0.96 (95% CI 0.88–1.00), respectively. The AUSROC (area under the SROC) curve was 0.89 (95%CI 0.75–1.03). When it comes to the prediction of disease progression, the overall sensitivity and specificity was 0.83 (95% CI 0.67–0.94) and 0.98 (95% CI 0.93–1.00), respectively. Moreover, a significant association also existed between the presence of ctDNA and worse progression-free survival (HR 2.63, 95% CI 1.27–5.43, $p = 0.009$), as well as overall survival (HR 2.92, 95% CI 1.53–5.57, $p = 0.001$).

Conclusions: The use of ctDNA in clinical practice for hematological malignancies is promising, as it may not only contribute to diagnosis, but could also predict the prognosis of patients so as to guide treatment. In the future, more studies are needed to realize the standardization of sequencing techniques and improve the detection sensitivity of exploration methods.

Keywords: circulating tumor DNA, hematological malignancies, lymphomas, multiple myeloma, myelodysplastic syndrome, leukemia, meta-analysis

INTRODUCTION

In recent years, significant progress in the diagnosis and treatment of hematological malignancies has been made. However, the current gold standard for disease diagnosis and monitoring, tissue or bone marrow (BM) biopsy, is invasive and painful. A further issue is that sampling a single tumor site during biopsy may not reveal all malignant clones (1).

Mandel and Metais first described the presence of DNA molecules in human plasma in 1948 (2). In 1994, Vasioukhin et al. described the presence of tumor-specific mutations in cell-free DNA (cfDNA) of patients with myelodysplastic syndrome (MDS) and acute myeloid leukemia (AML), demonstrating the significance of circulating tumor DNA (ctDNA) analysis in hematologic malignancies (3, 4). Unfortunately, due to the lack of sensitive and specific detection methods, the research on cfDNA is relatively behind. With the recent advent of new techniques, such as droplet digital polymerase chain reaction (ddPCR) and next-generation sequencing (NGS), tumor-derived fragmented DNA in the plasma or serum, known as ctDNA, has the ability to be one of the most sensitive, non-invasive biomarkers available for use in cancer patients (5). Compared with a classic biopsy, ctDNA is more convenient and presents minor procedural risk to the patient, with a less expensive price. And more importantly, ctDNA has been determined to have a half-time of 16 min to 2.5 h in circulation, which enables ctDNA analysis to be considered as a real-time snapshot of disease burden (6). In theory, ctDNA could also deliver more complete information regarding the patient's entire tumor burden, because the sample may represent all tumor DNA present in the circulation, without spatial limitations of the biopsy sampling of a single lesion within a single anatomic site (7).

Although many recent studies have focused on applications in hematological malignancies (8–13), the results are still unclear. Therefore, we performed a meta-analysis to estimate the clinical application value in patients with hematological malignancies.

METHODS

Search Strategy

We searched for studies in Pubmed, Embase, and Cochrane library with no restriction of publication date using key words "lymphomas AND ctDNA," "myeloma AND ctDNA," "myelodysplastic syndrome AND ctDNA," and "leukemia AND ctDNA."

Inclusion Criteria, Exclusion Criteria

Two reviewers evaluated potential articles independently, according to the inclusion and exclusion criteria mentioned below. Discrepancies were resolved by discussion until a consensus was reached.

Inclusion criteria: (1) retrospective and prospective observational cohort studies involving patients with lymphoma, multiple myeloma, myelodysplastic syndrome, or leukemia; (2) ctDNA was analyzed in patients; (3) information on the diagnostic, prognostic, or predictive value of ctDNA was provided; (4) prognostic studies had to report the results of a survival analysis in the form of a hazard ratio and 95 % confidence intervals; (5) a sample size≥5; (6) reported in English; and (7) participants were adults.

Exclusion criteria: (1) cell-free DNA without information of mutations; (2) circulating viral DNA; (3) lack of outcomes; and (4) conference abstracts, comments, reviews, case reports, or meta-analyses.

Data Extraction

Only full-text articles were taken into consideration. Extracted study characteristics included: first author, publication year, type of cancer, number of patients, ctDNA measurement method, and mutation evaluated in ctDNA. If the eligible studies provided survival data, hazard ration (HR) for overall survival (OS), progress-free survival (PFS), event-free survival (EFS), or disease progressing with 95% confidence interval (CI) they were extracted.

TABLE 1 | Results of diagnosis quality assessment of included studies according to the QUADAS-2 tool criteria.

Study	Risk of bias				Applicability concerns		
	Patients selection	Index text	Reference standard	Flow and time	Patients selection	Index text	Reference standard
Fontanilles, M.2017	L	L	L	L	L	L	L
Hickmann, A.K.2019	U	L	U	L	L	L	L
Mazzotti.C 2018	U	L	L	L	U	L	L
Sakata-Yanagimoto, M 2017	U	L	L	U	L	L	L
Watanabe, J. 2019 PCNSL	L	L	L	L	L	L	L

L: low risk of bias; H: high risk of bias; U: unclear risk of bias.

TABLE 2 | A study could be allocated one point for each of the seven criteria; in case of ambiguity, half a point was assigned.

Adapted REMARK criteria for quality assessment (1 point/criteria)	
1.	Case selection adequate (baselines from medical chart)
2.	States the marker examined and the aim of the study
3.	Reporting at least the following characteristics: disease stage, histology, and received treatment
4.	States the time and type of sampling (serum/plasma)
5.	States the assay methods used and provides a detailed protocol (at least cfDNA isolation, sequence method, and sequence depth)
6.	A clear description of the flow of patients through the study
7.	A clear description of the reasons for dropout

A study was included for further analysis when graded ≥ 5.5 points.

Abbreviations: ctDNA, circulating tumor DNA; BM, bone marrow; cfDNA, cell-free DNA; ddPCR, droplet digital polymerase chain reaction; NGS, next-generation sequencing; HR, hazard ration; OS, overall survival; PFS, progress-free survival; EFS, event-free survival; CI, confidence interval; PLR, positive likelihood ratios; NLR, negative likelihood ratios; DOR, diagnostic ratios; SROC, the summary receiver operating characteristic curve; EGFR, epidermal growth factor receptor; MRD, the minimal residual disease; MAF, the mutant allele fraction; MDS, myelodysplastic syndrome.

TABLE 3 | Prognostic studies were scored according to the criteria in **Table 2**.

Study	1	2	3	4	5	6	7	Total
Roschewski, M.2015	1	1	1	1	1	1	1	7
Assouline, S. E.2016	1	1	1	1	1	1	1	7
Kurtz, D. M.2018	1	0.5	1	1	0.5	1	1	6
Sarkozy, C.2017	1	1	1	1	0.5	1	1	6.5
Fontanilles, M. 2017	1	1	1	1	1	1	1	7
Hossain, N. M.2019	0.5	1	0.5	1	0.5	1	1	5.5
Qiong Li.2020	1	1	1	1	1	1	1	7

Studies' Quality Assessment

The results of diagnosis quality assessment were shown in **Table 1**. The quality of prognostic studies was assessed by an adapted version of the reporting recommendations for tumor marker prognostic studies (REMARK) criteria for biomarker studies (**Table 2**) (14). Detailed information on quality assessment about prognostic studies was shown in **Table 3**.

Statistical Analysis

Diagnostic variables, such as sensitivity, specificity, likelihood ratios [i.e., positive likelihood ratios (PLR) or negative likelihood ratios (NLR)], diagnostic ratios (DOR), and the summary receiver operating characteristic curve (SROC) were calculated and analyzed using the Meta-Disc software, version 1.4. The pooled HR and the 95% CIs for OS or PFS were analyzed by the Review Manager version 5.4 software. We used a random-effect model if significant heterogeneity was observed ($P < 0.05$ or $I^2 >$ 50%); if not, we would turn to a fixed-effect model.

RESULTS

A total of 996 articles were identified through the search (**Figure 1**). After screening, 273 duplicated studies were removed, and 674 studies were excluded based on their titles and abstracts. A further 39 studies were excluded for not fulfilling the inclusion criteria. Finally, a total of 11 studies were included in the meta-analysis. The details and main characteristics of included studies are summarized in **Table 4**.

ctDNA as Marker for Diagnosis in Hematological Malignancies

Five studies were pooled for the meta-analysis of diagnostic accuracy. As presented in **Figure 2**, the overall sensitivity and specificity was 0.51 (95% CI 0.38–0.64) and 0.96 (95% CI 0.88–1.00) respectively. The pooled PLR and NLR were 4.04 (95% CI 1.68–9.70) and 0.60 (95% CI 0.37–0.98), respectively. The area under the SROC was 0.89 and the DOR was 14.60 (95%CI 3.74–57.02).

ctDNA as Prognostic Marker in Hematological Malignancies

Three studies were pooled for the meta-analysis of disease progression prediction. As shown in **Figure 3**, the overall sensitivity and specificity was 0.83 (95% CI 0.67–0.94) and 0.98 (95% CI 0.93–1.00) respectively. The pooled PLR and NLR were 17.31 (95%CI 4.11–72.84) and 0.21 (95% CI 0.09–0.49), respectively. The DOR was 145.74 (95% CI 30.17–704.12).

Three articles with a total of 266 patients included analysis on the association of ctDNA and PFS in patients with hematological malignancies. A significantly worse PFS for ctDNA positive patients was observed(HR 2.63, 95% CI 1.27–5.43)(**Figure 4**). Moreover, there were four articles with 352 patients that included analysis on the association of ctDNA and OS with hematological malignancies. Patients who had ctDNA positive or higher ctDNA levels had a worse OS (HR 2.92, 95% CI 1.53–5.57) (**Figure 5**).

DISCUSSION

Since fragmented DNA was first found in the whole blood by Mandel and Metais, cfDNA and ctDNA have been applied in a variety of disciplines. For example, detection of ctDNA is an effective method to determine EGFR status in NSCLC, providing a more expedient measure to predict resistance to EGFR tyrosine kinase inhibitors and prognosis (25). A study showed that ctDNA monitoring may help identify hematologic cancer patients at risk for relapse in advance of established clinical parameters (8). However, the relationship between ctDNA and hematological malignancies remains unclear. Therefore, it is necessary to conduct comprehensive analysis illuminating the clinical utility of ctDNA in the diagnoses of patients with hematological malignancies and prognosis prediction.

Our pooled data have shown that the detection of ctDNA has an obvious advantage in hematological malignancies diagnosis specificity (specificity: 0.96, 95% CI 0.88–1.00). A phase 1 clinical trial which studied the clinical value of ctDNA in MDS showed that there was an excellent correlation ($r^2 = 0.84$; $P < 0.0001$) between the mutant allele fraction (MAF) of somatic mutations in BM and ctDNA across multiple matched time points (26). Another study on gene detection with 26 patients with MDS showed that the correlation of 52 somatic mutations detected in BM and ctDNA was also significant ($R^2 = 0.8272$, $P <$ 0.0001) (13). These results imply that mutations in ctDNA may represent somatic mutations in tumor cells. So in this regard, ctDNA testing is a good alternative to biopsy because of its non-invasive advantages. However, in terms of test sensitivity, the present evidence showed no superiority of ctDNA over biopsy (sensitivity: 0.51, 95% CI 0.38–0.64). Hematologic tumors are highly heterogeneous, with various gene mutations in a tumor,

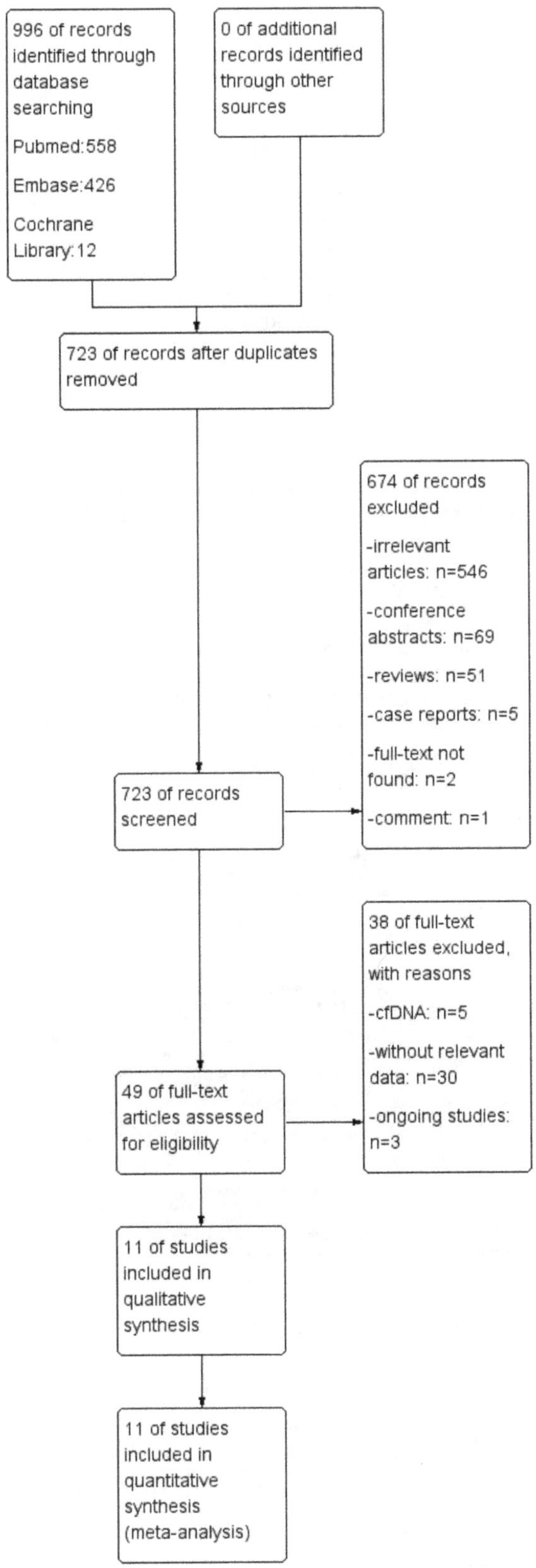

FIGURE 1 | Flow chartof selection process to enrolleligiblestudie.

which may be one of the main reasons for its lack of sensitivity. On the other hand, we pooled results of various tumors and mutations on account of the limited number of studies in our meta-analysis, which may lead to inaccurate results. Therefore, more accurate circulating gene targets need to be defined. To increase the sensitivity of ctDNA, there is a necessity to study the detection rate of ctDNA using a panel-based NGS approach, and panels should include the most-frequently mutated genes in tumor tissue.

The quantitative level of ctDNA has prognostic value for patients which could influence therapy choices (27, 28). Detection of ctDNA clearance during first-line chemotherapy can reflect tumor response to treatment, which may allow real-time adjustment of duration or intensity, or identification of patients at high risk of treatment failure (20). Similar to our results, studies by Herrera et al. also showed a correlation between ctDNA and disease progression as well as recurrence, whose multivariable model results show that detectable ctDNA was associated with increased risk of progression/death (HR 3.9, $P = 0.003$) and relapse/progression (HR 10.8, $P = 0.0006$) (29). Moreover, some studies indicated that detectable ctDNA was also associated with tumor volume, which means ctDNA is associated with tumor burden in patients (11, 24). Given the non-invasive nature and short half-life of ctDNA, its interim monitoring during therapy can provide a real-time assessment of tumor dynamics, allowing for an early indication of response or resistance to therapy. After treatment, ctDNA can be used for post-treatment monitoring. It can perform a similar function to surveillance imaging without the need for radiation exposure, which may potentially increase susceptibility to preclinical recurrence, and ultimately allow for early intervention (28, 30, 31). The study by Roschewski et.al. showed that patients developed detectable ctDNA a median of 3.5 months before clinical evidence of disease (20). Similarly, ctDNA detected relapse at a mean of 6 months before imaging detection in another study by Scherer et al. (32). These encouraging results suggest that ctDNA may help faster relapse detection, and allows subsequent therapy to be initiated before clinical progression. These findings will highly strengthen the value of ctDNA in clinical management of patients with hematological malignancies.

As is shown in our pooled data, the presence of ctDNA or higher levels of ctDNA is associated with a poorer PFS and OS. Sarkozy's study has a similar result to us, showing that patients with higher levels of ctDNA experienced a significantly shorter PFS than those with lower levels of ctDNA (median 15.3 months vs. not reached, $p = 0.004$) (23). Another study also showed that patients with detectable ctDNA have worse survival outcomes than those without (6). These results imply that ctDNA assessment could be a useful alternative endpoint for PFS and OS.

Several limitations in this study need to be addressed. Firstly, the lack of a well-accepted ctDNA gene target might contribute to the presence of bias. Secondly, due to the limited studies, we included little data which may lead to results' bias. Furthermore,

TABLE 4 | Major characteristics of enrolled studies.

No.	Study	Type of cancer	Number of patients	ctDNA measurement method	Mutation evaluated in ctDNA
1	Fontanilles, M. (14)	PCNSL	50	NGS	MYD88 c.T778C
2	Hickmann, A, K. (15)	PCNSL	6	NGS	MYD88, PIM1, BCL2, ETV6, KMT2D, LPHN3, PRDM1, CD79B, SOCS1, IRF4, MYC, FOXB1, LRP1B, HLA-B, LTF, EPHA5, EP400, SYNE1, BLNK, STAT3, FES, SEPT9, POLR3A, DPYD, TFE3, CSMD3, FAT1, KIT, MAGI1, TP53, ASXL1, SETD2, IDH2, MTRR, PBRM1, BCR, MN1, RNF213, TOP1, ATM, FANCM, CDKN1B, PAX5, FOXO1, MCL1, PTPRT, CARD11, PPM1D, DST, BCL10, TCL1A, FN1, HSP90AA1, NIN, SLCO1B1, HSP90AB1, ARID5B, ETS1, ERBB4, CCND2, HLA-C, ITGB2, EPHA3, BCL6, TBL1XR1, PCBP1, RECQL4, CREBBP, STAT4, MLLT3, KEAP1, BTK
3	Mazzotti,C. (16)	MM	37	NGS	IGH, IGK, IGL rearrangements
4	Sakata-Yanagimoto, M. (17)	PTCL	14	Targeted sequencing	G17V-RHOA
5	Watanabe, J. (18)	PCNSL	12	ddPCR	MYD88
6	Roschewski, M. (19)	DLBCL	126	NGS	VDJ rearrangements
7	Assouline, S. E. (20)	DLBCL	20	CAPP-seq and ddPCR	EZH2, MEF2B, CREBBP, EP300, MLL2, FAS, STAT6, TP53, MYD88, MLL3
8	Kurtz, D. M. (21)	DLBCL	217	CAPP-seq	ABCB11, ACTG1, AFF1, APC, B2M, BCHE, BCL10, BCL2, BCL6, BTG1, BTG3, BTK, CAPZA3, CARD11, CCND1, CCND3, DSEL, EGR1, EPHA7, RF1, IRF4, KRAS, LAMA1, MAP2K1, MC5R, MED12, MEF2B, PXDN, RASSF9, STAT6, ZFP42, ZMYM6, ZNF608, ZNF678, et al.
9	Sarkozy, C. (22)	FL	29	NGS	VDJ rearrangements
10	Hossain, N. M. (23)	DLBCL	6	NGS	immunoglobulin gene V(D)J rearrangements
11	Qiong, Li. (24)	ENTKL	65	NGS	ADAM3A, APC, ARID1A, ARID1B, ARID2, ASXL3, ATM, BCOR, BCORL1, CD28, CHD8, CREBBP, DDX3X, DNMT3A, EP300, EZH2, FYN, IDH2, IL2RG, JAK1, JAK3, KDM6A, KMT2A, KMT2D, MGA, NF1, NOTCH1, PRDM1, PTPN1, RHOA, SETD2, SOCS1, STAT3, STAT5B, STAT6, TET1, TET2, TNFRSF14, TP53, TRAF3, ZAP608

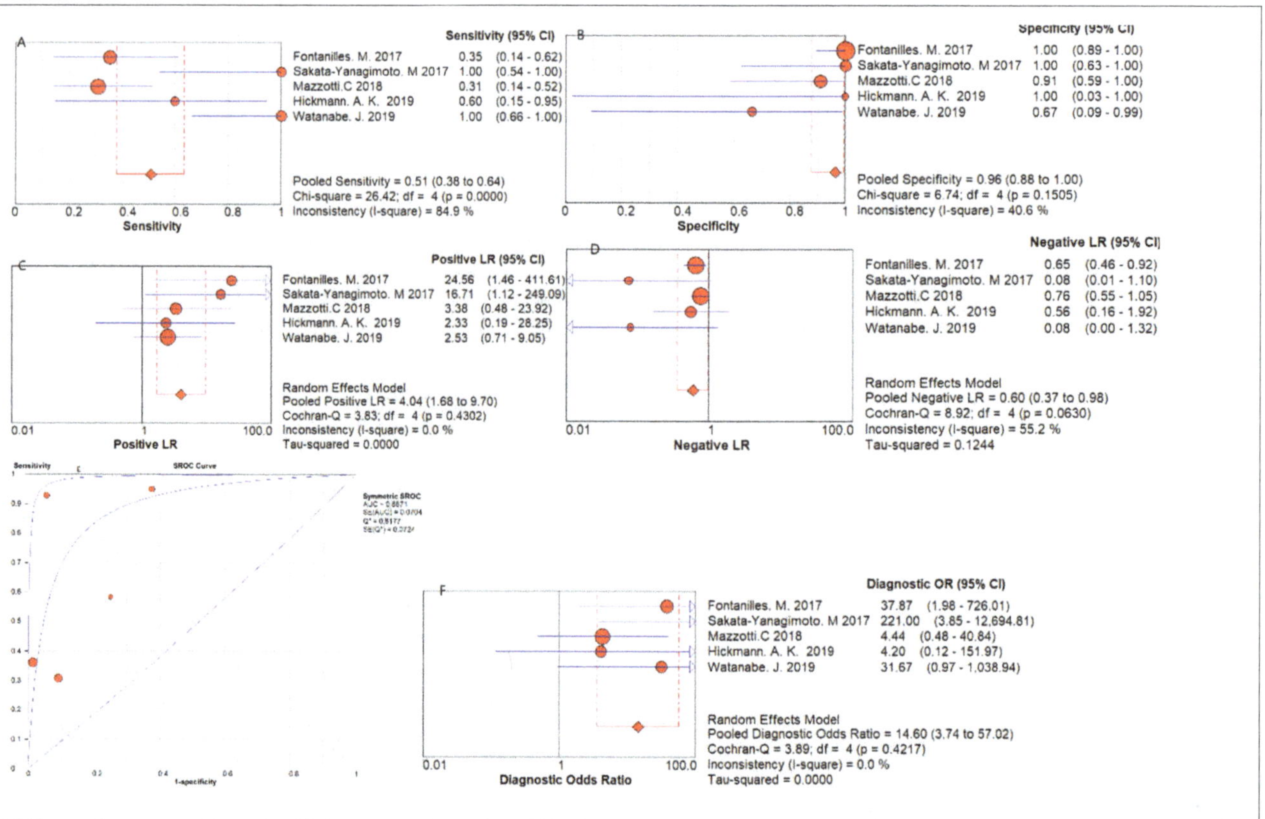

FIGURE 2 | Diagnostic accuracy forest plots. **(A)** Forest plots of overall sensitivity. **(B)** Forest plots of overall specificity. **(C)** Forest plots of positive likelihood ratio. **(D)** Forest plots of negative likelihood ratio. **(E)** Forest plots of SROC Curve. **(F)** Forest plots of diagnostic odds ratio.

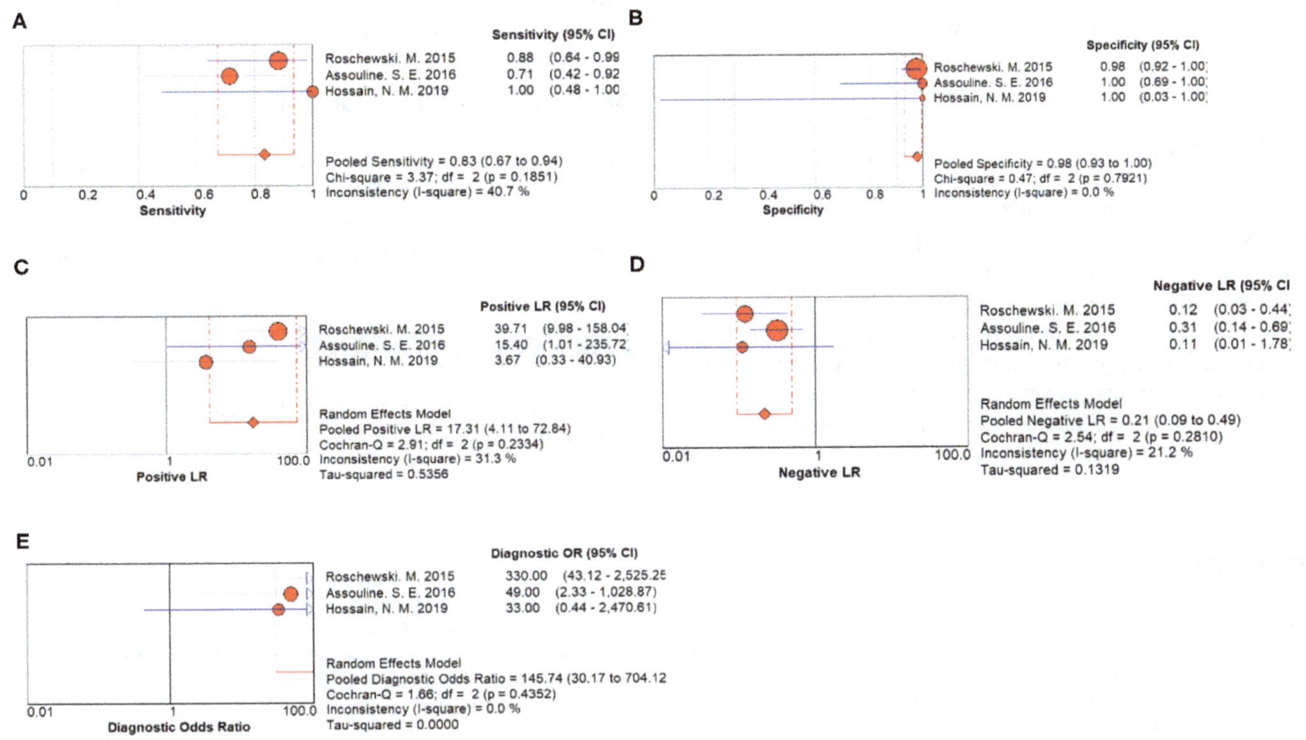

FIGURE 3 | Disease progression prediction forest plots. **(A)** Forest plots of overall sensitivity. **(B)** Forest plots of overall specificity. **(C)** Forest plots of positive likelihood ratio. **(D)** Forest plots of negative likelihood ratio. **(E)** Forest plots of diagnostic odds ratio.

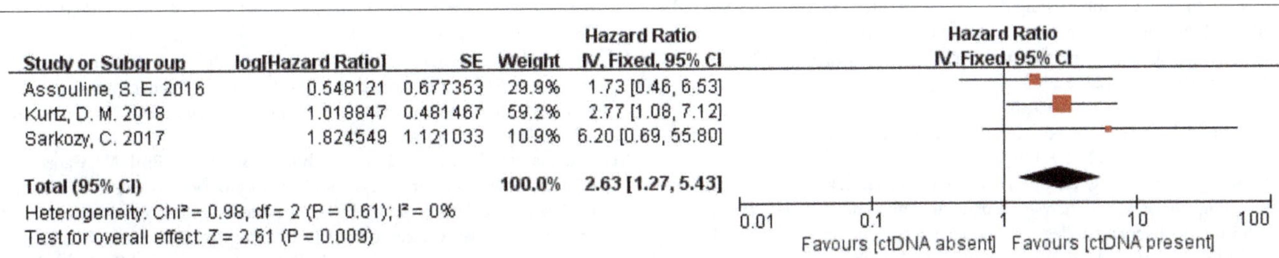

FIGURE 4 | Forest plot of a Fixed-effect meta-analysis of the prognostic role of ctDNA on progression-free survival.

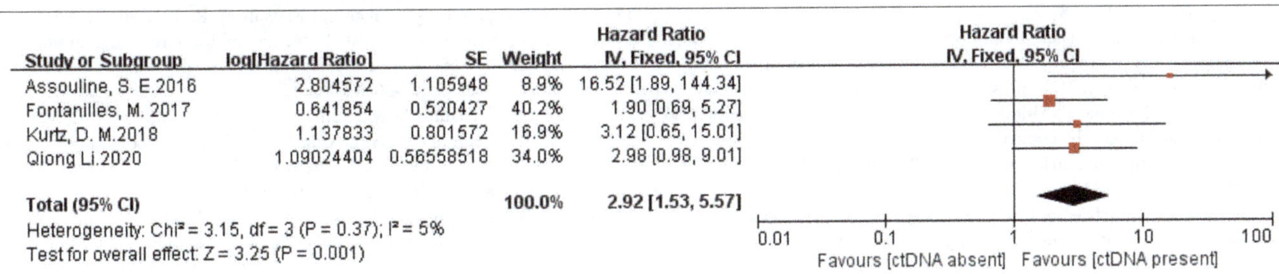

FIGURE 5 | Forest plot of a Fixed-effect meta-analysis of the prognostic role of ctDNA on overall survival.

the difference in detection method and materials, such as PCR primers or the equipment applied, is also an important source of study bias. Therefore, our conclusion might not be universal suitable.

Despite its preliminary nature, this study clearly indicated that the presence of ctDNA in hematological malignancies patients predicted unfavorable survival. Before its wide application in hematological malignancies patients, some concerns still need to be addressed, including more accurate molecule targets and more suitable detection techniques. In a word, more prospective studies with consistent and standardized methodology are needed to further resolve these problems.

CONCLUSIONS

In summary, our meta-analysis revealed that the presence of ctDNA is related to a worse prognosis in patients with hematological malignancies (lymphomas, multiple myeloma, myelodysplastic syndrome, or leukemia). Moreover, ctDNA is a potential diagnostic biomarker in hematological malignancies, although the low diagnostic accuracy is a point of concern. The specificity and non-invasive nature of ctDNA testing, as well as its ability to reflect the patient's tumor burden in real time, makes it a potential substitute for biopsy. In the future, more studies are needed to realize the standardization of sequencing techniques and explore methods to improve detection sensitivity.

AUTHOR CONTRIBUTIONS

XYT and HY collected and analyzed the data and wrote the paper. LC analyzed the data. YYZ revised the paper. CYS conceived and designed this study, analyzed the data, and wrote the paper. All authors read, reviewed, and approved the final manuscript.

ACKNOWLEDGMENTS

We would like to thank the researchers and study participants for their contributions.

REFERENCES

1. Kubaczkova V, Vrabel D, Sedlarikova L, Besse L, Sevcikova S. Cell-free DNA—minimally invasive marker of hematological malignancies. *Eur J Haematol.* (2017) 99:291–9. doi: 10.1111/ejh.12925
2. Mandel P, Metais P. The nucleic acids in blood plasma in humans. *C R Seances Soc Biol Fil.* (1948) 142:241–3.
3. Vasioukhin V, Anker P, Maurice P, Lyautey J, Lederrey C, Stroun M. Point mutations of the N-ras gene in the blood plasma DNA of patients with myelodysplastic syndrome or acute myelogenous leukaemia. *Br J Haematol.* (1994) 86:774–9. doi: 10.1111/j.1365-2141.1994.tb04828.x
4. Postel M, Roosen A, Laurent-Puig P, Taly V, Wang-Renault SF. Droplet-based digital PCR and next generation sequencing for monitoring circulating tumor DNA: a cancer diagnostic perspective. *Expert Rev Mol Diagn.* (2018) 18:7–17. doi: 10.1080/14737159.2018.1400384
5. Wan JCM, Massie C, Garcia-Corbacho J, Mouliere F, Brenton JD, Caldas C, et al. Liquid biopsies come of age: towards implementation of circulating tumour DNA. *Nat Rev Cancer.* (2017) 17:223–38. doi: 10.1038/nrc.2017.7
6. Merker JD, Oxnard GR, Compton C, Diehn M, Hurley P, Lazar AJ, et al. Circulating tumor DNA analysis in patients with cancer: American society of clinical oncology and college of american pathologists joint review. *J Clin Oncol.* (2018) 36:1631–41. doi: 10.1200/JCO.2017.76.8671
7. Nakamura S, Yokoyama K, Yusa N, Ogawa M, Takei T, Kobayashi A, et al. Circulating tumor DNA dynamically predicts response and/or relapse in patients with hematological malignancies. *Int J Hematol.* (2018) 108:402–10. doi: 10.1007/s12185-018-2487-2
8. Kis O, Kaedbey R, Chow S, Danesh A, Dowar M, Li T, et al. Circulating tumour DNA sequence analysis as an alternative to multiple myeloma bone marrow aspirates. *Nat Commun.* (2017) 8:15086. doi: 10.1038/ncomms15086
9. Nakamura S, Yokoyama K, Shimizu E, Yusa N, Kondoh K, Ogawa M, et al. Prognostic impact of circulating tumor DNA status post–allogeneic hematopoietic stem cell transplantation in AML and MDS. *Blood.* (2019) 133:2682–95. doi: 10.1182/blood-2018-10-880690
10. Chen F, Pang D, Guo H, Jiang X, Liu S, Huang L, et al. Clinicopathological characteristics and mutational profiling of adult t-cell lymphoblastic lymphoma in a chinese population. *Cancer Manage Res.* (2020) 12:3003–12. doi: 10.2147/CMAR.S242903
11. Long X, Xu Q, Lou Y, Li C, Gu J, Cai H, et al. The utility of non-invasive liquid biopsy for mutational analysis and minimal residual disease assessment in extramedullary multiple myeloma. *Br J Haematol.* (2020). 189:e45–8. doi: 10.1111/bjh.16440
12. Zhao P, Qin J, Liu W, Zhu Q, Fan T, Xiao H, et al. Using circulating tumor DNA to monitor myelodysplastic syndromes status. *Hematol Oncol.* (2019) 37:531–3. doi: 10.1002/hon.2649
13. Creemers A, Krausz S, Strijker M, van der Wel MJ, Soer EC, Reinten RJ, et al. Clinical value of ctDNA in upper-GI cancers: A systematic review and meta-analysis. *Biochim Biophys Acta Rev Cancer.* (2017). (1868). 394–403. doi: 10.1016/j.bbcan.2017.08.002
14. Fontanilles M, Marguet F, Bohers É, Viailly PJ, Dubois S, Bertrand P, et al. Non-invasive detection of somatic mutations using next-generation sequencing in primary central nervous system lymphoma. *Oncotarget.* (2017) 8:48157–68. doi: 10.18632/oncotarget.18325
15. Hickmann AK, Frick M, Hadaschik D, Battke F, Bittl M, Ganslandt O, et al. Molecular tumor analysis and liquid biopsy: A feasibility investigation analyzing circulating tumor DNA in patients with central nervous system lymphomas. *BMC Cancer.* (2019) 19:192. doi: 10.1186/s12885-019-5394-x
16. Mazzotti C, Buisson L, Maheo S, Perrot A, Chretien ML, Leleu X, et al. Myeloma MRD by deep sequencing from circulating tumor DNA does not correlate with results obtained in the bone marrow. *Blood Adv.* (2018) 2:2811–3. doi: 10.1182/bloodadvances.2018025197
17. Sakata-Yanagimoto M, Nakamoto-Matsubara R, Komori D, Nguyen TB, Hattori K, Nanmoku T, et al. Detection of the circulating tumor DNAs in angioimmunoblastic T- cell lymphoma. *Ann Hematol.* (2017) 96:1471–5. doi: 10.1007/s00277-017-3038-2
18. Watanabe J, Natsumeda M, Kanemaru Y, Okada M, Oishi M, Kakita A, et al. Comparison of circulating tumor DNA between body fluids in patients with primary central nervous system lymphoma. *Leuk Lymphoma.* (2019) 60:3587–9. doi: 10.1080/10428194.2019.1639169
19. Roschewski M, Dunleavy K, Pittaluga S, Moorhead M, Pepin F, Kong K, et al. Circulating tumour DNA and CT monitoring in patients with untreated

diffuse large B-cell lymphoma: a correlative biomarker study. *Lancet Oncol.* (2015) 16:541–549. doi: 10.1016/S1470-2045(15)70106-3

20. Assouline SE, Nielsen TH, Yu S, Alcaide M, Chong L, MacDonald D, et al. Phase 2 study of panobinostat with or without rituximab in relapsed diffuse large B-cell lymphoma. *Blood.* (2016) 128:185–94. doi: 10.1182/blood-2016-02-699520
21. Kurtz DM, Scherer F, Jin MC, Soo J, Craig AFM, Esfahani MS, et al. Circulating tumor DNA measurements as early outcome predictors in diffuse large B-cell lymphoma. *J Clin Oncol.* (2018) 36:2845–53. doi: 10.1200/JCO.2018.78.5246
22. Sarkozy C, Huet S, Carlton VE, Fabiani B, Delmer A, Jardin F, et al. The prognostic value of clonal heterogeneity and quantitative assessment of plasma circulating clonal IG-VDJ sequences at diagnosis in patients with follicular lymphoma. *Oncotarget.* (2017) 8:8765–74. doi: 10.18632/oncotarget.14448
23. Hossain NM, Dahiya S, Le R, Abramian AM, Kong KA, Muffly LS, et al. Circulating tumor DNA assessment in patients with diffuse large B-cell lymphoma following CAR T-cell therapy. *Leuk Lymphoma.* (2019) 60:503–506. doi: 10.1080/10428194.2018.1474463
24. Li Q, Zhang W, Li J, Xiong J, Liu J, Chen T, et al. Plasma circulating tumor DNA assessment reveals KMT2D as a potential poor prognostic factor in extranodal NK/T-cell lymphoma. *Biomark Res.* (2020) 8:27. doi: 10.1186/s40364-020-00205-4
25. Qiu M, Wang J, Xu Y, Ding X, Li M, Jiang F, et al. Circulating tumor DNA is effective for the detection of EGFR mutation in non-small cell lung cancer: a meta-analysis. *Cancer Epidemiol Biomarkers Prev.* (2015) 24:206–12. doi: 10.1158/1055-9965.EPI-14-0895
26. Yeh P, Dickinson M, Ftouni S, Hunter T, Sinha D, Wong SQ, et al. Molecular disease monitoring using circulating tumor DNA in myelodysplastic syndromes. *Blood.* (2017) 129:1685–1690. doi: 10.1182/blood-2016-09-740308
27. Hohaus S, Giachelia M, Massini G, Mansueto G, Vannata B, Bozzoli V, et al. Cell-free circulating DNA in Hodgkin's and non-Hodgkin's lymphomas. *Ann Oncol.* (2009) 20:1408–13. doi: 10.1093/annonc/mdp006
28. Galimberti S, Luminari S, Ciabatti E, Grassi S, Guerrini F, Dondi A, et al. Minimal residual disease after conventional treatment significantly impacts on progression-free survival of patients with follicular lymphoma: the FIL FOLL05 trial. *Clin Cancer Res.* (2014) 20:6398–6405. doi: 10.1158/1078-0432.CCR-14-0407
29. Herrera AF, Kim HT, Kong KA, Faham M, Sun H, Sohani AR, et al. Next-generation sequencing-based detection of circulating tumour DNA After allogeneic stem cell transplantation for lymphoma. *Br J Haematol.* (2016) 175:841–50. doi: 10.1111/bjh.14311
30. Pott C, Hoster E, Delfau-Larue MH, Beldjord K, Böttcher S, Asnafi V, et al. Molecular remission is an independent predictor of clinical outcome in patients with mantle cell lymphoma after combined immunochemotherapy: a European MCL intergroup study. *Blood.* (2010) 115:3215–3223. doi: 10.1182/blood-2009-06-230250
31. Armand P, Oki Y, Neuberg DS, Faham M, Cummings C, Klinger M, et al. Detection of circulating tumour DNA in patients with aggressive B-cell non-Hodgkin lymphoma. *Br J Haematol.* (2013) 163:123–6. doi: 10.1111/bjh.12439
32. Scherer F, Kurtz DM, Newman AM, Stehr H, Craig AFM, Esfahani MS, et al. Distinct biological subtypes and patterns of genome evolution in lymphoma revealed by circulating tumor DNA. *Sci Transl Med.* (2016) 8:364ra155. doi: 10.1126/scitranslmed.aai8545

19

PHF6 Mutations in Hematologic Malignancies

Jason H. Kurzer[1] *and Olga K. Weinberg*[2*]

[1] *Department of Pathology, Stanford University School of Medicine, Stanford, CA, United States,* [2] *Department of Pathology, UT Southwestern, Dallas, TX, United States*

***Correspondence:**
Olga K. Weinberg
Olga.Weinberg@UTSouthwestern.edu

Next generation sequencing has uncovered several genes with associated mutations in hematologic malignancies that can serve as potential biomarkers of disease. Keeping abreast of these genes is therefore of paramount importance in the field of hematology. This review focuses on *PHF6*, a highly conserved epigenetic transcriptional regulator that is important for neurodevelopment and hematopoiesis. *PHF6* serves as a tumor suppressor protein, with *PHF6* mutations and deletions often implicated in the development of T-lymphoblastic leukemia and less frequently in acute myeloid leukemia and other myeloid neoplasms. *PHF6* inactivation appears to be an early event in T-lymphoblastic leukemogenesis, requiring cooperating events, including *NOTCH1* mutations or overexpression of TLX1 and TLX3 for full disease development. In contrast, *PHF6* mutations tend to occur later in myeloid malignancies, are frequently accompanied by *RUNX1* mutations, and are often associated with disease progression. Moreover, *PHF6* appears to play a role in lineage plasticity within hematopoietic malignancies, with *PHF6* mutations commonly present in mixed phenotype acute leukemias with a predilection for T-lineage marker expression. Due to conflicting data, the prognostic significance of *PHF6* mutations remains unclear, with a subset of studies showing no significant difference in outcomes compared to malignancies with wild-type *PHF6*, and other studies showing inferior outcomes in certain patients with mutated *PHF6.* Future studies are necessary to elucidate the role *PHF6* plays in development of T-lymphoblastic leukemia, progression of myeloid malignancies, and its overall prognostic significance in hematopoietic neoplasms.

Keywords: PHF6, leukemia, tumor suppressor, T-ALL, AML

INTRODUCTION

Plant homeodomain (PHD) finger proteins consist of a family of epigenetic regulators that bind to a variety of targets, including both post-translationally modified and unmodified histones (1). The PHD finger protein, homeodomain finger protein 6 (*PHF6*), is a highly conserved, 365 amino acid, 41kDa protein, that was first identified in the X-linked neurodevelopmental disorder, Börjeson-Forssman-Lehmann syndrome (BFLS) (2, 3). *PHF6* contains two imperfect PHD-like zinc finger domains, two nuclear localization signals as well as a nucleolar localization sequence (**Figure 1**) (2, 4–6). Expression of PHF6 is found in almost all tissues, with particularly high expression in the brain/developing central nervous system as well as in all hematopoietic subpopulations (high levels

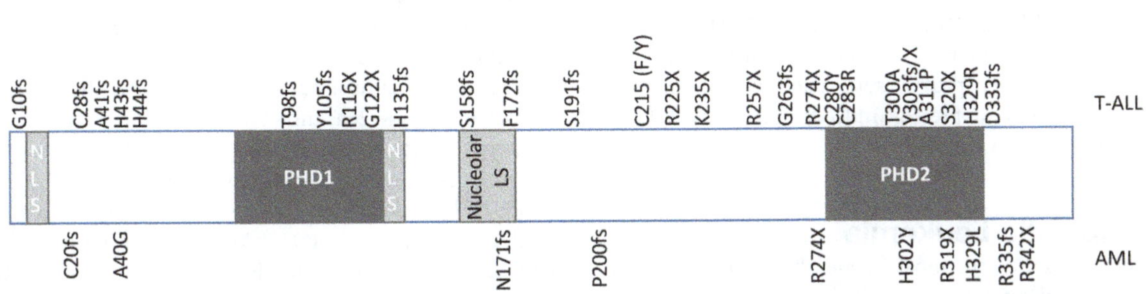

FIGURE 1 | Diagram of *PHF6*. *PHF6* has two imperfect PHD-like zinc finger domains (PHD1 and PHD2), two nuclear localization signals (NLS), and one nucleolar localization signal. Mutations originally identified in T-ALL by Van Vlierberghe et al. (4) are identified at the top of the diagram, whereas mutations originally identified in AML by Van Vliergerghe et al. (21) are identified at the bottom of the diagram.

in CD34+ precursor cells and B-cells; low levels in NK-cells and monocytes) implicating a role for *PHF6* in a variety of functions including neurogenesis and hematopoiesis (2, 7, 8).

FUNCTION OF *PHF6*

Supporting a fundamental role for *PHF6* in general development, *PHF6*-homozygous knockout mice die perinatally (9). However, scientists have also developed various knockout models in mice to explore the role of *PHF6* in hematopoiesis (8, 10–13). McRae et al. showed that germline deletion of murine *PHF6* is lethal in males whereas heterozygous females survived to adulthood (10). Using $Phf6^{lox/Y}$;$Tie\text{-}cre^{Tg/+}$ male mice with a *Phf6*-null mutation in hematopoietic and endothelial cells, McRae et al. showed an increase in $Lin^{-}c\text{-}Kit^{+}Sca\text{-}1^{+}$ (LSK) stem and progenitor cell-enriched populations, specifically the heterogeneous progenitor cell population (HPC-1), with an enrichment in cycling forms (10). Inactivation of *PHF6* at various stages of development results in increased embryologic proliferative properties of hematopoietic stem cells, but also an increased ability for *PHF6*-deficient neonatal and adult HSCs to repopulate the bone marrow in serial transplant assays (10–13). Studies suggest that this enhanced proliferative ability of *PHF6*-deleted HSCs results, at least in part, from IFN-α signaling, the inhibition of TNFα-associated growth suppressing genes, and perhaps upregulation of JAK1 signaling (10–12).

Wendorff et al. similarly showed that conditional knockout of *PHF6* displayed expansions of total immature hematopoietic LSK cells, but also showed increased multipotent MPP2, and MPP3 populations in 8-week-old mice, and no differences in the numbers of more mature myeloid progenitors, uncommitted lymphoid progenitors, or B-cell precursors (11). However, conditional knockout of *PHF6* does show a mild reduction in double-negative DN2 and DN3 thymic progenitors and decreased numbers of peripheral blood CD4 and CD8 positive T-cells in 8-week-old mice (10, 11, 13). Moreover, knockdown studies in cord blood and thymus-derived hematopoietic precursors showed that *PHF6* loss fosters a preferential differentiation of B-lymphocytes, reduced erythroid development, and accelerated T-cell development *via* downregulation of *NOTCH1* (8).

Like other PHD finger proteins, *PHF6* functions in chromatin-mediated regulation of gene expression. It is capable of binding double-stranded DNA, but not histones, *in vitro via* its atypical PHD2 domain (14). Co-immunoprecipitation experiments using antibodies to *PHF6*, reveal it interacts with constituents of the nucleosome remodeling deacetylase (NuRD) complex, including CHD_4, $HDAC_1$, and Rbb_4 (6, 15). The NuRD complex is a major ATP-dependent chromatin remodeling complex, implicated in nucleosome positioning and both repressing and activating genes involved in embryonic development (16). PHF6 has additionally been shown to bind to the PAF1 transcription elongation complex, regulating Neuroglycan C/Chondroitn sulfate proteoglycan 5 (NGC/CSPG5) and ultimately neuronal migration in murine cerebral cortex development (17). One consequence of *PHF6*-mediated transcription regulation includes the modulation of levels of the RNA Pol I preinitiation complex activator, upstream binding factor (UBF), thereby suppressing UBF-mediated rRNA transcription (5, 18).

Knockdown studies of PHF6 suggest a tumor suppressor role for the protein, as PHF6 deficiency in HeLa cell lines resulted in increased UBF protein levels, and increased DNA damage at the rDNA locus (5). Deficiency of PHF6 results in the formation of DNA-RNA hybrid (R-loops) and increased R-loop-dependent rDNA damage (5). Moreover, knockdown of *PHF6* interferes with the G2 checkpoint recovery of U2OS cells, leading to decreased DNA repair in response to ionizing radiation (19). These data implicate a tumor suppressor role for PHF6 resulting from regulating DNA damage response.

PHF6 AND HEMATOLOGIC DISEASE

Despite the discovery of *PHF6 via* its role in BFL syndrome and its prominent role in neurogenesis, mutations of *PHF6* have only been identified to date in hematologic malignancies (20). The first and most well-documented hematologic malignancy harboring mutations of *PHF6* is T-lymphoblastic leukemia (T-ALL), with fewer cases identified in acute myeloid leukemia (AML), and rarer cases identified in pre-malignant clonal hematopoiesis (4, 21–23). Mutations in hematologic malignancies include deletion, missense, frameshift, and nonsense mutations, which span the whole coding region, with missense mutations concentrated in the PHD2 domain (**Figure 1**) (4, 21, 24). The ultimate effect of these mutations is to inhibit PHF6 function or deplete its levels, and as such, provide supporting evidence that this protein serves as a tumor suppressor. Indeed, a patient with BFLS was noted to develop T-ALL (25).

T-Lymphoblastic Leukemia

The *PHF6* locus is one of the most frequently mutated genes in T-lymphoblastic leukemia (T-ALL). Inactivating mutations of *PHF6* have been identified in 5-16% of pediatric and 19-40% of adult patients with T-ALL and ~25% of adults with T-lymphoblastic lymphoma (T-LBL) with some groups identifying an association with *NOTCH1* mutations (67%-84.6% of *PHF6* mutated/deleted T-ALL with *NOTCH1* mutations versus 39.8% *PHF6* WT) (4, 26–38). Copy number alterations of *PHF6* in pediatric T-ALL has been reported to be between 13-14% (39, 40). The location of *PHF6* on chrX26.2 lead researches to speculate that such mutations may at least partially explain the 2-3 fold increased incidence of T-ALL in males, as *PHF6* mutations were originally found predominantly in male T-ALL patients (31.5% *vs* 2.6%) (4). Subsequent studies, however, have failed to show a gender preference (26–28, 33). Recently, *PHF6* mutations have additionally been found in up to 25% (3/12) of early T-cell precursor subtype of T-ALL (ETP), a form of T-ALL that frequently expresses myeloid-associated markers (41, 42).

The role *PHF6* plays in leukemogenesis is actively under investigation. Analyzing whole exome sequencing data from diagnostic and relapse leukemias, Wendorff et al. showed that somatic mutations of *PHF6* occur early in leukeomogenesis (11). Nevertheless, animal models have revealed that while *PHF6* mutations/deletions may be initial events, they are insufficient for tumor initiation without additional driver mutations. For example, Miyagi et al. did not observe leukemia development subsequent to serial transplantation of *PHF6*-deleted HSCs in mice (12). Likewise, no T-ALL tumors developed in a *PHF6*$^{+/-}$ zebrafish model (43).

Studies show that *PHF6* dysfunction cooperates with several other driver mutations. For example, inactivation of *PHF6* in hematopoietic progenitors has been reported to facilitate NOTCH1-induced T-ALL, potentially through increasing leukemia-initiating cells and development of a "leukemia stem cell transcriptional program" in lymphoblasts (11, 13). A study of 102 pediatric T-ALL cases in Taiwan showed that *PHF6* mutations frequently cooperate with *HOX11L2* overexpression and/or *WT1* mutations (44). In addition, *PHF6* mutations have been shown to be associated (at times in conjunction with *DNM2*) with T-ALLs that overexpress homeobox transcription factors, *TLX1* and *TLX3* (4, 32, 45). Indeed, ectopic expression of TLX3 in *PHF6*-deleted mice facilitated early onset leukemia and a *hTLX1;PHF6*$^{+/-}$ zebrafish model demonstrated fully penetrant early-onset leukemia development, underscoring the role of cooperation between these mutations in leukemogenesis (10, 43). Other associations include those with mutations in X-linked genes, *USP9X* and *MED1* as well as with *IL7R-JAK* pathway genes, *WT1*, *PTPN2* deletions, and *HOX11L2* overexpression (33, 34, 44, 46). In the setting of ETP, *PHF6* mutations frequently occur with mutations in *EZH2*, *EED*, and *SUZ12* (41). Finally, a network of miRNAs, including miR-19b, miR-20a/93, miR-26a, miR-92, and miR-223, have been shown to target multiple PHF6 and other T-ALL-associated tumor suppressors, and thus promote leukemia (47).

PHF6 has additionally been shown to interact with LMO2 to bind DNA *via* the LMO2/TAL1/LDB/GATA2 complex in T-ALL cell lines (48). The PHF6/LMO2/TAL1/LDB/GATA2 complex was shown to bind at DNA segments associated with hematopoietic or lymphoid organ development, hematopoiesis, as well as T-cell activation and differentiation (48).

While sample sizes are small, patients with T-ALL harboring *PHF6* mutations tend to be older, have been demonstrated to have lower white blood cell counts than other T-ALL patients, as well as lower hemoglobin and platelet levels, splenomegaly/lymphadenopathy, and have blasts with a tendency to express CD13 (26, 29, 37). Genomic analysis of matched diagnosis, germline (remission) and relapse DNA samples from 46 T-ALL cases reveals that *PHF6* alterations are found commonly at diagnosis, and persist at relapse (49). While mutations in *PHF6* have been implicated in increased resistance to prednisolone in T-ALL cell lines, the majority of studies have shown no correlation with *PHF6* mutations and overall survival in patients with T-ALL, and a potential favorable prognosis associated with T-LBL (4, 26, 27, 29, 50, 51). Nevertheless, one study of pediatric T-ALL found *PHF6* mutations/deletions predict an inferior overall survival upon multivariate analysis (44). Another study of Chinese adults found that the co-existence of *PHF6* and *NOTCH1* mutations in T-ALL conferred a shorter event-free survival and a poor prognosis (37). Further study is therefore required to assess the true prognostic significance of *PHF6* mutations in T-ALL.

Myeloid Neoplasms

The largest study of *PHF6* mutations in myeloid malignancies involved targeted sequencing of 1760 cases with myeloid neoplasms (24). This study revealed 54 patients with 62 somatic mutations of *PHF6* (24). With regard to disease burden, the percentage of blasts in the bone marrow tended to be higher in patients with myeloid neoplasms harboring *PHF6* mutations (24). As for cytogenetics, abnormal karyotypes showed no significant predilection for *PHF6* mutations, although +8, t (8;21), and complex karyotypes were abnormalities most often identified (24). At the molecular level, co-mutated genes associated with *PHF6* mutations included *RUNX1*, *U2AF1*, *SMC1A*, *ZRSR2*, *EZH2*, and *ASXL1*, whereas *PHF6* was found to be mutually exclusive with *SF3B1* (24). In contrast to T-ALL, mutations of *PHF6* tend to occur later in disease evolution, sometimes with different mutations in parallel clones (24).

Acute Myeloid Leukemia

Inactivating somatic *PHF6* mutations have been found in ~2-3% of AMLs (20, 21, 24, 28, 52, 53). Similar to T-ALL, a male predominance was initially reported but not further substantiated for AML identified with *PHF6* mutations (21, 24, 53). With respect to AML subtypes, *PHF6* mutations are found in 15% of AML with inv(3)(q21q26.2)/t(3;3)(q21;q26.2) and 15.4% of cases of AML with myelodysplasia related changes (MRC) (24, 54). Interestingly, a case report of AML with MRC harboring a *P2RY8-CRLF2* fusion was found to have gained a *PHF6* mutation upon transformation to AML, suggesting a potential role for *PHF6* in the transition of MDS to AML (55). Further evidence for *PHF6* mutations acquired secondarily and leading to progression of myeloid neoplasms was found in patients with germline mutations of *RUNX1*, where *PHF6* mutations were implicated in the transition to MDS in one patient and the transition to AML in the other (56, 57). Interestingly, *PHF6* has been shown to frequently co-occur with *RUNX1* in AML (58).

Despite *PHF6* mutations leading to inactivation of the protein, an analysis of *PHF6* expression levels in AML regardless of mutation status revealed that PHF6 protein levels are higher in patients with AML than normal controls, a finding seemingly at odds with its role as a tumor suppressor (59). Moreover, increased PHF6 levels correlated with an increased percentage of blasts, with a possible correlation with CD34 positivity (59). Decreased PHF6 protein expression correlated with longer overall survival than those with high expression levels (2 years versus 6 months) (59).

A study of 318 pediatric patients with *de novo* AML identified *PHF6* mutations in 6 (2%) cases with FAB subtypes of M0, M1, and M2 (53). The median age for this group was 12.6 years (versus 9.5 in wild type *PHF6 AML*), with 4 of 6 succumbing to the disease. Co-genetic abnormalities included *RUNX1/RUNX1T1* translocations, *NUP98/KDM5A* translocations, and mutations in *WT1*, *RAS*, *ETV6*, *TET2*, *IDH1*, and *BCORL1* (53). Measuring the expression level of PHF6 showed decreased PHF6 levels in patients with mutations compared to M0, M1, and M2 AML subtypes with wild-type *PHF6*, again supporting a tumor suppressor role for *PHF6* and providing at least some genetic context to the results found by Mousa et al. above (53, 59).

A study of 398 patients with AML younger than 60 years of age revealed *PHF6* to be associated with decreased overall survival in patients with intermediate-risk AML with wild-type FLT3-ITD (60). This implicates *PHF6* mutations as a potential prognostic marker to be used in intermediate-risk AML, although it should be noted that this finding has not been replicated by others (24). Interestingly, subdividing AML with MRC cases that are associated with complex karyotypes into typical (those harboring 5q, 7q and/or 17p abnormalities) and atypical (those without these abnormalities) shows that AML with atypical complex karyotypes tend to have *PHF6* mutations more frequently, *TP53* mutations less frequently, be younger, have a higher WBC and blast percentage, and higher complete remission and overall survival rates (61).

Myelodysplastic Syndrome

Animal models suggest a possible role for *PHF6* mutations in myelodysplastic syndrome (MDS), as aged mice with knocked-out *PHF6* exhibit megakaryocytic dysplasia and associated decreased platelet counts as well as extramedullary hematopoiesis (13). Nevertheless, *PHF6* mutations are relatively rare (~3%) in MDS (24, 62–64). The limited data indicate that *PHF6* mutations are found most frequently (5.3% of MDS cases) in the high-grade subtypes (MDS with excess blasts) (24). *PHF6* mutations tended to show low variant allele frequencies and acquisition in sub-clonal populations (24). The most frequent co-mutations were seen in ASXL1, RUNX1, TET2, and DNMT3A (64). A study of 21 MDS patients harboring *PHF6* mutations revealed 61.9% had normal karyotypes and no patients had complex karyotypes (64).

Myeloproliferative Neoplasms

PHF6 mutations are rarely identified in myeloproliferative neoplasms (MPN) (0.7%), occurring in only 1.6% of chronic myelogenous leukemia (24). A screen of 81patients with CML in myeloid blast crisis identified 2 male patients with *PHF6* mutations, with at least one patient showing no *PHF6* mutations in the preceding chronic phase (65). This finding raises the possibility that, similar to MDS, the accumulation of *PHF6* mutations might mediate progression of the disease. Relatedly, a review of 22 patients with *PHF6* mutations in myeloproliferative neoplasms at three institutions revealed an enrichment in cases with increased fibrosis and/or blast crisis (66). Other than JAK2, the most common co-mutations in these MPNs were *ASXL1*, and *TET2* with a median of 2.5 non JAK2 co-mutated genes (66).

With respect to mixed myelodysplastic syndrome/myeloproliferative neoplasm cases, *PHF6* mutations were seen in 4.7% of CMML patients (24). To date, no effect on survival has been seen in *PHF6*-mutation associated CMML patients (64).

B-Lymphoblastic Leukemia

Despite their prevalence in T-ALL, *PHF6* mutations have only rarely been identified in B-lymphoblastic leukemia (4, 41, 67). 50% of the rare *MEF2D*-rearranged B-ALL was found to have *PHF6* mutations (67). Intriguingly, use of a retrovirally-expressed shRNA screening library into a B-lymphobastic leukemia cell line revealed that knockdown of PHF6 levels inhibited cell growth and leukemia growth in transplanted models (68). Indeed, CRISPR-Cas9-mediated deletion of *PHF6* in a murine *BCR-ABL1*$^{+}$; *p19*$^{-/-}$; *mCherry*$^{+}$ B-ALL cell line resulted in delayed tumor formation after injection in immunocompetent mice compared to wild-type B-ALL cells (69). Moreover, *PHF6* KO B-ALL cells induced a malignancy closer in presentation to lymphoma than leukemia, with tumor cells showing reduced expression of CD19 and B220 and B-cell development genes (e.g., *Cd74*, *IL4ra*, *Lyn*, *Ly86*, and *BLK*), and upregulation of CD4 and T-cell signal transduction genes (69). These data therefore implicate PHF6 mutations as lineage specific with respect to tumorigenesis, and even implicate mutation of *PHF6* as a potential mediator of lineage plasticity in hematopoietic neoplasms.

Acute Leukemia of Ambiguous Lineage

The association of *PHF6* mutations with leukemias of ambiguous lineage further supports a role for these mutations in lineage plasticity. An analysis of 29 mixed phenotype acute leukemia cases at Memorial Sloan Kettering Cancer Center revealed *PHF6*

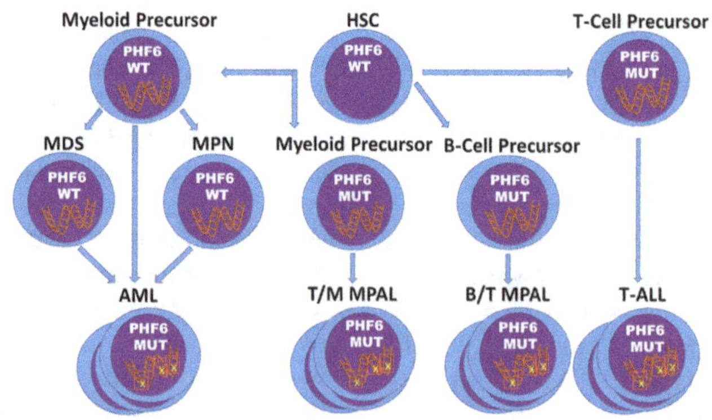

FIGURE 2 | Model of *PHF6* in Hematopoietic Malignancies. The timing and context of the acquisition of *PHF6* deletions/mutations appear to determine the fate of the resulting malignancy. In T-ALL, *PHF6* deletions/mutations arise early, but are insufficient for transformation into leukemia. In contrast, in myeloid neoplasms, *PHF6* deletions/mutations tend to develop later possibly leading to disease progression. Finally, acquisition of inactivating mutations of *PHF6* in myeloid or B-cell precursors may promote T-cell gene expression and eventual development of mixed phenotype acute leukemias.

(23%) and *DNMT3A* (23%) as the most common recurrent mutations (70). Mutations in *PHF6* and *DNMT3A* are mutually exclusive in MPAL, correlate with T-lineage marker expression (83% and 100%, respectively), and have higher relapse at 2 years (58% and 79%, respectively) compared to MPAL lacking these mutations (70).

In addition to T/M cases, Xiao et al. identified *PHF6* mutations in patients with T/B/M and T/B phenotypes (70). Similarly, Getta et al. found *PHF6* mutations in 3 of 16 MPAL patients with at least 2 of 3 patients of the MPAL, NOS subtype (B/T or B/T/M) (71). Furthermore, a review of 9 patients from multiple institutions identified *PHF6* mutations in 5 patients with B/T MPAL (56%) (72).

Similar to T-ALL, *PHF6* mutations are believed to be early events in MPAL, as Xiao et al. found every blast population isolated from selected cases showed nearly 100% VAF (70). Interestingly, *PHF6*-associated MPAL correlates with younger patients, higher hemoglobin and higher platelet values (70, 72).

Bond et al. performed an analysis of the transcriptional program of AMLs and T-ALLs and identified an expression program at the interface of these two diseases (73). Comparing T-ALL to T-ALL-like AMLs and AML-like T-ALLs, it was found that all T-ALLs with *PHF6* mutations were accompanied by *NOTCH1* mutations, whereas 3/5 *PHF6* mutated interface cases lacked *NOTCH1* mutations (73).

Interestingly, a study of acute undifferentiated leukemias found *PHF6* mutations in 7/16 cases of AUL, whereas only 1/25 cases of minimally differentiated AML harbored these mutations (74). Nevertheless, in the limited study, no clinical outcome differences were seen between the two groups (74).

DISCUSSION

The last two decades have elucidated a role for *PHF6* in neurodevelopment and hematopoiesis, and revealed it as a potent tumor suppressor with an exclusive tendency for hematologic malignancies (**Figure 2**). *PHF6* mutations are most common in T-ALL, and appear early in the disease course yet appear insufficient for leukemia development. Given the conflicting data regarding the prognostic significance of *PHF6* mutations in T-ALL, additional studies are necessary to clarify the role of *PHF6* inactivation in the disease course. It is likely that appropriately powered studies will need to assess its significance in specific patient cohorts.

In contrast to T-ALL, *PHF6* mutations are less frequent in myeloid malignancies. Of interest, these mutations are more frequently found later in the disease course at points of disease progression. Further work is therefore required to determine the mechanism by which *PHF6* pushes these neoplasms to a more aggressive disease, as well as to determine the overall prognostic significance of *PHF6* mutations in myeloid malignancies in general. If additional studies continue to show a role for *PHF6* mutations in disease progression, laboratories may wish to offer specific targeted analysis of *PHF6* for the monitoring of myeloid disease.

Finally, it is becoming clear that *PHF6* plays a role in lineage plasticity of hematopoietic malignancies, as *PHF6* mutations exist in T/Myeloid MPAL as well as MPAL, NOS (particularly B/T MPAL) and is frequently associated with early T-ALL which frequently shows myeloid marker expression. The underlying contextual factors, including cell of origin and cooperative gene mutations, remain to be elucidated to understand what drives a *PHF6*-associated malignancy to be T-lineage, myeloid lineage, or a combination of both.

AUTHOR CONTRIBUTIONS

OW conceived of the review subject matter and provided editorial review while JK primarily composed the manuscript. All authors contributed to the article and approved the submitted version.

REFERENCES

1. Musselman CA, Kutateladze TG. Handpicking Epigenetic Marks With PHD Fingers. *Nucleic Acids Res* (2011) 39:9061–71. doi: 10.1093/nar/gkr613
2. Lower KM, Turner G, Kerr BA, Mathews KD, Shaw MA, Gedeon AK, et al. Mutations in PHF6 Are Associated With Börjeson-Forssman-Lehmann Syndrome. *Nat Genet* (2002) 32:661–5. doi: 10.1038/ng1040
3. Todd MAM, Ivanochko D, Picketts DJ. PHF6 Degrees of Separation: the Multifaceted Roles of a Chromatin Adaptor Protein. *Genes* (2015) 6:325–52. doi: 10.3390/genes6020325
4. Van Vlierberghe P, Palomero T, Khiabanian H, Van der Meulen J, Castillo M, Van Roy N, et al. PHF6 Mutations in T-Cell Acute Lymphoblastic Leukemia. *Nat Genet* (2010) 42:338–42. doi: 10.1038/ng.542
5. Wang J, Leung JW, Gong Z, Feng L, Shi X, Chen J. PHF6 Regulates Cell Cycle Progression by Suppressing Ribosomal RNA Synthesis. *J Biol Chem* (2013) 288:3174–83. doi: 10.1074/jbc.M112.414839
6. Todd MAM, Picketts DJ. PHF6 Interacts With the Nucleosome Remodeling and Deacetylation (Nurd) Complex. *J Proteome Res* (2012) 11:4326–37. doi: 10.1021/pr3004369
7. Voss AK, Gamble R, Collin C, Shoubridge C, Corbett M, Gécz J, et al. Protein and Gene Expression Analysis of Phf6, the Gene Mutated in the Börjeson-Forssman-Lehmann Syndrome of Intellectual Disability and Obesity. *Gene Expr. Patterns GEP* (2007) 7:858–71. doi: 10.1016/j.modgep.2007.06.007
8. Loontiens S, Dolens A-C, Strubbe S, Van de Walle I, Moore FE, Depestel L, et al. Phf6 Expression Levels Impact Human Hematopoietic Stem Cell Differentiation. *Front Cell Dev Biol* (2020) 8:599472. doi: 10.3389/fcell.2020.599472
9. Cheng C, Deng P-Y, Ikeuchi Y, Yuede C, Li D, Rensing N, et al. Characterization of a Mouse Model of Börjeson-Forssman-Lehmann Syndrome. *Cell Rep* (2018) 25:1404–14.e6. doi: 10.1016/j.celrep.2018.10.043
10. McRae HM, Garnham AL, Hu Y, Witkowski MT, Corbett MA, Dixon MP, et al. PHF6 Regulates Hematopoietic Stem and Progenitor Cells and its Loss Synergizes With Expression of TLX3 to Cause Leukemia. *Blood* (2019) 133:1729–41. doi: 10.1182/blood-2018-07-860726
11. Wendorff AA, Quinn SA, Rashkovan M, Madubata CJ, Ambesi-Impiombato A, Litzow MR, et al. Phf6 Loss Enhances HSC Self-Renewal Driving Tumor Initiation and Leukemia Stem Cell Activity in T-ALL. *Cancer Discov* (2019) 9:436–51. doi: 10.1158/2159-8290.CD-18-1005
12. Miyagi S, Sroczynska P, Kato Y, Nakajima-Takagi Y, Oshima M, Rizq O, et al. The Chromatin-Binding Protein Phf6 Restricts the Self-Renewal of Hematopoietic Stem Cells. *Blood* (2019) 133:2495–506. doi: 10.1182/blood.2019000468
13. Hsu Y-C, Chen T-C, Lin C-C, Yuan C-T, Hsu C-L, Hou H-A, et al. Phf6-Null Hematopoietic Stem Cells Have Enhanced Self-Renewal Capacity and Oncogenic Potentials. *Blood Adv* (2019) 3:2355–67. doi: 10.1182/bloodadvances.2019000391
14. Liu Z, Li F, Ruan K, Zhang J, Mei Y, Wu J, et al. Structural and Functional Insights Into the Human Börjeson-Forssman-Lehmann Syndrome-Associated Protein PHF6 *. *J Biol Chem* (2014) 289:10069–83. doi: 10.1074/jbc.M113.535351
15. Liu Z, Li F, Zhang B, Li S, Wu J, Shi Y. Structural Basis of Plant Homeodomain Finger 6 (PHF6) Recognition by the Retinoblastoma Binding Protein 4 (RBBP4) Component of the Nucleosome Remodeling and Deacetylase (Nurd) Complex. *J Biol Chem* (2015) 290:6630–8. doi: 10.1074/jbc.M114.610196
16. Basta J, Rauchman M. The Nucleosome Remodeling and Deacetylase (Nurd) Complex in Development and Disease. *Transl Res J Lab Clin Med* (2015) 165:36–47. doi: 10.1016/j.trsl.2014.05.003
17. Zhang C, Mejia LA, Huang J, Valnegri P, Bennett EJ, Anckar J, et al. The X-Linked Intellectual Disability Protein PHF6 Associates With the PAF1 Complex and Regulates Neuronal Migration in the Mammalian Brain. *Neuron* (2013) 78:986–93. doi: 10.1016/j.neuron.2013.04.021
18. Todd MAM, Huh MS, Picketts DJ. The Sub-Nucleolar Localization of PHF6 Defines its Role in Rdna Transcription and Early Processing Events. *Eur J Hum Genet EJHG* (2016) 24:1453–9. doi: 10.1038/ejhg.2016.40
19. Warmerdam DO, Alonso-de Vega I, Wiegant WW, van den Broek B, Rother MB, Wolthuis RM, et al. PHF6 Promotes non-Homologous End Joining and G2 Checkpoint Recovery. *EMBO Rep* (2020) 21:e48460. doi: 10.15252/embr.201948460
20. Huether R, Dong L, Chen X, Wu G, Parker M, Wei L, et al. The Landscape of Somatic Mutations in Epigenetic Regulators Across 1,000 Paediatric Cancer Genomes. *Nat Commun* (2014) 5:3630. doi: 10.1038/ncomms4630
21. Van Vlierberghe P, Patel J, Abdel-Wahab O, Lobry C, Hedvat CV, Balbin M, et al. PHF6 Mutations in Adult Acute Myeloid Leukemia. *Leukemia* (2011) 25:130–4. doi: 10.1038/leu.2010.247
22. Yoshizato T, Dumitriu B, Hosokawa K, Makishima H, Yoshida K, Townsley D, et al. Somatic Mutations and Clonal Hematopoiesis in Aplastic Anemia. *N Engl J Med* (2015) 373:35–47. doi: 10.1056/NEJMoa1414799
23. Abelson S, Collord G, Ng SWK, Weissbrod O, Mendelson Cohen N, Niemeyer E, Barda N, et al. Prediction of Acute Myeloid Leukaemia Risk in Healthy Individuals. *Nature* (2018) 559:400–4. doi: 10.1038/s41586-018-0317-6
24. Mori T, Nagata Y, Makishima H, Sanada M, Shiozawa Y, Kon A, et al. Somatic PHF6 Mutations in 1760 Cases With Various Myeloid Neoplasms. *Leukemia* (2016) 30:2270–3. doi: 10.1038/leu.2016.212
25. Chao MM, Todd MA, Kontny U, Neas K, Sullivan MJ, Hunter AG, et al. T-Cell Acute Lymphoblastic Leukemia in Association With Börjeson-Forssman-Lehmann Syndrome Due to a Mutation in PHF6. *Pediatr Blood Cancer* (2010) 55:722–4. doi: 10.1002/pbc.22574
26. Grossmann V, Haferlach C, Weissmann S, Roller A, Schindela S, Poetzinger F, et al. The Molecular Profile of Adult T-Cell Acute Lymphoblastic Leukemia: Mutations in RUNX1 and DNMT3A Are Associated With Poor Prognosis in T-ALL. *Genes Chromosomes Cancer* (2013) 52:410–22. doi: 10.1002/gcc.22039
27. Wang Q, Qiu H, Jiang H, Wu L, Dong S, Pan J, et al. Mutations of PHF6 are Associated With Mutations of NOTCH1, JAK1 and Rearrangement of SET-NUP214 in T-Cell Acute Lymphoblastic Leukemia. *Haematologica* (2011) 96:1808–14. doi: 10.3324/haematol.2011.043083
28. Yoo NJ, Kim YR, Lee SH. Somatic Mutation of PHF6 Gene in T-Cell Acute Lymphoblatic Leukemia, Acute Myelogenous Leukemia and Hepatocellular Carcinoma. *Acta Oncol Stockh Swed* (2012) 51:107–11. doi: 10.3109/0284186X.2011.592148
29. Huh HJ, Lee SH, Yoo KH, Sung KW, Koo HH, Jang JH, et al. Gene Mutation Profiles and Prognostic Implications in Korean Patients With T-Lymphoblastic Leukemia. *Ann Hematol* (2013) 92:635–44. doi: 10.1007/s00277-012-1664-2
30. Chang Y-H, Yu C-H, Jou S-T, Lin C-Y, Lin K-H, Lu M-Y, et al. Targeted Sequencing to Identify Genetic Alterations and Prognostic Markers in Pediatric T-Cell Acute Lymphoblastic Leukemia. *Sci Rep* (2021) 11:769. doi: 10.1038/s41598-020-80613-6
31. Sentís I, Gonzalez S, Genescà E, García-Hernández V, Muiños F, Gonzalez C, et al. The Evolution of Relapse of Adult T Cell Acute Lymphoblastic Leukemia. *Genome Biol* (2020) 21:284. doi: 10.1186/s13059-020-02192-z
32. Liu Y, Easton J, Shao Y, Maciaszek J, Wang Z, Wilkinson MR, et al. The Genomic Landscape of Pediatric and Young Adult T-Lineage Acute Lymphoblastic Leukemia. *Nat Genet* (2017) 49:1211–8. doi: 10.1038/ng.3909
33. Spinella J-F, Cassart P, Richer C, Saillour V, Ouimet M, Langlois S, et al. Genomic Characterization of Pediatric T-Cell Acute Lymphoblastic Leukemia Reveals Novel Recurrent Driver Mutations. *Oncotarget* (2016) 7:65485–503. doi: 10.18632/oncotarget.11796
34. Vicente C, Schwab C, Broux M, Geerdens E, Degryse S, Demeyer S, et al. Targeted Sequencing Identifies Associations Between IL7R-JAK Mutations and Epigenetic Modulators in T-Cell Acute Lymphoblastic Leukemia. *Haematologica* (2015) 100:1301–10. doi: 10.3324/haematol.2015.130179
35. Zhang H-H, Wang H-S, Qian X-W, Fan C-Q, Li J, Miao H, et al. Genetic Variants and Clinical Significance of Pediatric Acute Lymphoblastic Leukemia. *Ann Transl Med* (2019) 7:296. doi: 10.21037/atm.2019.04.80
36. Richter-Pechańska P, Kunz JB, Hof J, Zimmermann M, Rausch T, Bandapalli OR, et al. Identification of a Genetically Defined Ultra-High-Risk Group in Relapsed Pediatric T-Lymphoblastic Leukemia. *Blood Cancer J* (2017) 7:e523. doi: 10.1038/bcj.2017.3
37. Li M, Xiao L, Xu J, Zhang R, Guo J, Olson J, et al. Co-Existence of PHF6 and NOTCH1 Mutations in Adult T-Cell Acute Lymphoblastic Leukemia. *Oncol Lett* (2016) 12:16–22. doi: 10.3892/ol.2016.4581
38. De Keersmaecker K, Atak ZK, Li N, Vicente C, Patchett S, Girardi T, et al. Exome Sequencing Identifies Mutation in CNOT3 and Ribosomal Genes

RPL5 and RPL10 in T-Cell Acute Lymphoblastic Leukemia. *Nat Genet* (2013) 45:186–90. doi: 10.1038/ng.2508

39. Teachey DT, Pui C-H. Comparative Features and Outcomes Between Paediatric T-Cell and B-Cell Acute Lymphoblastic Leukaemia. *Lancet Oncol* (2019) 20:e142–54. doi: 10.1016/S1470-2045(19)30031-2
40. Lejman M, Włodarczyk M, Styka B, Pastorczak A, Zawitkowska J, Taha J, et al. Advantages and Limitations of SNP Array in the Molecular Characterization of Pediatric T-Cell Acute Lymphoblastic Leukemia. *Front Oncol* (2020) 10:1184. doi: 10.3389/fonc.2020.01184
41. Zhang J, Ding L, Holmfeldt L, Wu G, Heatley SL, Payne-Turner D, et al. The Genetic Basis of Early T-Cell Precursor Acute Lymphoblastic Leukaemia. *Nature* (2012) 481:157–63. doi: 10.1038/nature10725
42. Noronha EP, Marques LVC, Andrade FG, Thuler LCS, Terra-Granado E, Pombo-de-Oliveira MS, et al. The Profile of Immunophenotype and Genotype Aberrations in Subsets of Pediatric T-Cell Acute Lymphoblastic Leukemia. *Front Oncol* (2019) 9:316. doi: 10.3389/fonc.2019.00316
43. Loontiens S, Vanhauwaert S, Depestel L, Dewyn G, Van Loocke W, Moore FE, et al. A Novel TLX1-Driven T-ALL Zebrafish Model: Comparative Genomic Analysis With Other Leukemia Models. *Leukemia* (2020) 34:3398–403. doi: 10.1038/s41375-020-0938-2
44. Yeh T-C, Liang D-C, Liu H-C, Jaing T-H, Chen S-H, Hou J-Y, et al. Clinical and Biological Relevance of Genetic Alterations in Pediatric T-Cell Acute Lymphoblastic Leukemia in Taiwan. *Pediatr Blood Cancer* (2019) 66:e27496. doi: 10.1002/pbc.27496
45. Seki M, Kimura S, Isobe T, Yoshida K, Ueno H, Nakajima-Takagi Y, et al. Recurrent SPI1 (PU.1) Fusions in High-Risk Pediatric T Cell Acute Lymphoblastic Leukemia. *Nat Genet* (2017) 49:1274–81. doi: 10.1038/ng.3900
46. Alcantara M, Simonin M, Lhermitte L, Touzart A, Dourthe ME, Latiri M, et al. Clinical and Biological Features of PTPN2-Deleted Adult and Pediatric T-Cell Acute Lymphoblastic Leukemia. *Blood Adv* (2019) 3:1981–8. doi: 10.1182/bloodadvances.2018028993
47. Mavrakis KJ, Van Der Meulen J, Wolfe AL, Liu X, Mets E, Taghon T, et al. A Cooperative Microrna-Tumor Suppressor Gene Network in Acute T-Cell Lymphoblastic Leukemia (T-ALL). *Nat Genet* (2011) 43:673–8. doi: 10.1038/ng.858
48. Stanulović VS, Binhassan S, Dorrington I, Ward DG, Hoogenkamp M. PHF6 Interacts With LMO2 During Normal Haematopoiesis and in Leukaemia and Regulates Gene Expression and Genome Integrity. *bioRxiv* (2020), 2020.08.18.255471. doi: 10.1101/2020.08.18.255471
49. Oshima K, Zhao J, Pérez-Durán P, Brown JA, Patiño-Galindo JA, Chu T, et al. Mutational and Functional Genetics Mapping of Chemotherapy Resistance Mechanisms in Relapsed Acute Lymphoblastic Leukemia. *Nat Cancer* (2020) 1:1113–27. doi: 10.1038/s43018-020-00124-1
50. Xiang J, Wang G, Xia T, Chen Z. The Depletion of PHF6 Decreases the Drug Sensitivity of T-Cell Acute Lymphoblastic Leukemia to Prednisolone. *Biomed Pharmacother Biomed Pharmacother* (2019) 109:2210–7. doi: 10.1016/j.biopha.2018.11.083
51. Kroeze E, Loeffen JLC, Poort VM, Meijerink JPP. T-Cell Lymphoblastic Lymphoma and Leukemia: Different Diseases From a Common Premalignant Progenitor? *Blood Adv* (2020) 4:3466–73. doi: 10.1182/bloodadvances.2020001822
52. Ding L, Ley TJ, Larson DE, Miller CA, Koboldt DC, Welch JS, et al. Clonal Evolution in Relapsed Acute Myeloid Leukaemia Revealed by Whole-Genome Sequencing. *Nature* (2012) 481:506–10. doi: 10.1038/nature10738
53. Rooij JDE de, van den Heuvel-Eibrink MM, van de Rijdt NKAM, Verboon LJ, de Haas V, Trka J, et al. PHF6 Mutations in Paediatric Acute Myeloid Leukaemia. *Br J Haematol* (2016) 175:967–71. doi: 10.1111/bjh.13891
54. Papaemmanuil E, Gerstung M, Bullinger L, Gaidzik VI, Paschka P, Roberts ND, et al. Genomic Classification and Prognosis in Acute Myeloid Leukemia. *N Engl J Med* (2016) 374:2209–21. doi: 10.1056/NEJMoa1516192
55. Aypar U, Taylor J, Garcia JS, Momeni-Boroujeni A, Gao Q, Baik J, et al. P2RY8-CRLF2Fusion-Positive Acute Myeloid Leukemia With Myelodysplasia-Related Changes: Response to Novel Therapy. *JCO Precis Oncol* (2020) 4:152–60. doi: 10.1200/PO.19.00294
56. Ng IK, Lee J, Ng C, Kosmo B, Chiu L, Seah E, et al. Preleukemic and Second-Hit Mutational Events in an Acute Myeloid Leukemia Patient With a Novel Germline RUNX1 Mutation. *Biomark Res* (2018) 6:16. doi: 10.1186/s40364-018-0130-2
57. Staňo Kozubík K, Radová L, Pešová M, Réblová K, Trizuljak J, Plevová K, et al. C-Terminal RUNX1 Mutation in Familial Platelet Disorder With Predisposition to Myeloid Malignancies. *Int J Hematol* (2018) 108:652–7. doi: 10.1007/s12185-018-2514-3
58. Desai P, Mencia-Trinchant N, Savenkov O, Simon MS, Cheang G, Lee S, et al. Somatic Mutations Precede Acute Myeloid Leukemia Years Before Diagnosis. *Nat Med* (2018) 24:1015–23. doi: 10.1038/s41591-018-0081-z
59. Mousa NO, Gado M, Assem MM, Dawood KM, Osman A, Mousa NO, et al. Expression Profiling of Some Acute Myeloid Leukemia - Associated Markers to Assess Their Diagnostic/Prognostic Potential. *Genet Mol Biol* (2021) 44(1). doi: 10.1590/1678-4685-gmb-2019-0268
60. Patel JP, Gado M, Assem MM, Dawood KM, Osman A, Mousa NO, et al. Prognostic Relevance of Integrated Genetic Profiling in Acute Myeloid Leukemia. *N Engl J Med* (2012) 366:1079–89. doi: 10.1016/j.yonc.2012.07.030
61. Mrózek K, Eisfeld A-K, Kohlschmidt J, Carroll AJ, Walker CJ, Nicolet D, et al. Complex Karyotype in *De Novo* Acute Myeloid Leukemia: Typical and Atypical Subtypes Differ Molecularly and Clinically. *Leukemia* (2019) 33:1620–34. doi: 10.1038/s41375-019-0390-3
62. Haferlach T, Nagata Y, Grossmann V, Okuno Y, Bacher U, Nagae G, et al. Landscape of Genetic Lesions in 944 Patients With Myelodysplastic Syndromes. *Leukemia* (2014) 28:241–7. doi: 10.1038/leu.2013.336
63. Yoshida K, Sanada M, Shiraishi Y, Nowak D, Nagata Y, Yamamoto R, et al. Frequent Pathway Mutations of Splicing Machinery in Myelodysplasia. *Nature* (2011) 478:64–9. doi: 10.1038/nature10496
64. Chien KS, Kanagal-Shamanna R, Naqvi K, Sasaki K, Alvarado Y, Takahashi K, et al. The Impact of PHF6 Mutations in Myelodysplastic Syndromes, Chronic Myelomonocytic Leukemia, and Acute Myeloid Leukemia. *Blood* (2019) 134:1436–6. doi: 10.1182/blood-2019-131188
65. Li X, Yao H, Chen Z, Wang Q, Zhao Y, Chen S. Somatic Mutations of PHF6 in Patients With Chronic Myeloid Leukemia in Blast Crisis. *Leuk Lymphoma* (2013) 54:671–2. doi: 10.3109/10428194.2012.725203
66. Kurzer JH, Nardi V, Ouseph M, Weinberg OK. Clinical and Genomic Characterization of Myeloproliferative Neoplasms Harboring PHF6 Mutations, Abstract 1411. *Abstr USCAP 2020 Hematop 1316-1502 Mod Pathol* (2020) 33:1328–9. doi: 10.1038/s41379-020-0475-6
67. Ohki K, Kiyokawa N, Saito Y, Hirabayashi S, Nakabayashi K, Ichikawa H, et al. Clinical and Molecular Characteristics of MEF2D Fusion-Positive B-Cell Precursor Acute Lymphoblastic Leukemia in Childhood, Including a Novel Translocation Resulting in MEF2D-HNRNPH1 Gene Fusion. *Haematologica* (2019) 104:128–37. doi: 10.3324/haematol.2017.186320
68. Meacham CE, Lawton LN, Soto-Feliciano YM, Pritchard JR, Joughin BA, Ehrenberger T, et al. A Genome-Scale *In Vivo* Loss-of-Function Screen Identifies Phf6 as a Lineage-Specific Regulator of Leukemia Cell Growth. *Genes Dev* (2015) 29:483–8. doi: 10.1101/gad.254151.114
69. Soto-Feliciano YM, Bartlebaugh JME, Liu Y, Sánchez-Rivera FJ, Bhutkar A, Weintraub AS, et al. PHF6 Regulates Phenotypic Plasticity Through Chromatin Organization Within Lineage-Specific Genes. *Genes Dev* (2017) 31:973–89. doi: 10.1101/gad.295857.117
70. Xiao W, Bharadwaj M, Levine M, Farnhoud N, Pastore F, Getta BM, et al. PHF6 and DNMT3A Mutations Are Enriched in Distinct Subgroups of Mixed Phenotype Acute Leukemia With T-Lineage Differentiation. *Blood Adv* (2018) 2:3526–39. doi: 10.1182/bloodadvances.2018023531
71. Getta BM, Roshal M, Zheng J, Park JH, Stein EM, Levine R, et al. Allogeneic Hematopoietic Stem Cell Transplantation With Myeloablative Conditioning Is Associated With Favorable Outcomes in Mixed Phenotype Acute Leukemia. *Biol Blood Marrow Transplant J Am Soc Blood Marrow Transplant* (2017) 23:1879–86. doi: 10.1016/j.bbmt.2017.06.026
72. Mi X, Griffin G, Lee W, Patel S, Ohgami R, Ok CY, et al. Genomic and Clinical Characterization of B/T Mixed Phenotype Acute Leukemia Reveals Recurrent Features and T-ALL Like Mutations. *Am J Hematol* (2018) 93:1358–67. doi: 10.1002/ajh.25256
73. Bond J, Krzywon A, Lhermitte L, Roumier C, Roggy A, Belhocine M, et al. A Transcriptomic Continuum of Differentiation Arrest Identifies Myeloid Interface Acute Leukemias With Poor Prognosis. *Leukemia* (2021) 35:724–36. doi: 10.1038/s41375-020-0965-z
74. Weinberg OK, Hasserjian RP, Baraban E, Ok CY, Geyer JT, Philip JKSS, et al. Clinical, Immunophenotypic, and Genomic Findings of Acute Undifferentiated Leukemia and Comparison to Acute Myeloid Leukemia With Minimal Differentiation: a Study From the Bone Marrow Pathology Group. *Mod Pathol Off J U S Can Acad Pathol Inc* (2019) 32:1373–85. doi: 10.1038/s41379-019-0263-3

20

Opportunities and Challenges for Gut Microbiota in Acute Leukemia

Tao Ma[1,2]*, Yan Chen*[2]*, Li-Juan Li*[1*†] *and Lian-Sheng Zhang*[1*†]

[1] *Department of Hematology, Lanzhou University Second Hospital, Lanzhou, China,* [2] *Department of Hematology, The Affiliated Hospital of Southwest Medical University, Luzhou, China*

Correspondence:
Li-Juan Li
doctorjuan@sina.com
Lian-Sheng Zhang
doctorzhanglsh@sina.com

Acute leukemia (AL) is a highly heterogeneous hematologic malignancy, and although great progress has been made in the treatment of AL with allogeneic hematopoietic stem cell transplantation (Allo-HSCT) and new targeted drugs, problems such as infection and GVHD in AL treatment are still serious. How to reduce the incidence of AL, improve its prognosis and reduce the side effects of treatment is a crucial issue. The gut microbiota plays an important role in regulating disease progression, pathogen colonization, and immune responses. This article reviews recent advances in the gut microbiota and AL pathogenesis, infection, treatment and its role in allo-HSCT.

Keywords: gut microbiota, acute leukemia, pathogenesis, GVHD, drugs, immunity, allo-HSCT

INTRODUCTION

Acute leukemia (AL), a kind of hematologic malignancy, mainly includes acute myeloid leukemia (AML) and acute lymphoblastic leukemia (ALL) (1). In 2018, a global survey of 36 cancers in 185 countries indicated that leukemia ranks fifteenth in cancer incidence and tenth in cancer deaths (2). The most common cancer in children is AL (3). More than 80% of children with ALL are long term survivors, compared with 20% to 40% of adults (4). In AML, the five-year survival rate is 40% for patients younger than 60, and only 10-20% for patients older than 60 (5). Cytotoxic chemotherapy, ionizing radiation, genetic mutations, benzene, and some blood system diseases (such as myelodysplastic syndrome, paroxysmal nocturnal hemoglobinuria) can lead to AL (6, 7). The specific pathogenesis of AL is not fully understood, and some types of AL are dangerous, ineffective and have a high mortality rate. Immune system plays an important role in the pathogenesis, progression and treatment of AL. AML patients have higher T regulatory cells (Tregs) and $CD8^+$ T cells compared to normal donors (8). However, AML patients have T-cell dysfunction, which is associated with immune escape of the disease (9). Moreover, Tregs are a major contributor to defective immune responses (10). In AML patients, increased Tregs can suppress effector T cells, and the more Tregs, the worse the treatment effect (11). Treatment with chimeric antigen receptor T-cell therapy is highly effective in patients with ALL, which is also associated with the immune system (12).

There are four major colonization sites of microorganisms in the human body: oral, vagina, skin, and gut (13). Gut microbiota colonize the newborn following birth (14). The gut microbiota is composed of native flora and transient flora in food intake (15). It is estimated that each individual's gut microbiome includes more than 100 different species (15). Gut microbiota has recently been recognized as an important factor in regulating disease progression, pathogen colonization, and immune responses (1, 13, 16), and the pathogenesis, progression, and treatment of AL have been linked to the immune system. Gut microbiota has also been linked to diabetes, Alzheimer's disease, tumor and so on (17–19). This review summarizes the progress of the interaction between gut microbiota and AL.

THE ROLE OF GUT MICROBIOTA IN THE PATHOGENESIS OF AL

The pathogenesis of AL is unclear. Greaves M propose a model for ALL, in which some children are born with pre-leukemic clones, but acquired infections cause key genetic mutations that develop into ALL (20). Some studies have found that newborns carry leukemia-related mutations, such as TCF3-PBX1 and ETV6-RUNX1 (21, 22). Exposure to infection promotes the occurrence of ALL in newborns carrying these genes (23, 24). In mice with PAX5 or ETV6-RUNX1, ALL was caused by a disruption in the microbiome caused by antibiotic treatment early in life, and the gut microbiome of PAX5-carrying mice differed from the wild type (25). A study enrolled 81 subjects, including 58 ALL patients and 23 healthy controls, using 16S rRNA quantitative arrays and bioinformatics analysis to examine their stool specimens (26). Many species of bacteria appeared significantly different in stool specimens from ALL patients compared to healthy controls, such as a significant enrichment of *Bacteroides clarus* in ALL (26). Whether gut microbiota disturbance can cause AL in humans needs further study.

Alterations in some gut microbiota species and metabolites may promote the development of leukemia. In a mouse model of leukemia, the proportion of bacteria with the function of converting dietary flavonoids in the small intestine of leukemic mice was increased (27). It has been suggested that maternal intake of bioflavonoids may lead to infant and young child leukemia (28). A national case-control study conducted in Denmark and found that infections of the gastrointestinal tract were associated with an increased risk of AML (29). So why does the occurrence of a gastrointestinal infection lead to an increased risk of developing AML? We assume that the imbalance of gut microbiota due to gastrointestinal infections causes immune disorders that lead to AML, but more studies are still needed to verify this.

The risk of AL increased significantly during childhood or adolescence after the cumulative dose of ionizing radiation (30). Ionizing radiation is the accepted cause of leukemia. A study found that mice that survived high doses of radiation had unique gut microbiota, with Lachnospiraceae and Enterococcaceae as the most abundant bacteria (31). Then, they collected stool samples from 21 leukemia patients who had received total body radiation before hematopoietic stem cell transplantation, patients with shorter duration of diarrhea (diarrhea less than 10 days) had more Lachnospiraceae and Enterococcaceae in their feces than patients with longer duration of diarrhea (diarrhea more than 10 days) (31). Lactobacillaceae also increased in patients with shorter duration of diarrhea, but there was no statistical significance (31). Bone marrow and small intestinal epithelial cells are highly sensitive to ionizing radiation, and they are the main site of radiation injury (32). Short-chain fatty acids (SCFAs), a metabolite of gut microbiota, reduces DNA damage and reactive oxygen species release in blood and gastrointestinal tissues during radiation damage (31). Fecal microbiota transplantation (FMT) improved the survival rate of irradiated animals, increased white blood cells, and improved gastrointestinal function (33). The gut microbiota plays a key role in host defenses against radiation, as well as protecting the hematopoietic and gastrointestinal systems.

Benzene is a widespread air pollutant and a component of gasoline, industrial emissions, automobile exhaust and tobacco smoke (34). Traffic-related benzene exposure can cause acute myeloid leukemia in children (35). A study of benzene exposure in mice showed that benzene exposure altered the gut microbiota, with increased level of Actinobacteria, and Helicobacter were observed in the stools of mice exposed to high doses of benzene, and increased level of Actinobacteria were significantly and negatively correlated with basic blood cells (white blood cell, red blood cell, and hemoglobin levels) (36). Whether gut microbiota plays a role in benzene causing leukemia remains to be studied.

It is well known that naïve helper T cells (Th0) can be transformed into Th1, Th2, Treg and Th17 cells etc. Th1 produces the cytokine interferon gamma (IFN-γ) that exerts anti-tumorigenic effects in the tumor microenvironment, while Th2/Treg produces the cytokines interleukin 4 (IL-4), IL-5, IL-10, etc. that mediate pro-tumorigenic effects (17). In some solid tumor models, depletion of the gut microbiota leaded to a significant increase in IFN-γ-producing T cells and a decrease in IL-17A and IL-10-producing T cells, thereby reduced tumor burden. However, this phenomenon was not present in mice lacking mature T and B cells, suggesting that the action of the gut microbiota on tumor cells required the active involvement of adaptive immunity (17). In innate and adaptive immunity, microbiota plays an important role in its maturation, development and functions (37).

There is no doubt that the development of AL is related to the dysregulation of the human immune system, and the gut microbiota also regulates the human immune system, which has been shown to be closely related to the development of pancreatic cancer, colon cancer and other tumors (38, 39). Whether the gut microbiota is also involved in the development of AL by modulating human immunity needs to be studied in more depth.

A NORMAL, DIVERSE GUT MICROBIOTA IS CRITICAL TO HUMAN IMMUNITY AND CAN PREDICT INFECTION IN PATIENTS WITH AL

Infection is a common symptom in patients with newly diagnosed AL. In addition, the bone marrow suppression that occurs after chemotherapy in AL patients is also prone to infection. Infection is an important cause of death in patients with AL (40, 41). Gut microbiota is strongly associated with host immune function and resistance to infection. It is essential for the host to maintain a healthy immune system (42). It has been shown that gut microbiota can produce inhibitory products to suppress vancomycin-resistant enterococci (43). The use of carbapenem antibiotics in the empirical treatment of fever due to neutropenia in patients with AL reduces gut microbiota diversity and increases colonization by vancomycin-resistant enterococci (44). SCFAs, a metabolite of gut microbiota, promote the differentiation of T lymphocytes into effector T cells and regulatory T cells by inhibiting histone deacetylase (45). SCFAs also significantly inhibited the activity and infectivity of E. coli and protected intestinal epithelial cells from damage caused by C. difficile toxins (45, 46). Treatment of mice with broad-spectrum antibiotics resulted in a decrease in the number of hematopoietic stem cells and pluripotent progenitor cells in their bone marrow, as well as a decrease in granulocytes and B cells in the bone marrow and an increase in CD8+ T cells (47). This is the result of broad-spectrum antibiotics interfering with the STAT1 signaling pathway by consuming the gut microbiota (47). The aromatic amino acid metabolite production pathway of intestinal gut symbiont Clostridium sporogenes produces 12 compounds, 9 of which accumulate in host serum, indolepropionic acid being one of them. A decrease in indolepropionic acid increases the number of immune cells in mice, including neutrophils, monocytes, and memory T cells, and mice with decreased indolepropionic acid have greater intestinal permeability and are more likely to trigger an inflammatory response in mice (48). A normal and diverse gut microbiota is essential for human immunity and resistance to infection.

Causes of gut microbiota dysbiosis in AL patients associated with antibiotic use, nutrition, and chemotherapy (49). A study used a 16s rRNA-based analysis of bacterial flora in oral and fecal specimens from 97 AML patients every two weeks from induction chemotherapy to neutrophil recovery. They found that fecal flora diversity and high levels of Porphyromonadaceae at the time of induction chemotherapy were positively associated with a low risk of infection (50). In AML patients who developed infection during induction chemotherapy, baseline fecal flora diversity was significantly lower than in patients who did not develop infection, and flora diversity gradually decreased over the course of induction chemotherapy (51). In a study of ALL, chemotherapy was also found to have an impact on the diversity of the gut microbiota, with a significant decrease in the relative abundance of certain bacterial groups (e.g., Bacteroidetes) and a significant increase in the relative abundance of other groups (e.g., Clostridiaceae and Streptococcaceae) following chemotherapy (52). In contrast to the findings of some studies (44), this study concluded that antibiotic use does not alter the diversity of the gut microbiota (52). However, it has also been suggested that vancomycin use significantly reduces gut microbial diversity in patients with ALL, while no correlation was found with piperacillin tazobactam, antifungal drugs and other antibiotics (53). Some investigators concluded that the composition, but not the diversity, of the gut microbiome prior to chemotherapy was an independent predictor of febrile neutropenia during chemotherapy. The predominance of Aspergillus phylum and Enterococcus (relative abundance ≥30%) predicted febrile neutropenia; Enterococcus (relative abundance ≥30%) and Streptococcaceae predominate in predicting diarrheal disease (52). Intestinal nutrition deficiency can lead to loss of intestinal epithelial barrier function and increased susceptibility to infection (54).

In a study evaluating the effect of probiotics on chemotherapy-induced gastrointestinal side effects in patients with AL, patients with AL were randomized to an oral Lactobacillus rhamnosus group and a control group. The primary endpoint was the incidence of gastrointestinal side effects, with significant reductions in nausea, vomiting, and abdominal distention ($P<0.05$) and a relative risk of diarrhea (0.5) in the oral probiotics group (55). Patients in the control group of this study did not take placebo and subjective error may occur. In a study of gut microbiota recovery in mice and humans, it was found that neither probiotics nor spontaneous recovery restored gut microbiota diversity after 4 weeks of disruption cessation with antibiotics. Importantly, probiotics significantly delayed recovery to baseline microbiome richness at all time points tested, compared to spontaneous recovery (56). However, gut microbiota diversity was indistinguishable to control after 8 days of fecal transplantation (56). The use of probiotics can only restore one or a few specific gut microbes, but not the function of a complex microbial community. Therefore, supplementation with one probiotic alone may have adverse effects on the host (49), or may even result in probiotic-induced infections. A patient who received autologous hematopoietic stem cell transplantation took probiotic-rich yogurt due to severe diarrhea, and a week later the patient developed infectious shock (57). Strain-specific PCR analysis showed that the pathogen was Lactobacillus rhamnosus GG, which was consistent with the probiotics in the yogurt (57). Another child with Philadelphia chromosome-positive ALL underwent chemotherapy and developed neutropenic fever with blood cultures suggestive of Bifidobacterium breve, which may be pathogenic when host immunity is reduced (58). In patients with AL, the diversity and composition of gut microbes correlate with whether or not an infection occurs or what type of infection occurs, and they are influenced by factors such as chemotherapy and antibiotics. Probiotics can reduce gastrointestinal symptoms such as diarrhea, but opportunistic infections with probiotics have also been reported in the presence of neutrophil deficiency.

The gut microbiota is closely related to the normal immunity of the organism (42). Among the infections present in patients with AL, the gut microbiota has been associated with diarrhea, neutropenic fever, and sepsis, and its diversity and composition are predictive of infection in patients (45–52, 59).

GUT MICROBIOTA AFFECTS A WIDE RANGE OF DRUGS USED TO TREAT AL

There is increasing evidence that host responses to chemotherapeutic agents can be influenced by the gut microbiota, primarily in terms of promoting drug efficacy; abrogation of anticancer effects; and modulation of toxicity (60). Gut microbiota regulates chemotherapeutic drugs through key mechanisms such as reduced diversity, ecological variation, translocation, immune regulation, metabolism, enzymatic degradation (60).

Cyclophosphamide (CTX) is commonly used to treat ALL, lymphoma, and other tumors. Viaud S et al. investigates the role of gut microbiota in CTX therapy through a mouse model (61). Non-myeloablative doses of CTX and adriamycin treated mice resulted in shortened small intestinal villi, disrupted epithelial barrier, and interstitial edema 48 hours after drug application (61). After the disruption of the intestinal barrier, some intestinal microorganisms are transferred to the mesenteric lymph nodes and spleen, and intestinal microorganisms including Lactobacillus johnsonii, Lactobacillus murinus and Enterococcus hirae can be cultured in these lymphoid organs (61). CTX treatment induces selective translocation of gut microbiota, for example, leading to reduced abundance of Lactobacillus and Enterococcus in the small intestine of mice. Some intestinal bacteria (Lactobacillus johnsonii, Lactobacillus murinus and Enterococcus hirae) stimulate the production of specific "pathogenic" T helper 17 (pT(H)17) cells. Killing these bacteria with antibiotics reduced the pT(H)17 response in tumor-bearing mice and made them resistant to CTX. Adoptive transplantation of pT(H)17 cells could recover the anti-neoplastic efficacy of CTX in part. In another study, calorie restriction was found to significantly enhance the gut microbiota with Lactobacillus and Trichinella, which are shown to relieve inflammation and improve intestinal barrier function. Calorie restriction reshapes stronger gut microbiota and may help reduce side effects of CTX (62).

Methotrexate (MTX) has the function of anticancer and immunosuppressive, and is one of the main drugs used in the treatment of ALL, central nervous system leukemia, and rheumatic immune system diseases (63–65). Common side effects of MTX include mucositis and intestinal damage (66, 67). MTX has significant effects on the amounts, diversity and major components of the mouse gut microbiota (68). MTX -treated mice showed reduced intestinal microbial diversity and changes in the composition of the gut microbiota, such as a dramatic decrease in the number of ruminal cocci and a dramatic increase in the number of members of the Lachnospiraceae (68). B. fragilis was significantly reduced by MTX treatment, and there was a tendency for the proliferation rate of B. fragilis to decrease with increasing M1 macrophage density (68). The mucosal muscle lesions seen in mtx-treated mice were significantly relieved by gavage with fragile B (68). Fragile B. markedly attenuated the MTX-induced increase in M1 macrophages, and the decrease in fragile B. in turn aggravated the MTX-induced macrophage imbalance, resulting in positive feedback, which led to intestinal tissue injury (68). Chronic long-term MTX exposure induced changes in the gut microbiota composition and function, with the relative abundance of the Firmicutes being higher than that of the Bacteroidetes at low doses of MTX, but the opposite at high doses of MTX. The relative abundance of the Firmicutes was positively correlated with the 48-h fecal excretion of 2,4-diamino-N-10-methylpteroic acid (DAMPA), a metabolite of MTX. Long-term exposure to MTX can alter the composition and function of the microbiome, which in turn affects its ability to detoxify MTX (69). MTX largely alters the human gut microbiota. Changes in gut flora and gene abundance were different between patients who responded to MTX and those who did not. MTX affects a variety of conserved human gut bacterial pathways, leading to reduced host immune activation (70).

PD-1 is a kind of immune checkpoint, PD-1 binding with PD-L1 will inhibit T cells and block the anti-tumor immune response. Anti-PD1 has been approved by FDA for the treatment of melanoma, non-small cell lung cancer, renal cell carcinoma and other tumors (71). In a mouse model, enhanced PD-1 expression on circulating CD8 T cells leads to the progression of AML (72). A phase II clinical trial of azacitidine combined with nivolumab in patients with relapsed/refractory AML obtained an encouraging result, with an overall response rate (ORR) of 33% (73). PD-1 inhibitors have promising applications in the treatment of AL, and the gut microbiota also interacts with PD-1 inhibitors. In a mouse model study of epithelial tumors, primary resistance of tumors to immune checkpoint inhibitors (ICIs) was found to be attributable to unusual composition of the gut microbiome, and the clinical benefit of ICIs in patients with late-stage cancer could be inhibited by antibiotics (74). Germ-free or antibiotic-treated mice receiving fecal microbiota transplantation (FMT) from patients with tumors that responded to ICIs improved the antitumor effects of PD-1 blockade, but FMT from patients with tumors that did not respond to ICIs had no such effect (74). Metagenomics of patient fecal samples revealed a correlation between the relative abundance of Akkermansia muciniphila and patient response to ICIs. Administration of oral supplementation of A. muciniphila to mice unresponsive to FMT restored the efficacy of PD-1 blockade in an interleukin-12-dependent manner (74). In another study of melanoma patients, researchers found that the effect of anti-pd-1 immunotherapy was associated with greater abundance of Bifidobacterium longum, Collinsella aerofaciens, and Enterococcus faecium in the patients' stools (75). Transplanting feces from patients who responded to anti-pd-1 into germ-free tumor-bearing mice enhanced the T-cell effect and improved tumor control (75). In a study of the gut microbiota of melanoma patients receiving PD-1 immunotherapy, investigators found that the diversity of the flora and the relative abundance of Ruminococcaceae family were significantly higher in patients who responded to PD-1 immunotherapy (76). In immunotherapy for liver cancer, researchers also found more taxa richness and higher gene counts in the stools of patients who responded to anti-PD-1 (77). Gut microbiota correlates with the efficacy of ICIs in a wide range of tumors, with higher diversity of gut microbes associated with better efficacy. Whether the efficacy of anti-PD-1 therapy in patients with AL is also associated with the gut microbiota needs to be urgently investigated.

There are no studies on the interaction of gut microbiota with drugs used to treat AML (e.g., erythromycin, cytarabine, etc.), which is a future direction to investigate the relevance of gut microbiota to AL therapeutic drugs.

THE PLACE OF GUT MICROBIOTA IN ALLO-HSCT: FOR BETTER OR FOR WORSE?

Allo-HSCT is currently one of the most effective treatments for AL (78). Allo-HSCT means that hematopoietic stem cells collected from a healthy donor are infused into a patient with leukemia, and the donor's immune cells can attack the leukemia cells to produce a graft-versus-leukemia (GVL) effect (79). The main side effect of allo-HSCT is graft-versus-host disease (GVHD) (79, 80). GVHD means that the immune cells of the donor attack the normal tissues of the patient, and the common organs are the skin, liver, and gastrointestinal tract, and the patient may present with diarrhea, vomiting, abdominal pain, jaundice, sclerosis of the skin, and other harmful manifestations (79). Acute graft-versus-host disease (aGVHD) occurs in 30-50% of all allo-HSCT patients, and chronic graft-versus-host disease (cGVHD) occurs in 35-50% of patients (81, 82). Prevention of GVHD includes the use of cyclosporine, tacrolimus, mycophenolate mofetil (MMF), methotrexate, etc (83). Despite the use of these drugs, many patients still develop GVHD, and glucocorticoids are an effective treatment for both aGVHD and cGVHD (83). But glucocorticoids can cause side effects such as osteoporosis, susceptibility to infection, increased blood sugar and blood pressure, necrosis of femoral head and so on. In summary, GVHD affects the quality of survival, mortality in allo-HSCT patients. Gut microbiota plays an important role in the development and treatment of GVHD (84).

Gut microbiota correlates with the development of GVHD. In 1974, van Bekkum DW et al. found that GVHD occurred in mice treated with lethal total body irradiation and allo-HSCT, with a mortality rate of 95% within 100 days, whereas mice treated similarly in a sterile state or given a colonization-resistant flora had almost no GVHD (85). This study confirmed in an animal model that the microbiome is associated with GVHD. In a study of mice, it was found that the gut microbiota diversity of mice with GVHD decreased significantly during the first 2 weeks of bone marrow transplantation, and in terms of changes in bacterial subgroups, the number of Lactobacillus increased significantly in the ileum, while the number of Clostridium and other Firmicutes decreased significantly (86). The authors also found that removal of Lactobacillus prior to bone marrow transplantation aggravated GVHD in mice and that reintroduction of a dominant species of Lactobacillus mediated protection against GVHD (86).

The presence of disruption of the gut microbiota early in bone marrow transplantation is also a potential risk factor for GVHD (86). We already know that SCFAs can reduce DNA damage in blood and gastrointestinal tissues during radiation damage (31), and SCFAs inhibit histone deacetylation (45). SCFAs mainly include formate, acetate, propionate and butyrate (87). Mathewson ND et al. analyzed SCFAs produced by the microbiome of allo-HSCT mice and found that only butyrate was significantly reduced in the intestinal tissues of transplanted recipients, resulting in reduced levels of histone deacetylation in small intestinal epithelial cells. In contrast, increasing the level of butyrate in the small intestine restored histone deacetylation, protected small intestinal epithelial cells, and reduced the severity of GVHD (88). The mechanism by which butyrate protects small intestinal epithelial cells may be through the regulation of histone deacetylation to increase anti-apoptotic genes. In butyrate-treated small intestinal epithelial cells, Bak1 and Bax were significantly reduced and the anti-apoptotic protein BCL-B was significantly increased (88). In the study of SCFAs and cGVHD, higher SCFAs (mainly butyrate and propionate) in the plasma of patients at 100 days post-transplantation were associated with decreased cGVHD (89). Golob JL et al. prospectively collected 669 stool samples from 66 allo-HSCT patients, once a week from pre-transplant to 100 days post-transplant. Their analysis revealed that the presence of Lachnospiraceae in stool was negatively associated with GVHD when neutrophils recovered after transplantation, whereas the presence of oral Actinobacteria and oral Firmicutes was positively associated with GVHD (90). A study by Han L et al. found more gut microbiota diversity in the non-aGVHD group than in the aGVHD group (91), they evaluated the gut microbiota to predict GVHD and found that Lachnospiraceae and Peptostreptococcaceae were negatively associated with GVHD, while Enterobacteriaceae were positively associated with aGVHD (91). Lachnospiraceae was negatively correlated with severe aGVHD, and levels of all major SFCAs were significantly decreased in patients with severe aGVHD, with a 75.8% decrease in acetate, a 95.8% decrease in propionate, and a 94.6% decrease in butyrate, while propionate levels were retained in patients with mild aGVHD. Butyrate was severely reduced in all gastrointestinal stages of aGVHD (92). Patients with ≤10% Lachnospiraceae in stool specimens at transplant pretreatment were significant contributors to overall mortality, and reduced gut microbiota diversity at day 10 post-transplant significantly increased the risk of GVHD (93). These studies all confirmed that abundant Lachnospiraceae and intact gut microbiota diversity were negatively correlated with GVHD (90–93). Lachnospiraceae-dominant gut microbiota mice also can withstand high doses of radiation (31), Lachnospiraceae and SCFA (propionate) are used to modulate host resistance to high doses of radiation by promoting hematopoiesis and gastrointestinal recovery (31).

Another product of the gut microbiota, indole, has also been shown to improve GVHD. Indole is produced by certain intestinal microflora (e.g., Escherichia coli, Lactobacillus, Bacteroides) (94). Indole-3-carbaldehyde (ICA) is an exogenous indole derivative. ICA upregulated genes associated with type I interferon (IFN1) responses, limited intestinal epithelial damage, reduced inflammatory cytokine production, and decreased GVHD pathology and GVHD mortality without affecting donor T cell-mediated graft-versus-leukemia responses (95). Although SCFAs and indoles, metabolites of the gut microbiota, have been shown to reduce the severity of GVHD, another circulating gut microbial metabolite, TMA N-oxide (TMAO), has been reported to enhance M1 macrophage polarization, and polarized inflammatory macrophages establish an environment for t helper type 1 (Th1) and Th17 responses, thereby increasing GVHD (96).

The use of broad-spectrum antibiotics can increase the severity of GVHD. In a mouse model of allo-HSCT, treatment with imipenem-cilastatin was found to disrupt intestinal microbiota and increase the severity of GVHD (mainly increased GVHD pathology in the colon) in mice with GVHD, resulting in increased mortality (97). However, if the mice did not develop GVHD, treatment with imipenem-cilastatin did not affect the survival of the mice (97). Why did the use of imipenem-cilastatin lead to increased severity of GVHD in mice? Further studies revealed that in these mice, donor effector CD4+ T cells (CD25+FoxP3-) and interleukin-23 (IL-23) were increased and granulocytes were infiltrated in their colon (97). AL patients treated with intensive chemotherapy and broad-spectrum antibiotics destroy the diversity of the intestinal microbiota (98). The use of autologous fecal microbiota transfer (AFMT) restores intestinal flora diversity and is safe for immunocompromised patients (98). Whether AFMT can improve GVHD requires further study.

Gut microbiota correlates with the prognosis of allo-HSCT. Kusakabe S et al. studied the gut microbiota of normal, autologous HSCT patients and allo-HSCT patients, and they found that in allo-HSCT patients with skewed microbiota had a higher frequency of more complications and death after transplantation than the subgroup with preserved microbiota composition (93). The diversity of the gut microbiota is an independent predictor of mortality in allo-HSCT patients, Taur Y collected stools from 80 allo-HSCT patients for analysis, and the percentage of patients maintaining high, intermediate, and low diversity of the gut microbiota was 26 (32.5%), 20 (25.0%), and 34 (42.5%), and their 3-year overall survival rates were 67%, 60% and 36%, respectively (99). Peled JU et al. analyzed 8767 stool samples from 1362 patients who received allo-HSCT from a total of four transplant centers in the United States, Germany, and Japan and found that higher gut microbiota diversity at the time of neutrophil engraftment was associated with lower patient mortality, patients with low gut microbiota diversity were positively associated with transplant-related mortality and a high risk of GVHD (100). A study on gut microbiota and pulmonary complications after allo-HSCT found that low gut microbiota diversity was associated with PCs occurring preengraftment, whereas γ-proteobacteria dominant gut flora was associated with PCs postengraftment (101). PCs postengraftment and γ-proteobacteria dominant gut flora were associated with mortality (101). In a study of a total of four bone marrow transplant centers from the United States, Japan, and Germany, the investigators defined Enterococcal dominance as having a relative genic abundance of ≥0.3 in any fecal sample (102). The incidence of Enterococcus dominance was high at all centers, with 441 of 1101 patients (40.1%) at Memorial Sloan Kettering Cancer Center (MSKCC) and 103 of 224 patients (46.0%) at the other 3 centers having E. faecium dominance between day -20 and day +80 of allo-HSCT (102). Early post-transplant (day 0 to + 21) Enterococcus dominance significantly reduced overall survival and increased GVHD-related mortality, increasing the risk of severe aGVHD (102). In a mouse model of allo-HSCT, an increase in Enterococcus in the feces of mice was also positively associated with GVHD, and the absence of lactose in the diet significantly reduced the colonization of Enterococcus after transplantation and attenuated GVHD (102). Lactose-free diets may be used in clinical settings to attenuate the growth of pathogens such as enterococci and improve clinical outcomes.

TABLE 1 | Mechanisms by which the gut microbiota affects GVHD.

Influence of gut microbiota on GVHD	Mechanisms	References
Lactobacillus shows improvement in GVHD	–	(86)
Disruption of gut microbiota diversity aggravates GVHD	–	(86, 91, 93)
Butyrate, a metabolite of the gut microbiota, attenuates GVHD	Butyrate improved IEC junctional integrity, decreased apoptosis	(88, 89)
Lachnospiraceae is negatively associated with GVHD	–	(90–93)
Indole, a metabolite of the gut microbiota, improves GVHD	Indole upregulates genes associated with IFN1 response, limits intestinal epithelial damage, reduces inflammatory cytokine production, and decreases GVHD pathology and GVHD mortality.	(95)
GVHD progression was induced by TMAO, a circulating gut microbial metabolite	TMAO enhances M1 macrophage polarization and establishes an environment for Th1 and Th17 responses	(96)
Antibiotic use alters the composition of the gut microbiota and increases GVHD	Loss of protective colonic mucosa and impairment of intestinal barrier function due to antibiotics	(97)
Obesity aggravates GVHD by affecting the gut microbiota	Obesity reduces the diversity of the gut microbiota and reduces Clostridiaceae abundance, leading to increased intestinal permeability, transintestinal transit of endotoxins, and radiation-induced gastrointestinal damage in mice	(107)
The microbiota controls MHC-II at the pre-transplant IEC	Microbiota depletion inhibits IL-12/23p40 production by ileal macrophages, IL-12/23p40 prevents upregulation of MHC class II cells on IECs and initiation of lethal GVHD in the gastrointestinal tract	(108)
The gut microbiota metabolite sensor G-protein-coupled receptor 43 (GPR43) attenuates gastrointestinal GVHD	GVHD protection by SCFAs requires GPR43-mediated ERK phosphorylation and activation of NLRP3 inflammasome in host non-hematopoietic target tissues	(109)

Interestingly, it has been shown that the relative abundance of Eubacterium hallii is higher in minimal residual disease (MRD)-negative multiple myeloma patients compared to MRD-positive patients (103). Whether the relative abundance of gut microbiota is associated with risk stratification of AL and MRD has not been studied, which warrants further research.

FMT is a treatment for multidrug-resistant bacteria colonization and GVHD in patients undergoing allo-HSCT. Battipaglia G et al. performed FMT in 10 patients colonized by multidrug resistance; eight of these patients were colonized by carbapenemase-producing bacteria and two by vancomycin-resistant enterococci; four of them underwent FMT before allo-HSCT and the other six underwent FMT after allo-HSCT; seven of the 10 patients achieved decolonization (104). We already know that disruption of gut microbiota diversity can exacerbate GVHD, but patients are in a state of severe immunosuppression after allo-HSCT, and performing FMT on them may be at potential risk for microbial infection. Kakihana K et al. performed FMT on one glucocorticoid-dependent and three glucocorticoid-resistant patients with gut aGVHD, and none of the patients experienced serious adverse effects (105). All four patients responded to FMT, with three complete responses and one partial response (105). DeFilipp Z et al. performed FMT on 13 patients at a median of 27 days (19-45) after allo-HSCT, and analysis of the patients' fecal microbiota composition and urinary 3-indoxyl sulfate concentration showed that FMT reconstructed the diversity of the patients' gut microbiota (106). We summarized recent studies on gut microbiota and GVHD (**Table 1**).

A study analyzing the gut microbiota of 541 patients undergoing allo-HSCT found that the cumulative incidence of recurrence/progression at 2 years was 19.8% and 33.8% in patients with and without Eubacterium limosum, respectively, with higher abundance of Eubacterium limosum being associated with fewer recurrences (110). Eubacterium limosum may serve as a biomarker for allo-HSCT to predict recurrence, and the exact mechanism by which it reduces recurrence needs to be confirmed by further studies.

In general, the gut microbiota may play an important role in the pathogenesis, progression and treatment of AL by influencing human immunity. The gut microbiota has been found to resist damage from radiation and benzene, which may cause AL. The gut microbiota is also closely related to the body's normal immunity, and in AL, the diversity of the gut microbiota is associated with multiple infections. When AL patients undergo chemotherapy, the gut microbiota is affected and, in turn, the gut microbiota affects the efficacy of multiple chemotherapeutic agents. The diversity of the gut microbiota and its metabolites are strongly associated with the occurrence of GVHD, mortality and relapse of allo-HSCT. More studies can be conducted in the future to focus on the relationship between the gut microbiota and AL, especially that the gut microbiota improves the treatment outcome and prognosis of AL patients by regulating human immunity.

AUTHOR CONTRIBUTIONS

TM and YC wrote the manuscript. L-JL and L-SZ wrote and critically revised the manuscript. All authors contributed to the article and approved the submitted version.

FUNDING

The present study was supported by grants from the National Natural Science Foundation of China (Grant No. 31660112); The Science and Technique Innovation Project of Lanzhou University Second Hospital (CY2017-ZD04 and CY2019-MS14); The Research Foundation of The Affiliated Hospital of Southwest Medical University (Grant No. 15015); The Research Foundation of Southwest Medical University (2017-ZRQN-092); and The Talent Innovation and Entrepreneurship Project of Lanzhou Science and Technology Bureau (2020-RC-48).

REFERENCES

1. Wen Y, Jin R, Chen H. Interactions Between Gut Microbiota and Acute Childhood Leukemia. *Front Microbiol* (2019) 10:1300. doi: 10.3389/fmicb.2019.01300
2. Bray F, Ferlay J, Soerjomataram I, Siegel RL, Torre LA, Jemal A. Global Cancer Statistics 2018: GLOBOCAN Estimates of Incidence and Mortality Worldwide for 36 Cancers in 185 Countries. *CA Cancer J Clin* (2018) 68 (6):394–424. doi: 10.3322/caac.21492 [Published Correction Appears in CA Cancer J Clin. 2020 Jul;70(4):313].
3. Steliarova-Foucher E, Colombet M, Ries LAG, Moreno F, Dolya A, Bray F, et al. International Incidence of Childhood Cancer, 2001-10: A Population-Based Registry Study. *Lancet Oncol* (2017) 18(6):719–31. doi: 10.1016/S1470-2045(17)30186-9 [Published Correction Appears in Lancet Oncol. 2017 Jun;18(6):e301].
4. Jabbour E, O'Brien S, Konopleva M, Kantarjian H. New Insights Into the Pathophysiology and Therapy of Adult Acute Lymphoblastic Leukemia. *Cancer* (2015) 121(15):2517–28. doi: 10.1002/cncr.29383
5. Yang X, Wang J. Precision Therapy for Acute Myeloid Leukemia. *J Hematol Oncol* (2018) 11(1):3. doi: 10.1186/s13045-017-0543-7
6. McNerney ME, Godley LA, Le Beau MM. Therapy-Related Myeloid Neoplasms: When Genetics and Environment Collide. *Nat Rev Cancer* (2017) 17(9):513–27. doi: 10.1038/nrc.2017.60
7. Short NJ, Rytting ME, Cortes JE. Acute Myeloid Leukaemia. *Lancet* (2018) 392(10147):593–606. doi: 10.1016/S0140-6736(18)31041-9
8. Williams P, Basu S, Garcia-Manero G, Hourigan CS, Oetjen KA, Cortes JE, et al. The Distribution of T-cell Subsets and the Expression of Immune Checkpoint Receptors and Ligands in Patients With Newly Diagnosed and Relapsed Acute Myeloid Leukemia. *Cancer* (2019) 125(9):1470–81. doi: 10.1002/cncr.31896
9. Le Dieu R, Taussig DC, Ramsay AG, Mitter R, Miraki-Moud F, Fatah R, et al. Peripheral Blood T Cells in Acute Myeloid Leukemia (AML) Patients at Diagnosis Have Abnormal Phenotype and Genotype and Form Defective Immune Synapses With AML Blasts. *Blood* (2009) 114(18):3909–16. doi: 10.1182/blood-2009-02-206946
10. Ustun C, Miller JS, Munn DH, Weisdorf DJ, Blazar BR. Regulatory T Cells in Acute Myelogenous Leukemia: Is it Time for Immunomodulation? *Blood* (2011) 118(19):5084–95. doi: 10.1182/blood-2011-07-365817
11. Szczepanski MJ, Szajnik M, Czystowska M, Mandapathil M, Strauss L, Welsh A, et al. Increased Frequency and Suppression by Regulatory T

Cells in Patients With Acute Myelogenous Leukemia. *Clin Cancer Res* (2009) 15(10):3325–32. doi: 10.1158/1078-0432.CCR-08-3010
12. Xu X, Sun Q, Liang X, Chen Z, Zhang X, Zhou X, et al. Mechanisms of Relapse After CD19 Car T-Cell Therapy for Acute Lymphoblastic Leukemia and Its Prevention and Treatment Strategies. *Front Immunol* (2019) 10:2664. doi: 10.3389/fimmu.2019.02664
13. Adak A, Khan MR. An Insight Into Gut Microbiota and Its Functionalities. *Cell Mol Life Sci* (2019) 76(3):473–93. doi: 10.1007/s00018-018-2943-4
14. Milani C, Duranti S, Bottacini F, Casey E, Turroni F, Mahony J, et al. The First Microbial Colonizers of the Human Gut: Composition, Activities, and Health Implications of the Infant Gut Microbiota. *Microbiol Mol Biol Rev* (2017) 81(4):e00036-17. doi: 10.1128/MMBR.00036-17
15. Sánchez B, Delgado S, Blanco-Míguez A, Lourenço A, Gueimonde M, Margolles A. Probiotics, Gut Microbiota, and Their Influence on Host Health and Disease. *Mol Nutr Food Res* (2017) 61(1):10.1002/mnfr.201600240. doi: 10.1002/mnfr.201600240
16. Pickard JM, Zeng MY, Caruso R, Núñez G. Gut Microbiota: Role in Pathogen Colonization, Immune Responses, and Inflammatory Disease. *Immunol Rev* (2017) 279(1):70–89. doi: 10.1111/imr.12567
17. Sethi V, Kurtom S, Tarique M, Lavania S, Malchiodi Z, Hellmund L, et al. Gut Microbiota Promotes Tumor Growth in Mice by Modulating Immune Response. *Gastroenterology* (2018) 155(1):33–37.e6. doi: 10.1053/j.gastro.2018.04.001
18. Jiang C, Li G, Huang P, Liu Z, Zhao B. The Gut Microbiota and Alzheimer's Disease. *J Alzheimers Dis* (2017) 58(1):1–15. doi: 10.3233/JAD-161141
19. Velmurugan G, Ramprasath T, Gilles M, Swaminathan K, Ramasamy S. Gut Microbiota, Endocrine-Disrupting Chemicals, and the Diabetes Epidemic. *Trends Endocrinol Metab* (2017) 28(8):612–25. doi: 10.1016/j.tem.2017.05.001
20. Greaves M. A Causal Mechanism for Childhood Acute Lymphoblastic Leukaemia [Published Correction Appears in Nat Rev Cancer. *Nat Rev Cancer* (2018) 18(8):471–84. doi: 10.1038/s41568-018-0015-6
21. Hein D, Dreisig K, Metzler M, Izraeli S, Schmiegelow K, Borkhardt A, et al. The Preleukemic TCF3-PBX1 Gene Fusion can be Generated In Utero and Is Present in ≈0.6% of healthy newborns. *Blood* (2019) 134(16):1355–8. doi: 10.1182/blood.2019002215
22. Schäfer D, Olsen M, Lähnemann D, et al. Five Percent of Healthy Newborns Have an ETV6-RUNX1 Fusion as Revealed by DNA-Based GIPFEL Screening. *Blood* (2018) 131(7):821–6. doi: 10.1182/blood-2017-09-808402
23. Rodríguez-Hernández G, Hauer J, Martín-Lorenzo A, Schäfer D, Bartenhagen C, García-Ramírez I, et al. Infection Exposure Promotes ETV6-RUNX1 Precursor B-Cell Leukemia Via Impaired H3k4 Demethylases. *Cancer Res* (2017) 77(16):4365–77. doi: 10.1158/0008-5472.CAN-17-0701
24. Martín-Lorenzo A, Hauer J, Vicente-Dueñas C, Auer F, González-Herrero I, García-Ramírez I, et al. Infection Exposure Is a Causal Factor in B-Cell Precursor Acute Lymphoblastic Leukemia as a Result of Pax5-Inherited Susceptibility. *Cancer Discov* (2015) 5(12):1328–43. doi: 10.1158/2159-8290.CD-15-0892
25. Vicente-Dueñas C, Janssen S, Oldenburg M, Auer F, González-Herrero I, Casado-García A, et al. An Intact Gut Microbiome Protects Genetically Predisposed Mice Against Leukemia. *Blood* (2020) 136(18):2003–17. doi: 10.1182/blood.2019004381
26. Liu X, Zou Y, Ruan M, Chang L, Chen X, Wang S, et al. Pediatric Acute Lymphoblastic Leukemia Patients Exhibit Distinctive Alterations in the Gut Microbiota. *Front Cell Infect Microbiol* (2020) 10:558799. doi: 10.3389/fcimb.2020.558799
27. Song Y, Gyarmati P. Microbiota Changes in a Pediatric Acute Lymphocytic Leukemia Mouse Model. *Microbiologyopen* (2020) 9(3):e982. doi: 10.1002/mbo3.982
28. Strick R, Strissel PL, Borgers S, Smith SL, Rowley JD. Dietary Bioflavonoids Induce Cleavage in the MLL Gene and may Contribute to Infant Leukemia. *Proc Natl Acad Sci USA* (2000) 97(9):4790–5. doi: 10.1073/pnas.070061297
29. Østgård LSG, Nørgaard M, Pedersen L, Østgård RD, Medeiros BC, Overgaard UM, et al. Autoimmune Diseases, Infections, Use of Antibiotics and the Risk of Acute Myeloid Leukaemia: A National Population-Based Case-Control Study. *Br J Haematol* (2018) 181(2):205–14. doi: 10.1111/bjh.15163
30. Little MP, Wakeford R, Borrego D, French B, Zablotska LB, Adams MJ, et al. Leukaemia and Myeloid Malignancy Among People Exposed to Low Doses (<100 mSv) of Ionising Radiation During Childhood: A Pooled Analysis of Nine Historical Cohort Studies. *Lancet Haematol* (2018) 5(8):e346–58. doi: 10.1016/S2352-3026(18)30092-9
31. Guo H, Chou WC, Lai Y, Liang K, Tam JW, Brickey WJ, et al. Multi-Omics Analyses of Radiation Survivors Identify Radioprotective Microbes and Metabolites. *Science* (2020) 370(6516):eaay9097. doi: 10.1126/science.aay9097
32. Ciorba MA, Riehl TE, Rao MS, Moon C, Ee X, Nava GM, et al. Lactobacillus Probiotic Protects Intestinal Epithelium From Radiation Injury in a TLR-2/cyclo-oxygenase-2-dependent Manner. *Gut* (2012) 61(6):829–38. doi: 10.1136/gutjnl-2011-300367
33. Cui M, Xiao H, Li Y, Zhou L, Zhao S, Luo D, et al. Faecal Microbiota Transplantation Protects Against Radiation-Induced Toxicity. *EMBO Mol Med* (2017) 9(4):448–61. doi: 10.15252/emmm.201606932
34. Loomis D, Guyton KZ, Grosse Y, El Ghissassi F, Bouvard V, Benbrahim-Tallaa L, et al. Carcinogenicity of Benzene. *Lancet Oncol* (2017) 18 (12):1574–5. doi: 10.1016/S1470-2045(17)30832-X
35. Houot J, Marquant F, Goujon S, Faure L, Honoré C, Roth MH, et al. Residential Proximity to Heavy-Traffic Roads, Benzene Exposure, and Childhood Leukemia-The GEOCAP Study, 2002-2007. *Am J Epidemiol* (2015) 182(8):685–93. doi: 10.1093/aje/kwv111
36. Sun R, Xu K, Ji S, Pu Y, Man Z, Ji J, et al. Benzene Exposure Induces Gut Microbiota Dysbiosis and Metabolic Disorder in Mice. *Sci Total Environ* (2020) 705:135879. doi: 10.1016/j.scitotenv.2019.135879
37. Macpherson AJ, Harris NL. Interactions Between Commensal Intestinal Bacteria and the Immune System. *Nat Rev Immunol* (2004) 4(6):478–85. doi: 10.1038/nri1373
38. Tilg H, Adolph TE, Gerner RR, Moschen AR. The Intestinal Microbiota in Colorectal Cancer. *Cancer Cell* (2018) 33(6):954–64. doi: 10.1016/j.ccell.2018.03.004
39. Li Q, Jin M, Liu Y, Jin L. Gut Microbiota: Its Potential Roles in Pancreatic Cancer. *Front Cell Infect Microbiol* (2020) 10:572492. doi: 10.3389/fcimb.2020.572492
40. Inaba H, Pei D, Wolf J, Howard SC, Hayden RT, Go M, et al. Infection-Related Complications During Treatment for Childhood Acute Lymphoblastic Leukemia. *Ann Oncol* (2017) 28(2):386–92. doi: 10.1093/annonc/mdw557
41. Bochennek K, Hassler A, Perner C, Gilfert J, Schöning S, Klingebiel T, et al. Infectious Complications in Children With Acute Myeloid Leukemia: Decreased Mortality in Multicenter Trial AML-BFM 2004. *Blood Cancer J* (2016) 6(1):e382. doi: 10.1038/bcj.2015.110
42. Chung H, Pamp SJ, Hill JA, Surana NK, Edelman SM, Troy EB, et al. Gut Immune Maturation Depends on Colonization With a Host-Specific Microbiota. *Cell* (2012) 149(7):1578–93. doi: 10.1016/j.cell.2012.04.037
43. Pultz NJ, Stiefel U, Subramanyan S, Helfand MS, Donskey CJ. Mechanisms by Which Anaerobic Microbiota Inhibit the Establishment in Mice of Intestinal Colonization by Vancomycin-Resistant Enterococcus. *J Infect Dis* (2005) 191(6):949–56. doi: 10.1086/428090
44. Ford CD, Coombs J, Stofer MG, Lopansri BK, Webb BJ, Ostronoff F, et al. Decrease in Vancomycin-Resistant Enterococcus Colonization Associated With a Reduction in Carbapenem Use as Empiric Therapy for Febrile Neutropenia in Patients With Acute Leukemia. *Infect Control Hosp Epidemiol* (2019) 40(7):774–9. doi: 10.1017/ice.2019.93
45. Zhang S, Dogan B, Guo C, Herlekar D, Stewart K, Scherl EJ, et al. Short Chain Fatty Acids Modulate the Growth and Virulence of Pathosymbiont Escherichia Coli and Host Response. *Antibiotics (Basel)* (2020) 9(8):462. doi: 10.3390/antibiotics9080462
46. Fachi JL, Felipe JS, Pral LP, da Silva BK, Corrêa RO, de Andrade MCP, et al. Butyrate Protects Mice From Clostridium Difficile-Induced Colitis Through an HIF-1-Dependent Mechanism. *Cell Rep* (2019) 27(3):750–761.e7. doi: 10.1016/j.celrep.2019.03.054
47. Josefsdottir KS, Baldridge MT, Kadmon CS, King KY. Antibiotics Impair Murine Hematopoiesis by Depleting the Intestinal Microbiota. *Blood* (2017) 129(6):729–39. doi: 10.1182/blood-2016-03-708594
48. Dodd D, Spitzer MH, Van Treuren W, Merrill BD, Hryckowian AJ, Higginbottom SK, et al. A Gut Bacterial Pathway Metabolizes Aromatic

Amino Acids Into Nine Circulating Metabolites. *Nature* (2017) 551 (7682):648–52. doi: 10.1038/nature24661

49. Rashidi A, Weisdorf DJ. Microbiota-Based Approaches to Mitigate Infectious Complications of Intensive Chemotherapy in Patients With Acute Leukemia. *Transl Res* (2020) 220:167–81. doi: 10.1016/j.trsl.2020.03.011
50. Galloway-Peña JR, Shi Y, Peterson CB, Sahasrabhojane P, Gopalakrishnan V, Brumlow CE, et al. Gut Microbiome Signatures Are Predictive of Infectious Risk Following Induction Therapy for Acute Myeloid Leukemia. *Clin Infect Dis* (2020) 71(1):63–71. doi: 10.1093/cid/ciz777
51. Galloway-Peña JR, Smith DP, Sahasrabhojane P, Ajami NJ, Wadsworth WD, Daver NG, et al. The Role of the Gastrointestinal Microbiome in Infectious Complications During Induction Chemotherapy for Acute Myeloid Leukemia. *Cancer* (2016) 122(14):2186–96. doi: 10.1002/cncr.30039
52. Hakim H, Dallas R, Wolf J, Tang L, Schultz-Cherry S, Darling V, et al. Gut Microbiome Composition Predicts Infection Risk During Chemotherapy in Children With Acute Lymphoblastic Leukemia. *Clin Infect Dis* (2018) 67 (4):541–8. doi: 10.1093/cid/ciy153
53. Nearing JT, Connors J, Whitehouse S, Van Limbergen J, Macdonald T, Kulkarni K, et al. Infectious Complications Are Associated With Alterations in the Gut Microbiome in Pediatric Patients With Acute Lymphoblastic Leukemia. *Front Cell Infect Microbiol* (2019) 9:28. doi: 10.3389/fcimb.2019.00028
54. Ralls MW, Demehri FR, Feng Y, Woods Ignatoski KM, Teitelbaum DH. Enteral Nutrient Deprivation in Patients Leads to a Loss of Intestinal Epithelial Barrier Function. *Surgery* (2015) 157(4):732–42. doi: 10.1016/j.surg.2014.12.004
55. Reyna-Figueroa J, Barrón-Calvillo E, García-Parra C, Galindo-Delgado P, Contreras-Ochoa C, Lagunas-Martínez A, et al. Probiotic Supplementation Decreases Chemotherapy-Induced Gastrointestinal Side Effects in Patients With Acute Leukemia. *J Pediatr Hematol Oncol* (2019) 41(6):468–72. doi: 10.1097/MPH.0000000000001497
56. Suez J, Zmora N, Zilberman-Schapira G, Mor U, Dori-Bachash M, Bashiardes S, et al. Post-Antibiotic Gut Mucosal Microbiome Reconstitution Is Impaired by Probiotics and Improved by Autologous Fmt. *Cell* (2018) 174(6):1406–23.e16. doi: 10.1016/j.cell.2018.08.047
57. Koyama S, Fujita H, Shimosato T, Kamijo A, Ishiyama Y, Yamamoto E, et al. Septicemia From Lactobacillus Rhamnosus GG, From a Probiotic Enriched Yogurt, in a Patient With Autologous Stem Cell Transplantation. *Probiotics Antimicrob Proteins* (2019) 11(1):295–8. doi: 10.1007/s12602-018-9399-6
58. Avcin SL, Pokorn M, Kitanovski L, Premru MM, Jazbec J. Bifidobacterium Breve Sepsis in Child With High-Risk Acute Lymphoblastic Leukemia. *Emerg Infect Dis* (2015) 21(9):1674–5. doi: 10.3201/eid2109.150097
59. Rashidi A, Kaiser T, Graiziger C, Holtan SG, Rehman TU, Weisdorf DJ, et al. Specific Gut Microbiota Changes Heralding Bloodstream Infection and Neutropenic Fever During Intensive Chemotherapy. *Leukemia* (2020) 34 (1):312–6. doi: 10.1038/s41375-019-0547-0
60. Alexander JL, Wilson ID, Teare J, Marchesi JR, Nicholson JK, Kinross JM. Gut Microbiota Modulation of Chemotherapy Efficacy and Toxicity. *Nat Rev Gastroenterol Hepatol* (2017) 14(6):356–65. doi: 10.1038/nrgastro.2017.20
61. Viaud S, Saccheri F, Mignot G, Yamazaki T, Daillère R, Hannani D, et al. The Intestinal Microbiota Modulates the Anticancer Immune Effects of Cyclophosphamide. *Science* (2013) 342(6161):971–6. doi: 10.1126/science.1240537
62. Liu T, Wu Y, Wang L, Pang X, Zhao L, Yuan H, et al. A More Robust Gut Microbiota in Calorie-Restricted Mice Is Associated With Attenuated Intestinal Injury Caused by the Chemotherapy Drug Cyclophosphamide. *mBio* (2019) 10(2):e02903–18. doi: 10.1128/mBio.02903-18
63. Sakura T, Hayakawa F, Sugiura I, Murayama T, Imai K, Usui N, et al. High-Dose Methotrexate Therapy Significantly Improved Survival of Adult Acute Lymphoblastic Leukemia: A Phase III Study by JALSG. *Leukemia* (2018) 32 (3):626–32. doi: 10.1038/leu.2017.283。
64. Larson RA. Managing CNS Disease in Adults With Acute Lymphoblastic Leukemia. *Leuk Lymphoma* (2018) 59(1):3–13. doi: 10.1080/10428194.2017.1326597
65. Friedman B, Cronstein B. Methotrexate Mechanism in Treatment of Rheumatoid Arthritis. *Joint Bone Spine* (2019) 86(3):301–7. doi: 10.1016/j.jbspin.2018.07.004
66. Kolli VK, Abraham P, Isaac B, Kasthuri N. Preclinical Efficacy of Melatonin to Reduce Methotrexate-Induced Oxidative Stress and Small Intestinal Damage in Rats. *Dig Dis Sci* (2013) 58(4):959–69. doi: 10.1007/s10620-012-2437-4
67. Ben-Lulu S, Pollak Y, Mogilner J, Bejar J, G Coran A, Sukhotnik I. Dietary Transforming Growth Factor-Beta 2 (TGF-β2) Supplementation Reduces Methotrexate-Induced Intestinal Mucosal Injury in a Rat. *PloS One* (2012) 7 (9):e45221. doi: 10.1371/journal.pone.0045221
68. Zhou B, Xia X, Wang P, Chen S, Yu C, Huang R, et al. Induction and Amelioration of Methotrexate-Induced Gastrointestinal Toxicity Are Related to Immune Response and Gut Microbiota. *EBioMedicine* (2018) 33:122–33. doi: 10.1016/j.ebiom.2018.06.029
69. Letertre MPM, Munjoma N, Wolfer K, Pechlivanis A, McDonald JAK, Hardwick RN, et al. A Two-Way Interaction Between Methotrexate and the Gut Microbiota of Male Sprague-Dawley Rats. *J Proteome Res* (2020) 19 (8):3326–39. doi: 10.1021/acs.jproteome.0c00230
70. Nayak RR, Alexander M, Deshpande I, Stapleton-Gray K, Rimal B, Patterson AD, et al. Methotrexate Impacts Conserved Pathways in Diverse Human Gut Bacteria Leading to Decreased Host Immune Activation. *Cell Host Microbe* (2021) 29(3):362–77.e11. doi: 10.1016/j.chom.2020.12.008
71. Farkona S, Diamandis EP, Blasutig IM. Cancer Immunotherapy: The Beginning of the End of Cancer? *BMC Med* (2016) 14:73. doi: 10.1186/s12916-016-0623-5
72. Zhou Q, Munger ME, Highfill SL, Tolar J, Weigel BJ, Riddle M, et al. Program Death-1 Signaling and Regulatory T Cells Collaborate to Resist the Function of Adoptively Transferred Cytotoxic T Lymphocytes in Advanced Acute Myeloid Leukemia. *Blood* (2010) 116(14):2484–93. doi: 10.1182/blood-2010-03-275446
73. Daver N, Garcia-Manero G, Basu S, Boddu PC, Alfayez M, Cortes JE, et al. Efficacy, Safety, and Biomarkers of Response to Azacitidine and Nivolumab in Relapsed/Refractory Acute Myeloid Leukemia: A Nonrandomized, Open-Label, Phase II Study. *Cancer Discovery* (2019) 9(3):370–83. doi: 10.1158/2159-8290.CD-18-0774
74. Routy B, Le Chatelier E, Derosa L, Duong CPM, Alou MT, Daillère R, et al. Gut Microbiome Influences Efficacy of PD-1-based Immunotherapy Against Epithelial Tumors. *Science* (2018) 359(6371):91–7. doi: 10.1126/science.aan3706
75. Matson V, Fessler J, Bao R, Chongsuwat T, Zha Y, Alegre ML, et al. The Commensal Microbiome Is Associated With Anti-PD-1 Efficacy in Metastatic Melanoma Patients. *Science* (2018) 359(6371):104–8. doi: 10.1126/science.aao3290
76. Gopalakrishnan V, Spencer CN, Nezi L, Reuben A, Andrews MC, Karpinets TV, et al. Gut Microbiome Modulates Response to Anti-PD-1 Immunotherapy in Melanoma Patients. *Science* (2018) 359(6371):97–103. doi: 10.1126/science.aan4236
77. Zheng Y, Wang T, Tu X, Huang Y, Zhang H, Tan D, et al. Gut Microbiome Affects the Response to Anti-PD-1 Immunotherapy in Patients With Hepatocellular Carcinoma. *J Immunother Cancer* (2019) 7(1):193. doi: 10.1186/s40425-019-0650-9
78. Lee CJ, Savani BN, Mohty M, Gorin NC, Labopin M, Ruggeri A, et al. Post-Remission Strategies for the Prevention of Relapse Following Allogeneic Hematopoietic Cell Transplantation for High-Risk Acute Myeloid Leukemia: Expert Review From the Acute Leukemia Working Party of the European Society for Blood and Marrow Transplantation. *Bone Marrow Transplant* (2019) 54(4):519–30. doi: 10.1038/s41409-018-0286-2
79. Fredricks DN. The Gut Microbiota and Graft-Versus-Host Disease. *J Clin Invest* (2019) 129(5):1808–17. doi: 10.1172/JCI125797
80. Ferrara JL, Levine JE, Reddy P, Holler E. Graft-Versus-Host Disease. *Lancet* (2009) 373(9674):1550–61. doi: 10.1016/S0140-6736(09)60237-3
81. Sarantopoulos S, Cardones AR, Sullivan KM. How I Treat Refractory Chronic Graft-Versus-Host Disease. *Blood* (2019) 133(11):1191–200. doi: 10.1182/blood-2018-04-785899
82. Zeiser R, Blazar BR. Acute Graft-versus-Host Disease - Biologic Process, Prevention, and Therapy. *N Engl J Med* (2017) 377(22):2167–79. doi: 10.1056/NEJMra1609337
83. Jacobsohn DA, Vogelsang GB. Acute Graft Versus Host Disease. *Orphanet J Rare Dis* (2007) 2:35. doi: 10.1186/1750-1172-2-35

84. Staffas A, Burgos da Silva M, van den Brink MR. The Intestinal Microbiota in Allogeneic Hematopoietic Cell Transplant and Graft-Versus-Host Disease. *Blood* (2017) 129(8):927–33. doi: 10.1182/blood-2016-09-691394 [published correction appears in Blood. 2017 Apr 13;129(15):2204].
85. van Bekkum DW, Roodenburg J, Heidt PJ, van der Waaij D. Mitigation of Secondary Disease of Allogeneic Mouse Radiation Chimeras by Modification of the Intestinal Microflora. *J Natl Cancer Inst* (1974) 52(2):401–4. doi: 10.1093/jnci/52.2.401
86. Jenq RR, Ubeda C, Taur Y, Menezes CC, Khanin R, Dudakov JA, et al. Regulation of Intestinal Inflammation by Microbiota Following Allogeneic Bone Marrow Transplantation. *J Exp Med* (2012) 209(5):903–11. doi: 10.1084/jem.20112408
87. Morrison DJ, Preston T. Formation of Short Chain Fatty Acids by the Gut Microbiota and Their Impact on Human Metabolism. *Gut Microbes* (2016) 7 (3):189–200. doi: 10.1080/19490976.2015.1134082
88. Mathewson ND, Jenq R, Mathew AV, Koenigsknecht M, Hanash A, Toubai T, et al. Gut Microbiome-Derived Metabolites Modulate Intestinal Epithelial Cell Damage and Mitigate Graft-Versus-Host Disease. *Nat Immunol* (2016) 17(5):505–13. doi: 10.1038/ni.3400 [published correction appears in Nat Immunol. 2016 Sep 20;17 (10):1235].
89. Markey KA, Schluter J, Gomes ALC, Littmann ER, Pickard AJ, Taylor BP, et al. The Microbe-Derived Short-Chain Fatty Acids Butyrate and Propionate Are Associated With Protection From Chronic GVHD. *Blood* (2020) 136(1):130–6. doi: 10.1182/blood.2019003369
90. Golob JL, Pergam SA, Srinivasan S, Fiedler TL, Liu C, Garcia K, et al. Stool Microbiota at Neutrophil Recovery Is Predictive for Severe Acute Graft vs Host Disease After Hematopoietic Cell Transplantation. *Clin Infect Dis* (2017) 65(12):1984–91. doi: 10.1093/cid/cix699
91. Han L, Zhao K, Li Y, Han H, Zhou L, Ma P, et al. A Gut Microbiota Score Predicting Acute Graft-Versus-Host Disease Following Myeloablative Allogeneic Hematopoietic Stem Cell Transplantation. *Am J Transplant* (2020) 20(4):1014–27. doi: 10.1111/ajt.15654
92. Payen M, Nicolis I, Robin M, Michonneau D, Delannoye J, Mayeur C, et al. Functional and Phylogenetic Alterations in Gut Microbiome Are Linked to Graft-Versus-Host Disease Severity. *Blood Adv* (2020) 4(9):1824–32. doi: 10.1182/bloodadvances.2020001531
93. Kusakabe S, Fukushima K, Maeda T, Motooka D, Nakamura S, Fujita J, et al. Pre- and Post-Serial Metagenomic Analysis of Gut Microbiota as a Prognostic Factor in Patients Undergoing Haematopoietic Stem Cell Transplantation. *Br J Haematol* (2020) 188(3):438–49. doi: 10.1111/bjh.16205
94. Lee JH, Wood TK, Lee J. Roles of Indole as an Interspecies and Interkingdom Signaling Molecule. *Trends Microbiol* (2015) 23(11):707–18. doi: 10.1016/j.tim.2015.08.001
95. Swimm A, Giver CR, DeFilipp Z, Rangaraju S, Sharma A, Ulezko Antonova A, et al. Indoles Derived From Intestinal Microbiota Act Via Type I Interferon Signaling to Limit Graft-Versus-Host Disease. *Blood* (2018) 132(23):2506–19. doi: 10.1182/blood-2018-03-838193
96. Wu K, Yuan Y, Yu H, Dai X, Wang S, Sun Z, et al. The Gut Microbial Metabolite Trimethylamine N-Oxide Aggravates GVHD by Inducing M1 Macrophage Polarization in Mice. *Blood* (2020) 136(4):501–15. doi: 10.1182/blood.2019003990
97. Shono Y, Docampo MD, Peled JU, Perobelli SM, Velardi E, Tsai JJ, et al. Increased GVHD-related Mortality With Broad-Spectrum Antibiotic Use After Allogeneic Hematopoietic Stem Cell Transplantation in Human Patients and Mice. *Sci Transl Med* (2016) 8(339):339ra71. doi: 10.1126/scitranslmed.aaf2311
98. Malard F, Vekhoff A, Lapusan S, Isnard F, D'incan-Corda E, Rey J, et al. Gut Microbiota Diversity After Autologous Fecal Microbiota Transfer in Acute Myeloid Leukemia Patients. *Nat Commun* (2021) 12(1):3084. doi: 10.1038/s41467-021-23376-6
99. Taur Y, Jenq RR, Perales MA, Littmann ER, Morjaria S, Ling L, et al. The Effects of Intestinal Tract Bacterial Diversity on Mortality Following Allogeneic Hematopoietic Stem Cell Transplantation. *Blood* (2014) 124 (7):1174–82. doi: 10.1182/blood-2014-02-554725
100. Peled JU, Gomes ALC, Devlin SM, Littmann ER, Taur Y, Sung AD, et al. Microbiota as Predictor of Mortality in Allogeneic Hematopoietic-Cell Transplantation. *N Engl J Med* (2020) 382(9):822–34. doi: 10.1056/NEJMoa1900623
101. Harris B, Morjaria SM, Littmann ER, Geyer AI, Stover DE, Barker JN, et al. Gut Microbiota Predict Pulmonary Infiltrates After Allogeneic Hematopoietic Cell Transplantation. *Am J Respir Crit Care Med* (2016) 194(4):450–63. doi: 10.1164/rccm.201507-1491OC
102. Stein-Thoeringer CK, Nichols KB, Lazrak A, Docampo MD, Slingerland AE, Slingerland JB, et al. Lactose Drives Enterococcus Expansion to Promote Graft-Versus-Host Disease. *Science* (2019) 366(6469):1143–9. doi: 10.1126/science.aax3760
103. Pianko MJ, Devlin SM, Littmann ER, Chansakul A, Mastey D, Salcedo M, et al. Minimal Residual Disease Negativity in Multiple Myeloma Is Associated With Intestinal Microbiota Composition. *Blood Adv* (2019) 3 (13):2040–4. doi: 10.1182/bloodadvances.2019032276
104. Battipaglia G, Malard F, Rubio MT, Ruggeri A, Mamez AC, Brissot E, et al. Fecal Microbiota Transplantation Before or After Allogeneic Hematopoietic Transplantation in Patients With Hematologic Malignancies Carrying Multidrug-Resistance Bacteria. *Haematologica* (2019) 104(8):1682–8. doi: 10.3324/haematol.2018.198549
105. Kakihana K, Fujioka Y, Suda W, Najima Y, Kuwata G, Sasajima S, et al. Fecal Microbiota Transplantation for Patients With Steroid-Resistant Acute Graft-Versus-Host Disease of the Gut. *Blood* (2016) 128(16):2083–8. doi: 10.1182/blood-2016-05-717652
106. DeFilipp Z, Peled JU, Li S, Mahabamunuge J, Dagher Z, Slingerland AE, et al. Third-Party Fecal Microbiota Transplantation Following allo-HCT Reconstitutes Microbiome Diversity. *Blood Adv* (2018) 2(7):745–53. doi: 10.1182/bloodadvances.2018017731
107. Khuat LT, Le CT, Pai CS, Shields-Cutler RR, Holtan SG, Rashidi A, et al. Obesity Induces Gut Microbiota Alterations and Augments Acute Graft-Versus-Host Disease After Allogeneic Stem Cell Transplantation. *Sci Transl Med* (2020) 12(571):eaay7713. doi: 10.1126/scitranslmed.aay7713
108. Koyama M, Mukhopadhyay P, Schuster IS, Henden AS, Hülsdünker J, Varelias A, et al. Mhc Class Ii Antigen Presentation by the Intestinal Epithelium Initiates Graft-Versus-Host Disease and Is Influenced by the Microbiota. *Immunity* (2019) 51(5):885–898.e7. doi: 10.1016/j.immuni.2019.08.011
109. Fujiwara H, Docampo MD, Riwes M, Peltier D, Toubai T, Henig I, et al. Microbial Metabolite Sensor GPR43 Controls Severity of Experimental GVHD. *Nat Commun* (2018) 9(1):3674. doi: 10.1038/s41467-018-06048-w
110. Peled JU, Devlin SM, Staffas A, Lumish M, Khanin R, Littmann ER, et al. Intestinal Microbiota and Relapse After Hematopoietic-Cell Transplantation. *J Clin Oncol* (2017) 35(15):1650–9. doi: 10.1200/JCO.2016.70.3348

Permissions

All chapters in this book were first published by Frontiers; hereby published with permission under the Creative Commons Attribution License or equivalent. Every chapter published in this book has been scrutinized by our experts. Their significance has been extensively debated. The topics covered herein carry significant findings which will fuel the growth of the discipline. They may even be implemented as practical applications or may be referred to as a beginning point for another development.

The contributors of this book come from diverse backgrounds, making this book a truly international effort. This book will bring forth new frontiers with its revolutionizing research information and detailed analysis of the nascent developments around the world.

We would like to thank all the contributing authors for lending their expertise to make the book truly unique. They have played a crucial role in the development of this book. Without their invaluable contributions this book wouldn't have been possible. They have made vital efforts to compile up to date information on the varied aspects of this subject to make this book a valuable addition to the collection of many professionals and students.

This book was conceptualized with the vision of imparting up-to-date information and advanced data in this field. To ensure the same, a matchless editorial board was set up. Every individual on the board went through rigorous rounds of assessment to prove their worth. After which they invested a large part of their time researching and compiling the most relevant data for our readers.

The editorial board has been involved in producing this book since its inception. They have spent rigorous hours researching and exploring the diverse topics which have resulted in the successful publishing of this book. They have passed on their knowledge of decades through this book. To expedite this challenging task, the publisher supported the team at every step. A small team of assistant editors was also appointed to further simplify the editing procedure and attain best results for the readers.

Apart from the editorial board, the designing team has also invested a significant amount of their time in understanding the subject and creating the most relevant covers. They scrutinized every image to scout for the most suitable representation of the subject and create an appropriate cover for the book.

The publishing team has been an ardent support to the editorial, designing and production team. Their endless efforts to recruit the best for this project, has resulted in the accomplishment of this book. They are a veteran in the field of academics and their pool of knowledge is as vast as their experience in printing. Their expertise and guidance has proved useful at every step. Their uncompromising quality standards have made this book an exceptional effort. Their encouragement from time to time has been an inspiration for everyone.

The publisher and the editorial board hope that this book will prove to be a valuable piece of knowledge for researchers, students, practitioners and scholars across the globe.

List of Contributors

Patrizia Leone, Eleonora Malerba, Rossella Fasano, Alessio Buonavoglia, Fabrizio Pappagallo, Angelo Vacca and Vito Racanelli
Department of Biomedical Sciences and Human Oncology, University of Bari Medical School, Bari, Italy

Antonio Giovanni Solimando and Nicola Silvestris
Department of Biomedical Sciences and Human Oncology, University of Bari Medical School, Bari, Italy
Department of Medical Oncology, IRCCS Istituto Tumori "Giovanni Paolo II" of Bari, Bari, Italy

Valli De Re
Bio-Proteomics Facility, Department of Translational Research, Centro di Riferimento Oncologico di Aviano (CRO) IRCCS, Aviano, Italy

Antonella Argentiero
Department of Medical Oncology, IRCCS Istituto Tumori "Giovanni Paolo II" of Bari, Bari, Italy

Michela Frenquelli
B-cell Neoplasia Unit, Division of Experimental Oncology, IRCCS San Raffaele Scientific Institute, Milan, Italy
Functional Genomics of Cancer Unit, Division of Experimental Oncology, IRCCS San Raffaele Scientific Institute, Milan, Italy

Alessandro Barbato, Fabrizio Puglisi and Daniela Cambria
Department of Clinical and Experimental Medicine, University of Catania, Catania, Italy

Tianzeng Chen and Maria Moscvin
Division of Hematology, Department of Medicine, Brigham and Women's Hospital, Boston, MA, United States

Giada Bianchi
Division of Hematology, Department of Medicine, Brigham and Women's Hospital, Boston, MA, United States
Harvard Medical School, Boston, MA, United States

Giovanni Tonon
Functional Genomics of Cancer Unit, Division of Experimental Oncology, IRCCS San Raffaele Scientific Institute, Milan, Italy
Center for Omics Sciences (COSR), IRCCS San Raffaele Scientific Institute, Milan, Italy

Grazia Scandura, Enrico La Spina and Francesco Di Raimondo
Department of General Surgery and Medical-Surgical Specialties, University of Catania, Catania, Italy

Giuseppe Alberto Palumbo and Cesarina Giallongo
Department of Medical, Surgical Sciences and Advanced Technologies G.F. Ingrassia, University of Catania, Catania, Italy

Giacomo Lazzarino
Saint Camillus International University of Health and Medical Sciences, Rome, Italy

Daniele Tibullo
Department of Biotechnological and Biomedical Sciences, University of Catania, Catania, Italy

Alessandra Romano
Department of Surgery and Medical Specialties, University of Catania, Catania, Italy

Tyler Moser-Katz, Nisha S. Joseph, Madhav V. Dhodapkar and Lawrence H. Boise
Department of Hematology and Medical Oncology, Winship Cancer Institute, Emory University, Atlanta, GA, United States

Kelvin P. Lee
Department of Immunology, Roswell Park Cancer Institute, Buffalo, NY, United States

Zheng Yan, Shuna Yao, Yanyan Liu, Haiying Wang, Junfeng Chu, Shuang Zhao and Zhihua Yao
Department of Internal Medicine, Affiliated Cancer Hospital of Zhengzhou University and Henan Cancer Hospital, Zhengzhou, China

Jianbo Zhang
Department of Pathology, Affiliated Cancer Hospital of Zhengzhou University and Henan Cancer Hospital, Zhengzhou, China

Peng Li
The PET-CT Center of Henan Province, Affiliated Cancer Hospital of Zhengzhou University and Henan Cancer Hospital, Zhengzhou, China

Leona Yamamoto, Annamaria Gulla and Kenneth Carl Anderson
Division of Hematologic Malignancy, Department of Medical Oncology, Jerome Lipper Multiple Myeloma Center, Dana-Farber Cancer Institute, Harvard Medical School, Boston, MA, United States

Nicola Amodio
Department of Experimental and Clinical Medicine, Magna Graecia University of Catanzaro, Catanzaro, Italy

Yue Song and Wenting Song
Department of Oncology, The First Affiliated Hospital of Zhengzhou University, Zhengzhou, China
The Academy of Medical Science of Zhengzhou University, Zhengzhou, China
Lymphoma Diagnosis and Treatment Center of Henan Province, Zhengzhou, China

Wei Song
Department of Pathology, The Affiliated Cancer Hospital of Zhengzhou University, Henan Cancer Hospital, Zhengzhou, China

Zhaoming Li, Jiwei Li and Mingzhi Zhang
Department of Oncology, The First Affiliated Hospital of Zhengzhou University, Zhengzhou, China,
Lymphoma Diagnosis and Treatment Center of Henan Province, Zhengzhou, China

Yibo Wen
The Academy of Medical Science of Zhengzhou University, Zhengzhou, China

Qingxin Xia
Department of Pathology, The Affiliated Cancer Hospital of Zhengzhou University, Henan Cancer Hospital, Zhengzhou, China

Heather Fairfield, Samantha Costa, Carolyne Falank and Connor S. Murphy
Center for Molecular Medicine, Maine Medical Center Research Institute, Scarborough, ME, United States,
School of Medicine, Tufts University, Boston, MA, United States
Graduate School of Biomedical Science and Engineering, University of Maine, Orono, ME, United States

Mariah Farrell and Anastasia D'Amico
Center for Molecular Medicine, Maine Medical Center Research Institute, Scarborough, ME, United States
School of Medicine, Tufts University, Boston, MA, United States
Biology Department, University of Southern Maine, Portland, ME, United States

Heather Driscoll
Biology Department, Norwich University, Northfield, VT, United States

Michaela R. Reagan
Center for Molecular Medicine, Maine Medical Center Research Institute, Scarborough, ME, United States
School of Medicine, Tufts University, Boston, MA, United States
Graduate School of Biomedical Science and Engineering, University of Maine, Orono, ME, United States,
Biology Department, University of Southern Maine, Portland, ME, United States

Alexander J. Ambinder, Kelly Norsworthy, Daniela Hernandez, Laura Palau, Bogdan Paun, Richard J. Jones, B. Douglas Smith and Gabriel Ghiaur
Department of Oncology, Sidney Kimmel Comprehensive Cancer Center, Johns Hopkins University School of Medicine, Baltimore, MD, United States

Amy Duffield
Department of Pathology, Johns Hopkins University School of Medicine, Baltimore, MD, United States

Rosh Chandraratna and Martin Sanders
IO Therapeutics, Santa Ana, CA, United States

Ravi Varadhan
Division of Biostatistics and Bioinformatics, Johns Hopkins/Sidney Kimmel Comprehensive Cancer Center, Baltimore, MD, United States

Yun Wang, Fang Hu, Jin-yuan Li, Si-liang Chen and Yang Liang
Sate key Laboratory of Oncology in South China, Sun Yat-sen University Cancer Center, Collaborative Innovation Center for Cancer Medicine, Guangzhou, China
Department of Hematologic Oncology, Sun Yat-sen University Cancer Center, Guangzhou, China

Run-cong Nie
Sate key Laboratory of Oncology in South China, Sun Yat-sen University Cancer Center, Collaborative Innovation Center for Cancer Medicine, Guangzhou, China
Department of Gastric Surgery, Sun Yat-sen University Cancer Center, Guangzhou, China

Yan-yu Cai and Ling-ling Shu
Sate key Laboratory of Oncology in South China, Sun Yat-sen University Cancer Center, Collaborative Innovation Center for Cancer Medicine, Guangzhou, China
Department of VIP Region, Sun Yat-sen University Cancer Center, Guangzhou, China

De-jun Deng
Department of Oncology and Hematology, Shenzhen Luohu District Hospital of Traditional Chinese Medicine, Shenzhen, China

Jing-bo Xu
Department of Hematology, The Fifth Affiliated Hospital of Sun Yat-sen University, Zhuhai, China

Yan Zhang
Department of Hematology, The First Affiliated Hospital, College of Medicine, Zhejiang University, Hangzhou, China
Department of Hematology, Huzhou Central Hospital, Affiliated Cent Hospital of Huzhou University, Huzhou, China

Yanlong Zheng, Yuanfei Shi, Huafei Shen, Mingyu Zhu, Xiujin Ye, Jie Jin and Wanzhuo Xie
Department of Hematology, The First Affiliated Hospital, College of Medicine, Zhejiang University, Hangzhou, China

Lihong Shou
Department of Hematology, Huzhou Central Hospital, Affiliated Cent Hospital of Huzhou University, Huzhou, China

Rodrigo Carlini Fernando, Fabrício de Carvalho and Gisele Wally Braga Colleoni
Department of Experimental and Clinical Oncology, Discipline of Hematology and Hemotherapy, Federal University of São Paulo, UNIFESP, São Paulo, Brazil

Adriana Franco Paes Leme
Laboratory of Mass Spectrometry, Laboratory of National Biosciences, LNBio, National Council for Research in Energy and Materials (CNPEM), Campinas, Brazil

Cirino Botta, Massimo Gentile and Ernesto Vigna
Hematology Unit, Hematology and Oncology Department, "Annunziata" Hospital of Cosenza, Cosenza, Italy
Biotechnology Research Unit, Hematology and Oncology Department, "Annunziata" Hospital of Cosenza, Cosenza, Italy

Nadia Caruso, Sabrina Bossio and Francesca Storino
Biotechnology Research Unit, Hematology and Oncology Department, "Annunziata" Hospital of Cosenza, Cosenza, Italy

Giuseppe Console and Massimo Martino
Stem Cell Transplant Program, Clinical Section, Department of Hemato-Oncology and Radiotherapy, "Grande Ospedale Metropolitano Bianchi-Melacrino-Morelli", Reggio Calabria, Italy

Francesco Mendicino and Eugenio Lucia
Hematology Unit, Hematology and Oncology Department, "Annunziata" Hospital of Cosenza, Cosenza, Italy

Rosellina Morelli
Medicine Department, "Annunziata" Hospital of Cosenza, Cosenza, Italy

Pierpaolo Correale
Medical Oncology Unit, Department of Hemato-Oncology and Radiotherapy, "Grande Ospedale Metropolitano Bianchi-Melacrino-Morelli", Reggio Calabria, Italy

Fortunato Morabito
Biotechnology Research Unit, Hematology and Oncology Department, "Annunziata" Hospital of Cosenza, Cosenza, Italy
Hematology Department and Bone Marrow Transplant Unit, Cancer Care Center, Augusta Victoria Hospital, East Jerusalem, Israel

Roberta Chirillo, Ilenia Aversa, Anna Di Vito, Alessandro Salatino, Anna Martina Battaglia, Alessandro Sacco, Maddalena Adriana Di Sanzo, Barbara Quaresima and Camillo Palmieri
Department of Experimental and Clinical Medicine, "Magna Græcia" University of Catanzaro, Catanzaro, Italy

Maria Concetta Faniello and Flavia Biamonte
Department of Experimental and Clinical Medicine, "Magna Græcia" University of Catanzaro, Catanzaro, Italy
Department of Experimental and Clinical Medicine, Research Center of Biochemistry and Advanced Molecular Biology, "Magna Græcia" University of Catanzaro, Catanzaro, Italy

Francesco Costanzo
Department of Experimental and Clinical Medicine, Research Center of Biochemistry and Advanced Molecular Biology, "Magna Græcia" University of Catanzaro, Catanzaro, Italy
Interdepartmental Center of Services (CIS), "Magna Græcia" University of Catanzaro, Catanzaro, Italy

Tao Pan
Department of Lymphoma & Hematology, Hunan Cancer Hospital, The Affiliated Cancer Hospital of Xiangya School of Medicine, Central South University, Changsha, China
The Third Xiangya Hospital, Central South University, Changsha, China

Yizi He, Huan Chen, Yajun Li, Ruolan Zeng, Yilang Zuo, Liping Qin and Hui Zhou
Department of Lymphoma & Hematology, Hunan Cancer Hospital, The Affiliated Cancer Hospital of Xiangya School of Medicine, Central South University, Changsha, China

Junfei Pei
Department of Gastrointestinal Surgery, First Hospital of Jilin University, Changchun, Jilin, China

Jiliang Xia
Hunan Province Key Laboratory of Tumor Cellular & Molecular Pathology, Cancer Research Institute, Hengyang School of Medicine, University of South China, Hengyang, China

Siwei Chen and Ling Xiao
Department of Histology and Embryology of School of Basic Medical Science, Central South University, Changsha, China

Melinda A. Biernacki and Marie Bleakley
Clinical Research Division, Fred Hutchinson Cancer Research Center, Seattle, WA, United States
Department of Medicine, University of Washington, Seattle, WA, United States

Marie Bleakley
Clinical Research Division, Fred Hutchinson Cancer Research Center, Seattle, WA, United States
Department of Pediatrics, University of Washington, Seattle, WA, United States

Xiangyu Tan, Han Yan, Lei Chen and Yuyang Zhang
Department of Hematology, Union Hospital, Tongji Medical College, Huazhong University of Science and Technology, Wuhan, China

Chunyan Sun
Department of Hematology, Union Hospital, Tongji Medical College, Huazhong University of Science and Technology, Wuhan, China
Collaborative Innovation Center of Hematology, Huazhong University of Science and Technology, Wuhan, China

Jason H. Kurzer
Department of Pathology, Stanford University School of Medicine, Stanford, CA, United States

Olga K. Weinberg
Department of Pathology, UT Southwestern, Dallas, TX, United States

Tao Ma
Department of Hematology, Lanzhou University Second Hospital, Lanzhou, China
Department of Hematology, The Affiliated Hospital of Southwest Medical University, Luzhou, China

Yan Chen
Department of Hematology, The Affiliated Hospital of Southwest Medical University, Luzhou, China

Li-Juan Li and Lian-Sheng Zhang
Department of Hematology, Lanzhou University Second Hospital, Lanzhou, China

Index

www.ingramcontent.com/pod-product-compliance
Lightning Source LLC
LaVergne TN
LVHW082211200926
848484LV00008B/2241
* 9 7 9 8 8 8 7 4 0 3 3 1 1 *